Harrison's

PRINCIPLES OF INTERNAL MEDICINE

Eleventh Edition

COMPANION HANDBOOK

Editors

EUGENE BRAUNWALD, A.B., M.D., M.A. (Hon.), M.D. (Hon.) Hersey Professor of the Theory and Practice of Physic and Herrman Ludwig Blumgart Professor of Medicine, Harvard Medical School; Chairman, Department of Medicine, Brigham and Women's and Beth Israel Hospitals, Boston

KURT J. ISSELBACHER, A.B., M.D.
Mallinckrodt Professor of Medicine, Harvard Medical School; Director, Cancer Center, and Chief, Gastrointestinal Unit, Massachusetts General Hospital, Boston

ROBERT G. PETERSDORF, A.B., M.D., M.A. (Hon.), D.Sc. (Hon.), M.D. (Hon.), L.H.D. (Hon.)
President, Association of American Medical Colleges, Washington, D.C.

JEAN D. WILSON, M.D.
Professor of Internal Medicine, The University of Texas Health Science Center, Dallas

JOSEPH B. MARTIN, M.D., Ph.D., F.R.C.P.(C), M.A. (Hon.) Julieanne Dorn Professor of Neurology, Harvard Medical School; Chief, Neurology Service, Massachusetts General Hospital, Boston

ANTHONY S. FAUCI, M.D.
Chief, Laboratory of Immunoregulation and Director, National Institute of Allergy and Infectious Diseases, National Institutes of Health, Bethesda

Harrison's
PRINCIPLES OF INTERNAL MEDICINE
Eleventh Edition

COMPANION HANDBOOK

Editors

EUGENE BRAUNWALD

KURT J. ISSELBACHER

ROBERT G. PETERSDORF

JEAN D. WILSON

JOSEPH B. MARTIN

ANTHONY S. FAUCI

McGRAW-HILL BOOK COMPANY

New York St. Louis San Francisco Auckland Bogotá Caracas Colorado Springs Hamburg Lisbon London Madrid Mexico Milan Montreal New Delhi Oklahoma City Panama Paris San Juan São Paulo Singapore Sydney Tokyo Toronto

NOTICE

Medicine is an ever-changing science. As new research and clinical experience broaden our knowledge, changes in treatment and drug therapy are required. The editors and the publisher of this work have made every effort to ensure that the drug dosage schedules herein are accurate and in accord with the standards accepted at the time of the publication. Readers are advised, however, to check the product information sheet included in the package of each drug they plan to administer to be certain that changes have not been made in the recommended dose or in the contraindications for administration. This recommendation is of particular importance in regard to new or infrequently used drugs.

Harrison's
Principles of Internal Medicine
Eleventh Edition
Companion Handbook

1234567890 DOCDOC 894321098

ISBN 0-07-07264-7

This book was set in Sabon by Monotype Composition Company. The editors were J. Dereck Jeffers and Eileen J. Scott; the production supervisor was Elaine Gardenier; the designer was Jules Perlmutter.
R. R. Donnelley & Sons Company was printer and binder.

Library of Congress Cataloging-in-Publication Data

Harrison's principles of internal medicine, eleventh edition. Companion handbook.

An extension of: Harrison's principles of internal medicine. 11th ed. © 1987.
I. Internal medicine. I. Harrison, Tinsley Randolph, Date . II. Braunwald, Eugene, Date . III. Principles of internal medicine. 11th ed. [DNLM: 1. Internal Medicine. WB 115 P957 1987 Suppl.]
RC46.P895 1987 Suppl. 616 87-16880
ISBN 0-07-07264-7

ABBREVIATED CONTENTS

CONTENTS

SECTION I
IMPORTANT SYMPTOMS AND SIGNS

SECTION II
INFECTIOUS DISEASES

SECTION III

CARDIOVASCULAR DISEASE

SECTION IV

RESPIRATORY DISEASE

SECTION V

RENAL DISEASE

SECTION VI
GASTROINTESTINAL DISEASES

SECTION VII
ALLERGY, CLINICAL IMMUNOLOGY, AND RHEUMATOLOGY

SECTION VIII
HEMATOLOGY AND ONCOLOGY

SECTION IX
ENDOCRINOLOGY AND METABOLISM

SECTION X

DERMATOLOGY

SECTION XI

NEUROLOGY

SECTION XII

PSYCHIATRY

SECTION XIII
NUTRITION

SECTION XIV
MEDICAL EMERGENCIES

SECTION XV

SECTION XVI

LIST OF CONTRIBUTORS

Numbers in parentheses indicate the chapters for which each contributor is responsible.

EUGENE BRAUNWALD, A.B., M.D., M.A.(Hon.), M.D.(Hon.) (2, 62, 183, 189)
Hersey Professor of the Theory and Practice of Physic and Herrman Ludwig Blumgart Professor of Medicine, Harvard Medical School; Chairman, Department of Medicine, Brigham and Women's and Beth Israel Hospitals, Boston

ANTHONY S. FAUCI, M.D. (25, 73, 107–121, 130–133, 169, 185, 190)
Chief, Laboratory of Immunoregulation and Director, National Institute of Allergy and Infectious Diseases, National Institutes of Health, Bethesda

LAWRENCE S. FRIEDMAN, M.D. (18, 20, 95, 96, 98, 100, 103–106)
Assistant Professor of Medicine, Jefferson Medical College, Thomas Jefferson University, Philadelphia

KURT J. ISSELBACHER, A.B., M.D. (3, 15, 17, 98)
Mallinckrodt Professor of Medicine, Harvard Medical School; Director, Cancer Center, and Chief, Gastrointestinal Unit, Massachusetts General Hospital, Boston

LEE M. KAPLAN, M.D. (3, 17, 19, 99, 102)
Instructor in Medicine, Harvard Medical School; Assistant in Medicine, Massachusetts General Hospital, Boston

WALTER KOROSHETZ, M.D. (8, 9, 155, 158, 170, 172, 173, 177, 188)
Instructor, Department of Neurology, Harvard Medical School; Department of Neurology, Massachusetts General Hospital, Boston

LEONARD S. LILLY, M.D. (12, 14, 56–61, 64–70)
Assistant Professor of Medicine, Harvard Medical School; Associate Physician, Brigham and Women's Hospital, Boston

JOSEPH B. MARTIN, M.D., Ph.D., F.R.C.P.(C), M.A.(Hon.) (1, 4, 5, 153, 163, 175)
Julieanne Dorn Professor of Neurology, Harvard Medical School; Chief, Neurology Service, Massachusetts General Hospital, Boston

NORMAN S. NISHIOKA, M.D. (15, 97, 101)
Instructor in Medicine, Harvard Medical School; Assistant in Medicine, Massachusetts General Hospital, Boston

ROBERT G. PETERSDORF, M.D., M.A.(Hon.), D.Sc.(Hon.), M.D.(Hon.), L.H.D.(Hon.) (6, 184, 186, 187)
President, Association of American Medical Colleges, Washington, D.C.

JEFFREY J. POPMA, M.D. (16, 23, 24, 134–146, 178–182)
Fellow in Cardiology, The University of Texas Health Science Center, Dallas

SHARON L. REED, M.D. (26–55, 63, 76, 90, 159, 160)
Assistant Professor of Medicine in Residence, Division of Infectious Diseases, U.C.S.D. Medical Center, San Diego

M. ELIZABETH ROSS, M.D., Ph.D. (7, 152, 157, 164, 165, 166, 171, 174)
Instructor, Department of Neurology, Harvard Medical School; Department of Molecular Biology, Massachusetts General Hospital, Boston

WILLIAM S. SAWCHUK, M.D. (147–150)
Medical Staff, Laboratory of Cellular Oncology, National Cancer Institute, Bethesda

ROBERT I. TEPPER, M.D. (122–129)
Instructor in Medicine, Harvard Medical School; Assistant in Medicine, Massachusetts General Hospital, Boston

KENNETH TYLER, M.D. (151, 154, 156, 161, 162, 167, 168, 176)
Assistant Professor of Neurology, Department of Microbiology and Molecular Genetics, Harvard Medical School, Boston

J. WOODROW WEISS, M.D. (10, 11, 71, 72, 74, 75, 77–83)
Assistant Professor of Medicine, Harvard Medical School; Associate Physician, Beth Israel Hospital, Boston

MARK E. WILLIAMS, M.D. (13, 21, 22, 84–89, 91–94)
Instructor in Medicine, Harvard Medical School; Assistant in Medicine, Beth Israel Hospital, Boston

JEAN D. WILSON, M.D. (16, 23, 24, 134–146, 178–182)
Professor of Internal Medicine, The University of Texas Health Science Center, Dallas

K. RANDALL YOUNG, Jr., M.D. (25, 73, 107–121, 130–133, 169, 185, 190)
Medical Staff Fellow, Laboratory of Immunoregulation, National Institute of Allergy and Infectious Diseases, Bethesda

PREFACE

Most medical students and many residents are often overwhelmed by the sheer quantity of medical information potentially applicable to the diagnosis and treatment of their patients. The editors and authors summarize this vast amount of information in *Harrison's Principles of Internal Medicine,* which is thoroughly revised and updated every three to four years. Although *Harrison's* represents a distillate of the broad field of internal medicine, along with its deep roots in the basic sciences, the total information presented in the book grows steadily, along with the base of useful medical knowledge.

While it would be ideal to have a copy of *Harrison's* in one's pocket at all times, the sheer bulk and weight of the book make this impossible. The editors, with the aid of a few selected contributors, have now condensed the clinical portions of *Harrison's* into this pocket-sized *Companion Handbook* which residents and students can use on their trek through the inpatient, outpatient, and emergency services of a teaching hospital. The *Companion Handbook* consists of brief summaries of the key features of the principal diseases of patients which trainees are likely to encounter on a medical service. The blank pages interspersed in the book are to allow recording of additional information obtained during rounds and conferences to supplement the text. Following the text is a glossary spelling out the abbreviations used throughout the book.

It is important to point out that the *Companion Handbook* should not and cannot be a replacement for a textbook of internal medicine. Rather it is an extension of the Eleventh Edition of *Harrison's.* Each brief chapter in the *Companion Handbook* is referenced to the appropriate chapter(s) in *Harrison's.* The *Companion Handbook* is meant to be used when the resident or student requires a brief introduction to or reminder of an aspect of clinical internal medicine but does not have immediate access to or the time to consult *Harrison's.* Since the quantity of material presented is too brief to stand on its own, it is recommended that the relevant subjects in *Harrison's* be consulted as soon as time permits. Thus, we consider the two books, Harrison's and the *Companion Handbook*, as a single educational package.

Since this is the first edition of the *Companion Handbook*, the editors would be grateful to the readers for their comments concerning its usefulness.

THE EDITORS

SECTION I
IMPORTANT SYMPTOMS AND SIGNS

1 PAIN AND ITS MANAGEMENT

Pain is the most common symptom of disease. Its management depends on determining its cause and alleviating triggering and potentiating factors.

ORGANIZATION OF PAIN PATHWAYS (See HPIM-11, Fig. 3-1.) Pain-producing (nociceptive) sensory stimuli in skin and viscera activate nerve endings of bipolar neurons of spinal dorsal root or cranial nerve ganglia. After synapse in cord or medulla, crossed ascending pathways reach thalamus and are projected to cortex. An indirect multisynaptic afferent system connects with brainstem reticular formation and projects to intralaminar and medial thalamic nuclei and limbic system. Pain transmission is regulated at level of dorsal horn by descending bulbospinal pathways that contain serotonin, norepinephrine, and several neuropeptides.

Agents that modify pain perception may act to reduce tissue inflammation (corticosteroids, NSAIDs, prostaglandin synthesis inhibitors), to interfere with pain transmission (narcotics), or to enhance descending modulation (tricyclic antidepressants). Anticonvulsants may alter aberrant pain sensations arising from neurogenic sources, e.g., demyelination of peripheral nerves.

EVALUATION Pain may be of *somatic* (skin, deep tissues, joints, muscles) or *neuropathic* (injury to nerves, spinal cord pathways, or thalamus) origin. Characteristics of each are summarized in Table 1-1.

Sensory symptoms and signs in neuropathic pain are described by the following definitions: *neuralgia:* pain in distribution of a single nerve, as in trigeminal neuralgia; *dysesthesia:* spontaneous

TABLE 1-1 **Characteristics of somatic and neuropathic pain**

Somatic pain:
- Nociceptive stimulus usually evident.
- Usually well localized; visceral pain may be referred.
- Similar to other somatic pains in patient's experience.
- Relieved by anti-inflammatory or narcotic analgesics.

Neuropathic pain:
- No obvious nociceptive stimulus.
- Often poorly localized.
- Unusual, dissimilar from somatic pain.
- Only partially relieved by narcotic analgesics.

Modified from Maciewicz R, Martin JB: HPIM-11, p. 15.

TABLE 1-2 **Drugs used to relieve pain**

Nonnarcotic analgesics: equivalent doses and intervals

Generic name	Dose, mg	Interval
Aspirin	750–1250	q 3 h
Phenacetin	750–1000	q 3 h
Acetaminophen	600–800	q 3 h
Phenylbutazone	200–400	q 4 h
Indomethacin	50–75	q 4 h
Ibuprofen	200–400	q 4 h
Naproxen	250–500	q 4 h
Nefopam	60–120	q 4 h

Narcotic analgesics compared to 10 mg morphine sulfate (MS)

Generic name	IM dose, mg	PO dose, mg	Differences from MS
Oxymorphine	1	6	None
Hydromorphine	1.5	7.5	Shorter acting
Levorphanol	2	4	Good PO-IM potency
Heroin	4		Short-acting
Methadone	10	20	Good PO-IM potency
Morphine	10	60	
Oxycodone	15	30	Short-acting
Meperidine	75	300	None
Pentazocine	60	180	Agonist-antagonist
Codeine	130	200	More toxic

Anticonvulsants

Generic name	PO dose, mg	Interval
Phenytoin	100	q 6–8 h
Carbamazepine	200	q 6 h
Clonazepam	1	q 6 h

Antidepressants

Generic name	PO dose, mg	Range, mg/day
Doxepin	200	75–400
Amitriptyline	150	75–300
Imipramine	200	75–400
Nortriptyline	100	40–150
Desipramine	150	75–300
Amoxapine	200	75–300
Trazodone	150	50–600

Reproduced from Maciewicz R, Martin JB: HPIM-11, p. 16.

background pain of aching, burning quality; *hyperalgesia* and *hyperesthesia:* exaggerated responses to nociceptive or touch stimulus, respectively; *allodynia:* perception of nonnociceptive stimulus as painful, as when vibration evokes painful sensation. Reduced pain perception is called *hypalgesia* or, when absent, *analgesia*. *Causalgia* is continuous severe burning pain with indistinct boundaries and accompanying sympathetic nervous system dysfunction (sweating, vascular, skin, and hair changes—sympathetic dystrophy) which occurs after injury to a peripheral nerve.

MANAGEMENT Acute somatic pain: Usually effectively treated with nonnarcotic analgesic agents (Table 1-2). Narcotic analgesics are usually required for relief of severe pain.

Neuropathic pain: Often chronic; management is particularly difficult. The following drugs, in combination with careful assessment of underlying factors that contribute to pain (depression, "compensation neurosis"), may be beneficial:

1 *Anticonvulsants:* In patients with neuropathic pain and little or no evidence of sympathetic dysfunction; diabetic neuropathy, trigeminal neuralgia (tic douloureux).

2 *Antisympathetic agents:* In patients with causalgia and sympathetic dystrophy, surgical or chemical sympathectomy may be tried (see HPIM-11, Chap. 3).

3 *Tricyclic antidepressants:* Pharmacologic effects include facilitation of monamine neurotransmitters by inhibition of transmitter reuptake. Are useful in management of patients with chronic pain, postherpetic neuralgia, atypical facial pain (see Chap. 4), chronic low back pain (see Chap. 5).

For more detailed discussion of this topic, see Maciewicz R, Martin JM: Pain: Pathophysiology and Management, Chap. 3 in HPIM-11, p. 13

---

2 CHEST PAIN

There is little correlation between the severity of chest pain and the seriousness of its cause.

POTENTIALLY SERIOUS CAUSES

MYOCARDIAL ISCHEMIA **Angina pectoris:** Substernal pressure, squeezing, constriction, with radiation typically to left arm; usually on exertion, especially after meals or with emotional arousal. Characteristically relieved by rest and nitroglycerin.
Acute myocardial infarction: Similar to angina but more severe, of longer duration (≥30 min), and not immediately relieved by rest or nitroglycerin. S_3 and S_4 common.

PULMONARY EMBOLISM May be substernal or lateral, pleuritic in nature, and associated with hemoptysis, tachycardia, hypoxemia.

AORTIC DISSECTION Very severe, in center of chest, a "ripping quality," radiates to back, not affected by changes in position. May be associated with weak or absent peripheral pulses.

MEDIASTINAL EMPHYSEMA Sharp, intense, localized to substernal region; often associated with audible crepitus.

ACUTE PERICARDITIS Usually steady, crushing, substernal; often has pleuritic component aggravated by cough, deep inspiration, supine position, and relieved by sitting upright; one-, two-, or three-component friction rub often audible.

PLEURISY Due to inflammation; less commonly tumor and pneumothorax. Usually unilateral, knifelike, superficial, aggravated by cough and respiration.

LESS SERIOUS CAUSES

COSTOCHONDRAL PAIN In anterior chest, usually sharply localized, may be brief and darting or a persistent dull ache. Can be reproduced by pressure on chondrosternal and/or costochondral junctions. In Tietze's syndrome (costochondritis), joints are swollen, red, and tender.

CHEST WALL PAIN Due to strain of muscles or ligaments from excessive exercise or rib fracture from trauma; accompanied by local tenderness.

ESOPHAGEAL PAIN Deep thoracic discomfort; may be accompanied by dysphagia and regurgitation.

EMOTIONAL DISORDERS Prolonged ache or dartlike, brief, flashing pain; associated with fatigue, emotional strain.

OTHER CAUSES

(1) Cervical disk; (2) osteoarthritis of cervical or thoracic spine; (3) abdominal disorders: peptic ulcer, hiatus hernia, biliary colic;

(4) tracheobronchitis, pneumonia; (5) diseases of the breast (inflammation, tumor); (6) intercostal neuritis (herpes zoster)

APPROACH TO PATIENT

- Obtain a meticulous history of the behavior of pain, what precipitates it and what relieves it.
- When localized pain can be reproduced by pressure, it usually originates from chest wall.
- Electrocardiogram *during* chest pain helpful in diagnosis of ischemia (ST segments may be elevated or depressed).
- Workup for angina (Chap. 65) in patients with episodic pain.
- Serum enzymes and evolution of ECG are diagnostic of myocardial infarction (Chap. 64) in patients with prolonged pain.
- Echogram or CT scan of aorta in patients with sudden, severe pain helpful in diagnosis of aortic dissection (Chap. 69).
- Esophageal pH, acid perfusion test, and barium esophagram useful in diagnosis of esophageal pain (Chap. 95).
- CXR for pleurisy, pneumonia, mediastinal emphysema, pneumothorax.

For more detailed discussion of this topic, see Braunwald E: Chest Discomfort and Palpitation, Chap. 4, in HPIM-11, p. 17

3 ABDOMINAL PAIN

Numerous causes, ranging from acute, life-threatening emergencies to chronic functional disease and disorders of several organ systems can generate abdominal pain. Evaluation of acute pain requires rapid assessment of likely causes and early initiation of appropriate therapy. A more detailed and leisurely approach to diagnosis may be followed in less acute situations. Table 3-1 lists the common causes of abdominal pain.

EVALUATION

History: Extremely important. Physical examination may be unrevealing or misleading; laboratory and radiologic exams delayed or unhelpful. Table 3-2 lists major components of history taking for evaluation of abdominal pain.

TABLE 3-1 **Common etiologies of abdominal pain**

Mucosal or muscle inflammation in hollow viscera: Acid-peptic disease (ulcers, erosions, inflammation), hemorrhagic gastritis, gastroesophageal reflux, appendicitis, diverticulitis, cholecystitis, cholangitis, inflammatory bowel diseases (Crohn's, ulcerative colitis, Behçet's), infectious gastroenteritis, or colitis

Visceral spasm or distention: Intestinal obstruction (adhesions, tumor, intussusception), appendiceal obstruction with appendicitis, irritable bowel syndrome (muscle hypertrophy and spasm), acute biliary obstruction, pancreatic ductal obstruction (chronic pancreatitis, stone), ureteral obstruction (kidney stone, blood clot), fallopian tubes (tubal pregnancy)

Vascular disorder: Mesenteric thromboembolic disease (arterial or venous), arterial dissection or rupture (e.g., aortic aneurysm), occlusion from external pressure or torsion (e.g., volvulus, hernia, tumor, intussusception), hemoglobinopathy (esp. sickle cell anemia)

Distention or inflammation of visceral surfaces: Hepatic capsule (hepatitis, hemorrhage, tumor, Budd-Chiari syndrome), renal capsular distention (tumor, infection, infarction, venous occlusion), splenic capsular distention (hemorrhage, abscess, infarction), pancreas (pancreatitis, pseudocyst, abscess), ovary (hemorrhage, ectopic pregnancy, abscess)

Peritoneal inflammation: Bacterial infection (perforated viscus, pelvic inflammatory disease, infected ascites), intestinal infarction, chemical irritation, pancreatitis, perforated viscus (esp. stomach and duodenum, mittelschmerz), reactive inflammation (neighboring abscess, incl. diverticulitis, pleuropulmonary infection or inflammation), serositis (collagen-vascular diseases, familial Mediterranean fever)

Abdominal wall disorders: Trauma, hernias, muscle inflammation or infection, hematoma (trauma, anticoagulant therapy), traction from mesentery (e.g., adhesions)

Toxins: Lead poisoning, black widow spider bite

Metabolic disorders: Uremia, ketoacidosis (diabetic, alcoholic), Addisonian crisis, porphyria, angioneurotic edema (C_1 esterase deficiency)

Neurologic: Tabes dorsalis, herpes zoster, causalgia, compression or inflammation of spinal roots, (e.g., arthritis, herniated disk, tumor, abscess), psychogenic

Referred pain: From heart, lungs, esophagus, genitalia

TABLE 3-2 Important historical aspects of abdominal pain

- Onset and duration of pain:
  - Acute vs. long-standing
  - Sudden vs. insidious
  - Steady vs. intermittent
- Location of pain:
  - Diffuse vs. localized
  - Referred sites of pain
- Quality of pain:
  - Mild vs. severe vs. *catastrophic*
  - Dull, sharp, gnawing, crampy, colicky, etc.
- Precipitants and relievers of pain:
  - Relationship to time of day
  - Relationship to food intake:
    - Temporal
    - Type of food
  - Relationship to medications or other therapies
  - Effect of movement or position:
    - Relation to breathing or coughing
    - Effect of physical activity
  - Relationship to urination or bowel movements
  - Relationship to menstrual cycle or menarche
- Changes in pain characteristics since onset
- Associated symptoms:
  - Syncope or light-headedness
  - Fever, chills, or diaphoresis
  - Nausea, vomiting, dysphagia, or early satiety
  - Constipation or diarrhea
  - Dysuria or urinary frequency
  - Vaginal or penile discharge
  - Evidence of coagulopathy or hemorrhage
  - Weight loss
  - Icterus (jaundice)
- Underlying or predisposing conditions:
  - Hypertension
  - Ethanol, smoking, illicit drugs, or other medications
  - Family history

Type and location of abdominal pain provide rough guide to nature of disease. Visceral pain (due to distention of a hollow viscus) localizes poorly and is often perceived in the midline. Intestinal pain tends to be crampy; when originating proximal to the ileocecal valve, it usually localizes above and around the umbilicus. Pain of colonic origin is perceived in the hypogastrium and lower quadrants. Pain from biliary or ureteral obstruction often causes patients to writhe in discomfort. Somatic pain (due to peritoneal inflammation) is usually sharper and more precisely localized to the diseased region (e.g., acute appendicitis, capsular distention of liver, kidney, or spleen), exacerbated by movement, causing patients to remain still. Pattern of radiation may be helpful: right shoulder (hepatobiliary origin), left shoulder (splenic), mid-back (pancreatic), groin (genitourinary).

Physical examination: Evaluate abdomen for prior trauma or surgery, current trauma; abdominal distention, fluid, or air; direct, rebound, and referred tenderness; liver and spleen size; masses, bruits, altered bowel sounds, hernias, arterial masses. Rectal examination for masses, tenderness, blood (gross or occult). Pelvic examination in women is essential. General examination: evaluate for evidence of hemodynamic instability, acid-base disturbances, nutritional deficiency, coagulopathy, arterial occlusive disease, stigmata of liver disease, cardiac dysfunction, lymphadenopathy, and skin lesions.

Routine laboratory and radiologic studies: Choices depend on clinical setting. Generally include CBC, serum electrolytes, arterial blood gases, coagulation parameters, serum glucose, and biochemical tests of liver, kidney, and pancreatic function; chest radiographs to determine the presence of diseases involving heart, lung, mediastinum, and pleura; ECG is helpful to exclude referred pain from cardiac disease; plain abdominal radiographs to evaluate bowel displacement, intestinal distention, fluid and gas pattern, free peritoneal air, liver size, and abdominal calcifications (e.g., gallstones, renal stones, chronic pancreatitis).

Special studies: May include abdominal ultrasonography (most helpful to visualize biliary ducts, gallbladder, liver, and kidneys); gastrointestinal barium contrast radiographs (barium swallow, upper GI series, small bowel follow-through, barium enema, enteroclysis); upper GI endoscopy, sigmoidoscopy, or colonoscopy; CT or MRI, cholangiography, angiography, and radionuclide scanning. In selected cases, biopsy of the liver, pancreas, or abdominal mass; laparoscopy; and sometimes exploratory laparoscopy; and sometimes exploratory laparotomy are required.

ACUTE, CATASTROPHIC ABDOMINAL PAIN

Intense abdominal pain of acute onset or pain associated with syncope, hypotension, or toxic appearance of patient, necessitates rapid yet orderly evaluation. Consider obstruction, perforation or rupture of hollow viscera, dissection or rupture of major blood vessels (esp. aortic aneurysm), upper GI bleeding, abdominal sepsis, ketoacidosis, and adrenal crisis.

Brief history and physical exam should focus on presence of hypothermia, hyperventilation, cyanosis, direct or rebound abdominal tenderness, pulsating abdominal mass, abdominal bruits, ascites, rectal blood, rectal or pelvic tenderness, evidence of coagulopathy. Useful laboratory studies include hematocrit (may be normal with acute hemorrhage or elevated with dehydration), WBC, arterial blood gases, serum electrolytes, BUN, creatinine, glucose, lipase or amylase, and urinalysis. Radiologic studies should include supine and upright abdominal films (left lateral decubitus view if upright unobtainable) to evaluate bowel caliber and presence of free peritoneal air, cross-table lateral film to assess aortic diameter. Abdominal paracentesis (or peritoneal lavage in cases of trauma) to detect evidence of bleeding or spontaneous peritonitis. Abdominal ultrasound (when readily available) to disclose evidence of abscess, cholecystitis, or hematoma.

Immediate therapy should include intravenous fluids, correction of life-threatening acid-base disturbances, and assessment of need for emergent surgery; careful follow-up with frequent reexamination (when possible, by the same examiner) is essential. Narcotic analgesics may best be withheld pending establishment of diagnosis and therapeutic plan, since masking of diagnostic signs may delay needed intervention.

For more detailed discussion of this topic, see Silen W: Abdominal Pain, Chap. 5, in HPIM-11, p. 23

4 HEADACHE AND FACE PAIN

GENERAL CONSIDERATIONS

Headache is a common complaint, often chronic or recurrent, signifying either vascular (migraine) or tension (muscle contraction) origin. Recurrent headache may be generalized in either tension or common migraine or unilateral. In the latter case it may be stereotyped in presentation (classical migraine, cluster migraine, trigeminal neuralgia).

CLASSICAL MIGRAINE Onset in childhood, adolescence, or early adulthood; positive family history; more common in females, with unilateral (right or left) throbbing pain. Nausea and vomiting occur early; visual scotomata and scintillations may occur. Usually lasts a few hours. May be triggered by wine, cheese, chocolate, contraceptives, stress, exercise, or travel.

COMMON MIGRAINE Unilateral headache, alternating sides, with nausea, but rarely with vomiting or visual complaints. More common in women. More gradual onset than classic migraine and may become generalized, persisting for hours or days. Commonly combined with or fades into typical tension (muscle contraction) headache.

CLUSTER MIGRAINE Retroorbital or temporal, unilateral (often recurrent on same side), nocturnal pain, 90% in men. Develops rapidly and is very severe; accompanied by lacrimation, nasal and conjunctival congestion, and periorbital edema. No visual complaints. Pain lasts 20–60 min and may recur at same time of night or several times each 24 h over several weeks. A pain-free period of months or years is then followed by another "cluster" of headaches. Cerebral berry aneurysm may cause unilateral retroorbital eye pain.

CHRONIC MUSCLE CONTRACTION (TENSION) HEADACHES Onset in adolescence or young adulthood; nonfamilial, bilateral, generalized; often bifrontal, bitemporal, or suboccipital. Pain is felt as pressure or tight band, but may be throbbing. Nausea and vomiting are rare; no lacrimation or nasal congestion. Tends to occur late in day; persists for hours or days. Often associated with situational or occupational stress, depression, or chronic anxiety.

BENIGN INTRACRANIAL HYPERTENSION Obese women under 40: vomiting and papilledema, increased CSF pressure without focal neurologic signs, and normal CT or MRI.

SPECIAL CONSIDERATIONS

HEADACHES WITH ONSET AFTER AGE 50 Should alert to possibility of *cranial (temporal) arteritis* (elevated sedimentation rate, tender temporal arteries), *brain tumor*, personality change, vomiting, papilledema, *subdural hematoma,* recent fall, altered consciousness.

TRIGEMINAL NEURALGIA Stabbing, lancinating pain lasting 10–30 s, unilateral location, most commonly mandibular or (less often) maxillary division of trigeminal nerve. Pain occurs after age 50. Trigger point in gum or cheek may prevent eating. Neurologic exam normal. Similar pain in younger person may indicate multiple sclerosis, aneurysm or vascular anomaly, trigeminal neuroma.

POSTHERPETIC (ZOSTER) NEURALGIA Follows herpetic eruptions of ophthalmic, maxillary, or (rarely) mandibular division of trigeminal nerve. May be accompanied by sensory loss—*anesthesia dolorosa.* Management is very difficult.

ATYPICAL FACIAL PAIN Not restricted to a cranial nerve distribution; generalized; sometimes associated with temporomandibular (TMJ) dysfunction. The latter is commonly overdiagnosed by dentists.

PRINCIPLES OF TREATMENT

Establish clinical diagnosis.

MIGRAINE Manage acute attack with ergotamines or analgesics. Prophylaxis in patients with frequent recurrences includes modification of trigger factors—diet, stress.

ACUTE MIGRAINE Treat early with ergotamine 1 mg PO, repeated q 30 min up to 4–6 tablets (6 mg per day or 12 mg per week maximum). (Cafergot contains caffeine 100 mg; Wigraine: caffeine 100 mg; Bellergal: caffeine 0.1 mg, phenacetin 130 mg; Bellergal-S: ergotamine 0.6 mg, belladonna 0.2 mg, phenobarb. 40 mg.) Ergotamine 0.2 mg may be given rectally for more acute effect.
Prophylaxis: (Table 4-1) A number of options exist; frequently need to be given as successive trials to determine most effective drug. Treat patients who experience more than two or three severe attacks each month. Bellergal 1 or 2 tablets daily, propranolol 40 mg tid or qid, amitriptyline 150 mg qhs (start gradually), or calcium

TABLE 4-1 **Prophylaxis of migraine**

Drug	Daily dose range	Side effects
Ergonovine	0.4–2.0 mg	Nausea, abdominal pain
Bellergal	1–4 tabs	Nausea, sedation
Propranolol	40–320 mg	Lethargy, insomnia, constipation
Amitriptyline	25–150 mg	Sedation, dry mouth
Cyproheptadine	12–24 mg	Sedation, weight gain
Phenelzine	15–75 mg	Insomnia, postural dizziness
Methysergide	2–8 mg	Nausea, abdominal cramps, insomnia, *retroperitoneal fibrosis*
Calcium channel blockers (verapamil, nifedipine under investigation)		

channel blockers. Methysergide may be used in otherwise refractory patients (2 mg q 8 h), but never for more than 4–6 mos because of retroperitoneal fibrosis.

TENSION HEADACHES Acetaminophen, aspirin, or Fiorinal.

TEMPORAL ARTERITIS Prednisone in doses sufficient to lower ESR to normal.

For more detailed discussion of this topic, see Adams RD, Martin JB: Headache, Chap. 6, in HPIM-11, p. 26

---

5 LOW BACK PAIN

Pain in the lower back is a common complaint. It may be acute or chronic; may arise from lesions of spinal column or nerve roots or be referred from deeper structures (kidney, pancreas, colon, retroperitoneal tumors).

ETIOLOGY

ACUTE LOW BACK PAIN Acute strain: Clear evidence by history of acute trauma; localized pain with paraspinal muscular spasm, restriction of movements, no radiation of pain to groin or legs.

Vertebral fractures: Usually result from flexion injury or fall onto legs; may occur with minimal or no trauma in patients with bone disease, osteoporosis, Cushing's disease, hyperparathyroidism, multiple myeloma, metastatic bone disease, Paget's disease.

Lumbar intervertebral disk protrusion: Most common site is L_5–S_1, then L_4–L_5, rarely L_3–L_4 or higher. Clinical findings include backache, abnormal posture, and limitation of movement. Nerve root involvement is indicated by radiating radicular pain, usually unilateral, sensory disturbances (paresthesias, hyperesthesia, or hypalgesia), and impairment of ankle jerk (S_1 or S_2 root). Localizing signs are summarized in Table 5-1. Herniation of an intervertebral disk usually affects the root below the level of the disk; i.e., L_4–L_5 disk affects L_5 root, L_5–S_1 disk affects S_1 root. Bladder or bowel symptoms suggest lesion in conus medullaris of spinal cord or in cauda equina.

Facet syndromes: Entrapment of nerve roots at sites of exit from spinal canal may cause radicular pain unrelated to disk disease. Unilateral facet syndrome, which most often affects L_5 root, is caused by enlarged superior or inferior facet with narrowing of intervertebral canal or foramen.

Epidural abscess: Occurs most commonly in thoracic region; may cause acute back pain with tenderness to percussion or pressure on spinous process. Requires rapid diagnosis and surgical treatment if spinal cord compression is found.

Hip disease: Can cause pain that radiates to buttocks and leg as far as *knee*.

CHRONIC LOW BACK PAIN Osteoarthritis: Also called lumbar spondylosis due to degenerative disease of lumbar vertebrae with bony spurs, narrowing of lumbar canal, impingement on nerve roots. Lumbosacral pain with neurologic symptoms on walking (numbness, paresthesia, or weakness in both legs) suggests syndrome of *intermittent claudication of spinal cord.* Diagnosis is confirmed by CT or MRI or by metrizamide myelography.

Ankylosing spondylitis: Presents in young men with low back pain radiating to thighs; 90% are positive for HLA-B27 antigen. Limitation of movement and morning stiffness are followed by limitation of chest expansion, progressive kyphosis, and flexion

TABLE 5-1 **Symptoms and signs of disk protrusion**

Symptoms and signs	L_3–L_4 (L_4 root)	L_4–L_5 (L_5 root)	L_5–S_1 (S_1 root)
Radicular pain, paresthesias, and/or sensory loss	Medial leg + arch of foot	Dorsum of foot and great toe	Lateral leg, foot and sole, 4th and 5th toes
Weakness or muscle atrophy	Quadriceps	Peroneals and extensor hallcis longus	Gastrocnemius, extensor digitorum brevis
Reflex change	Decreased knee jerk	No change	Decreased ankle jerk
Straight leg raising	May be positive with extension in prone position (reversed)	Positive	Positive

of thoracic spine. Radiologic hallmarks are destruction and obliteration of the sacroiliac joints and formation of "bamboo" spine. Similar patterns of restricted movements of lower spine may occur in psoriatic arthritis, Reiter's syndrome, and chronic inflammatory bowel disease.

Neoplastic, metastatic, metabolic diseases: Metastatic carcinoma (breast, lung, prostate, thyroid, kidney, GI tract), multiple myeloma, and lymphoma should be excluded by radiologic studies, CT, MRI, or myelography.

Osteomyelitis: From pyogenic bacteria (usually staphylococcus) or Tbc; should be considered and excluded by ESR, bone x-rays, tuberculin skin tests.

Intradural tumors: Neurofibromas, meningiomas, and lipomas may cause chronic pain before neurologic findings appear.

REFERRED PAIN FROM VISCERAL DISEASE Pelvic diseases refer pain to sacral region; lower abdominal diseases, to the lumbar region L_3–L_5; and upper abdominal diseases, to lower thoracic and upper lumbar region T_{10}–L_2. Characteristically, no local signs or stiffness of back; full range of movement of back does not augment pain.

1 Peptic ulcer and tumors of stomach, duodenum, or pancreas, particularly with retroperitoneal involvement, may cause T_{10}–L_2 back pain.

2 Ulcerative colitis, diverticulitis, and tumors of colon may cause low back pain.

3 Chronic pelvic inflammatory disease, endometriosis, or carcinoma of the ovary or uterus in women may cause low back pain. In men, chronic prostatitis and prostate carcinoma need to be excluded.

4 Renal disease can cause pain in costovertebral angle.

5 Aortic dissecting aneurysm can cause thoracic-lumbar pain.

MANAGEMENT

Careful attention should be given to onset, duration, location, factors that exacerbate or alleviate. Examination should include abdomen and pelvic regions, movements of spine, and evidence of neurologic dysfunction. In acute pain, plain radiographs are rarely helpful except after trauma. CT, MRI, and lumbar myelography are used to assess spondylosis, acute herniated disk, and tumor. Chronic pain should be assessed by ESR, serum acid phosphatase, carcinoembryonic antigen, and x-ray studies.

For more detailed discussion of this topic, see Mankin HJ, Adams RD: Pain in the Back and Neck, Chap. 7, in HPIM-11, p. 34

---

6 CHILLS AND FEVER

GENERAL CONSIDERATIONS

Causes of fever

• All infections • Mechanical trauma • Many neoplastic diseases (particularly metastatic to liver or lymphomas) • Hematopoietic disorders (hemolytic episodes) • Vascular accidents (myocardial, cerebral infarction) • Immune diseases (connective-tissue, drug fevers) • Acute metabolic disorders (gout, porphyria, thyroid crisis)

Accompaniments of fever

• Systemic symptoms (headache, back pain, myalgia) • Chills (differentiate true *shaking* chill from chilly sensations; chills may be evoked by antipyretics) • Herpes labialis (common in pneumococcal, streptococcal, and meningococcal infections) • Delirium (common in old age, alcoholism) • Convulsions (watch for in children)

Management of fever

• Do not lower temperature unless very high (heat stroke, delirium, seizures, heart failure) • Cooling blankets; sponging with cool saline • Immersion in ice water if temperature reaches 108°F • If antipyretics (aspirin 0.3–0.6 g or acetaminophen 0.5 g) are used, do so around clock (q 2–3 h) to mitigate sweats, abrupt fall in temperature, and compensatory chills with more fever • Steroids are potent antipyretics; use with caution to prevent abrupt fall in temperature • NSAIDs useful in fever due to neoplasia

Diagnostic considerations

• Fever patterns rarely of diagnostic value • In U.S., fever usually due to common diseases • Most febrile illness of short duration

Clues to infections of abrupt onset

• High fever ± chills • Respiratory Sx • Severe malaise • Nausea, vomiting, diarrhea • Acute enlargement of lymph nodes or spleen • Meningeal signs • WBC ≥ 12,000 or ≤ 5000 • Dysuria, frequency, flank pain

Fever of unknown origin: prolonged, undiagnosed fever

• Temperature ≥ 101°F for ≥ 3 weeks • Undiagnosed after 1 week of extensive studies • Rigid criteria eliminate common infections, easily diagnosed diseases, and tandem diseases (myocardial infarction followed by thrombophlebitis followed by pulmonary emboli)

DISEASES CAUSING PROLONGED FEVERS

Infections

• Abscesses • Mycobacterial infections (usually extrapulmonary; watch for *Mycobacterium avium-intracellulare* in AIDS) • Renal infections (usually complicated by stone or obstruction) • Other bacterial: sinusitis, vertebral osteomyelitis, infected IV catheters • SBE (rare cause of fever of unknown origin) • Iatrogenic (watch for IV lines, infected bandages or casts, wounds) • Viral, rickettsial, and chlamydial infections (rare in U.S. in immunocompetent individuals) • Parasitic (obtain travel history)

Neoplasms
• Lymphomas of all types • Malignant histiocytosis • Leukemias (telltale cells usually absent at onset) • Solid tumors (usually metastatic to liver) • Atrial myxomas • Renal cell carcinoma

Connective tissue diseases
• Systemic lupus erythematosus • Rheumatic fever (now rare) • Rheumatoid arthritis (usually juvenile without joint changes) • Granulomas (nonpulmonary sarcoid, regional enteritis, granulomatous hepatitis)

Miscellaneous
• Drug fever (often multiple drugs) • Multiple pulmonary emboli • Cryptic hematomas • Nonspecific pericarditis • Familial Mediterranean fever (ethnic origin; peritonitis; pleuritis; pericarditis; well between episodes; renal failure secondary to amyloidosis now rare; responds to colchicine 0.6 mg 2–3 times per day) • Psychogenic fever (habitual hyperthermia 99–100.5°F; young women; psychoneurosis; do not do extensive workup) • Factitious fever (malingerers; young women with professional/medical background; prove by personally being in room with thermometer in place; note dissociation of pulse and temperature; refractory to psychotherapy)

Undiagnosed
• Some patients' fever is steroid suppressible • Rarely life-threatening

DIAGNOSTIC PROCEDURES

Routine
• Must individualize workup • Careful Hx and PE • Hematology, chemistry, and immunologic battery rarely diagnostic • Microbiology; avoid repeated (more than 6) blood cultures; look at Gram and acid-fast bacillus smears; culture for anaerobes (do not withold therapy if otherwise indicated) • Skin tests rarely helpful

Imaging
• Chest x-rays most helpful; other films only if signs or symptoms warrant • Ultrasonography (best for kidneys and RUQ diseases) • Radionuclide scans (technetium liver and spleen scans helpful in RUQ and LUQ diseases; gallium: too many false positives or negatives; indium 111 helpful for abscesses) • CT scans (best for abscesses, nodes, tumors, hematomas)

Biopsies
• Abnormal-appearing tissues better than blind biopsy • Bone marrow if patient is anemic • Liver: low yield unless function tests abnormal • Lymph node useful except for inguinal nodes

Exploratory laparotomy: Only if there are clinical, laboratory, or imaging clues.

Therapeutic trials: Only useful if specific (INH or rifampin for tuberculosis, but not multiple antibiotics).
Prognosis generally favorable: Repeated history, physical, and chart reviews (not lab tests) may lead to diagnosis that was missed originally.

For more detailed discussion of this topic, see Petersdorf RG, Root RK: Chills and Fever, Chap. 9, in HPIM-11, p. 50

---

7 SYNCOPE AND SEIZURES

SYNCOPE Defined as generalized weakness, with loss of postural tone, inability to stand upright, and loss of consciousness. Begins with a sense of "feeling bad," with dimming vision, ringing in ears, or sweating. May occur so rapidly that there is no warning. Patient appears pale and ashen, with faint pulse. Complete loss of consciousness may be averted if subject can promptly lie down. Once horizontal, cerebral perfusion is no longer hindered by gravity. Pulse then becomes stronger, color returns to face, and consciousness is regained.

FAINTNESS A lack of strength with sensation of impending loss of consciousness.

FEATURES DISTINGUISHING SYNCOPE FROM SEIZURE Seizures may occur day or night, regardless of patient's posture; syncope rarely occurs when recumbent (exception: Stokes-Adams attack). Pallor is invariable in syncope, whereas cyanosis or plethora may occur in seizure. Seizures are often heralded by an aura of localizing significance. Injury from falling is common in seizure, rare in syncope. Unconsciousness usually lasts longer in seizure than in syncope; return to alertness is usually slow after a seizure, prompt with syncope. Urinary incontinence is common in seizure, rare in syncope. Repeated spells of unconsciousness (several per day or per month) in a young person suggest seizure rather than syncope. These points, when taken as a group and supplemented by EEG findings characteristic of seizure, provide the basis on which to distinguish syncope from seizure.

ETIOLOGY OF SYNCOPE Most often due to processes resulting in reduced cerebral blood flow: (1) inadequate vasoconstrictor mechanisms (vasovagal, postural hypotension, primary autonomic insufficiency, pharmacologic or surgical sympathectomy, diseases of central and peripheral nervous system); (2) hypovolemia (acute blood loss, Addison's disease); (3) reduction of venous return (Valsalva, cough, micturition); (4) reduced cardiac output due to mechanical obstruction, atrial myxoma, pulmonary embolism, myocardial infarction, congestive failure, or cardiac tamponade; (5) arrhythmias, complete AV block, ventricular fibrillation, or tachycardia; or (6) extracranial vascular insufficiency (vertebrobasilar or bilateral carotid disease). Episodic weakness and disturbance of consciousness also can occur with hypoxia, anemia, hyperventilation, or hypoglycemia.

For detailed discussion of this topic, see Adams RD, Martin JB: Faintness, Syncope, and Seizures, Chap. 12, in HPIM-11, p. 64

8 DIZZINESS AND VERTIGO

Patients use the term *dizziness* to describe any of several unusual head sensations or to complain of gait unsteadiness. With a careful history, the patient's symptoms can be placed into more specific neurologic categories, of which faintness and vertigo are most important.

DEFINITIONS Faintness: A symptom of insufficient blood oxygen or, rarely, glucose supply to the brain. Usually described as light-headedness followed by visual blurring and postural swaying. Occurs with hyperventilation, hypoglycemia, and prior to a syncopal event (Chap. 7). Light-headedness also can occur as an aura before a seizure. Chronic light-headedness is a common somatic complaint in patients with depression.
Vertigo: The illusion of self or environmental movement, most commonly a sensation of spinning. Physiologic vertigo is due to unfamiliar head movement or visual-proprioceptive-vestibular mismatch, i.e., seasickness, height vertigo, visual vertigo. True vertigo almost never occurs in the presyncopal state.
Pathologic vertigo: Caused by abnormalities of visual, somatosensory, or vestibular inputs, most commonly the latter. Frequently accompanied by nausea, postural unsteadiness, and gait ataxia. May be caused by peripheral (labyrinth or eighth nerve) or central (CNS) lesions. The distinction is prognostically important.

PERIPHERAL VERTIGO Usually severe, accompanied by nausea and emesis. Tinnitus, a feeling of ear fullness or hearing loss, may occur. Patient may be pale and diaphoretic. Jerk nystagmus almost always present. The nystagmus is unidirectional, horizontal with a torsional component, and has its fast phase to side of normal ear. It is inhibited by visual fixation. Patient senses spinning motion in direction of slow phase and falls or mispoints to that side. Usually no other neurologic abnormalities.
Etiology: Peripheral vertigo is common and usually episodic because central compensatory mechanisms ultimately diminish it. *Labyrinthitis* (postviral) is a common cause and may present as an acute attack followed by persistent benign positional vertigo. Severe bilateral vestibular lesions can cause chronic symptoms. Common causes of persistent vertigo include recent head trauma, Ménière's disease (recurrent vertigo accompanied by tinnitus and deafness), and acoustic neuroma. The latter also may cause facial weakness and facial sensory loss due to involvement of cranial nerves V and VII. Drug toxicity (streptomycin, gentamicin, neomycin) can cause peripheral vestibulopathy. Psychogenic vertigo should be suspected in patients with chronic incapacitating vertigo who also have agorophobia, a normal neurologic exam, and no nystagmus.

CENTRAL VERTIGO Identified by associated abnormal neurologic signs such as dysarthria, diplopia, paresthesia, headache, weakness, limb ataxia. The nystagmus can take almost any form, i.e., vertical, multidirectional, but is often purely horizontal without a torsional component. Central nystagmus is not inhibited by fixation. Central vertigo may be chronic or mild and is less likely to be accompanied by tinnitus or hearing loss. It usually is a sign of brainstem dysfunction and may be due to demyelinating, vascular, or neoplastic disease. Rarely it occurs as a manifestation of epilepsy.

EVALUATION The dizzy patient usually requires provocative tests to reproduce the symptoms. Valsalva maneuver, hyperventilation, or postural changes may reproduce faintness. Rapid rotation of the patient in a swivel chair may reproduce vertigo. Benign positional vertigo is identified by positioning the head of a recumbent patient in extension over the edge of the bed with movements to the appropriate side to elicit vertigo and nystagmus. If patient does not exhibit characteristic signs of peripheral vertigo or shows other neurologic abnormalities, then prompt evaluation for central pathology is indicated, i.e., CT or MRI scan of the brainstem, electronystagmography, evoked potential tests, or vertebrobasilar angiography.

TREATMENT For acute vertigo, bed rest and vestibular suppressant drugs such as antihistamines (meclizine, dimenhydrinate, promethazine), anticholinergics (scopolamine), or hypnotics. Ménière's may respond to a low-salt diet with a diuretic. A mild exercise program is prescribed for patients with a prolonged episode of peripheral vertigo to induce central compensatory mechanisms. Patients with central vertigo should be carefully evaluated for potentially life-threatening brainstem lesions.

For more detailed discussion of this topic, see Daroff RB: Dizziness and Vertigo, Chap. 14, in HPIM-11, p. 76

9 CONFUSION, STUPOR, AND COMA

Consciousness disorders are common in medical practice. Assessment of consciousness abnormalities should determine whether there is a change in *level* of consciousness (drowsy, stuporous, comatose) or *content* of consciousness (confusion, perseveration, hallucinations). *Confusion* is a lack of clarity in thinking with inattentiveness; *stupor,* a state in which vigorous stimuli are needed to elicit a response; *coma,* a condition of unresponsiveness. Patients in such states are usually seriously ill and etiologic factors must be assessed.

APPROACH TO PATIENT

1 Support the patient's vital functions.
2 Administer glucose, thiamine, and naloxone if etiology is not clear.
3 Utilize history, examination, and laboratory and radiologic information to rapidly establish the cause of the disorder.
4 Provide the appropriate medical or surgical treatment.

HISTORY Patient should be aroused, if possible, and questioned regarding use of insulin, narcotics, anticoagulants, other prescription drugs, suicidal intent, recent trauma, headache, epilepsy, significant medical problems, and preceding symptoms. Witnesses and family members should be interrogated, often by phone. History of sudden headache followed by loss of consciousness suggests intracranial hemorrhage; preceding vertigo, nausea, diplopia, ataxia, hemisensory disorder suggest basilar insufficiency; palpitations and faintness suggest cardiac arrhythmia.

IMMEDIATE ASSESSMENT Vital signs should be evaluated, and appropriate support initiated. Blood should be drawn for glucose, Na, K, Ca, BUN, ammonia, alcohol, liver transaminase levels; also screen for presence of toxins. Fever, especially with petechial rash, should suggest meningitis; spinal fluid should be examined and antibiotics given without delay.

NEUROLOGIC EVALUATION Focuses on establishing patient's best level of function and uncovering signs that enable a specific diagnosis. Although confused states may occur with unilateral cerebral lesions, stupor and coma are signs of bihemispheral dysfunction or damage to midbrain-tegmentum (reticular activating system).

Responsiveness: Stimuli of increasing intensity are used to gauge degree of unresponsiveness. A shout, shake, or mild or heavy noxious stimuli may be needed to elicit a verbal or motor response. The stimulus and response should be recorded to assess progress. Motor responses may be purposeful or reflexive. Spontaneous flexion of elbows with leg extension, termed *decortication,* accompanies severe damage to contralateral hemisphere above midbrain. Extension of elbows, wrists, and legs, termed *decerebration,* suggests damage to diencephalon or midbrain.

Pupils: In patients with coma, equal, round, reactive pupils exclude midbrain damage as cause and suggest a metabolic abnormality. Pinpoint pupils occur in narcotic overdose (except meperidine, which causes midsize pupils). Small pupils also occur with hydrocephalus and thalamic or pontine damage. A unilateral, enlarged, often oval, poorly reactive pupil is caused by midbrain lesions or compression of third cranial nerve, as occurs in transtentorial herniation. Bilaterally dilated, unreactive pupils indicate severe bilateral midbrain damage, anticholinergic overdose, or ocular trauma.

Eye movements: Spontaneous and reflex eye movements should be examined for limitations of ocular movement, involuntary movements, and misalignment of ocular axes. Intermittent horizontal divergence is common in drowsiness. An *adducted* eye at rest with impaired ability to turn eye laterally indicates an abducens (VI) nerve palsy, common in raised intracranial pressure or pontine damage. The eye with a dilated, unreactive pupil often is *abducted* at rest and cannot turn fully in a medial direction due to third nerve dysfunction, as occurs with transtentorial herniation. Vertical separation of ocular axes occurs in pontine or cerebellar lesions. Involuntary, brisk downward and slow upward movements of globes are called *ocular bobbing* and indicate bilateral pontine damage. The converse, slow downward and brisk upward movements, termed *ocular dipping,* suggests diffuse anoxic cortical injury. Oculocephalic reflex is tested by observing eye movements in response to lateral rotation of head (significant neck injury is a contraindication). Loose movement of eyes with this *doll's head maneuver* occurs in bihemispheric dysfunction. In comatose patients with an intact brainstem, raising head to 60° above the horizontal and irrigating external auditory canal with cold water causes tonic deviation of gaze to irrigated ear. In conscious patients, it causes nystagmus, vertigo, and emesis. Doll's head maneuver and *cold caloric*–induced eye movements allow accurate diagnosis of gaze or cranial nerve palsies in patients who do not move their eyes purposefully.

Respiration: Respiratory pattern may suggest site of neurologic damage. Cheyne-Stokes (periodic) breathing occurs in bihemispheral dysfunction and is common in metabolic encephalopathies. Respiratory patterns composed of gasps or apneustic breathing are indicative of lower brainstem damage; patients usually require intubation and ventilatory assistance.

Other: Comatose patient's best motor and sensory function should be assessed by testing reflex responses to noxious stimuli; carefully note any asymmetric responses, which suggest a focal lesion. If possible, patient with disordered consciousness should have gait examined. Ataxia may be the prominent neurologic finding in a stuporous patient with a cerebellar mass.

RADIOLOGIC EXAMINATION Lesions causing raised intracranial pressure commonly cause impaired consciousness. CT scans of the brain are often abnormal in coma but are not usually diagnostic in patients with metabolic encephalopathy, meningitis, early infarction, early encephalitis, diffuse anoxic injury, or drug overdose. Postponing appropriate therapy in these patients while awaiting a CT scan may be deleterious. Patients with disordered consciousness due to high intracranial pressure can deteriorate rapidly; emergent CT study is necessary to confirm presence of mass effect and to guide surgical consideration. CT scan is normal in some patients with subarachnoid hemorrhage; the diagnosis then rests on clinical history combined with RBC in spinal fluid. Cerebral angiography is frequently necessary to establish basilar artery insufficiency as cause of coma in patients with brainstem signs.

Brain death: This results from total cessation of cerebral function and blood flow at a time when cardiopulmonary function continues but is dependent on ventilatory assistance. EEG is isoelectric at high gain, patient is unresponsive, brainstem reflexes are absent, drug toxicity and hypothermia are excluded. Diagnosis should be made only if the state persists for some agreed upon period, 6–24 hours. Demonstration of apnea requires that the P_{CO_2} be high enough to stimulate respiration.

For more detailed discussion of this topic, see Ropper AH, Martin JB: Coma and Other Disorders of Consciousness, Chap. 21, in HPIM-11, p. 114

---

10 DYSPNEA AND PULMONARY EDEMA

DYSPNEA

Definition: An uncomfortable awareness of breathing; intensity can be quantified by establishing the amount of physical exertion necessary to produce the sensation.

CAUSES **Heart disease:** Dyspnea is due to ↑ pulmonary capillary pressure, left atrial hypertension, and sometimes fatigue of respiratory muscles. Vital capacity and lung compliance are ↓ and airway resistance ↑. Begins as exertional breathlessness → orthopnea → paroxysmal nocturnal dyspnea and dyspnea at rest. Diagnosis depends on recognition of heart disease, e.g., Hx of MI, presence of S_3, S_4 murmurs, cardiomegaly, jugular vein distention, hepatomegaly, and peripheral edema (see Chap. 58).

Obstructive disease of the airways: May occur with obstruction anywhere from extrathoracic airways to lung periphery. Acute dyspnea with difficulty *inhaling* suggests *upper* airway obstruction. Physical exam may reveal inspiratory stridor and retraction of supraclavicular fossae. Acute intermittent dyspnea with expiratory wheezing suggests reversible intrathoracic obstruction due to asthma. Chronic, slowly progressive exertional dyspnea characterizes emphysema and CHF.

Diffuse parenchymal lung diseases: Many parenchymal lung diseases, ranging from sarcoidosis to the pneumoconioses, may cause dyspnea. Dyspnea is usually related to exertion early in the course of the illness. Physical exam typically reveals late tachypnea and inspiratory rales.

Pulmonary embolism (See Chap. 77): Repeated discrete episodes of dyspnea may occur with recurrent pulmonary emboli, but others describe slowly progressive dyspnea without abrupt worsening; tachypnea is frequent. Finding of deep venous thrombosis often absent in chronic pulmonary embolism.

Disease of the chest wall or respiratory muscles: Severe kyphoscoliosis may produce chronic dyspnea, often with chronic cor pulmonale. The spinal deformity must be severe before respiratory function is compromised. Pts with bilateral diaphragmatic paralysis appear normal while standing, but complain of severe orthopnea and display paradoxical abnormal respiratory movement when supine.

APPROACH TO PATIENT Elicit a description of the amount of physical exertion necessary to produce the sensation and whether it varies under different conditions.

- If acute upper airway obstruction is suspected, lateral neck films or a fiberoptic exam of upper airway may be helpful. Patient should be accompanied by a physician adept in all aspects of airway management during the evaluation. With chronic upper airway obstruction the respiratory flow-volume curve may show inspiratory cutoff of flow, suggesting variable extrathoracic obstruction.

- Dyspnea due to emphysema is reflected in a reduction in expiratory flow rates (FEV_1).
- Patients with intermittent dyspnea due to asthma may have normal pulmonary function if tested when asymptomatic.
- Patients with dyspnea due to both cardiac and pulmonary diseases may report orthopnea. Paroxysmal noctural dyspnea occurring after awakening from sleep is characteristic of CHF.
- Dyspnea of chronic obstructive lung disease tends to develop more gradually than that of heart disease.
- PFTs should be performed in pts in whom the etiology is not clear.
- Management depends on elucidating etiology.

PULMONARY EDEMA (PE)

Results either from elevations of hydrostatic pressures in the pulmonary capillaries or from increased permeability of the pulmonary alveolar-capillary membrane.

Cardiogenic PE: Results from increased mean intracapillary pressure. In early stages, physical exam reveals tachypnea, and arterial blood gas measurements demonstrate reductions of both P_{O_2} and P_{CO_2}. As interstitial fluid accumulates, tachypnea increases, gas exchange worsens, and radiographic findings such as Kerley B lines and blurring of vascular margins appear. Pts with cardiogenic PE often have a history of orthopnea. When alveolar edema is present, bilateral rales are evident, the patient may perspire and appears anxious. Late, severe hypoxemia develops, often with hypercapnia.

Treatment: See Chap. 58.

Noncardiogenic PE: Caused by disruption or increased permeability of the alveolar-capillary membrane which may occur in response to sepsis, aspiration, pancreatitis, environmental toxic insults, and following cardiopulmonary bypass. As extravascular lung water accumulates, pts develop tachypnea and severe dyspnea. In contrast to cardiogenic PE, these pts may *not* experience orthopnea. ABGs show hypoxemia and hypocapnia. Hypercapnia occurs very late.

Other forms of PE: While PE due to high altitude exposure and CNS disorders probably results from hydrostatic factors, these pts resemble those with noncardiogenic PE.

Treatment: Remove cause; also see treatment of ARDS (Chap. 83).

For more detailed discussion of this topic, see Ingram RH Jr, Braunwald E: Dyspnea and Pulmonary Edema, Chap. 26, in HPIM-11, p. 141

---

11 COUGH AND HEMOPTYSIS

COUGH

Produced by inflammatory, mechanical, chemical, and thermal stimulation of cough receptors.

ETIOLOGY **Inflammatory:** Edema and hyperemia of airways and alveoli due to laryngitis, tracheitis, bronchitis, bronchiolitis, pneumonitis, lung abscess.
Mechanical: Inhalation of particulates (dust) or compression of airways (pulmonary neoplasms, foreign bodies, granulomas, bronchospasm).
Chemical: Inhalation of irritant fumes, including cigarette smoke.
Thermal: Inhalation of cold or very hot air.

DIAGNOSIS Specific cause may be suggested by duration: e.g., acute suggests viral and bacterial infections; chronic suggests postnasal drip. Character may suggest anatomic site: e.g., "barking"—epiglottal infection; "brassy"—tracheal or large airway infection; wheezing cough—bronchospasm, asthma, nocturnal cough, CHF; with meals—tracheoesophageal fistula; precipitated by change in position—lung abscess.

Physical exam should look for stridor (upper airway obstruction), wheezing (bronchospasm), and inspiratory crackles (interstitial fibrosis/edema). *CXR* may show neoplasm, infection, or interstitial disease. *Pulmonary function studies* may show obstruction or restriction. *Sputum exam* may reveal infection or neoplasm. Any change in character of a chronic "cigarette cough" should result in detailed evaluation for neoplasm.

COMPLICATIONS (1) Syncope, due to transient decrease in venous return; (2) rupture of an emphysematous bleb with pneumothorax; (3) rib fractures—may occur in otherwise normal individuals.

THERAPY Definitive treatment requires identification of a specific cause. Cough productive of sputum should not be suppressed. Mild suppression with codeine is appropriate for painful, dry, debilitating cough.

HEMOPTYSIS

Includes both streaked sputum and coughing up of gross blood.

ETIOLOGY (Table 11-1) Determine that blood comes from respiratory tract. Often frothy, may be preceded by desire to cough. Bronchitis and bronchiectasis are most common causes. Neoplasm may be cause, particularly in smokers and when hemoptysis is persistent. Pulmonary thromboembolism, infection, CHF are other causes.

DIAGNOSIS History may suggest diagnosis: chronic hemoptysis in otherwise asymptomatic young woman suggests bronchial

TABLE 11-1 Causes of hemoptysis

Inflammatory:
- Bronchitis
- Bronchiectasis
- Tuberculosis
- Lung abscess
- Pneumonia, particularly *Klebsiella*

Neoplastic:
- Lung cancer: squamous cell, adenocarcinoma, oat cell
- Bronchial adenoma

Other:
- Pulmonary thromboembolism
- Left ventricular failure
- Mitral stenosis
- Traumatic, including foreign body and lung contusion
- Primary pulmonary hypertension; AV malformation; Eisenmenger's syndrome; pulmonary vasculitis, including Wegener's granulomatosis and Goodpasture's syndrome; idiopathic pulmonary hemosiderosis; and amyloid
- Hemorrhagic diathesis, including anticoagulant therapy

Reproduced from Tisi GM, Braunwald E: HPIM-11, p. 140.

adenoma; recurrent hemoptysis in pts with chronic copious sputum production suggests bronchiectasis; hemoptysis, weight loss, and anorexia in a smoker suggest carcinoma; acute pleuritic chest pain suggests infarction.

Physical exam may provide diagnostic information: localized wheeze suggests endobronchial tumor; diffuse wheezing suggests bronchitis; pleural friction rub may accompany infarction or pneumonia. *Other tests* should include CXR and, in all pts in a high-risk group for bronchogenic carcinoma, bronchoscopy.

THERAPY Scant hemoptysis requires no therapy other than that directed at the underlying condition. Substantial hemoptysis should be treated with bed rest and cough suppression. Massive hemoptysis (≥600 mL/day) is life-threatening, requiring intensive monitoring and immediate availability of endotracheal intubation. Selective intubation to isolate a focal bleeding site in one lung may be necessary. Massive hemoptysis from cavitary TBC, lung abscess, and lung cancer have a particularly high mortality. Surgery and selective bronchial artery embolization are lifesaving in selected cases.

For more detailed discussion of this topic, see Tisi GM, Braunwald E: Cough and Hemoptysis, Chap. 25, in HPIM-11, p. 138

12 CYANOSIS

The circulating quantity of reduced hemoglobin is elevated (>5 g/dL) resulting in bluish discoloration of the skin and/or mucous membranes.

CENTRAL CYANOSIS Results from arterial desaturation.

1 *Impaired pulmonary function:* Poorly ventilated alveoli or impaired oxygen diffusion; most frequent in pneumonia, pulmonary edema, and chronic obstructive pulmonary disease.

2 *Anatomic vascular shunting:* Shunting of desaturated venous blood into the arterial circulation may result from congenital heart disease or pulmonary AV fistula.

3 *Decreased inspired O_2:* Cyanosis may develop at ascents to altitudes >8000 ft.

4 *Abnormal hemoglobins:* Methemoglobinemia, sulfhemoglobinemia, and mutant hemoglobins with low oxygen affinity (see HPIM-11, Chap. 288).

PERIPHERAL CYANOSIS Occurs with normal arterial O_2 saturation with increased extraction of O_2 from capillary blood caused by decreased localized blood flow. Vasoconstriction due to cold exposure, decreased cardiac output (in shock states, Chap. 14), and peripheral vascular disease with arterial obstruction or vasospasm (Chap. 70).

APPROACH TO PATIENT

- Inquire about congenital heart disease or exposure to chemicals that result in abnormal hemoglobins.
- Examine nailbeds, lips, and mucous membranes for cyanosis; clubbing of fingers and toes may be present.
- Examine chest for evidence of pulmonary disease, pulmonary edema, or murmurs associated with congenital heart disease.
- If cyanosis is localized to an extremity, evaluate for peripheral vascular obstruction.
- Obtain arterial blood gas to measure systemic O_2 saturation. Repeat while patient inhales 100% O_2; if saturation fails to increase to >95%, intravascular shunting of blood bypassing the lungs is likely (e.g., right-to-left intracardiac shunts).
- To look for mutant hemoglobins carry out electrophoresis.

For more detailed discussion of this topic, see Braunwald E: Cyanosis, Hypoxia, and Polycythemia, Chap. 27, in HPIM-11, p. 145

13 EDEMA

DEFINITION Soft-tissue swelling due to abnormal expansion of interstitial fluid volume. Edema fluid is a plasma transudate that accumulates when movement of fluid from vascular to interstitial space is favored. Since detectable diffuse edema in the adult reflects a gain of ≥ 3 L, renal retention of salt and water is necessary for edema to occur. Distribution of edema can be an important guide to cause.

Localized edema: Limited to a particular organ or vascular bed; easily distinguished from generalized edema. Unilateral extremity edema is usually due to venous or lymphatic obstruction. Stasis edema of a paralyzed lower extremity also may occur. Allergic reactions and superior vena caval obstruction are causes of localized facial edema. Bilateral lower extremity edema may have localized causes; e.g., inferior vena caval obstruction, compression due to ascites, abdominal mass. Ascites (fluid in peritoneal cavity) and hydrothorax (in pleural space) are other forms of localized edema.

Generalized edema: Fluid accumulation in all areas of the body. Lower extremity swelling, more pronounced after standing, and pulmonary edema are usually cardiac in origin. Periorbital edema may be noted on awakening; often results from renal disease. Ascites and edema of lower extremities and scrotum occur with cirrhosis or CHF. In the latter, diminished cardiac output and effective arterial blood volume result in both increased venous pressure and renal Na retention; the latter is due to renal vasoconstriction, intrarenal blood flow redistribution, and secondary hyperaldosteronism.

In *cirrhosis,* arteriovenous shunts lower effective renal perfusion resulting in Na retention. Ascites accumulates when ↑ intrahepatic vascular resistance produces portal hypertension. Reduced serum albumin and increased abdominal pressure promote lower extremity edema.

In *nephrotic syndrome,* massive renal loss of albumin lowers plasma oncotic pressure, promoting fluid transudation into interstitium; lowering of effective blood volume stimulates renal Na retention.

In acute or chronic *renal failure,* edema occurs if Na intake exceeds kidney's ability to excrete Na secondary to marked reductions in glomerular filtration. Severe *hypoalbuminemia* (<2.5 dL) of any cause (e.g., nephrosis, nutritional deficiency states, chronic liver disease) may lower plasma oncotic pressure sufficiently to cause edema.

Less common causes of generalized edema: *idiopathic edema,* a syndrome of recurrent rapid weight gain and edema in women of reproductive age; *hypothyroidism,* in which myxedema is typically located in pretibial region; *drugs* such as steroids, estrogens, and vasodilators; *pregnancy; refeeding* after starvation.

TABLE 13-1 **Diuretics for edema**

Drug	Strength	Common Dose	Comments
Distal, K-losing:			
Hydrochlorothiazide	25, 50 mg	25–200 mg	First choice; causes hypokalemia; need GFR > 25 mL/min
Chlorthalidone (Hygroton)	25, 50, 100 mg	100 mg qd or qod	Long-acting (up to 72 h); hypokalemia; need GFR > 25 mL/min
Metolazone (Zaroxylin)	1 mg	1–10 mg qd	Long-acting; hypokalemia; effective with low GFR
Loop:			
Furosemide (Lasix)	20, 40, 80 mg	40–120 mg qd or bid	Short-acting; potent; effective with low GFR
Bumetanide	0.5, 1 mg	0.5–2 mg qd or bid	May be used if allergic to furosemide
Ethacrynic acid (Edecrin)	25, 50 mg	50–200 mg qd	Longer-acting; side effects at high doses
Distal, K-sparing:			
Spironolactone (Aldactone)	25 mg	25–100 mg qid	Hyperkalemia; acidosis; blocks aldosterone; gynecomastia, impotence, amenorrhea; onset takes 2–3 days; not if GFR < 25 mL/min
Amiloride (Midamor)	5 mg	5–10 mg qd or bid	Hyperkalemia; once daily; less potent than spironolactone
Triamterene (Dyazide)	50, 100 mg	100 mg bid	Hyperkalemia; less potent than spironolactone; renal stones

TABLE 13-2 **Complications of diuretics**

Common	Uncommon
Volume depletion	Interstitial nephritis (thiazides, furosemide)
Prerenal azotemia	Pancreatitis (thiazides)
Potassium depletion	Loss of hearing (loop diuretics) (?)
Hyponatremia (thiazides)	Hematologic abnormalities (thiazides)
Metabolic alkalosis	
Hypercholesterolemia	
Hyperglycemia (thiazides)	
Hyperkalemia (K-sparers)	
Hypomagnesemia	
Hyperuricemia	
Hypercalcemia (thiazides)	
GI complaints	
Rash (thiazides)	

TREATMENT Begin cautiously, since effective blood volume may be low. Except in pulmonary edema (Chap. 58), edema fluid should be mobilized slowly. Management should address underlying disorder.

Dietary Na restriction may prevent further edema formation. Bed rest enhances response to salt restriction in CHF and cirrhosis. Supportive stockings are also useful. If severe hyponatremia (Na < 132 meq/L) is present, water intake should also be reduced. Diuretics are required (Table 13-1). Indications: marked peripheral edema, pulmonary edema, CHF, inadequate dietary salt restriction. Side effects are listed in Table 13-2. Weight loss should be limited to less than 1 kg per day. Metolazone may be added for loop diuretic–resistant patients. Intestinal edema may impair absorption of oral diuretics. When desired weight is achieved, doses of diuretics should be reduced.

In *CHF* (Chap. 58), overdiuresis may result in a fall in cardiac output and prerenal azotemia. Diuretic-induced hypokalemia may predispose to digitalis toxicity.

In *cirrhosis,* spironolactone is the diuretic of choice, but may produce acidosis and hyperkalemia. Thiazides or small doses of loop diuretics also may be required. Renal failure may result from volume depletion. Severe hyponatremia and hypokalemia (with worsening encephalopathy) are commonly observed.

In *nephrotic syndrome,* albumin infusion should be limited to very severe cases, such as patients with hypotension, as rapid renal excretion prevents any sustained rise in serum albumin.

For more detailed discussion of this topic, see Braunwald E: Edema, Chap. 28, in HPIM-11, p. 149

14 SHOCK

DEFINITION Condition of severe impairment of tissue perfusion. Rapid recognition and treatment are essential to prevent irreversible organ damage. Common etiologies are listed in Table 14-1.

CLINICAL MANIFESTATIONS Hypotension (systolic BP < 90), tachycardia, tachypnea, pallor, restlessness, and altered sensorium; signs of intense peripheral vasoconstriction; weak pulses; cold clammy extremities (*note:* in septic shock, extremities are warm). Oliguria (<20 mL/h) and metabolic acidosis common.

APPROACH TO PATIENT

Tissue perfusion must be restored immediately (see below); also obtain history for underlying cause, including

- Known cardiac disease (coronary disease, CHF, pericarditis)
- Recent fever or infection (leading to sepsis)
- Drugs, i.e., excess diuretics or antihypertensives
- Predisposing conditions for pulmonary embolism (Chap. 77)
- Possible bleeding from any site, particularly GI tract.

TABLE 14-1 **Causes of shock**

Hypovolemia:
- Hemorrhage (external or internal)
- Dehydration:
  - Vomiting or diarrhea
  - Diuretic overusage
  - Diabetes (mellitus or insipidus)
  - Impaired fluid intake
- Severe burns
- Internal sequestration (pancreatitis, ascites, intestinal obstruction)

Cardiovascular:
- Myocardial infarction
- Severe congestive heart failure
- Arrhythmias
- Critical aortic stenosis with heart failure
- Acute valvular regurgitation (mitral, aortic)
- Massive pulmonary embolism
- Cardiac tamponade
- Aortic dissection

Loss of vascular tone:
- Sepsis
- Anaphylaxis
- Spinal cord injury
- Drug overdoses

Uncommon (often unsuspected):
- Addison's disease (adrenocortical insufficiency)
- Myxedema (severe hypothyroidism)

PHYSICAL EXAMINATION

- Jugular veins are flat in hypovolemic shock; jugular venous distention (JVD) suggests cardiogenic shock; JVD in presence of paradoxical pulse may reflect cardiac tamponade (Chap. 67).
- Look for evidence of CHF (Chap. 58), murmurs of aortic stenosis, acute regurgitation (mitral or aortic), ventricular septal defect.
- Check for asymmetry of pulses (aortic dissection).
- Tenderness or rebound in abdomen may indicate peritonitis or pancreatitis; high-pitched bowel sounds suggest intestinal obstruction. Perform stool guaiac to rule out GI bleeding.

LABORATORY Obtain hematocrit, WBC, electrolytes. If actively bleeding, check platelet count, PT, PTT, DIC screen. If sepsis suspected, draw blood cultures and obtain Gram stain and cultures of sputum, urine, and other suspected sites.

Obtain ECG (myocardial ischemia or acute arrhythmia), chest x-ray (CHF, tension pneumothorax, aortic dissection). Echocardiogram may be helpful (cardiac tamponade, CHF). Central venous pressure or pulmonary capillary wedge (PCW) pressure measurements may be necessary to distinguish cardiogenic from hypovolemic shock: mean PCW < 6 mmHg suggests hypovolemia; PCW > 20 mmHg suggests left ventricular failure.

TREATMENT

Aimed at rapid improvement of tissue hypoperfusion and respiratory impairment:

- Serial measurements of BP (intraarterial line preferred), heart rate, ECG, urine output, blood studies: Hct, electrolytes, creatinine, BUN, ABGs, urine Na concentration ($<$20 meq/L suggests volume depletion). Continuous monitoring of CVP and/or pulmonary artery pressure (with serial PCW pressures).
- Augment systolic BP to $>$100 mmHg: (1) reverse Trendelenburg position (supine with foot of bed elevated on "shock block"); (2) IV volume infusion unless PCW > 20 mmHg (saline to start, then whole blood, dextran, or packed RBCs, depending on Hct; give vasopressors with excessive vasodilation, vasodilators with excessive vasoconstriction, but only if systolic pressure > 90 mmHg); maintain PCW < 18 mmHg ($<$20 in acute MI); (3) vasoactive drugs are used after intravascular volume is optimal; inotropic agents in CHF.
- Use 100% oxygen (mask or nasal cannula).
- Identify and treat underlying cause of shock. Treatment of cardiogenic shock in myocardial infarction is discussed in Chap. 64.

For more detailed discussion of this topic, see Braunwald E, Williams GH: Alterations in Arterial Pressure and the Shock Syndrome, Chap. 29, in HPIM-11, p. 153

---

15 NAUSEA AND VOMITING

DEFINITIONS **Nausea** refers to the imminent desire to vomit.
Vomiting refers to the forceful expulsion of gastric contents through the mouth.
Retching refers to labored rhythmic respiratory activity that precedes emesis.
Regurgitation refers to expulsion of gastric contents in the absence of nausea and abdominal diaphragmatic muscular contraction.

PATHOPHYSIOLOGY Gastric contents are propelled into the esophagus when there is relaxation of the gastric fundus and gastroesophageal sphincter followed by a rapid increase in intra-abdominal pressure produced by contraction of the abdominal and diaphragmatic musculature. Increased intrathoracic pressure results in further movement of the material to the mouth. Reflex elevation of the soft palate and closure of the glottis protect the nasopharynx and trachea and complete the act of vomiting. Vomiting is controlled by two brainstem areas: vomiting center and chemoreceptor trigger zone.

ETIOLOGY Nausea and vomiting are manifestations of a large number of disorders. Clinical classification:

1 Acute abdominal emergency: appendicitis, acute cholecystitis, acute intestinal obstruction, acute peritonitis
2 Chronic indigestion: peptic ulcer disease, aerophagia
3 Infections: bacterial, viral, and parasitic infections of GI tract; systemic infection not involving GI tract directly, especially in children
4 Uremia
5 CNS disorders: Increased intracranial pressure results in vomiting, often of a projectile nature. Labyrinthine disorders that underlie vertigo are often associated with nausea and vomiting.
6 Cardiac: acute myocardial infarction (especially inferior MI) and heart failure
7 Endocrine disorders: diabetic ketoacidosis, adrenal insufficiency, pregnancy
8 Medicines/toxins: Nausea is a common side effect of many medications and toxins. Enterotoxins produced by bacteria cause food poisoning.
9 Psychogenic: emotional upset, anorexia, bulimia
10 GI hemorrhage: Blood in the stomach from any cause can result in nausea and vomiting.

EVALUATION The history, including careful drug history, and character of the vomitus can be helpful; e.g., feculent emesis implies distal intestinal obstruction or gastrocolic fistula; projectile vomiting suggests increased intracranial pressure. Plain radiographs can suggest diagnoses such as intestinal obstruction. Upper GI series assesses motility of proximal GI tract as well as mucosa. Other studies may be indicated; e.g., gastric emptying scans (diabetic gastroparesis), CT scan of the brain.

COMPLICATIONS Rupture of the esophagus (Boerhaave's syndrome), hematemesis from a mucosal tear (Mallory-Weiss syndrome), dehydration, metabolic alkalosis, hypokalemia, and aspiration pneumonitis.

TREATMENT Depends on specific etiology. Antiemetic medications which inhibit cerebral dopaminergic receptors (phenothiazine derivatives, metoclopramide) can be effective in controlling nausea and vomiting.

For more detailed discussion of this topic, see Isselbacher KJ: Anorexia, Nausea, and Vomiting, Chap. 34, in HPIM-11, p. 173

---

16 WEIGHT LOSS AND WEIGHT GAIN

Changes in weight may involve body fluid or tissue mass. Rapid fluctuations of weight over days suggest loss or gain of fluid, whereas long-term changes usually involve body mass and reflect the balance of caloric intake and expenditure.

WEIGHT GAIN Fluid accumulation can be due to congestive heart failure, cirrhosis of the liver, nephrosis, or renal disease. The most common cause of increased tissue mass is endogenous obesity, usually from overeating. The history may be misleading, and excess intake should be documented by calorie counts. Secondary causes of obesity include Cushing's syndrome, hypothyroidism, hypogonadism, and insulin-secreting tumors. Rarely, neoplasms of the CNS such as craniopharyngiomas cause a central drive to overeat. Congenital disorders such as Prader-Willi and Laurence-Moon-Biedl syndromes cause obesity early in life.

WEIGHT LOSS In the absence of dieting, weight loss has more import than weight gain. Weight loss in the setting of an increased appetite suggests accelerated metabolism or loss of calories in the urine or stool. Thyrotoxicosis causes enhanced energy expenditure from increase in metabolic rate and physical activity. Weight loss in pheochromocytoma is due to catecholomine-mediated hypermetabolism. Diabetes mellitus typically causes polyuria, polydipsia, polyphagia, and weight loss. Initial weight loss is secondary to osmotic diuresis, but subsequent loss of body mass reflects caloric wastage in the urine (glycosuria). Malabsorption with steatorrhea, as in sprue, chronic pancreatitis, or cystic fibrosis, and chronic diarrhea of diverse causes also may cause weight loss despite increased food intake.

Weight loss with a diminished appetite is due to the inadequacy of intake for metabolic needs and suggests occult malignancy. The search for malignancy should include GI tract, pancreas, liver, lymphoma, and leukemia. Weight loss and anorexia also can be due to hidden infection such as tuberculosis, fungal disease, amebic abscess, and bacterial endocarditis. The mechanism involves both anorexia and acceleration of cellular metabolic demands. Adrenal insufficiency rarely causes weight loss due to a diminished appetite, as may anorexia nervosa, depressive states, and schizophrenia.

For more detailed discussion of this topic, see Foster DW: Gain and Loss in Weight, Chap. 35, in HPIM-11, p. 175

17 DIARRHEA, CONSTIPATION, AND MALABSORPTION SYNDROMES

NORMAL GASTROINTESTINAL FUNCTION

ABSORPTION OF FLUID AND ELECTROLYTES Fluid delivery to GI tract 8–10 L/day, including 2 L ingested; most is absorbed in small bowel. Colonic absorption normally 500–2000 mL, with capacity for 6 L/day if required. Water absorption passively follows active transport of Na^+ and Cl^-. Additional transport mechanisms include Cl^-/HCO_3^- exchange, H^+, K^+, and HCO_3^- secretion and Na^+-glucose cotransport.

NUTRIENT ABSORPTION (1) Proximal small intestine: iron, Ca, folate, fats (triglycerides hydrolyzed to fatty acids by pancreatic lipase and colipase), proteins (after hydrolysis by pancreatic and intestinal peptidases), carbohydrates (after hydrolysis by amylases and disaccharidases); triglycerides absorbed as micelles after solubilization by bile salts; amino acids and dipeptides absorbed via specific carriers; sugars absorbed by active transport; (2) distal small intestine: B_{12}, bile salts; (3) colon: water, electrolytes.

INTESTINAL MOTILITY Allows propulsion of intestinal contents from stomach to anus and separation of components to facilitate nutrient absorption. Propulsion is controlled by neural, myogenic, and hormonal mechanisms; mediated by migrating motor complex, an organized wave of neuromuscular activity which originates in the distal stomach during fasting and migrates slowly down the small intestine. Colonic motility is mediated by local peristalsis to propel feces. Defecation is effected by relaxation of internal anal sphincter in response to rectal distention, with voluntary control by contraction of external anal sphincter.

DIARRHEA

PHYSIOLOGY Formally defined as stool weight greater than 200 g/day on low-fiber (Western) diet; *diarrhea* also frequently used to connote loose or watery stools. Mediated by one or more of the following mechanisms:

Osmotic diarrhea: Nonabsorbed solutes increase intraluminal oncotic pressure, causing outpouring of water; usually ceases with fasting; stool osmolal gap greater than 40. Causes include disaccharidase (e.g., lactase) deficiencies, lactulose ingestion, polyvalent laxative abuse. Lactase deficiency either primary (more prevalent in blacks and Asians, usually presenting in early adulthood) or secondary (from gastroenteritis, celiac or tropical sprue, or kwashiorkor).

Secretory diarrhea: Active ion secretion causes obligatory water loss; diarrhea usually watery, often profuse, unaffected by fasting; stool Na^+ and K^+ elevated with osmolal gap less than 40. Causes include cholera and toxigenic *E. coli* (increased cAMP; decreased cGMP), Zollinger-Ellison syndrome (excess gastrin production), vasoactive intestinal peptide (VIP)-producing tumors, carcinoid tumors (histamine and serotonin), medullary thyroid carcinoma (prostaglandins and serotonin), systemic mastocytosis, basophilic leukemia, distal colonic villous adenomas (direct secretion of electrolyte-rich fluid).

Exudative: Inflammation, necrosis, and sloughing of colonic mucosa; may include component of secretory diarrhea due to prostaglandin release by inflammatory cells; stools usually contain polymorphonuclear leukocytes as well as occult or gross blood. Causes include bacterial infections (e.g., *Campylobacter, Salmonella, Shigella, Yersinia,* invasive *E. coli,* gonorrhea, *Chlamydia*), colonic parasites (e.g., *Entamoeba histolytica, Giardia, Cryptosporidia*), idiopathic inflammatory bowel disease, diverticulitis, radiation enterocolitis, and intestinal ischemia.

Altered intestinal motility: Alteration of coordinated control of intestinal propulsion; diarrhea often intermittent or alternating with constipation. Causes include diabetes mellitus, adrenal insufficiency, hyperthyroidism, collagen-vascular diseases, parasitic infections, gastrin and VIP hypersecretory states, amyloidosis, drugs (esp. magnesium-containing laxatives), primary neurologic dysfunction (e.g., Parkinson's disease), and irritable bowel syndrome. Blood in intestinal lumen is cathartic, and major upper GI bleeding leads to diarrhea from increased motility.

Decreased absorptive surface: Usually arises from surgical manipulation (e.g., extensive bowel resection or rearrangement) which leaves inadequate absorptive surface for fluid and electrolyte absorption; occurs spontaneously from enteroenteric fistulas (esp. gastrocolic).

EVALUATION **History:** Must be distinguished from fecal incontinence, change in stool caliber, rectal bleeding, and small, frequent, but otherwise normal stools. Alternating diarrhea and constipation suggests fixed colonic obstruction or irritable bowel disease. Sudden, acute course is typical of infections, including diverticulitis, and drug-induced diarrhea and may be initial presentation of inflammatory bowel disease. A longer, more insidious course suggests malabsorption, inflammatory bowel disease, metabolic or endocrine disturbance, pancreatic insufficiency, laxative abuse, ischemia, neoplasm (hypersecretory state or partial obstruction), or irritable bowel syndrome. Parasitic and certain forms of bacterial enteritis also can produce chronic symptoms. Particularly foul-smelling or oily stool suggests fat malabsorption. Fecal impaction may cause apparent diarrhea because only liquids pass partial obstruction.

Physical examination: Signs of dehydration often prominent in acute diarrhea. Fever and abdominal tenderness suggest infection or inflammatory disease but are often absent in viral enteritis. Evidence of malnutrition suggests chronic course. Certain signs are frequently associated with specific deficiency states secondary to malabsorption (e.g., cheilosis with riboflavin deficiency, glossitis with B_{12}, folate deficiency).

Stool examination: Culture for bacterial pathogens, measurement of *Clostridium* toxin, and examination for ova and parasites important components of evaluation of patients with severe, protracted, or bloody diarrhea. Presence of blood (fecal occult blood test) or leukocytes (Wright's stain) suggests inflammation (e.g., IBD, infection, or ischemia). Gram's stain of stool can be diagnostic of *Staphylococcus, Campylobacter,* or *Candida* infection. Steatorrhea (determined with Sudan III stain of stool sample or 72-h quantitative fecal fat analysis) suggests malabsorption or pancreatic insufficiency. Measurement of Na^+ and K^+ levels in fecal water helps to distinguish osmotic from other types of diarrhea [stool osmolal gap $\approx (\text{osmol})_{\text{serum}} - (Na^+ + K^+)_{\text{stool}}$].
Laboratory studies: CBC may indicate anemia (acute or chronic blood loss or malabsorption of iron, folate, or B_{12}), leukocytosis (inflammation), eosinophilia (parasitic, neoplastic, and inflammatory bowel diseases). Serum levels of Ca, albumin, iron, cholesterol, folate, and B_{12}, serum iron-binding capacity, and prothrombin time can provide evidence of intestinal malabsorption.
Other studies: Sigmoidoscopy or colonoscopy useful in the diagnosis of colitis (esp. pseudomembranous and ischemic); it may not allow distinction between infectious and noninfectious (esp. ulcerative) colitis. Barium contrast x-ray studies may suggest malabsorption (thickened bowel folds), inflammatory bowel disease (ileitis or colitis), tuberculosis, diverticulitis, neoplasm, intestinal fistula, or motility disorders. D-Xylose absorption test a convenient screen for small bowel absorptive function. Small-bowel biopsy especially useful for evaluating intestinal malabsorption. Specialized studies include Schilling test (B_{12} absorption), lactose H_2 breath test (carbohydrate malabsorption), [^{14}C]xylose and lactulose H_2 breath tests (bacterial overgrowth), glycocholic breath test (ileal malabsorption), triolein breath test (fat malabsorption), and bentiromide and secretin tests (pancreatic insufficiency).

TREATMENT Varies widely depending on etiology (refer to individual sections dealing with specific diseases). Symptomatic therapy includes vigorous hydration, electrolyte replacement, binders of osmotically active substances (e.g., kaolin-pectin), and opiates to decrease bowel motility (e.g., loperamide, diphenoxylate); opiates may be contraindicated in infectious or inflammatory causes of diarrhea.

MALABSORPTION SYNDROMES

Table 17-1 lists common causes of intestinal malabsorption. Protein-losing enteropathy is associated with several causes of malabsorption; it is associated with hypoalbuminemia and can be detected by measuring stool α_1-antitrypsin or radiolabeled albumin levels.

CONSTIPATION

Decrease in frequency of stools or difficulty in defecation; may result in abdominal pain, distention, and fecal impaction, with

TABLE 17-1 Common causes of malabsorption

Maldigestion: Chronic pancreatitis, cystic fibrosis, pancreatic carcinoma
Bile salt deficiency: Cirrhosis, cholestasis, bacterial overgrowth (blind loop syndromes, intestinal diverticula, hypomotility disorders), impaired ileal reabsorption (resection, Crohn's disease), bile salt binders (cholestyramine, calcium carbonate, neomycin)
Inadequate absorptive surface: Massive intestinal resection, gastrocolic fistula, jejunoileal bypass
Lymphatic obstruction: Lymphoma, Whipple's disease, intestinal lymphangiectasia
Vascular disease: Constrictive pericarditis, right-sided heart failure, mesenteric vascular disease
Mucosal disease: Inflammatory diseases (Crohn's disease, infectious enteritis, radiation enteritis, eosinophilic enteritis, ulcerative jejunitis, mastocytosis, tropical sprue), infiltrative disorders (amyloidosis, scleroderma, lymphoma, collagenous sprue), biochemical abnormalities (gluten-sensitive enteropathy, disaccharidase deficiency, hypogammaglobulinemia, abetalipoproteinemia), endocrine disorders (diabetes mellitus, hypoparathyroidism, adrenal insufficiency, hyperthyroidism, Zollinger-Ellison syndrome, carcinoid syndrome)

consequent obstruction or, rarely, perforation. A frequent and often subjective complaint. Contributory factors may include inactivity, low-roughage diet, and inadequate allotment of time for defecation.

SPECIFIC CAUSES Altered colonic motility due to neurologic dysfunction (diabetes mellitus, spinal cord injury, multiple sclerosis, Hirschsprung's disease, chronic idiopathic intestinal pseudoobstruction, idiopathic megacolon), scleroderma, drugs (esp. anticholinergic agents, opiates), hypothyroidism, Cushing's syndrome, hypokalemia, hypercalcemia, dehydration, mechanical causes (colorectal tumors, diverticulitis, volvulus, hernias, intussusception), and anorectal pain (from fissures, hemorrhoids, abscesses, or proctitis) leading to retention, constipation, and fecal impaction.

TREATMENT In absence of identifiable cause, constipation may improve with reassurance, exercise, increased dietary roughage, and increased fluid intake. Specific therapies include removal of bowel obstruction (fecolith, tumor), discontinuance of nonessential hypomotility agents (esp. aluminum-containing antacids, opiates). For symptomatic relief, magnesium-containing agents or other cathartics are occasionally needed. With severe hypo- or dysmotility or in presence of opiates, osmotically active agents (e.g., oral lactulose, intestinal lavage solutions) and mineral oil (orally or as enema) are most effective.

For more detailed discussion of this topic, see Goldfinger SE: Constipation, Diarrhea, and Disturbances of Anorectal Function, Chap. 36, in HPIM-11, p. 177

18 GASTROINTESTINAL BLEEDING

PRESENTATION

1 *Hematemesis:* Vomiting of blood or altered blood ("coffee grounds"); indicates bleeding proximal to ligament of Treitz.

2 *Melena:* Altered (black) blood per rectum (≥ 100 mL blood required for one melenic stool); usually indicates bleeding proximal to ligament of Treitz, but may be as distal as ascending colon; pseudomelena may be caused by iron, bismuth, licorice, beets, blueberries, charcoal.

3 *Hematochezia:* Bright red or maroon rectal bleeding; usually implies bleeding beyond ligament of Treitz, but may be due to rapid upper GI bleeding (≥ 1000 mL).

4 *Positive fecal occult blood test* (see Chap. 125).

5 *Iron deficiency anemia* (see Chap. 122).

Hemodynamic changes: Orthostatic hypotension >10 mmHg; usually indicates >20% reduction in blood volume (± syncope, light-headedness, nausea, sweating, thirst).
Shock BP < 100mmHg systolic; usually indicates > 30% reduction in blood volume (± pallor, cool skin).
Laboratory changes: Hematocrit may not reflect extent of blood loss because of delayed equilibration with extravascular fluid. Mild leukocytosis and thrombocytosis and elevated BUN are common in upper GI bleeding.
Adverse prognostic signs: Age > 60, presentation with shock, rebleeding, endoscopic stigmata of recent bleeding [e.g., "visible vessel" in ulcer base (see below)].

UPPER GI BLEEDING

CAUSES Common: Peptic ulcer, gastritis (alcohol, aspirin, NSAIDs stress), esophagitis, Mallory-Weiss tear (mucosal tear at gastroesophageal junction due to retching), gastroesophageal varices.
Less common: Swallowed blood (nosebleed); esophageal, gastric, or intestinal neoplasm; anticoagulant and fibrinolytic therapy; hypertrophic gastropathy (Ménétrier's disease); aortic aneurysm; aortoenteric fistula (from aortic graft); AV malformation; telangiectases (Osler-Rendu-Weber syndrome); vasculitis; connective-tissue disease (pseudoxanthoma elasticum, Ehlers-Danlos syndrome); blood dyscrasias; neurofibroma; amyloidosis; hemobilia (biliary origin).

EVALUATION Only *after* hemodynamic resuscitation (see below).

- History and physical examination: Drugs, prior ulcer, bleeding history, family history, features of cirrhosis or vasculitis, etc.
- Nasogastric aspirate for blood if upper source not clear from history; may be falsely negative if bleeding has ceased.

- Upper endoscopy: Accuracy > 90%; allows visualization of bleeding site and possibility of therapeutic intervention; mandatory for suspected varices, aortoenteric fistulas; preferable to radiography for suspected ulcer to identify "visible vessel" (protruding artery in ulcer crater), which connotes high (~50%) risk of rebleeding.
- Upper GI barium radiography: Accuracy ~80%; acceptable alternative to endoscopy in resolved or chronic low-grade bleeding.
- Selective mesenteric arteriography: When brisk bleeding precludes adequate endoscopic examination.
- Radioisotope scanning (e.g., ^{99m}Tc tagged to red blood cells or albumin): Used primarily as screening test to assess feasibility of arteriography in intermittent bleeding of unclear origin.

LOWER GI BLEEDING

CAUSES Anal lesions (hemorrhoids, fissures), rectal trauma, proctitis, colitis (ulcerative colitis, Crohn's disease, infectious colitis, ischemic colitis), colonic polyps, colonic carcinoma, angiodysplasia (vascular ectasia), diverticulosis, intussusception, solitary ulcer, blood dyscrasias, vasculitis, connective-tissue disease, neurofibroma, amyloidosis, anticoagulation.

EVALUATION

- History and physical examination.
- Anoscopy and sigmoidoscopy: Exclude hemorrhoids, fissure, ulcer, proctitis, neoplasm.
- Nasogastric aspirate (if any suspicion of upper GI source, best to do upper endoscopy).
- Barium enema: No role in active bleeding.
- Arteriography (requires bleeding rate > 0.5 mL/min; may require prestudy radioisotope bleeding scan as above): Defines site of bleeding or abnormal vasculature.
- Colonoscopy: Often impossible if bleeding is massive.
- Surgical exploration (last resort).

BLEEDING OF OBSCURE ORIGIN Often small-bowel source. Consider small-bowel enteroclysis x-ray (careful barium radiography via peroral intubation of small bowel), Meckel's scan, or exploratory laporotomy with intraoperative enteroscopy.

MANAGEMENT

- Venous access; central venous line for major bleed; monitor vital signs, urine output, hemoglobin (fall may lag). Gastric lavage of unproven benefit, but clears stomach before endoscopy.
- Type and cross match blood (6 units for major bleed).
- Surgical standby.
- Support blood pressure with isotonic fluids (normal saline), albumin in cirrhotics, then packed red blood cells when available (whole blood if massive bleeding); maintain Hct ≥ 25–30.
- Fresh frozen plasma and vitamin K (10 mg SC or IV) in cirrhotics with coagulopathy.

- IV calcium if serum calcium falls (due to citrated blood).
- Empiric drug therapy (antacids, cimetidine) of unproven benefit; experimental—IV somatostatin; estrogen in patients with chronic renal failure and vascular ectasias.
- Specific measures: *Varices:* IV vasopressin (0.4–0.9 U/min), Blakemore-Sengstaken tube tamponade, endoscopic sclerosis; *ulcer with visible vessel:* endoscopic electro- or laser coagulation; *gastritis:* embolization or vasopressin infusion of left gastric artery; *diverticulosis:* mesenteric arteriography with intraarterial vasopressin; *angiodysplasia:* colonoscopic electro- or laser coagulation.
- Indications for emergency surgery: Uncontrolled or prolonged bleeding, severe rebleeding, aortoenteric fistula.

For more detailed discussion of this topic, see Isselbacher KJ, Richter JM: Hematemesis, Melena, and Hematochezia, Chap. 37, in HPIM-11, p. 180

---

19 JAUNDICE, HEPATOMEGALY, AND LIVER TESTS

JAUNDICE

Definition: Yellow skin pigmentation caused by elevation in serum bilirubin level. *Icterus* refers to similar pigmentation in sclerae, which is often more easily discernible. Jaundice and icterus become clinically evident at a serum bilirubin level of 2–2.5 mg/dL (approximately twice normal); yellow skin discoloration also occurs with elevated serum carotene levels, but there is no pigmentation of the sclerae.

BILIRUBIN METABOLISM Bilirubin is the major breakdown product of hemoglobin released from senescent erythrocytes. Initially it is bound to albumin, transported into the liver, conjugated to a water-soluble form (glucuronide) by glucuronyl transferase, excreted into the bile, and converted to urobilinogen in colon. Urobilinogen is mostly excreted in the stool; a small portion is reabsorbed and excreted by the kidney. Bilirubin can only be filtered by the kidney in its conjugated form (measured as the "direct" fraction); thus increased direct serum bilirubin level is associated with bilirubinuria. Increased bilirubin production and excretion (even without hyperbilirubinemia, as in hemolysis) produce elevated urinary urobilinogen levels.

ETIOLOGY Hyperbilirubinemia occurs as a result of (1) overproduction, (2) decreased hepatic uptake, (3) decreased hepatic conjugation (required for excretion), or (4) decreased biliary excretion (see Table 19-1). Disorders of liver transport mechanisms are often associated with pruritus, possibly from deposition of bile salts in skin; these include all causes of *conjugated* hyperbilirubinemia except Dubin-Johnson and Rotor syndromes and benign familial cholestasis (in which only bilirubin excretion is affected).

HEPATOMEGALY

Definition: Generally a span of greater than 12 cm in the right midclavicular line or a palpable left lobe in the epigastrium. It is important to exclude low-lying liver (e.g., with chronic obstructive pulmonary disease and lung hyperinflation) and other right upper quadrant masses. Independent assessment of size best obtained from ultrasound examination or radionuclide liver scan. Contour and texture are important: focal enlargement or rocklike consistency suggests tumor; tenderness suggests inflammation (e.g., hepatitis) or rapid enlargement (e.g., right-sided heart failure, Budd-Chiari syndrome, fatty infiltration). Cirrhotic livers are usually firm and nodular, often enlarged until late in course. Pulsations usually connote tricuspid regurgitation. Arterial bruit or hepatic rub suggests tumor. Portal hypertension is occasionally associated with continuous venous hum (see Table 19-2).

TABLE 19-1 **Causes of hyperbilirubinemia**

Predominantly unconjugated (indirect-reacting) bilirubin:

Overproduction of bilirubin pigments: Intravascular hemolysis, hematoma resorption, ineffective erythropoiesis (bone marrow)

Decreased hepatic uptake: Sepsis, prolonged fasting, right-sided heart failure, drugs (e.g., rifampin, probenecid)

Decreased conjugation: Severe hepatocellular disease (e.g., hepatitis, cirrhosis), sepsis, drugs (e.g., chloramphenicol), inherited glucuronyl transferase deficiency (Gilbert's syndrome, Crigler-Najjar syndrome type II, or Crigler-Najjar syndrome type I)

Predominantly conjugated (direct-reacting) bilirubin:

Impaired hepatic excretion: Hepatocellular disease (e.g., drug-induced, viral, or ischemic hepatitis, cirrhosis), drug-induced cholestasis (e.g., oral contraceptives, methyltestosterone), sepsis, inherited disorders (Dubin-Johnson syndrome, Rotor syndrome, cholestasis of pregnancy, benign familial recurrent cholestasis)

Biliary obstruction: Biliary cirrhosis (primary or secondary), sclerosing cholangitis, mechanical obstruction (e.g., stone, tumor, stricture)

Modified from Isselbacher KJ, HPIM-11, p. 186.

BLOOD TESTS OF LIVER FUNCTION

Used to evaluate functional status of liver and to discriminate among different types of liver disease (e.g., inflammatory, infiltrative, biliary obstruction). (See Table 19-3.)

Bilirubin: Provides indication of hepatic uptake, metabolic (conjugation), and excretory functions; conjugated fraction (direct-reacting) distinguished from unconjugated by chemical assay.

Aminotransferases: Aspartate aminotransferase (AST; SGOT) and alanine aminotransferase (ALT; SGPT); sensitive indicators of liver cell integrity; greatest elevations seen in hepatocellular necrosis (e.g., viral hepatitis, toxic liver injury, ischemic hepatitis); milder abnormalities in cholestatic and infiltrative disease; ALT more specific measure of liver injury, since AST also found in striated muscle; ethanol-induced liver injury often produces more prominent elevation of AST than ALT.

TABLE 19-2 **Important causes of hepatomegaly**

Vascular congestion: Right-sided heart failure (including tricuspid valve disease), Budd-Chiari syndrome

Infiltrative disorders: Fatty liver (e.g., ethanol abuse, diabetes, parenteral hyperalimentation, pregnancy), lymphoma or leukemia, extramedullary hematopoiesis, amyloidosis, granulomatous hepatitis (e.g., TBC, sarcoidosis, CMV), hemochromatosis, Gaucher's disease, glycogen storage diseases

Inflammatory disorders: Viral hepatitis, drug-induced hepatitis, cirrhosis

Tumors: Hepatocellular carcinoma, metastatic cancer, focal nodular hyperplasia, hepatic adenoma

Cysts (e.g., polycystic disease)

Modified from Isselbacher KJ, HPIM-11, p. 188.

TABLE 19-3 **Patterns of liver test abnormalities**

Test	Type of liver disease			
	Hepato-cellular	Obstructive	Ischemic	Infiltrative
AST, ALT*	↑ ↑ ↑	↑	↑ – ↑ ↑ ↑	N– ↑
Alkaline phosphatase	↑ – ↑ ↑	↑ ↑ ↑	↑ – ↑ ↑	↑ – ↑ ↑ ↑
5′-Nucleotidase	↑ – ↑ ↑	↑ ↑ ↑	↑	↑ – ↑ ↑ ↑
Bilirubin	↑ – ↑ ↑ ↑	↑ – ↑ ↑ ↑	N– ↑	N
Prothrombin time	↑ – ↑ ↑ ↑	N†	N– ↑ ↑	N
Albumin	N– ↓ ↓ ↓	N‡	N– ↓	N

* In *acute complete obstruction,* serum transaminases may rise rapidly and dramatically, but return to near normal levels after 1–3 days even in the presence of continued obstruction.
† May increase with prolonged biliary obstruction and secondary biliary cirrhosis.
‡ May decrease with prolonged biliary obstruction and secondary biliary cirrhosis.
Note: N, normal; ↑, elevated; ↓, decreased. (Modified from Podolsky DK, Isselbacher KJ, HPIM-11, p. 1315.)

Lactate dehydrogenase (LDH): Less specific measure of hepatocellular integrity with little value in evaluation of liver disease.
Alkaline phosphatase: Sensitive indicator of cholestasis (more sensitive than serum bilirubin) and liver infiltration; mild elevations in other forms of liver disease; limited specificity because of wide tissue distribution; elevations also seen in childhood, pregnancy, and bone diseases; tissue-specific isoenzymes can be distinguished by differences in heat stability (liver enzyme activity stable under conditions which destroy bone enzyme activity).
5′-Nucleotidase (5′-NT): Pattern of elevation in hepatobiliary disease similar to alkaline phosphatase; has greater specificity for liver disorders; used to confirm suspected liver source of isolated elevation in serum alkaline phosphatase.
γ-Glutamyltranspeptidase: Correlates with serum alkaline phosphatase activity; greater sensitivity for liver disease, but also elevated in pancreatic, renal, pulmonary, and cardiac disorders.
Prothrombin time (PT) (see also Chap. 127): Measure of clotting factor activity; prolongation results from clotting-factor deficiency or inactivity; all clotting factors except factor VIII are synthesized in the liver, and deficiency commonly results from widespread liver necrosis, as in hepatitis, toxic injury, or cirrhosis; clotting factors II, VII, IX, X function only in the presence of the fat-soluble vitamin K; PT prolongation from fat malabsorption distinguished from hepatic disease by rapid response to vitamin K replacement.
Albumin: Decreased serum levels result from decreased hepatic synthesis (chronic liver disease or prolonged malnutrition) or excessive losses in urine or stool; insensitive indicator of acute hepatic dysfunction, since serum half-life is 2 to 3 weeks; in pts with chronic liver disease, degree of hypoalbuminemia correlates with severity of dysfunction.

Globulin: Mild polyclonal hyperglobulinemia often seen in chronic liver diseases; marked elevation frequently seen in the autoimmune, idiopathic form of chronic active hepatitis.
Ammonia: Elevated blood levels result from deficiency of hepatic detoxification pathways and portal-systemic shunting, as in fulminant hepatitis, hepatotoxin exposure, and severe portal hypertension (e.g., from cirrhosis); for many (but not all) pts, blood ammonia level correlates with degree of portal-systemic encephalopathy; asterixis correlates with encephalopathy more accurately, but does not distinguish among several metabolic causes, including hepatic dysfunction, uremia, and hypercarbia.

HEPATOBILIARY IMAGING PROCEDURES

Used in evaluation of jaundice, hepatomegaly, and liver biochemical test abnormalities.
Ultrasonography: Rapid, noninvasive examination of abdominal structures; no radiation exposure; images and interpretation strongly dependent on expertise of examiner; particularly valuable for detecting biliary duct dilatation and gallbladder stones; much less sensitive for intraductal stones; most sensitive means of detecting ascites; relatively insensitive for detecting hepatic masses but excellent for discriminating solid from cystic structures; useful in directing percutaneous needle biopsies of suspicious lesions; imaging improved by presence of ascites but severely hindered by bowel gas.
Computed tomography (CT): Particularly useful for detecting, differentiating, and directing percutaneous needle biopsy of abdominal masses, cysts, and lymphadenopathy; imaging enhanced by intestinal or intravenous contrast dye and unaffected by intestinal gas; relatively insensitive for detecting gallstones or biliary dilatation.
Magnetic resonance imaging (MRI): Holds promise for most sensitive detection of hepatic masses and cysts; allows easy differentiation of hemangiomas from other hepatic tumors; most accurate noninvasive means of assessing hepatic and portal vein patency.
Radionuclide scanning: Using various radiolabeled compounds, different scanning methods allow sensitive assessment of biliary excretion (HIDA, PIPIDA, DESIDA scans), parenchymal changes (technetium sulfur colloid liver/spleen scan), and selected inflammatory and neoplastic processes (gallium scan); HIDA and related scans particularly useful for assessing biliary patency and excluding cholecystitis; colloid scans and CT have similar sensitivity for detecting liver tumors and metastases; colloid scans provide most accurate assessment of spleen size and can provide strong indirect evidence for cirrhosis and portal hypertension; combination of colloidal liver and lung scans sensitive for detecting right subphrenic (suprahepatic) abscesses.
Cholangiography: Most sensitive means of detecting biliary ductal calculi, biliary tumors, and sclerosing cholangitis; may be performed via endoscopic (transampullary) or percutaneous (transhepatic) route with equal efficacy.

Angiography: Most accurate means of determining portal pressures and assessing patency and direction of flow in portal and hepatic veins; highly sensitive for detecting small vascular lesions and hepatic tumors (esp. primary hepatocellular carcinoma); "gold standard" for differentiating hemangiomas from solid tumors; only means of studying vascular anatomy in preparation for complicated hepatobiliary surgery (e.g., portal-systemic shunting, biliary reconstruction).

For more detailed discussion of these topics, see Isselbacher KJ; Jaundice and Hepatomegaly, Chap. 38, and Podolsky DK, Isselbacher KJ; Diagnostic Procedures in Liver Disease, Chap. 245, in HPIM-11, pp. 183 and 1315

---

20 ASCITES

DEFINITION

Accumulation of fluid within the peritoneal cavity. Small amounts may be asymptomatic; increasing amounts cause abdominal distention and discomfort, anorexia, nausea, early satiety, heartburn, frank pain, and respiratory distress.

DETECTION **Physical examination** (detects no less than several 100 mL): Bulging flanks, fluid wave, shifting dullness, "puddle sign" (dullness over dependent abdomen with patient on hands and knees). May be associated with penile or scrotal edema, umbilical herniation, pleural effusion.
Ultrasonography/CT: Very sensitive; able to distinguish fluid from cystic masses.

EVALUATION Diagnostic paracentesis (50–100 mL) essential. Evaluation includes inspection, protein, cell count and differential, lactate dehydrogenase, amylase, pH, lipids, culture, cytology. Rarely, laparoscopy or even exploratory laparotomy may be required.

DIFFERENTIAL DIAGNOSIS (More than 90% of cases due to cirrhosis, neoplasm, CHF, TBC).

1 *Diseases of peritoneum:* Infections (bacterial, TBC, fungal, parasitic), neoplasms, vasculitis, miscellaneous (Whipple's disease, familial Mediterranean fever, endometriosis, starch peritonitis, etc.).
2 *Diseases not involving peritoneum:* Cirrhosis, CHF, Budd-Chiari syndrome, hypoalbuminemia (nephrotic syndrome, protein-losing enteropathy, malnutrition), miscellaneous (myxedema, ovarian diseases, pancreatic disease, chylous ascites).

Alternative classifications (frequent exceptions): *Exudative* (protein > 2.5 g/dL or serum-ascites albumin gradient < 1.1): infection, neoplasm, pancreatitis, vasculitis. *Transudative* (protein < 2.5 g/dL or serum-ascites albumin gradient > 1.1); cirrhosis, nephrosis, CHF.

REPRESENTATIVE FLUID CHARACTERISTICS (See Table 20-1.)

CIRRHOTIC ASCITES

PATHOGENESIS (1) Portal hypertension, (2) hypoalbuminemia, (3) increased hepatic lymph formation, (4) renal sodium retention—secondary to hyperaldosteronism, increased sympathetic nervous activity (renin-angiotensin production), increased renal production of prostaglandins; role of atrial natriuretic factor as yet unclear.

TREATMENT Maximum mobilization ≃ 700 mL/day (peripheral edema may be mobilized faster).

TABLE 20.1

Cause	Appearance	Protein, g/dL	Cell count, per mm³		Other
			RBC	WBC	
Cirrhosis	Straw-colored	<2.5	Low	<250	—
Neoplasm	Straw-colored, hemorrhagic, mucinous, or chylous	>2.5	Often high	>1000 (>50% lymphs)	+ Cytology
Bacterial peritonitis	Turbid or purulent	>2.5	Low	>250 polys	+ Gram's stain, culture
Tuberculous peritonitis	Clear, hemorrhagic, or chylous	>2.5	Occ. high	>1000 (>70% lymphs)	+ AFB stain, culture
CHF	Straw-colored	Variable	Low	<1000 (mesothelial)	—
Pancreatitis	Turbid, hemorrhagic, or chylous	>2.5	Variable	Variable	Increased amylase

1 Initially bed rest, rigid salt restriction (400 mg Na/day).
2 Fluid restriction of 1–1.5 L only if hyponatremia.
3 Diuretics if no response after 1 week: spironolactone (mild, potassium-sparing, aldosterone-antagonist) 100 mg/day PO increased by 100 mg q 4–5 d to maximum of 600 mg/day; furosemide 40–80 mg/day PO or IV in addition to spironolactone if necessary (greater risk of hepatorenal syndrome, encephalopathy).
4 Monitor weight, urinary sodium and potassium, serum electrolytes and creatinine.
5 Repeated large-volume paracentesis (1–2 L) with IV infusions of albumin may be acceptable alternative to diuretic therapy for initial management of massive ascites, especially if peripheral edema is also present.
6 In rare refractory cases, consider peritoneovenous (LeVeen, Denver) shunt (high complication rate—occlusion, infection, DIC) or side-to-side portacaval shunt (high mortality rate in end-stage cirrhotic patient).

COMPLICATIONS **Spontaneous bacterial peritonitis:** Suspect in cirrhotic patient with ascites and fever, abdominal pain, worsening ascites, ileus, hypotension, worsening jaundice, or encephalopathy; suggested by ascitic fluid PMN cell count > 250/mm^3 or ascitic pH < blood pH; confirmed by positive culture (usually Enterobacteriaceae, group D streptococci, *Streptococcus pneumoniae, Streptococcus viridans*). Initial treatment: Cefotaxime 2 g IV q 6 h or ampicillin 2 g IV q 6 h + tobramycin 1.75 mg/kg IV q 8 h (adjust for renal function); treat 10–14 days or until ascitic PMN count < 250/mm^3.

Hepatorenal syndrome: Progressive renal failure characterized by azotemia, oliguria with urinary sodium concentration < meq/L, hypotension, and lack of response to volume challenge. May be spontaneous or precipitated by bleeding, excessive diuresis, paracentesis, or drugs (aminoglycosides, NSAIDs). Thought to result from altered renal hemodynamics and decreased urinary prostaglandin levels. Treatment: Trial of plasma expansion; no definitive therapy. Prognosis poor.

For more detailed discussion of this topic, see Glickman RM, Isselbacher KJ: Abdominal Swelling and Ascites, Chap. 39, in HPIM-11, p. 188

21 ABNORMALITIES IN URINARY FUNCTION

AZOTEMIA Retention of nitrogenous waste normally cleared by the kidney, with marked (>50%) reduction in GFR; ↑ plasma creatinine (Cr) and urea (BUN).

OLIGURIA Urine output less than the amount sufficient to remove waste products. When maximally concentrated, 400–500 mL urine must be formed to excrete the daily osmolar load. Smaller volumes result in azotemia.

ANURIA Less than 100 mL urine daily. Bilateral urinary obstruction and renal arterial occlusion are important treatable causes. Also may be due to cortical necrosis, crescentic glomerulonephritis, and severe acute tubular necrosis.

APPROACH TO PATIENT WITH OLIGURIA OR ANURIA (Table 21-1) Consider *prerenal* azotemia, due to hypovolemia or CHF. Also consider postrenal failure due to lower urinary tract obstruction. Acute intrinsic renal failure (Chap. 85) is the cause in the remainder.

PROTEINURIA An important indicator of renal parenchymal disease. Normal urine contains <150 mg protein/24 h. Concentrated urine may contain trace to 1+ proteinuria by dipstick.

TABLE 21-1 **Approach to the oliguric patient**

1 Obtain Hx for volume depletion, i.e., prerenal oliguria (diarrhea, diuresis, poor intake) or postrenal factors (bladder, prostate, anticholinergic or opioid drugs, recent catheter).
2 Evaluate PE for prerenal (low BP, tachycardia, flat neck veins, poor skin turgor) or postrenal (large bladder, CVA tenderness, pelvic mass) factors.
3 Search for potential causes of ARF (hypotension, nephrotoxins, sepsis, systemic disease).
4 Obtain urine tests:

	Prerenal	ARF	Postrenal*
U_{Na} (meq/L)	<20	>40	Variable
U_{osmol}(mosmol/kg)	>500	<350	Variable
FENA†	<1	>1	Variable
Urinalysis	Normal	Muddy brown casts	Crystals, WBCs, RBCs, bacteria
U/P Cr	>40	>20	Variable

5 Echo to rule out obstruction.
6 Fluid challenge if prerenal cause is suspected

* In acute obstruction values resemble prerenal.

$$\dagger \text{ FENA} = \frac{U_{Na}\text{ (meq/L)}}{S_{Na}\text{ (meq/L)}} \times \frac{S_{Cr}\text{ (mg/dL)}}{U_{Cr}\text{ (mg/dL)}} \times 100$$

where FENA = fraction of filtered Na which is excreted; U = urine; S = serum.

False-positive dipstick for protein may occur in alkaline urine. Dipstick will not detect light-chain proteinuria or small proteins from damaged renal tubules.

Conditions causing mild proteinuria (<1 g/day) include CHF, hypertensive nephrosclerosis, and polycystic kidney disease; also, orthostatic proteinuria, vigorous exercise, and fever. Interstitial nephritis, analgesic abuse, sickle cell anemia, and some glomerulonephritides are typically associated with moderate (1–3.5 g/day) proteinuria. Massive proteinuria (>3.5 g/day) with hypoalbuminemia, edema, and hyperlipidemia is characteristic of the nephrotic syndrome (Chap. 88).

Evaluation: Proteinuria due to activity or upright posture can be excluded by collection of first morning specimens. Renal biopsy is frequently necessary in moderate or severe cases.

HEMATURIA **Definition:** The presence of RBCs (>1–2 per hpf) or gross blood in the urine; RBCs are present in spun sediment. The dipstick does *not* distinguish among intact RBCs, Hb, and myoglobin. *Hemoglobinuria* may be due to lysis of red cells in hypotonic urine or to filtered plasma Hb. *Myoglobinuria* originates from circulating myoglobin from injured muscle. Both hemoglobinuria and myoglobinuria have + dipstick with negative sediment.

Hematuria may originate at any site from glomerulus to urethra. Concomitant proteinuria and impaired renal function suggest a renal parenchymal source. RBC casts support a diagnosis of glomerulonephritis.

Isolated hematuria (without RBC casts or proteinuria) suggests bleeding from a site between renal pelvis and urethra, such as neoplasm of urinary tract, TBC, renal calculi, trauma, papillary necrosis, analgesic nephropathy, hemoglobinopathies, IgA nephropathy, prostatitis, and acute cystitis. Menstrual contamination may be mistaken for hematuria in the female.

Diagnosis: Exclude coagulation disorders, UTI, TBC, and sickle cell disease. The *pattern* of hematuria may suggest a specific source, e.g., bladder (hematuria throughout voiding), urethra (hematuria at start of voiding), or prostate (terminal hematuria). IVP, ultrasound, and cystoscope are often useful.

If renal disease is evident, serologic tests (ANA, complement, hepatitis B, VDRL) should be performed. A renal biopsy may be required to make a specific diagnosis.

POLYURIA A daily urine volume > 3 L/day; reflects renal water loss due either to an increase in obligatory excretion or a decrease in tubular reabsorption of water (Table 21-2).

Obligate water loss is due to increased intake in *primary polydypsia,* a psychogenic disorder associated with other mental illness and occurring most often in middle-aged females. Diuretic or cathartic abuse is frequently present. Obligate water loss also may be due to *solute diuresis* after infusion of glucose, saline, or mannitol; glucosuria in the poorly controlled diabetic; and urea from high-protein feedings. Polyuria is also observed in the recovery phase of acute tubular necrosis, after renal transplantation, in salt-

TABLE 21-2 **Major causes of polyuria**

Obligate water excretion	Decreased water reabsorption
Psychogenic polydipsia	Central DI:
Solute diuresis:	Idiopathic
Glucose	Hypophysectomy
Saline	Head trauma
Diabetes mellitus	Tumors
Protein feeding	Sarcoid
Contrast agents	Infection
Recovery ATN	Nephrogenic DI:
Renal transplant	Hypokalemia
Salt-wasting nephropathy	Hypercalcemia
Postobstruction	Obstructive uropathy
Diuretics	Analgesic abuse
	Pyelonephritis
	Drugs

wasting conditions, following relief of urinary obstruction, and in diuretic abuse.

Decreased tubular reabsorption of water is due to *diabetes insipidus* (DI). Causes are inadequate secretion of vasopressin (central DI) (see Chap. 89) or renal tubular unresponsiveness to the hormone (nephrogenic DI). Nephrogenic DI may be congenital but is usually acquired, due to tubulointerstitial diseases (obstructive uropathy, hypercalcemia, hypokalemia, analgesic abuse, pyelonephritis) or to drugs (lithium, ethanol, propoxyphene, diphenylhydantoin, methoxyflurane).

Polydipsia and DI are best evaluated by water deprivation test and administration of exogenous vasopressin. Polydypsic patients will concentrate their urine to 600–800 mosmol, not lose weight during water deprivation, and have little further response to vasopressin. Patients with complete central DI will lose weight and continue to form a dilute urine, which improves with vasopression. Patients with nephrogenic DI will lose weight and elaborate a dilute urine during water deprivation, with little further improvement after vasopressin. Responses may overlap among milder cases of these disorders.

For more detailed discussion of this topic, see Coe FL: Alterations in Urinary Function, Chap. 40, in HPIM-11, p. 191

SODIUM (Na)

HYPONATREMIA (Serum Na <135 meq/L) Due to excess body H_2O relative to Na and occurs in conditions in which total extracellular fluid Na may be normal, ↑, or ↓. Hypoosmolality is present unless non-Na solutes are ↑↑, as in diabetes, severe hyperlipidemia, or in severe hyperproteinemic states, such as multiple myeloma.

Hypovolemic hyponatremia results when Na losses, usually from GI tract, exceed losses of H_2O, often associated with partial volume replacement with H_2O and/or impaired H_2O diuresis. Clinical features reflect volume depletion; urinary Na <10 meq/L, except when vomiting produces metabolic alkalosis and obligates renal $NaHCO_3$ losses. Hypovolemic hyponatremia may also result from renal losses (diuretics, Addison's disease, or osmotic diuresis); urinary Na >20 meq/L.

Hypervolemic hyponatremia occurs when increase in total body H_2O exceeds increase of Na; may occur in severe CHF, cirrhosis, and nephrotic syndrome. Urinary Na <10 meq/L except in renal failure.

Euvolemic hyponatremia occurs in syndrome of inappropriate ADH secretion (SIADH), in which excessive ADH-mediated H_2O reabsorption causes dilutional hyponatremia, urine is relatively hypertonic to plasma, urinary Na losses associated with normal renal and adrenal function. Common causes are ectopic production of ADH by tumors (e.g., oat cell cancer of lung), endogenous overproduction due to pulmonary diseases (pneumonia, abscess, TBC, positive end expiratory pressure), CNS disorders (tumors, meningitis, encephalitis, trauma, subarachnoid hemorrhage, stroke), and stressful conditions. Drugs may impair water excretion by releasing ADH (e.g., morphine, tricyclics, cyclophosphamide, nicotine), or enhancing its action (NSAIDs), or both (sulfonylureas). Hypothyroidism and cortisol deficiency may also cause euvolemic hyponatremia.

Symptoms include confusion, anorexia, lethargy, disorientation, and cramps. When Na drops abruptly to <120 meq/L, seizures, hemiparesis, and coma may develop.

Treatment: First, assess volume status. Hypovolemic pts should receive normal saline (hypertonic saline when Na <120 meq/L). Any mineralocorticoid deficiency should be corrected. In hypervolemic hyponatremia H_2O intake should be restricted. Further improvement may occur with appropriate treatment of CHF, albumin infusion in nephrosis, or cautious use of diuretics and sometimes albumin in cirrhosis. Pts with SIADH require H_2O restriction; demeclocycline, which induces nephrogenic diabetes insipidus (DI) may be helpful.

HYPERNATREMIA (Serum Na >150 meq/L) Due to deficit of H_2O relative to Na. May result from: (1) loss of H_2O, usually insensible losses (from skin or lungs) that are not replaced; or *renal* losses due to DI caused by head injury, or neurosurgery; (2) H_2O losses exceeding Na losses: (a) with fever, burns, or exposure to high temperature; or (b) from renal losses during osmotic diuresis, as in severe hyperglycemia, in which urine is hypo- or isotonic with Na >20 meq/L; (3) Na excess may occur in pts who ingest NaCl or are resuscitated with hypertonic $NaHCO_3$.

Symptoms include altered mental status, twitching, seizures, coma. Acute severe (>160 meq/L) hypernatremia dehydrates cerebral cells and may rupture cerebral vessels, causing irreversible neurologic sequelae, and substantial mortality.

Treatment: Normalize osmolality by replacing H_2O slowly. Hypovolemic hypernatremia is initially treated with isotonic saline until volume is repleted, then with 0.45% saline. When manifestations of hypertonicity predominate, therapy may be initiated with hypotonic saline. Hypervolemic hypernatremia is best treated with hypotonic fluids and loop diuretics or, in renal failure, dialysis. Pts with central DI should receive aqueous vasopressin or the intranasal analogue, desmopressin. In pts with partial central DI, chlorpropamide may suffice. Nephrogenic DI frequently responds to thiazides and Na restriction.

POTASSIUM

EXTERNAL K BALANCE This is determined by oral intake and renal excretion. 90% of K intake is excreted by the kidney, most secreted by the distal nephron, a process augmented by aldosterone, high cell K content, and alkalosis. Factors which modulate *internal K balance* include insulin, beta-2-adrenergic agonists, and alkalosis which promote K uptake by cells. Acidosis shifts K out of cells.

HYPOKALEMIA (K < 3.5 meq/L) (Fig. 22-1A) May result from: (1) inadequate intake and/or (2) excessive losses: (a) GI (vomiting, nasogastric suction, diarrhea, villous adenoma, and laxative abuse) and associated alkalosis, secondary hyperaldosteronism, and bicarbonaturia; (b) renal losses of K may result from alkalosis of any cause, from diuretics (except K-sparing agents), from osmotic diuresis, as in hyperglycemia, primary and secondary hyperaldosteronism, renal tubular disorders, drugs (amphotericin, gentamicin, and carbenicillin) and Mg depletion; (3) hypokalemia due to *internal* imbalance may occur when cellular uptake of K from extracellular fluid is increased, as in alkalosis, after insulin therapy, or in periodic paralysis.

Clinical features: Muscle weakness, ileus, polyuria, and ECG changes (U-waves, ↑ Q-T interval, and flat T-waves). Severe hypokalemia causes flaccid paralysis and cardiac arrest.

The cause of hypokalemia is usually evident on presentation. Inadequate intake or diarrhea is suggested when urinary K excretion <25 meq/day. Greater urinary K losses suggest vomiting, current diuretic use, or renal tubular losses. Presence of acidemia suggests diarrhea, renal tubular acidosis, or diabetic ketoacidosis. Mineralocorticoid excess is suggested by increased renal K losses and hypertension.

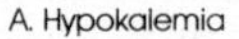

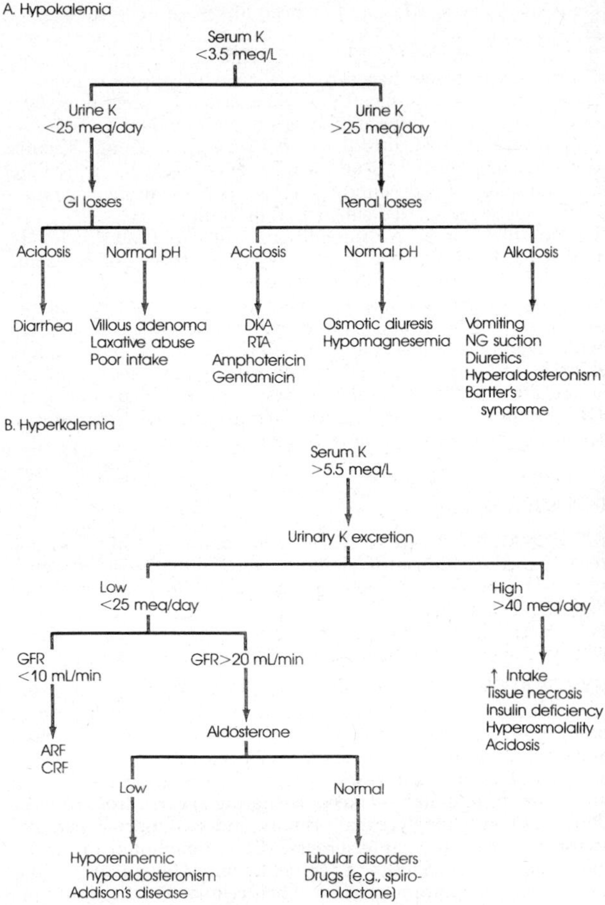

A. Hypokalemia

- Serum K <3.5 meq/L
  - Urine K <25 meq/day → GI losses
    - Acidosis → Diarrhea
    - Normal pH → Villous adenoma, Laxative abuse, Poor intake
  - Urine K >25 meq/day → Renal losses
    - Acidosis → DKA, RTA, Amphotericin, Gentamicin
    - Normal pH → Osmotic diuresis, Hypomagnesemia
    - Alkalosis → Vomiting, NG suction, Diuretics, Hyperaldosteronism, Bartter's syndrome

B. Hyperkalemia

- Serum K >5.5 meq/L → Urinary K excretion
  - Low <25 meq/day
    - GFR <10 mL/min → ARF, CRF
    - GFR>20 mL/min → Aldosterone
      - Low → Hyporeninemic hypoaldosteronism, Addison's disease
      - Normal → Tubular disorders, Drugs (e.g., spironolactone)
  - High >40 meq/day → ↑ Intake, Tissue necrosis, Insulin deficiency, Hyperosmolality, Acidosis

NG = nasogastric; DKA = diabetic ketoacidosis; RTA = renal tubular acidosis

FIG. 22-1 *Evaluation of potassium disorders.*

Treatment with dietary supplements, using KCl, suffices in mild cases. In edematous pts on diuretics, dietary supplementation and addition of K-sparing agents (e.g., aldactone) are useful. GI losses should be replaced with IV KCl (≤20 meq/h). Severe symptomatic hypokalemia requires larger doses (20–40 meq/h), with cardiac monitoring and frequent plasma K levels. Hypokalemia with digitalis toxicity also requires urgent correction.

HYPERKALEMIA (Serum K >5.5 meq/L) (Fig. 22-1B) May be due to *impaired K excretion,* as in oliguric acute renal failure, in chronic renal failure when GFR <10 mL/min, when dietary K is excessive, and/or with administration of K-sparing diuretics.
Hyporeninemic hypoaldosteronism occurs in diabetes mellitus and the elderly. Acidosis and mild renal failure are frequent concomitants. Hypoaldosteronism also causes hyperkalemia in Addison's disease, in pts treated with NSAIDs, angiotensin converting enzyme inhibitors, heparin, and cyclosporine. Renal K retention is also provoked by spironolactone, triamterene, and amiloride.

Hyperkalemia due to *internal K imbalance* (release of K from cells) occurs in acidosis and in diabetics with deficient insulin-mediated K uptake. Cellular necrosis may release excess K into the circulation, from muscle (e.g., rhabdomyolysis), tumor cells (tumor lysis syndrome), and RBCs (hemolytic states). Arginine HCl, used to correct metabolic acidosis, may elevate serum K in pts with renal and/or liver failure.

The most important *clinical effects* of hyperkalemia are cardiac conduction changes (Figure 22-2) and arrhythmias, which are exaggerated by ↓ Na, ↓ Ca, acidosis, and ↑ Mg. Hyperkalemia may also cause an ascending muscle weakness.
Treatment is shown in Table 22-1.

FIG. 22-2 *Diagrammatic ECGs at normal and high serum K. Peaked T waves (precordial leads) are followed by diminished R wave, wide QRS, prolonged P-R, loss of P wave, and ultimately a sine wave.*

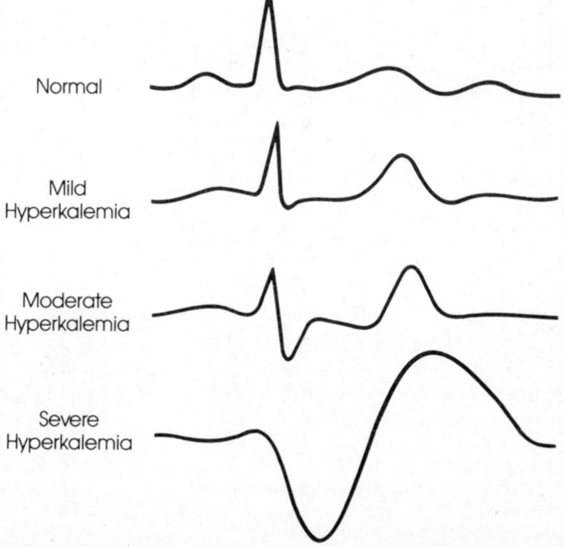

TABLE 22-1 **Management of hyperkalemia**

Treatment	Indication	Dose	Onset	Duration	Mechanism	Note
Calcium gluconate*	K > 6.5 meq/L with advanced ECG changes	10 mL of 10% solution IV over 2–3 min	1–5 min	30 min	Lowers threshold potential. Antagonizes cardiac and neuromuscular toxicity of hyperkalemia.	Fastest action. Monitor ECG. Repeat in 5 min if abnormal ECG persists. Hazardous in presence of digitalis. Correct hyponatremia if present. Follow with other treatment for K.
Insulin + Glucose	Moderate hyperkalemia, peaked T waves only	10 U reg, IV + 50 mL, 50% IV	15–45 min	4–6 h	Moves K into cells.	Glucose unnecessary if blood sugar elevated. Repeat insulin q 15 min with glucose infusion if needed.
$NaHCO_3$	Moderate hyperkalemia	90 meq (2 ampules, IV push over 5 min)	Immediate	Short	Moves K into cells.	Most effective when acidosis is present. Of more risk in CHF or hypernatremia. Beware of hypocalcemic tetany.
Kayexalate + Sorbitol	Moderate hyperkalemia	Oral: 30 g, with 50 mL 20% Sorbitol; Rectal: 50 g in 200 mL 20% Sorbitol enema, retain 45 min	1 h	4–6 h	Removes K.	Each gram Kayexalate removes about 1 meq K orally or about 0.5 meq K rectally. Repeat every 4 h. Use with caution in CHF.
Furosemide	Moderate hyperkalemia, serum creatinine < 3 mg%	20–40 mg IV push	15 min	4 h	Kaliuresis.	Most useful if inadequate K excretion contributes to hyperkalemia.
Dialysis	Hyperkalemia with renal failure		Immediate after start-up	Variable	Removes K.	Hemodialysis most effective. Also improves acidosis.

* Calcium chloride may be preferable in presence of circulatory instability or liver impairment.

ACID-BASE DISORDERS (Figure 22-3)

Regulation of normal pH (7.35–7.45) depends on lungs and kidneys. By the Henderson-Hasselbach equation, pH may be considered a function of the ratio of HCO_3 (regulated by the kidney) to P_{CO_2} (regulated by the lungs.) The HCO_3/P_{CO_2} relationship is useful in classifying disorders of acid-base balance. *Acidosis* is due to gain of acid or loss of alkali; causes may be metabolic (fall in serum HCO_3) or respiratory (rise in P_{CO_2}). *Alkalosis* is due to loss of acid or addition of base, and is either metabolic (↑ serum HCO_3) or respiratory (↓ P_{CO_2}).

To limit the change in pH, metabolic disorders evoke an immediate compensatory response in ventilation; compensation to respiratory disorders by the kidneys takes days. *Simple* acid-base disorders consist of one primary disturbance and its compensatory response. In *mixed* disorders, a combination of primary disturbances is present.

FIG. 22-3 *Nomogram, showing bands for uncomplicated respiratory or metabolic acid-base disturbances in intact subjects. Each "confidence" band represents the mean ±2 SD for the compensatory response of normal subjects or patients to a given primary disorder. Ac = acute; chr = chronic, resp = respiratory; met = metabolic; acid = acidosis; alk = alkalosis. (From Levinsky NG: HPIM-11, p. 209; modified from Arbus GS: Can Med Assoc J 109:291, 1973.)*

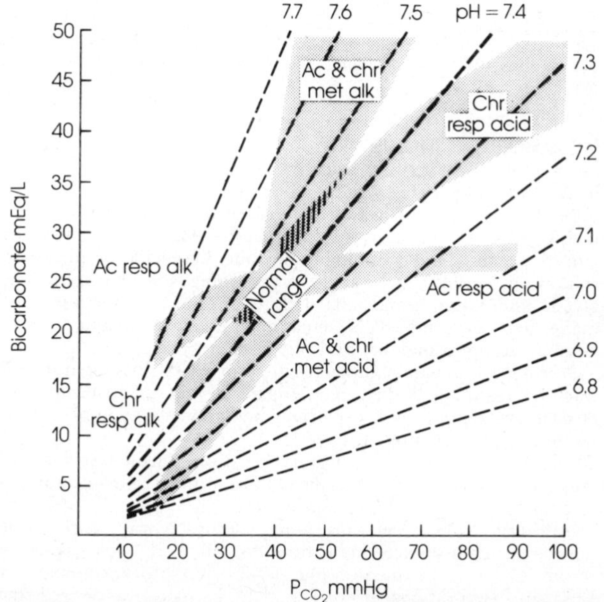

TABLE 22-2 **Metabolic acidosis**

Non-anion gap acidosis		Anion gap acidosis	
Cause	Clue	Cause	Clue
Diarrhea	Hx; ↓ K	DKA	Hyperglycemia, ketones
Enterostomy	Drainage	RF	Uremia, ↑ BUN, ↑ CR
RTA		Lactic acidosis	Clinical setting + ↑ serum lactate
Proximal	↓ K	Alcoholic ketoacidosis	Hx; weak + ketones; + osm gap
Distal	↓ K; UpH > 5.5	Starvation	Hx; mild acidosis; + ketones
Dilutional	Volume expansion	Salicylates	Hx; tinnitus; high serum level; + ketones
Ureterosigmoidostomy	Obstructed ileal loop	Methanol	large AG; retinitis; + toxic screen; + osm gap
Hyperalimentation	Amino acid infusion	Ethylene glycol	RF, CNS; + toxic screen; crystalluria; + osm gap
Acetazolamide NH_4Cl Lysine HCl Arginine HCl	Hx of administration of these agents		

RTA = renal tubular acidosis; UpH = urinary pH; DKA = diabetic ketoacidosis; RF = renal failure; AG = anion gap; osm gap = osmolar gap

METABOLIC ACIDOSIS The low HCO_3 results from the addition of (organic or inorganic) acids or loss of HCO_3. The *causes* of metabolic acidosis are categorized by the anion gap, which equals $Na - (Cl + HCO_3)$ (Table 22-2). *Increased* anion gap acidoses (>12 meq/L) are due to addition of acid (other than HCl) and unmeasured anions to the body. Etiologies include ketoacidosis (diabetes, starvation, alcohol), lactic acidosis, poisoning (salicylates, ethylene glycol, and ethanol) and renal failure. Specific diagnoses may be made by measuring BUN, creatinine, glucose, lactate, serum ketones, serum osmolality and obtaining a toxic screen.

Normal anion gap acidoses result from HCO_3 loss from the GI tract or from the kidney, e.g., renal tubular acidosis, urinary obstruction, rapid volume expansion, and administration of NH_4Cl, lysine HCl, or arginine HCl.

Clinical features include hyperventilation, cardiovascular collapse, and a variety of nonspecific symptoms ranging from anorexia to coma.

Treatment depends on cause and severity. Always correct the underlying disturbance. Indications for alkali therapy include a serum HCO_3 <15 meq/L, pH <7.2, circulatory collapse, or Kussmaul respirations. If correction to 18 meq/L is desired, the

HCO_3 deficit can be calculated as body wt (kg) × 0.50 × (18 − actual serum HCO_3). Replace half in 12 h; remainder in next 24 h.

Chronic acidosis is treated when HCO_3 <15 meq/L or symptoms or anorexia or fatigue are present. Na citrate may be more palatable than oral $NaHCO_3$.

METABOLIC ALKALOSIS A primary increase in serum HCO_3. Most cases originate with loss of acid from the stomach or kidney and volume contraction. Less commonly, HCO_3 administered or derived from endogenous lactate is the cause and is maintained when renal HCO_3 reabsorption continues. In vomiting, Cl loss reduces its availability for renal reabsorption with Na. Enhanced Na avidity due to volume depletion then accelerates HCO_3 reabsorption, and sustains the alkalosis. Urine Cl is typically low (<10 meq/L) (Table 22-3). Alkalosis may also be maintained by hypermineralocorticoidism, due to the direct enhancement of H secretion and HCO_3 reabsorption. Severe K depletion may also cause metabolic alkalosis by increased HCO_3 reabsorption; urine Cl >20 meq/L.

Vomiting and nasogastric drainage cause HCl and volume loss, kaliuresis, and alkalosis. Diuretics are a common cause of alkalosis due to volume contraction, Cl depletion, and hypokalemia. Pts with chronic pulmonary disease, high P_{CO_2} and serum HCO_3 levels, whose ventilation is acutely improved, may develop alkalosis.

Excessive mineralocorticoid activity due to Cushing's syndrome (worse in ectopic ACTH or primary hyperaldosteronism) causes metabolic alkalosis not associated with volume or Cl depletion and not responsive to NaCl. Severe K depletion also causes metabolic alkalosis.

Diagnosis: The Cl on a random urine is useful (Table 22-3) unless diuretics have been administered.

Therapy: Correct the underlying cause. In cases of Cl depletion, administer NaCl; and in hypokalemia, add KCl. Pts with adrenal hyperfunction require treatment of the underlying disorder.

Severe alkalosis may require, in addition, treatment with acidifying agents such as NH_4Cl, HCl, or acetazolamide. The initial amount of H needed should be calculated from 0.5 × (body wt in kg) × (serum HCO_3 − 24).

RESPIRATORY ACIDOSIS Characterized by CO_2 retention due to ventilatory failure. Causes include sedatives, stroke, chronic pulmonary disease, airway obstruction, severe pulmonary edema, neuromuscular disorders, and cardiopulmonary arrest.

TABLE 22-3 **Metabolic alkalosis**

NaCl responsive (low U_{Cl})	NaCl resistant (high U_{Cl})
Vomiting	Primary hyperaldosteronism
Nasogastric suction	Cushing's syndrome
Diuresis	Severe K depletion
Post-hypercapneic	Bartter's syndrome

Symptoms include confusion, asterixis, and obtundation.
Therapy: The goal is to improve ventilation, through pulmonary toilet and reversal of bronchospasm. Intubation may be required in severe acute cases. Acidosis due to hypercapnia is usually mild.

RESPIRATORY ALKALOSIS. Excessive ventilation causes a primary reduction in CO_2 and ↑ pH and is observed in pneumonia, pulmonary edema, interstitial lung disease, asthma. Pain and psychogenic causes are common; other causes include fever, hypoxemia, sepsis, delirium tremens, salicylates, hepatic failure, mechanical overventilation, and CNS lesions. Severe respiratory alkalosis may cause seizures, tetany, cardiac arrhythmias, or loss of consciousness.
Therapy should be directed at the underlying disorders. In psychogenic cases, sedation or a rebreathing bag may be required.

"MIXED" DISORDERS In many circumstances, more than a single acid-base disturbance exists. Examples include combined metabolic and respiratory acidosis in pts with cardiogenic shock; metabolic alkalosis and acidosis in pts with vomiting and diabetic ketoacidosis; and metabolic acidosis with respiratory alkalosis in pts with sepsis. The diagnosis may be clinically evident or suggested by relationships between the P_{CO_2} and HCO_3 which are markedly different from those found in simple disorders.

In simple anion-gap acidosis, anion gap increases in proportion to fall in HCO_3. When increase in anion gap occurs despite a normal HCO_3, simultaneous anion-gap acidosis and metabolic alkalosis are suggested. When fall in HCO_3 due to metabolic acidosis is proportionately larger than increase in anion gap, mixed anion gap and non-anion gap metabolic acidosis is suggested.

For more detailed discussion of this topic, see Levinsky NG: Fluids and Electrolytes, Chap. 41, and Levinsky NG: Acidosis and Alkalosis, Chap. 42, in HPIM-11, pp. 198 and 208

---

23 SEXUAL DYSFUNCTION IN WOMEN

Women commonly seek medical advice because of sexual problems that are at the interface of medicine and sociology. In each instance it is essential that the medical contribution to the problem be identified and, if possible, corrected. These sexual complaints can be separated into three broad categories.

FAILURE OF SATISFACTION FROM SEXUAL CONTACT This is the most common complaint and is usually termed *frigidity* (i.e., failure of sexual arousal) or *anorgasmia* (i.e., failure to achieve orgasm). Diagnosis must be made with caution; e.g., omission of foreplay or coitus shorted by premature ejaculation would preclude diagnosis of anorgasmia.

Normal sexual arousal causes vasocongestion of the vagina, labia minora, and clitoris and results in vaginal lubrication in preparation for intromission. Healthy vaginal tissue and appropriate sexual stimuli (tactile, visual, auditory, and olfactory) are prerequisites for vasocongestion and vaginal transudation. Estrogen deprivation after surgical or natural menopause causes vaginal atrophy and decreased vaginal lubrication. Appropriate hormone replacement enhances vaginal lubrication and sexual enjoyment (see Chap. 141). Impairment of neurologic function (such as diabetes mellitus) or of the circulation (such as atherosclerosis) may impair sexual arousal, similar to their effects on erectile function in men. Likewise, drugs that impair male sexual function have similar adverse effects on sexual arousal in women (see Table 24-1). Indeed, all causes of erectile failure in men can probably also inhibit sexual arousal of women.

Nevertheless, failure of arousal also may be due to psychological causes. Such problems include misinformation or feelings of guilt about previous trauma such as incest, rape, or unwanted pregnancy. Women who have had hysterectomies or mastectomies may consider themselves incomplete. Anxiety, depression, fatigue, or interpersonal conflict may prevent normal vaginal lubrication. Such problems are approached by attempting to identify and reduce the stresses.

PAINFUL INTERCOURSE, OR DYSPAREUNIA This is the second most common sexual complaint and may affect all sexual contacts or be intermittent. It is usually organic in cause, and the diagnosis of functional dyspareunia is one of exclusion. The usual cause is vaginitis, including *Trichomonas,* fungus, and yeast infections; nonspecific vaginitis; herpes vaginitis; and *E. coli* vaginitis. Pelvic infections may cause pain due to active infection itself or from scarring secondary to previous inflammation. Other pelvic causes of dyspareunia include malignant and nonmalignant tumors, disorders of adjacent viscera (urethra, bladder, lower sigmoid, and rectum), and orthopedic problems (e.g., subluxation of pelvis). Other causes include atrophic vaginitis secondary to estrogen lack in postmenopausal women, allergic reactions, infections of Skene's or Bartholin's glands, vulvitis, hymenal obstruction, episiotomy scarring, or postirradiation vaginitis.

VAGINISMUS This is involuntary tightening of the vaginal musculature, and it precludes intercourse and sometimes prevents examination by the physician. Vaginismus is a conditioned response to previous organic or psychogenic trauma such as negative conditioning to sex during childhood, traumatic sexual experiences, or phobias about pelvic examinations, pregnancy, or venereal diseases. Treatment is directed toward elimination of the conditioned response through progressive vaginal dilation by the patient in conjunction with psychotherapy.

For more detailed discussion of this topic, see Carr BR, Wilson JD: Disturbances of Menstruation and Sexual Function in Women, Chap. 43, in HPIM-11, p. 214

---

24 IMPOTENCE IN MEN

Impotence may involve loss of sexual desire, inability to obtain or maintain an erection, premature ejaculation, absence of emission, or inability to achieve orgasm.

CAUSES

Such complaints can be due to systemic disease such as diabetes mellitus, to drug therapy (see Table 24-1), or to abnormalities of urogenital tract or endocrine system.

TABLE 24-1 **Some organic causes of erectile impotence in men**

Endocrine causes:	Penile diseases:
Testicular failure (primary or secondary)	Previous priapism
Hyperprolactinemia	Penile trauma
Drugs:	Peyronie's disease
Antihistamines	Neurologic diseases:
Antihypertensives	Anterior temporal lobe lesions
Anticholinergics	Diseases of the spinal cord
Antidepressants	Loss of sensory input
Antipsychotics	Disease of nervi erigentes
Tranquilizers	Vascular disease
Drugs of habituation or addiction	

ANDROGEN DEFICIENCY Because androgens have a major influence on male sexual desire, impotence due to pituitary or testicular disease is invariably accompanied by a loss of sexual desire. The level of testosterone required to maintain libido is less than the amount necessary for maintenance of the prostate and seminal vesicles, and absence of emission is also a common feature of hypogonadism. The diagnosis of androgen deficiency is confirmed by measurement of serum testosterone, gonadotropins, and semen volume. Hyperprolactinemia may cause impotence by uncertain mechanisms.

ERECTILE IMPOTENCE This is more commonly not due to endocrine disease. Drug causes include antihistamines, antihypertensives, anticholinergics, psychogenic agents, and drugs of addiction. Neurologic causes include spinal cord disorders, diabetic neuropathy, tabes dorsalis, and damage to parasympathetic nerves following surgical procedures such as prostatectomy. Vascular insufficiency causes impotence when blood flow into penis is insufficient to produce (or maintain) erectile state.

RETROGRADE EJACULATION This may occur following surgery on the bladder neck or develop spontaneously in men with autonomic nervous system neuropathy. Demonstration of sperm in postcoital urine will establish diagnosis. Drugs such as guanethidine, phenoxybenzamine, and phetolamine primarily impair ejaculation rather than erection or sex drive. If libido, erection, and ejaculation are normal, the absence of orgasm is almost always due to psychogenic causes.

DISEASES OF THE PENIS Such diseases as Peyronie's disease or priapism also can cause impotence. Priapism, a persistent painful erection, often unrelated to sexual activity, results from clotting within penile vascular network. The process disrupts the vascular network and can lead to fibrosis and impotence.

ANXIETY OR DEPRESSION The most common cause of prolonged impotence. Psychological and organic causes can usually be distinguished on the basis of history. If there is a history of turgid erections at any time (often on early awakening), the efferent neurologic and circulatory systems are intact and the dysfunction is probably due to a psychogenic cause. If the history of nocturnal erections is questionable, nocturnal penile tumescence can be measured with the use of a strain gauge attached to a recorder. Alternatively, the penis can be wrapped with gummed, perforated paper; failure to break the perforation on three successive nights suggests the absence of nocturnal erections.

WORKUP

Having deduced an organic cause, the *history* should be probed for drugs, diabetes mellitus, peripheral neuropathy or bladder dysfunction, and intermittent claudication (Table 24-1). Testes should be palpated for size and asymmetry; if testicular length is less than 3.5 cm, hypogonadism should be considered. Evidences of feminization include gynecomastia and abnormal body hair distribution. Pulses should be palpated, including the penile pulse, which can be felt by pressing both corpora between thumb and forefinger and palpating to either side of the midline. If a vascular cause is suspected, a Doppler procedure or arteriography should be performed.

The *neurologic exam* should measure anal sphincter tone, perineal sensation, and bulbocavernosus reflex. This reflex is elicited by squeezing the glans penis and noting the degree of anal sphincter constriction. Examination for peripheral neuropathy should include assessment of distal muscle strength, tendon reflexes in the legs, and vibratory, position, tactile, and pain sensation. Laboratory evaluation is of minimal value. Measurement of serum testosterone in the absence of feminization or hypogonadism is seldom helpful.

THERAPY

Except in hypogonadal men, medical therapy with androgens offers little more than placebo benefit. If a prolactin-secreting pituitary tumor is present, either surgical removal or treatment with bromocriptine usually results in return of potency. Surgical therapy may be useful in the treatment of decreased potency related to aortic disease; however, potency can be lost after aortic surgery if the nerve supply to the penis is damaged. In patients with depressive illnesses, measures directed at their alleviation may restore sexual potency, and sexual counseling, education, and psychotherapy are beneficial in alleviating psychogenic causes. Implantation of a penile prothesis may be successful in the treatment of refractory impotence, as in patients with diabetes mellitus.

For more detailed discussion of this topic, see Walsh PC, Wilson JD: Impotence and Infertility in Men, Chap. 44, in HPIM-11, p. 217

---

25 LYMPHADENOPATHY AND SPLENOMEGALY

LYMPH NODE STRUCTURE AND FUNCTION

Lymph nodes are peripheral lymphoid organs populated by many cell types and connected to the circulation by afferent and efferent lymphatic vessels and postcapillary venules. Fibroblasts and fibroblast-derived reticular cells are supporting cells. Tissue macrophages, dendritic cells, and Langerhans cells are important antigen-presenting cells. Lymphoid follicles consist chiefly of B-lymphocytes. Primary lymphoid follicles are aggregates of IgM- and IgD-bearing B cells as well as $T4^+$ helper (inducer) T lymphocytes and arise prior to antigenic stimulation. Secondary lymphoid follicles result from antigenic stimulation and contain an inner zone (germinal center) of activated B cells, macrophages, reticular cells, and $T4^+$ helper T cells. Interfollicular zones and paracortical areas are populated largely by T lymphocytes.

Juxtaposition of large numbers of macrophages, dendritic cells, Langerhans cells, and lymphocytes allows the lymph node to serve its major function as specialized structure for interaction of these cell types in efficient generation of cellular and humoral immune responses.

Lymph node enlargement can be due to (1) an increase in number of benign lymphocytes and macrophages during response to antigens, (2) infiltration of inflammatory cells during infections involving the node (lymphadenitis), (3) malignant proliferation of lymphocytes or macrophages arising in the node, (4) infiltration by metastatic malignant cells, or (5) infiltration by metabolite-laden macrophages in various storage diseases.

DISEASES ASSOCIATED WITH LYMPHADENOPATHY

For a complete list, see HPIM-11, Table 55-1, p. 274.

Infectious diseases

- Viral infections: Infectious hepatitis, mononucleosis syndromes, AIDS and AIDS-related complex, rubella, varicella zoster virus
- Bacterial infections: Streptococci, staphylococci, *Salmonella, Brucella, Francisella tularensis, Listeria monocytogenes, Pasteurella pestis, Haemophilus ducreyi,* cat-scratch disease
- Fungal infections
- Chlamydial infections
- Mycobacterial infections: TBC, leprosy
- Parasitic infections
- Spirochetal diseases

Immunologic diseases

- Rheumatoid arthritis, SLE, dermatomyositis
- Serum sickness
- Drug reactions: Diphenylhydantoin, hydralazine, allopurinol
- Angioimmunoblastic lymphadenopathy

Malignant diseases

- Hematologic: Hodgkin's disease, non-Hodgkin's lymphomas, acute and chronic leukemias
- Metastatic tumors to lymph nodes

Endocrine diseases: Hyperthyroidism
Lipid storage diseases: Gaucher's and Niemann-Pick diseases
Miscellaneous diseases: Giant follicular lymph node hyperplasia, sinus histiocytosis, dermatopathic lymphadenitis, sarcoidosis, amyloidosis, mucocutaneous lymph node syndrome (Kawasaki's disease), multifocal Langerhans cell (eosinophilic) granulomatosis

EVALUATION OF PATIENT

In normal adults, inguinal lymph nodes may be easily palpable, from 0.5–2 cm in size. Smaller nodes may be palpable elsewhere due to past infections. Enlargment requires investigation when one or more new nodes present ≥ 1 cm in diameter and not known to arise from a previously recognized cause. Important factors: (1) patient's age, (2) physical characteristics of node, (3) node locations, and (4) clinical setting associated with the lymphadenopathy.

CLINICAL APPROACH TO PATIENT

1 Complete history and physical exam, with special attention to defining presence and extent of adenopathy and any systemic or localizing symptoms/signs.
2 If adenopathy is regional, search for infection or malignancy.
3 Laboratory studies (when appropriate): CBC, cultures of blood and other sites, CXR, PPD and control skin testing, serologies (fungal, viral, parasitic, VDRL).
4 If adenopathy persists and remains unexplained, perform lymph node biopsy. Tissue should be processed for histologic examination, cultured for appropriate organisms, and frozen for lymphocyte studies and staining for other cell types.

SPLEEN STRUCTURE AND FUNCTION

The spleen is a lymphoreticular organ that serves at least four major functions: (1) major organ of immune system, involved in generation of cell-mediated and humoral responses to antigens, and major site of removal of microorganisms and particulate antigens from blood; (2) instrumental in sequestration and removal of normal and abnormal blood cells; (3) helps regulate portal blood flow; and (4) may be major site of extramedullary hematopoiesis in states of marrow stress or replacement.

DISEASES ASSOCIATED WITH SPLENIC ENLARGEMENT

For complete list, see HPIM-11, Table 55-2, p. 276.
Infections: Mononucleosis, septicemia, endocarditis, TBC, parasites, AIDS, viral hepatitis, splenic abscess, histoplasmosis.
Disordered immunoregulation: RA, SLE, immune hemolytic anemias, immune thrombocytopenias and neutropenias.

Disordered splenic blood flow: Portal or splenic venous hypertension with resultant splenic congestion.
Abnormal erythrocytes: Spherocytosis, sickle cell disease (before autosplenectomy occurs), ovalocytosis, thalassemia.
Infiltrative diseases: Benign and malignant.
Miscellaneous: Idiopathic splenomegaly, thyrotoxicosis, iron-deficiency anemia, sarcoidosis, berylliosis.

EVALUATION OF PATIENT

Normal-sized spleen is about 12 cm in length and 7 cm in width; located along tenth left rib in midaxillary line; inaccessible to palpation when normal in size and shape. Dullness can be percussed between ninth and eleventh ribs with patient lying on right side. Palpation best performed with patient lying to the right and inspiring deeply.

CLINICAL APPROACH TO PATIENT

1 Careful history and physical exam, with special attention to characterizing illness as acute or chronic, obtaining evidence of associated signs/symptoms, and defining size of spleen.
2 When necessary or appropriate, imaging techniques may prove useful: ^{99m}Tc-colloid liver/spleen scan, CT, abdominal ultrasound.
3 Cultures, CBC, serologies, PPD and control skin tests, mononucleosis screen (heterophile antibody and EBV titers).
4 Blood smear for cellular morphology and parasites; bone marrow aspiration and biopsy.
5 Occasionally, laparotomy and splenectomy may be necessary for the diagnosis of persistent unexplained splenomegaly.

For more detailed discussion of this topic, see Haynes BF: Enlargement of Lymph Nodes and Spleen, Chap. 55, in HPIM-11, p. 272

SECTION II
INFECTIOUS DISEASES

26 DIAGNOSTIC METHODS

MICROSCOPIC EXAMINATION

Direct examination: Useful to diagnose *Borrelia* (relapsing fever) or *Plasmodium* (malaria) in blood smears.

Wet mounts

• Darkfield of genital lesions for syphilis. • Superficial mycoses (tinea versicolor) from skin scrapings, hair, or nails in drop of 10% KOH. • Diagnosis of systemic fungal infection (*Cryptococcus* in CSF, coccidioidomycosis spherules in sputum). • Stool or duodenal drainage for protozoa (amebiasis, giardiasis, cryptosporidiosis). • Stool for helminthic infections (ascariasis, trichuriasis, strongyloidiasis, hookworm). • Blood smears for filariasis (microfilariae), sleeping sickness (trypanosomes).

Stains

• Gram's stain check for contaminating epithelial cells at low power under oil (blue: gram-positive; pink: gram-negative). • Acid-fast (Ziehl-Neelsen, Kinyoun) to diagnose TBC, *Cryptosporidium* in stool, *Nocardia* (mineral acid instead of acid-alcohol). • Giemsa for *Chlamydia* from eye, urethra, cervix. • Wright's or methenamine silver for *Pneumocystis carinii* • Romanowsky for *Plasmodium, Leishmania.* • Trichrome iron hematoxylin for intestinal protozoa.

Other stains

Fluorescent antibody tests for herpes simplex or rabies on brain tissue; *Legionella* on lung tissue, pleural fluid, or sputum; influenza, parainfluenza, or respiratory syncytial virus on nasal epithelial cells.

OTHER DETECTION METHODS

Counterimmunoelectrophoresis (CIE): very sensitive test to detect pneumococcal, meningococcal, group B streptococcal, or *H. influenzae* antigens in CSF.

CULTURES

Collection

• Clean skin with 70% isopropyl alcohol and then iodophor; preferably transport to lab within 1 h. • Aspirates in syringe with air expressed. • Swabs in transport media except group A Streptococci may be in dry sterile test tube.

Upper respiratory tract

• Cultures seldom useful except when looking for specific pathogen (*S. pyogenes, Bordatella pertussis, Corynebacterium diphtheriae,* meningococci, or gonococci). • Single throat swab 90% positive for streptococcal pharyngitis. • Throat cultures not indicated if no fever or cervical lymphadenopathy (<5% +).

Lower respiratory tract

• Should also culture blood. • More likely to have lower tract flora if <10 epithelial cells and >25 leukocytes per low-power field. • Bronchoscopy with brush biopsy may be used for anaerobic cultures. • Transtracheal aspiration (only in severe infection or unsatisfactory expectorated sputum); 20% may have respiratory pathogen without clinical pneumonia. Risks: hemoptysis, subcutaneous and mediastinal emphysema, vagal discharge; contraindicated with bleeding diathesis. • Percutaneous needle aspiration: high yield, 5% risk of pneumothorax.

Urine

• Periurethral cleaning important in females; first 25 mL discarded. • Should refrigerate if not to lab within 1 h (can be held 4–6 h). • Single specimen of $>10^5$ organisms/mL in male and 2 specimens in female suggest infection but $\geq 10^2$ in symptomatic dysuric women and $\geq 10^3$ in symptomatic men suggestive (may have lower counts if on antibiotics or specimens by catheterization or suprapubic aspiration). • Even slight growth significant with suprapubic collection. • With indwelling catheter, should disinfect catheter and collect directly with sterile needle and syringe. • Gram's stain of unspun urine suggestive of infection if >1 bacterium per 20 oil fields. • Never culture Foley drainage bag or tips.

Blood cultures

• Should culture all febrile patients with rigors, serious illness, possible endocarditis or vascular infection, or immunosuppression. • Optimal: 3 blood cultures of 10–30 mL 1 h apart. • With previous antibiotics, can add penicillinase to rule out endocarditis (6 cultures over 2 days). • Avoid collection from femoral vein, through indwelling intravascular cannula, or arterial blood cultures.

Cerebrospinal fluid

• Collect minimum of 2 mL for glucose (with simultaneous blood sugar), total protein, cell counts, cultures. • With negative Gram's stain, consider CIE or particle agglutination.

Gastrointestinal tract

• Fecal cultures can detect diarrhea caused by *Salmonella, Shigella, Arizona, Vibrio parahemolyticus, Yersinia enterocolitica, Campylobacter jejuni, Clostridium difficile.* • If not cultured in 1 h, preserve in phosphate-buffered glycerol.

Exudates and body fluids

• Optimal collection of pus by syringe and needle aspiration through disinfected skin. • Sinus should be cultured through sterile plastic catheter but curettings or biopsy more definitive.

Skin, soft tissue

• Usually heavily contaminated with normal flora, so should aspirate with syringe or culture punch biopsy. • Culture intravenous catheter tip (last 5 cm) after disinfecting skin to diagnose infected line.

Viral

• Throat swabs must be placed in buffered, high-protein transport medium. • CSF cultures in patients with meningitis or encephalitis. • Stool cultures for enteroviruses or adenoviruses. • Urine cultures for rubella and cytomegalovirus. • Pericardial fluid to diagnose myocarditis or pericarditis. • Buffy coat cultures for herpes and CMV infections. • Brain biopsy culture best to diagnose herpes encephalitis.

For more detailed discussion of this topic, see Plorde JJ: The Diagnosis of Infectious Diseases, Chap. 83, in HPIM-11, p. 459

---

27 INFECTIONS IN THE COMPROMISED HOST

Infections associated with common defects in inflammatory or immunologic response

Host defect	Examples of diseases or therapies associated with defects	Common etiologic agents of infections
Inflammatory response:		
Neutropenia	Hematologic malignancies	Gram-negative bacilli
	Cytotoxic chemotherapy	*Staphylococcus aureus*
	Aplastic anemia	*Candida* species *Aspergillus* species
Chemotaxis	Chédiak-Higashi syndrome	*Staphylococcus aureus* *Streptococcus pyogenes*
	Job's syndrome	*Staphylococcus aureus* *Haemophilus influenzae*
	Protein-calorie malnutrition	Gram-negative bacilli
Phagocytosis (cellular)	Systemic lupus erythematosus	*Streptococcus pneumoniae*
	Chronic myelogenous leukemia	*Haemophilus influenzae*
	Megaloblastic anemia	
Microbicidal defect	Chronic granulomatous disease	Catalase-positive bacteria and fungi: Staphylococci *Escherichia coli* *Klebsiella* species *Pseudomonas aeruginosa* *Candida* species *Aspergillus* species
	Chédiak-Higashi syndrome	*Staphylococcus aureus* *Streptococcus pyogenes*
Complement system:		
C3	Congenital	*Staphylococcus aureus*
	Liver disease	*Streptococcus pneumoniae*
	Systemic lupus erythematosus	*Pseudomonas* species *Proteus* species
C5	Congenital	*Neisseria* species Gram-negative rods
C6, C7, C8	Congenital	*Neisseria meningitidis*
	Systemic lupus erythematosus	*Neisseria gonorrhoeae*
Alternate pathway	Sickle cell disease	*Streptococcus pneumoniae*
	Splenectomy	Salmonella species

(*continued*)

Infections associated with common defects in inflammatory or immunologic response (continued)

Host defect	Examples of diseases or therapies associated with defects	Common etiologic agents of infections
Immune response:		
T-lymphocyte deficiency	Thymic aplasia Thymic hypoplasia Hodgkin's disease Sarcoid Lepromatous leprosy	*Listeria monocytogenes* *Mycobacterium* species *Candida* species *Aspergillus* species *Cryptococcus neoformans* *Herpes simplex* *Herpes zoster*
	AIDS	*Pneumocystis carinii* Cytomegalovirus *Herpes simplex* *Mycobacterium avium intracellulare* *Cryptococcus neoformans* *Candida* species
T lymphocyte	Mucocutaneous candidiasis	*Candida* species
	Purine nucleoside phosphorylase deficiency	Fungi Viruses
B-cell deficiency/dysfunction	Bruton's X-linked agammaglobulinemia	*Streptococcus pneumoniae* Other streptococci
	Agammaglobulinemia	*Haemophilus influenzae*
	Chronic lymphocytic leukemia	*Neisseria meningitidis* *Staphylococcus aureus*
	Multiple myeloma	*Streptococcus pneumoniae* *Staphylococcus aureus* *Klebsiella pneumoniae* *Escherichia coli* *Giardia lamblia*
	Dysglobulinemia	*Pneumocystis carinii* Enteroviruses
	Selective IgM deficiency	*Streptococcus pneumoniae* *Haemophilus influenzae* *Escherichia coli*
	Selective IgA deficiency	*Giardia lamblia* Viral hepatitis *Streptococcus pneumoniae* *Haemophilus influenzae*

(*continued*)

Infections associated with common defects in inflammatory or immunologic response (continued)

Host defect	Examples of diseases or therapies associated with defects	Common etiologic agents of infections
Mixed T- and B-cell deficiency/dysfunction	Common variable hypogammaglobulinemia	*Pneumocystis carinii* Cytomegalovirus *Streptococcus pneumoniae* *Haemophilus influenzae* Various other bacteria
	Ataxia-telangiectasia	*Streptococcus pneumoniae* *Haemophilus influenzae* *Staphylococcus aureus* Rubella *Giardia lamblia*
	Severe combined immunodeficiency	*Candida albicans* *Pneumocystis carinii* Varicella Rubella Cytomegalovirus
	Wiskott-Aldrich	Infections seen in T- and B-cell abnormalities

Reproduced from Masur H, Fauci AS, HPIM-11, p. 468.

For more detailed discussion of this topic, see Masur H, Fauci AS; Infections in the Compromised Host, Chap. 84, in HPIM-11, p. 466

Important pathogens

• Gram-negative bacilli, especially in urinary tract; reservoirs in hospital environment; acquire and transfer antibiotic resistance by plasmids (R factors). • *Staphylococcus aureus:* Some strains in Europe and North America resistant to all β-lactam antibiotics. • Enterococcus: Nosocomial urinary tract infections; wound pathogen in patients who received broad-spectrum cephalosporins. • Opportunistic infections by low-virulence organisms: *S. epidermidis,* JK diphtheroid, fungi (*Aspergillus, Candida*).

Urinary tract infections

• Up to 40% of hospital-acquired infections, especially with indwelling catheters. • To prevent, should use indwelling catheters only for bladder obstruction or close monitoring of fluids; change after 5 to 7 days.

Wound infections

• Usually patient's flora introduced at the time of surgery. • Risk factors: Operations involving contaminated sites (bowel, vagina), lengthy surgery, foreign bodies, hematomas, advanced age, poor nutritional status, diabetes, renal failure, corticosteroid therapy. • Early infections (24–48 h): Usually group A *Streptococcus* or *Clostridium* spp. • Staphylococcal infections: 4–6 days after surgery. • Gram-negative bacilli and anaerobic bacteria: At least 1 week. • Prophylactic antibiotics should be given immediately preoperatively and for only 24 to 48 h after surgery (especially colon surgery and vaginal hysterectomy).

Pneumonia

• Leading cause of mortality from hospital-acquired infections. • Especially gram-negative bacilli and *S. aureus* acquired by aspiration. • Risk factors: Obtundation with ineffective cough and gag reflex, underlying pulmonary disease or congestive heart failure with impaired pulmonary clearance mechanisms, respiratory tract instrumentation. • Prevention: Positioning obtunded patients in a swimmer's position, treatment of congestive heart failure.

Bacteremia

• Vascular cannulas infected by *S. epidermidis, S. aureus,* gram-negative bacilli, enterococci, *Candida* most important. • IV fluids (5% dextrose) may be contaminated by *Enterobacter, Klebsiella, Serratia, Pseudomonas cepacia, Citrobacter freundii.* • Prevention: Stainless steel needles preferable; avoid use of legs; sterile insertion; change every 48 to 72 h.

Other

• Hepatitis B infection risk for hospital personnel who handle blood specimens and patients on dialysis or who receive blood products. Prevent with blood and needle precautions, labeling all blood and tissues from infected patients; hepatitis B immunization for hospital personnel at risk; prompt immunization with hepatitis

B immune globulin after exposure. • AIDS: Blood and secretion precautions to protect other patients and hospital personnel. • Legionnaire's disease: Can be prevented by hyperchlorination or superheating of hospital tap water. • *Clostridium difficile* colitis: Enteric precautions for infected patients.

For more detailed discussion of this topic, see Gardner P, Arnow PM: Hospital-Acquired Infection, Chap. 85, in HPIM-11, p. 470

---

29 SEPTIC SHOCK

Definition

• Inadequate tissue perfusion following bacteremia, usually with gram-negative enteric bacilli, due to release of bacterial toxins (endotoxin). • Most frequently caused by *Escherichia coli, Klebsiella-Enterobacter, Proteus, Pseudomonas, Serratia, Neisseria meningitidis, Bacteroides* spp.; may be associated with gram-positive infections with staphylococci, pneumococci, and streptococci.

Complications

• Coagulation defects: Consumption of clotting factors (DIC), especially with decrease in factors II, V, and VIII, fibrinogen and platelets; fibrinolysis measured as fibrin split products; clinical bleeding rare but may develop capillary thrombi in lungs. • Respiratory failure: Most important cause of death, ARDS. • Renal failure: Oliguria occurs early and may progress to acute tubular necrosis. • Cardiac failure: Due to release of depressant factor.

Clinical manifestations

• Usually abrupt chills, fever, nausea, vomiting, diarrhea, prostration; with shock are also tachycardia, tachypnea, hypotension. • May develop only unexplained hypotension, increasing confusion, disorientation, or hyperventilation.

Laboratory findings

• Usually elevated hematocrit, leukocytosis, and decreased platelet count, but may be normal. • BUN and creatinine are elevated; if urine osmolality < 400 and urine/plasma osmolality < 1.5, more likely to be renal failure than volume depletion. • Electrolytes: $\uparrow Na^+$, $\downarrow Cl^-$, $\downarrow HCO_3^-$, $\uparrow$ lactate. • Early respiratory alkalosis with later metabolic acidosis.

Treatment

• Need to monitor CVP or pulmonary wedge pressure, pulse pressure for stroke volume, cutaneous vasoconstriction, hourly urine output. • Ventilatory support if $P_{O_2} < 70$ mmHg. • Volume: Replace with blood (if anemic), plasma, or colloids; dextrose-saline better than lactate; HCO_3^- to increase blood pH to 7.2 to 7.3; may require 8 to 12 liters over several hours; should continue vigorous fluid replacement even if oliguria develops, by diuresis with furosemide to keep CVP 10–12 cmH_2O, pulmonary artery pressure 16–18 cmH_2O. • Antibiotics: Culture blood and potential sites of infection; if cause unknown, begin treatment with both gentamicin (or tobramycin) and cephalosporin or semisynthetic penicillin. • Surgery: Septic foci (abscesses, infarcted or necrotic bowel, inflamed gallbladder, infected uterus, pyonephrosis) must be removed or drained. • Vasoactive drugs: Dopamine started at 2–5 μg/kg/min and increased until urine flow and blood pressure respond (about 20 μg/kg/min, predominantly alpha-receptor stimulant and may get vasoconstriction of renal and splanchnic circulation); isoproterenol has direct vasodilating effect plus cardiac inotropic effect at 2–8 μg/min. • Diuretics: Once volume is replaced, furosemide given to keep hourly urine greater than 30–40 mL/h. • Glucocorticoids: May be beneficial early; methylprednisolone (30 mg/kg) or dexamethasone (3 mg/kg); then repeated in 4 h.

For more detailed discussion of this topic, see Dale DC, Petersdorf RG: Septic Shock, Chap. 86, in HPIM-11, p. 476

30 ANTIBIOTIC THERAPY

TABLE 30-1 Antimicrobial therapy

Drug	Organism/disease
Penicillins:	
Natural penicillins:	
Penicillin G	Pneumococcal pneumonia
	Gonorrhea
	Syphilis—primary *S. viridans* endocarditis Pneumococcal and meningococcal meningitis
Penicillin VK	Streptococcal pharyngitis
Aminopenicillins:	
Ampicillin	Shigellosis
	Enterococcal endocarditis
Amoxacillin	UTI, bronchitis Otitis media with sensitive organisms
Penicillinase-resistant penicillins:	
Nafcillin	Sensitive *S. aureus* and *S. epidermidis* infections: endocarditis osteomyelitis, abscesses
Dicloxacillin	Superficial *Staph.* infections
Carboxy penicillins:	
Ticarcillin	Serious *Pseudomonas* infections
Indanyl carbenicillin	*Pseudomonas* UTI or prostatitis only
Ureido penicillins:	
Azlocillin	*Pseudomonas* infections
Mezlocillin	*Pseudomonas* infections
Piperacillin	*Pseudomonas* infections
Cephalosporins:	
1st generation:	
Cefazolin	Active against *S. pneumoniae, S. aureus, S. epidermidis,* ~ 80% of *E. coli, P. mirabilis;* prophylactic for surgery

Dosage	Comments
600,000 U procaine IM bid	Dose adjustment needed for $C_{cr} < 30$ mL/min
2.4 million U procaine IM × 2 + 1.0 g probenecid PO	3 million U → 115 μg/mL blood, 300 μg/mL urine, 6 μg/mL CSF
2.4 million U benzathine IM	Other sensitive organisms: *Erysipelothrix, Listeria monocytogenes, Pasteurella multocida, Streptobacillus, Spirillum, Fusospirochetes, Actinomyces israelii*
2 million U IV g 2 h*	
250 mg PO qid × 10 days	60% absorbed; 0.25 g → 2 μg/mL blood, 300 μg/mL urine
500 mg PO qid × 5 days*	0.25 g PO → 1.5 μg/mL blood, urine 50μg/mL
2 g q 6 h + gentamicin, 1 mg/kg q 8 h or streptomycin 1 g IM bid × 6 wks	90% rash with mono; 1 g IV → 35 μg/mL blood, 500 μg/mL urine, 10 μg/mL bile
500 mg PO tid*	2 × oral absorption of ampicillin and should replace except for *Shigella*; 0.5 g → peak blood 10 μg/mL, urine 1000 μg/mL
4–9 g/day	1.0 g IV → 70 μg/mL blood, 2 μg/mL CSF
0.25 g PO qid	0.5 g → 15 μg/mL blood
200–300 mg/kg qd divided q 4–6 h*	3.0 g IV → 190 μg/mL blood, > 2000 μg/mL urine, 50 μg/mL bile; 4.7 meq NA/g can precipitate CHF; high dose can precipitate hypokalemia, prolonged bleeding times
382 mg (1 tablet) PO qid × 7 days	1 g → 15 μg/mL blood, 600 μg/mL urine
3–4.5 g q 6 h†	3.0 g IV → 190 μg/mL blood; > 2000 μg/mL urine, 50 μg/mL bile; less accumulation in renal failure than ticarcillin
3–4.5 g q 6 h†	Same levels as azlocillin, more active against streptococci
3–4.5 g q 6 h†	Most active against *Pseudomonas*
0.5–1 g q 6–8 h†	1.0 g IV → 110 μg/mL blood, > 1000 μg/mL urine, 50 μg/mL bile

(*continued*)

TABLE 30-1 Antimicrobial therapy (continued)

Drug	Organism/disease
Cephalexin/cephradine	Minor staphylococcal infections
Cefaclor	Respiratory infection
2nd generation:	
Cefuroxime	*H. influenzae, S. pneumoniae, N. meningitidis* meningitis in children and young adults
Cefoxitin	Mixed aerobic and anaerobic infections; prophylaxis for abdominal surgery Penicillinase-producing *Neisseria*
3rd generation:	
Cefotaxime	Meningitis due to group B *Streptococcus, E. coli, H. influenzae, N. meningitidis, S. pneumoniae* infections with Enterobacteriaciae
Ceftizoxime	Gram-negative meningitis
Ceftriaxone	Gram-negative meningitis; most gram-positive (except *S. faecalis*) and gram-negative infections (except *Pseudomonas*, anaerobes)
Cefoperazone	Active against most gram-positive, Enterobacteriaceae, and *Pseudomonas* infections
Ceftazidime	Very active against *Pseudomonas* and Enterobacteriaceae
Other β-lactams:	
Imipenem	Active against aerobic gram-positive cocci, including *S. faecalis*; anaerobic species, including *B. fragilis*
Aztreonam	Active against aerobic gram-negative bacteria only
Aminoglycosides:	
Streptomycin	TBC Tularemia, plaque, brucellosis *S. faecalis* endocarditis
Gentamicin	Aerobic gram-negative infections
Tobramycin	More active against *Pseudomonas*
Amikacin	

(*continued*)

Dosage	Comments
0.25–0.5 g tid–qid†	0.25 g → 8 μg/mL blood, 500 μg/mL urine
0.25–0.5 g q 8 h (adults)	—
750 mg q 8 hr to 3 g q 6 h IV†	0.75 g IV → 40 μg/mL blood, > 1000 μg/mL urine, 10–30 μg/mL bile, 1–10 μg/mL CSF
1–2 g q 6–8 hr†	—
2 g IM + probenecid 1 g PO	1.0 g IV → 70 μg/mL blood, 1000 μg/mL urine, 100 μg/mL bile
1 g q 6–8 h to 2 g q 4 h†	1.0 g IV → 80 μg/mL blood, > 1000 μg/mL urine, 15 μg/mL bile, 10 μg/mL CSF
1 g q 6–8 h to 2 g q 4 h†	1.0 g IV → 80 μg/mL blood, > 1000 μg/mL urine, 30 μg/mL bile, 1–10 μg/mL CSF
1 g qd to 2 g bid†	1 g → 150 μg/mL blood, > 1000 μg/mL urine, 200 μg/mL bile, 1–30 μg/mL CSF; may be given as once-daily IM injection
1–2 g IV q 12 h†	2.0 g IV → 250 μg/mL blood; disulfiram reactions
1–2 g q 8–12 h†	1 g IV → 80 μg/mL blood, >1000 μg/mL urine, 5–10 μg/mL bile
0.5–1 g q 6 h†	0.5 g IV → 30 μg/mL blood, 100 μg/mL urine, 10 μg/mL bile Administered with dehydropeptidase inhibitor, cilastatin to prevent hydrolysis
0.5–2 g q 6–12 h†	1 g IV → 160 μg/mL blood, >1000 μg/mL urine, 5–10 μg/mL bile
1 g IM twice weekly	—
1 g IM qd	—
2 mg/kg loading; then 1.5–2 mg/kg q 8 h†	1.5 g mg/kg → 6 μg/mL blood, 50 μg/mL urine, 2 μg/mL bile Should measure serum levels: 5–10 μg/mL peak, 1–2 μg/mL trough All aminoglycosides may cause nephrotoxicity and ototoxicity
2 mg/kg loading; then 1.5–2 mg/kg q 8 h†	Same levels
8 mg/kg loading; then 5 mg/kg q 8 h†	Less drug resistance but use should be restricted

TABLE 30-1 Antimicrobial therapy (continued)

Drug	Organism/disease
Tetracyclines:	
Tetracycline	*Rickettsia, Chlamydia, Mycoplasma, Brucella*
Doxycycline	*Rickettsia, Chlamydia, Mycoplasma, Brucella*
Other:	
Vancomycin	Active against all gram-positive methicillin-resistant staphylococcal infections *S. faecalis* endocarditis in penicillin-allergic; infections in hemodialysis Pseudomembranous colitis
Chloramphenicol	Anaerobic bacteria, Rocky mountain spotted fever, meningitis with *H. influenzae, S. pneumoniae, H. meningitidis*
Erythromycin	Streptococcal infections in penicillin-allergic, *Mycoplasma* Legionella
Clindamycin	Most *Strep, Staph,* and anaerobic infections
Rifampin	Staphylococci with second drug TBC Meningococcal prophylaxis
Metronidazole	Anaerobic infections Pseudomembranous colitis *Trichomonas vaginitis* Amebic liver abscess, colitis
Sulfadiazine	Toxoplasmosis
Trimethoprim-sulfamethoxazole	UTI, bronchitis, *Shigella* *Pneumocystis carinii*

*Minor adjustments necessary in renal failure.

†Major adjustments necessary in renal failure.

‡Adjustment for creatinine clearance: $C_{cr} = \frac{(140 - \text{age}) \times \text{wt (kg)}}{\text{Cr (mg/dL)} \times 72}$.

For $C_{cr} < 100$ mL/min, dose given q 8 h multiplied by $C_{cr} \times 0.0.1$

Dosage	Comments
250–500 mg PO qid†	0.25 g PO → 2.2 μg/mL blood, 100 μg/mL urine, 15 μg/mL bile; absorption ↓ by milk, antacids
100 mg PO bid	Avoid in pregnant women, children; 100 mg → 2.5 μg/mL blood, 100 μg/mL urine, 15 μg/mL bile
0.5–1.0 g q 8–12 h†	0.5 g IV → 30 μg/mL blood, 100 μg/mL urine, 3 μg/mL bile
0.5 g q 8 h + aminoglycoside	—
125 mg PO qid × 10 days	—
0.25–0.75 g IV or PO q 6 h	1 g IV → 15 μg/mL blood, 100 μg/mL urine, 3 μg/mL bile, 10 μg/mL CSF; levels after oral dose equivalent to IV; 1 in 25,000 develop aplastic anemia; ↑ half-life of tolbutamide, phenytoin, warfarin
250–500 mg PO qid	0.25 g PO → 1.4 μg/mL blood
500 mg–1 g IV q 6 h	1 g IV → 10 μg/mL blood; ↑ blood levels of theophylline
150–450 mg PO g 6 h; 150–900 mg IV q 6 h	Adjust dose for hepatic failure; 600 mg IV → 15 μg/mL blood
600 mg PO qd (10 mg/kg)	8 mg/kg → 10 μg/mL blood, 50 μg/mL urine, 100 μg/mL bile, 0.5 μg/mL CSF; red discoloration of urine and tears; ↓ effect of steroids and birth control pills
600 mg PO qd (10 mg/kg)	
600 mg qd × 2	
500 mg IV q 6–8 h	Disulfiram reaction with alcohol
250–500 mg PO qid × 14 days	—
2.0 gm PO	Potentiation of warfarin
750 mg PO tid × 5–10 days	Should not be used in pregnancy
75–100 mg/kg qd in 4 doses	All sulfas can cause rash, fever, jaundice, hemolysis in G6PD-deficient, agranulocytosis, leukopenia
1 double-strength (DS) bid	Displace warfarin, methotrexate and chlorpropamide from albumin
20 mg trimethoprim + 100 mg sulfamethoxazole/kg/day (4 amps = 2 DS q 6 h)	

TABLE 30-2 Antiviral therapy

Infection	Antiviral drug	Administration
Influenza A (prophylaxis)	Amantadine	Oral
	or	
	rimantadine	Oral
Influenza A (therapy)	Amantadine	Oral
	or	
	rimantadine	Oral
Respiratory syncytial virus	Ribavirin	Aerosol
Herpes simplex encephalitis	Acyclovir	IV
	or	
	vidarabine	IV
Neonatal herpes simplex	Vidarabine	IV
	or	
	acyclovir	IV
Genital herpes simplex: primary infection	Acyclovir	IV
		Oral
		Topical
Genital herpes simplex: recurrent infections (therapy)	Acyclovir	Oral

Modified from Dolin R, HPIM-11, p. 670.

Dosage	Comment
Adults: 200 mg per day for period at risk Children ≤ 9 yrs: 4.4–8.8 mg/kg per day not to exceed 150 mg per day	Needs to be administered for the duration of the outbreak. Dosage should be reduced in renal failure and in the elderly. Can be administered along with vaccine.
As above	Not yet licensed by FDA. May be better tolerated than amantadine.
As above for 5–7 days	Both amantadine and rimantadine are effective in uncomplicated influenza. Neither drug has been demonstrated to be effective in complicated influenza (e.g., pneumonia).
As above for 5–7 days	Under study for treatment of complicated influenza in placebo-controlled trials.
Administered continuously by small-particle aerosol from a reservoir containing 20 mg/mL for 3–6 days	Utilized for treatment of infants and young children hospitalized with RSV pneumonia and bronchiolitis.
10 mg/kg every 8 h for 10 days	Acyclovir is the drug of choice for this infection on the basis of comparative trials vs. vidarabine. Optimal results are obtained when therapy is initiated early in illness.
15 mg/kg per day as a continuous infusion for 12 h for 10 days	
30 mg/kg per day given as a continuous infusion over 12 h per day for 10 days	Vidarabine reduces mortality, but severe morbidity is frequent. Currently being compared with acyclovir in a clinical trial.
10 mg/kg every 8 h for 10 days.	
5 mg/kg every 8 h for 5–10 days	IV route is preferred if infection is of sufficient severity to warrant hospitalization, or if neurologic complications are present.
200 mg 5 times per day for 10 days	Preferred route of administration for patients who do not warrant hospitalization. Adequate hydration should be maintained.
5% ointment; 4–6 applications per day for 7–10 days	Largely supplanted by oral therapy. May be of use in pregnant women in order to avoid systemic therapy. Systemic symptoms and untreated areas are not affected.
200 mg 5 times per day for 5 days	Clinical effect is modest and is enhanced if therapy is initiated early. No effect on subsequent recurrence rates.

For more detailed discussion of these topics, see Neu HC: Chemotherapy for Infections, Chap. 88, in HPIM-11, p. 485, and Dolin R: Principles of Antiviral Chemotherapy, Chap. 129, in HPIM-11, p. 668

31 PREVENTION OF INFECTION BY IMMUNIZATION

IMMUNIZATION

PRINCIPLES

- Inactivated vaccines can be given simultaneously at separate sites.
- Multiple doses of live vaccine should be separated by at least 1 month; live vaccine should be delayed 3 months after passive immunization.

TABLE 31-1 **Active immunization in adults**

	Type of vaccine
All adults:	
Tetanus and diphtheria	Adsorbed toxoid
Poliomyelitis	Live attenuated
	Formalin-inactivated
Measles, mumps, rubella	Live attenuated
Women of childbearing age:	
Rubella vaccine	Live attenuated
Postpubertal males:	
Mumps	Live attenuated
Persons at high risk of acquiring disease or developing complications of disease:	
Influenza vaccine	Inactivated
Pneumococcal polysaccharide vaccine	Purified tetradecavalent polysaccharide vaccine
Hepatitis B vaccine	Inactivated subunit vaccine

(*continued*)

- Live vaccines are contraindicated in immunosuppressed, febrile, or pregnant patients.

ACTIVE IMMUNIZATION See Table 31-1.

PASSIVE IMMUNIZATION See Table 31-2.

For more detailed discussion of this topic, see Corey L, Petersdorf RG: Prevention of Infection: Immunization and Antimicrobial Prophylaxis, Chap. 92, in HPIM-11, p. 524

Administration and frequency*	Comments
IM at least every 10 years	Usually administered together as Td vaccine
Oral polio vaccine (OPV)	Preferred for routine use and during epidemics
Inactivated polio vaccine (IPV)	Selective use in unimmunized adults
SC once	All adults born after 1957 should have measles—see text for specific recommendations re: mumps and rubella vaccine
SC once	Only to women who are antibody (HI) negative and if pregnancy can be prevented for 3 months post-vaccination
SC once	Prevention of orchitis in susceptible seronegative males
SC yearly	Directed at reducing morbidity and mortality in those at risk of complications of influenza, e.g., chronic heart and lung disease and those over 65 years
SC once	Same population as influenza vaccine, functional or surgical asplenia, agammaglobulinemia, cirrhosis, multiple myeloma, and nephrotic syndrome
3 doses IM at 0, 1, and 3 months	High-risk groups for acquisition of hepatitis B, including household contacts of hepatitis B patients, patients requiring a large volume of clotting factors, illicit drug users, homosexual men, and selected medical and dental personnel

TABLE 31-1 Active immunization in adults (continued)

	Type of vaccine
Populations exposed to localized outbreaks:	
Meningococcal vaccine	Purified capsular polysaccharide
Haemophilus influenzae type B	Purified capsular polysaccharide
Measles vaccine	Live attenuated
BCG vaccine	Live attenuated
Adenovirus vaccine	Live attenuated bivalent (types 4 and 7)
Typhoid vaccine	Inactivated bacilli
Rubella vaccine	Live attenuated
Travelers to foreign countries:	
Smallpox	Live vaccinia virus
Yellow fever	Live attenuated
Cholera	Phenol-inactivated suspension of *Vibrio cholerae*
Typhoid	Inactivated bacilli
Plague	Formaldehyde-inactivated *Yersinia pestis*
Poliomyelitis	Oral or inactivated polio vaccine

Modified from Corey L, Petersdorf RG, HPIM-11, pp. 526–527.

Administration and frequency*	Comments
SC once	Control of localized epidemics and adjunct to chemoprophylaxis in household contacts
SC once	Routine use in children 18–24 months of age; younger adults at high risk of getting the disease
SC once	Control of outbreaks usually among adolescents or young adults
SC or intradermally, once	Used in groups with excessive risk of new infection with tuberculosis or individuals persistently exposed to sputum-positive tuberculosis
PO once	Used only for military recruits
SC in two doses	Household contact of documented *Salmonella typhi* carrier
SC once	Control of outbreaks among adolescents and young adults (must screen pubertal females with HI test prior to vaccination)
Intradermally, every 3–5 years	No indications for smallpox vaccine in civilians
SC once per 10 years	Administered at yellow fever vaccination centers
SC approximately every 6 months	Only 50% effective and not effective in decreasing transmission of disease
SC in half doses 4 weeks apart	70–90% efficacy in "normal" exposure
Primary series = three IM doses. First dose 1 mL; second dose 4 weeks later, 0.2 mL; third dose 5 months later, 0.2 mL	Agricultural workers who reside in plague-endemic areas
See text	Immunized adults should receive a complete primary series or at least 2 doses of IPV 1 month apart; if not, then a single dose of OPV is recommended; for high-risk travel, a single dose of OPV or IPV is recommended

TABLE 31-2 Passive immunization

Disease	Preparation
Hepatitis A	ISG, human
Hepatitis B	Human hepatitis B immunoglobulin ISG, human
Vaccinia immunoglobulin	Human VIG
Herpes zoster	Human varicella-ZIG
Diphtheria	Diphtheria antitoxin, horse
Tetanus	Human tetanus immunoglobulin (TIG)
Rabies	Human rabies immunoglobulin Equine antirabies globulin
Pertussis	Pertussis immunoglobulin, human
Measles	ISG, human
Rubella	ISG, human
Botulism	Horse serum, trivalent AB
Snake bite	Polyvalent crotaline antivenom (pit vipers)
Spider bite	Equine

Reproduced from Corey L, Petersdorf RG, HPIM-11, p. 531.

Route and dose	Comments
IM (0.02–0.06 ml/kg)	Household contacts
IV (100 mg/kg)	
IM (0.06 mL/kg: two doses 4 weeks apart) IM (0.05 mL/kg: two doses 4 weeks apart)	HBIG is preferred prophylaxis for direct parenteral exposure (needle stick) or mucous-membrane contact in susceptibles; if unavailable, ISG should be given. HBIG should be administered to neonates born to mothers with hepatitis B.
IM (0.3 mL/kg)	Use in eczema vaccinatum, disseminated vaccinia, vaccinia in pregnancy
IM (125 U per 10 kg, up to 625 U)	Prevention and amelioration of varicella in susceptible immunosuppressed patients
IM or IV (10,000–100,000 U)	Dose dependent on extent of membrane and degree of toxicity; may also be used in unimmunized household contacts
IM (250 U)	When given with tetanus toxoid, use separate syringes and sites
One-half locally and one-half IM (20 IU/kg)	Used for postexposure prophylaxis with both tissue culture and duck embryo rabies vaccine
One-half locally and one-half IM (40 IU/kg)	Same as above
IM (1.5 mL, repeat in 5–7 days)	No studies suggest efficacy in susceptible infants
IM (0.2 mL/kg or 20–30 mL)	Susceptible household contacts less than 1 year old, exposed susceptible pregnant females, or immunodeficient persons
IM (20–30 mL)	Exposed susceptible pregnant females who will not consider termination
One-half IM and one-half IV (8–32 mL)	Use only therapeutically; greatest efficacy in type E
IV (dose function of severity of bite)	—
IM (2.5 mL)	*Latrodectus* (black widow spider) poisoning

SEXUALLY TRANSMITTED DISEASES

APPROACH

Male urethritis

- Diagnose by ≥5 WBC per oil field of discharge.
- PMNs with intracellular gram-negative diplococci → *N. gonorrhoeae* (confirm by culture); treat with amoxicillin 3.0 g + 1.0 g probenecid PO + 0.5 g tetracycline qid × 7 days; always treat sexual partners.
- PMNs only—culture or antigen detection for *Chlamydia*; treat with tetracycline 0.5 g PO qid or doxycycline 100 mg bid × 7 days.

Epididymitis

- Rule out testicular torsion (Doppler exam or ^{99m}Tc scan), tumor, trauma.
- Pts up to 35 years of age—usually *C. trachomatis*; treat with doxycycline 100 mg bid × 10 days.
- *N. gonorrhoeae*; treat with ceftriaxone 250 mg IM.
- Older men or following urinary tract instrumentation—*E. coli* or *Pseudomonas*—mild: treat with Septra DS 1 bid; severe: tobramycin or gentamicin 1.5 mg/kg then 1.0 mg/kg q 8 h IV.

Lower GU tract infection in women

- Cystitis: ≥20 WBC/400× field spun midstream urine; $\geq 10^2$ bacteria/mL on culture.
- Urethritis: pyuria and symptoms with negative urine cultures, probably chlamydial.
- Vaginitis: *T. vaginalis*—profuse, yellow, purulent discharge, motile trophozoites on wet mount; treat with 2.0 g metronidazole PO; bacterial vaginosis—vaginal malodor with ↑ white or gray discharge, "clue cells" on wet-mount; treat with metronidazole 500 mg bid × 7 days; candidiasis—marked vulvar itching with thick white discharge, fungal elements on 10% KOH; treat with intravaginal miconazole or clotrimazole 100 mg qd × 7 days.

Mucopurulent cervicitis

- Yellowish discharge from cervical os with ≥ 10 PMN/oil field.
- ~50% chlamydial, but also treat for gonococcal cervicitis (GC) (see male urethritis)

Ulcerative genital lesions

- Exclude syphilis by dark-field exam and VDRL.
- Painful vesicles or pustules: culture for herpes.
- Painful, nonvesicular ulcer: culture for herpes or chancroid.
- Painless ulcerative lesions: test for syphilis.
- Treatment: If herpes and syphilis ruled out and lesions persist, consider ceftriaxone 250 mg IM or erythromycin 500 mg qid or Septra DS 1 bid × 7 days.

Proctitis, proctocolitis, enteritis

- Proctitis: tenesmus, constipation, anorectal pain, mucopurulent or bloody rectal discharge; HSV and LGV (*C. trachomatis*); culture for *N. gonorrhoeae*.
- Proctocolitis and enterocolitis: in homosexual men, especially *Campylobacter* and *Shigella*.
- Enteritis: diarrhea, abdominal bloating, cramps without anorectal symptoms; in homosexuals, *Giardia lamblia, Campylobacter, Shigella, E. histolytica*.

Acute arthritis

- Gonococcal arthritis-dermatitis syndrome; most common in sexually active; culture from synovial fluid, blood, skin lesions, or CSF; diagnosis: (1) culture + from mucosal site or from sex partner, (2) typical pustular or hemorrhagic skin lesions on extremities, and (3) prompt response to antibiotics; treat with penicillin G 10 million U qd until improved, then ampicillin 500 mg qid for 7–10 days total; penicillinase-producing or penicillin-allergic: cefoxitin or cefotaxime 4–6 g IV qd or ceftriaxone 1–2 g IV qd × 7–10 days.
- Reiter's syndrome: 80% HLA-B27 +; *C. trachomatis* most often associated with sporadic form; others: *Shigella, Campylobacter, Salmonella, Yersinia, N. gonorrhoeae*; diagnose by acute, noninfectious arthritis persisting at least 1 month; ↑ sacroiliitis; acute conjunctivitis or uveitis, painless ulcers of oral mucosa, circinate balanitis, keratoderma blenorrhagicum.

PELVIC INFLAMMATORY DISEASE

Clinical manifestations

- Tuberculous salpingitis: abnormal vaginal bleeding, pain, infertility; 50% postmenopausal; diagnose by endometrial biopsy → granulomas and/or positive culture.
- Nontuberculous salpingitis: evolves from cervicitis → endometritis → salpingitis (bilateral lower abdominal and pelvic pain); IUD-associated; cervical motion tenderness, uterine fundal and adnexal tenderness; gonococcal or chlamydial PID onset at time of menses, younger age, and presence of mucopurulent cervicitis.
- Perihepatitis and periappendicitis.

Diagnosis

- Associations: onset with menses, recent abnormal menstrual bleeding, IUD, previous salpingitis, exposure to male with urethritis.
- Laparoscopy most specific.
- Endometrial biopsy with plasma cell endometritis sensitive.
- Culture endocervical swabs, endocervical aspiration, culdocentesis, specimens at laparoscopy for *Chlamydia* and GC.

Treatment

- Exclude surgical emergencies (appendicitis, ectopic pregnancy); rule out pelvic abscess.

- Treatment regimens: doxycycline 100 mg q 12 h + cefoxitin 2 g q 6 h IV for 48 h after defervesence, then doxycycline 100 mg PO bid for 14 days total; clindamycin 600 mg q 6 h + gentamicin 2.0 mg/kg, then 1.5 mg/kg q 8 h for at least 4 days, then clindamycin 450 mg PO qid for 14 days total.
- Outpatients: cefoxitin 2 g IM + doxycycline 100 mg bid × 14 days with reevaluation in 48–72 h.
- Examine all sexual partners; remove IUD.

GONOCOCCAL INFECTIONS

Clinical manifestations

- Males: incubation 2 to 7 days; complications uncommon with therapy (epididymitis, inguinal lymphadenitis, fistulas); rectal GC in homosexuals with pain, pruritus, tenesmus, bloody, mucopurulent rectal discharge; pharyngeal infection frequently asymptomatic.
- Females: acute uncomplicated → dysuria, frequency, increased vaginal discharge, infection extends from endocervix to fallopian tubes in 15%; acute inflammation of Bartholin's glands usually unilateral.
- Children: during childbirth; conjunctiva, pharynx, respiratory tract, or anal canal may be infected; 1% silver nitrate drops prophylaxis for ophthalmia.
- Disseminated gonococcal infection (DGI): two-thirds of women at time of menses; present with gonococcemia (fever, polyarthralgias, papular, petechial, or necrotic skin lesions, tenosynovitis of several asymmetrical joints) or septic arthritis (purulent arthritis in usually one joint).

Diagnosis: Gram's stain of urethral or endocervical exudate diagnostic with gram-negative diplococci within PMNs, but need to confirm with culture on Thayer-Martin medium with ↑ CO_2.

Treatment

- Should check VDRL and follow-up cultures for GC 3–7 days after therapy in all patients.
- Uncomplicated infection in adult: amoxicillin 3.0 g or ampicillin 3.5 g PO + probenicid 1.0 g PO or ceftriaxone 250 mg IM, then tetracycline 0.5 g PO qid × 7 days.
- Treatment failures, penicillinase-producing (PPNG): spectinomycin 2.0 g (not pharyngeal infection) or ceftriaxone 250 mg IM.
- Disseminated gonococcal infection: penicillin G 10 million U qd IV at least 3 days, then ampicillin 0.5 g qid or amoxicillin 0.5 g tid for 7 days total.

SYPHILIS

Clinical manifestations

- Primary syphilis: single painless papule → eroded and indurated; usually on penis, cervix, or labia, but rectum or mouth also;

painless inguinal lymphadenopathy within 1 week; chancre heals in 4–6 weeks.

- Secondary: skin—bilateral, symmetrical pink, nonpruritic macules on trunk and extremities; intertriginous area—broad, moist, pink or gray lesions (condylomata lata, very infectious); mucous patches—painless silver-gray erosion with red periphery in mouth or on genitals; constitutional symptoms ±.
- Latent syphilis: positive VDRL, normal CSF and physical exam; early <1 year, late latent >1 year.
- Symptomatic neurosyphilis: meningovascular—stroke syndrome or headache, vertigo, insomnia, psychological abnormalities; general paresis—20 years incubation, ↓ memory, ↑ reflexes, Argyll-Robertson pupils; tabes dorsalis (25–30 years)—demyelinization of posterior columns with ataxic wide-based gait, bladder disturbances, areflexia, trophic joint degeneration, optic atrophy.
- Cardiovascular syphilis: aortitis, aortic regurgitation, saccular aneurysm of ascending and transverse aortic arch.
- Gummas.
- Congenital syphilis.

Diagnosis

- Dark-field exam of all cutaneous lesions and saline aspirates of lymph nodes of secondary disease; repeat on three successive days before considering negative.
- Nontreponemal serology: VDRL, RPR (rapid plasma reagin); used for initial screening and titers; fall in titer correlates with response to therapy; approximately one-third negative in primary or late (false positives in acute infections).
- Treponemal tests to confirm diagnosis of syphilis in patient with positive VDRL or RPR.
- Asymptomatic neurosyphilis: CSF exam necessary in any seropositive patient with neurologic signs or untreated syphilis or > 1 year's duration; CSF VDRL very specific.

Treatment

- Early syphilis: primary, secondary, or early latent—Benzathine penicillin 1.2 million U × 2, tetracycline 2 g qd × 15 if allergic; penicillin treatment for GC adequate.
- Latent, late and unknown (late latent with normal CSF, cardiovascular, gummas)—2.4 million U benzathine penicillin every week × 3.
- Neurosyphilis (asymptomtic or symptomatic): procaine penicillin 2.4 million U IM qd × probenecid 500 mg PO qid × 10 days, then benzathine penicillin 2.4 million U weekly × 3; allergic: tetracycline 2 g PO qd × 30.
- Pregnant: treat with penicillin according to stage.
- Jarisch-Herxheimer reaction: fevers, chills, myalgias, headache, mild hypotension 2–8 h after treatment; treat with aspirin and bed rest.

- Follow-up: follow quantitative VDRL at 1, 3, 6, 12 months; should re-treat if does not ↓ 4-fold in 1 year; repeat LP in neurosyphilis q 3–6 mos. × 3 years.

CHLAMYDIAL INFECTIONS (See Chap. 53.)

Lymphogranuloma venereum (LGV)

- Clinical: primary lesion (painless vesicle or papule) → painful inguinal adenopathy and/or draining fistulas with fever, chills, meningesmus; proctitis in homosexual men (mucopurulent rectal discharge with tenesmus).
- Diagnosis: culture from aspirated bubo, rectum, urethra, cervix; complement fixation (CF) titer ≥ 1:64 suggestive.
- Treatment: tetracycline 0.5 g qid × 3 weeks; aspirate fluctuant buboes to prevent rupture.

For more detailed discussion of these topics, see Holmes KK, Handsfield HH: Sexually Transmitted Diseases, Chap. 90, p. 506; Holmes KK: Pelvic Inflammatory Disease, Chap. 91, p. 519; Holmes KK: Gonococcal Infections, Chap. 104, p. 576; Ronald AR, Plummer FA: Chancroid, Chap. 110, p. 608; Holmes KK: Donovanosis (Granuloma Inguinale), Chap. 111, p. 609; Holmes KK, Lukehart SA: Syphilis, Chap. 122, p. 639; and Stamm WE, Holmes KK: Chlamydial Infections, Chap. 150, p. 759, in HPIM-11

---

33 INFECTIOUS DIARRHEAS

NONINVASIVE BACTERIAL PATHOGENS

Enterotoxigenic *E. coli*

- Epidemiology: causes majority of traveler's diarrhea in S. America, Africa, and Asia.
- Clinical: 24–72 h incubation; mild, watery diarrhea to severe cholera-like; occasional low fever; vomiting in <50%.
- Treatment: fluid replacement; antibiotics may decrease duration of illness (tetracycline 7.5 mg/kg qid × 2 days, trimethoprim/sulfamethoxazole 160/800 (DS) mg bid × 5 days); symptomatic relief with bismuth subsalicylate 60 mL qh × 4; prophylaxis: doxycycline 100 mg qd or Septra 1 DS qd.

Clostridium perfringens

• Epidemiology: incubation 6–12 h after ingestion of contaminated meat, poultry, or legumes; rarely lasts >24 h. • Treatment: fluid replacement; no antibiotics.

Staphylococcus aureus

• Ingestion of preformed enterotoxin. • Epidemiology: institutional outbreaks; short incubation (2–4 h); short duration (<10 h); high attack rates (>75%). • Clinical: prominent vomiting. • Treatment: fluid replacement.

Bacillus cereus Diarrheal syndrome like staphylococcal; treatment: fluids.

INVASIVE PATHOGENS

Campylobacter jejuni

• Epidemiology: second to *Giardia* for waterborne outbreaks in U.S.; raw milk, contaminated water. • Clinical: incubation 2–6 days with fever, cramping abdominal pain, diarrhea; lasts 2–5 days (up to 3–4 weeks); associated with acute reactive arthritis. • Diagnosis: culture from stool at 42°C on special media. • Treatment: erythromycin 30 mg/kg qd may shorten course. • *C. fetus* especially associated with bacteremia in patients with chronic renal, hepatic, neoplastic, or alcoholic disease; requires 4 weeks of gentamicin because of infection of intravascular sites.

Vibrio parahemolyticus

• Epidemiology: present in coastal waters worldwide, but especially in Japan with ingestion of raw seafood. • Clinical: incubation 6–48 h; moderately severe abdominal cramps; chills and fever in about half; lasts ~24 h. • Diagnosis: stool with many PMNs; culture. • Treatment: fluids.

Vibrio mimicus: Acute diarrheal illness, especially following raw oyster ingestion along Gulf Coast.

Invasive *E. coli:* Rare in U.S., E. Europe, S.E. Asia; symptoms similar to *Shigella* (see below) except less vomiting and shorter duration; treatment: symptomatic.

Cytotoxic *E. coli:* Epidemiology: strain 0157:H7, undercooked meat, especially hamburger.

Salmonella typhi (typhoid fever)

- Epidemiology: ingestion of contaminated food, water, or milk; humans only reservoir; ↑ risk of infection with malnutrition, prior antibiotic therapy.
- Clinical: average incubation 10 days (3–60); insidious onset with headache, malaise, anorexia, fever for 2–3 weeks; rose spots (2–4 mm erythematous macules upper abdomen); ↑ liver and spleen by second week; fever abates after third week.
- Complications: intestinal hemorrhage or perforation, localized infection (meningitis, chondritis, periostitis, osteomyelitis, arthritis, pyelonephritis), relapse, chronic carriage.
- Diagnosis: leukopenia; 90% positive BC (first week); 75% positive stool culture (third week); 3% stools positive >1 year; serology less specific.
- Treatment: if sensitive, chloramphenicol 50 mg/kg qd orally (divided q 6–8 h) →30 mg/kg qd when afebrile for 2 weeks or ampicillin 1 g q 6 h IV or Septra 1 DS bid × 2 weeks; life-threatening toxemia—prednisone 60 mg or dexamethasone 3 mg/kg tapered over 24 to 48 h; chronic carriers: normal gallbladder—ampicillin 6 g PO qd + probenecid 1g PO qd × 6 weeks; cholecystectomy if abnormal gallbladder plus ampicillin 2–3 weeks.

Other salmonella

- Epidemiology: acquired by ingestion of contaminated drink or food (especially egg or egg products); ↑ risk with antacids, antimotility drugs, antibiotics, immunosuppression, AIDS, sickle cell.
- Gastroenteritis.
- Enteric or paratyphoid fever: clinically indistinguishable from typhoid fever.
- Bacteremia: usually prolonged; BC intermittently +; 1/4 local infection; associated with *Schistosoma* infections
- Local pyogenic infections: with or without previous gastroenteritis or bacteremia; localization at site of preexisting disease—aneurysms, bone adjacent to aortic aneurysms, hematomas, tumors.
- Diagnosis: stool or BC.
- Treatment: antibiotics not indicated for gastroenteritis (may prolong excretion) unless documented bacteremia, prolonged fever, >50 years old with aneurysms or vascular prostheses; treat with chloramphenicol 3 g qd for at least 2 weeks; other: ampicillin (if sensitive), Septra.

Shigellosis

- Epidemiology: *S. sonnei* most common in U.S.; *S. dysenteriae* in developing countries; increased in children <10 years old, in day-care centers, in homosexuals.

- Clinical: symptoms 1–7 days after exposure; mild watery diarrhea to severe dysentery; severity increased in infants, elderly, *S. dysenteriae* type 1; without treatment, fever resolves in 3–4 days, diarrhea up to 1–2 weeks.
- Diagnosis: WBC normal to increased; stool cultures.
- Treatment: fluid replacement; antibiotics decrease fever, carriage; Septra 1 DS bid × 5–6 days; ampicillin 50 mg/kg qd if sensitive; antimotility drugs contraindicated.

Cholera

- Epidemiology: Ganges delta, S.E. Asia, coastal Texas and Louisiana; epidemics waterborne.
- Clinical: incubation 12–48 h, then abrupt onset of watery, painless diarrhea, severe vomiting → severe dehydration.
- Diagnosis: direct plating of stool on TCBS (thiosulfate-citrate-bile salt-sucrose) agar.
- Treatment: fluid replacement IV or oral (20 g glucose + 2.5 g $NaHCO_3$ + 3.5 g NaCl + 1.5 g KCl per liter H_2O); tetracycline 500 mg q 6 h × 2 days.

VIRAL GASTROENTERITIS

Rotavirus: Most important cause of severe dehydrating diarrhea in children under 3 years of age worldwide; up to 25% of traveler's diarrhea.

Norwalk and related viruses: Occurs year-round; a third of epidemics of nonbacterial diarrhea in developed countries; cause of food- and waterborne epidemics.

ACUTE PROTOZOAL DIARRHEAS

(see Chap. 54)

For more detailed discussion of these topics, see Carpenter CCJ: Acute Infectious Diarrheal Diseases and Bacterial Food Poisonings, Chap. 89, p. 502; Guerrant RL: *Salmonella* Infections, Chap. 107, p. 592; Pearson RD, Guerrant RL: Shigellosis, Chap. 108, p. 599; Carpenter CCJ: Cholera, Chap. 115, p. 618; and Greenberg HB: Viral Gastroenteritis, Chap. 140, p. 707, in HPIM-11

---

34 PNEUMOCOCCAL INFECTIONS

PNEUMOCOCCAL PNEUMONIA

Manifestations

• Distribution usually segmental or lobar in adults, but may be patchy bronchopneumonia. • Often preceded by coryza, followed by abrupt shaking chill, fever with subsequent severe pleuritic pain, and cough. • If untreated, high fever and cough continue for 7–10 days with defervescence; abdominal distention and herpes labialis frequent complications. • Physical exam: Tactile fremitus may be ↑ early but ↓ with consolidation, tubular breath sounds, fine crepitant rales. • Defervescence usually within 12–36 h of instituting therapy, but may take up to 4 days.

Complications

• Atelectasis can occur before or during treatment with sudden recurrence of pleuritic pain; usually clears with coughing and deep breathing, but bronchoscopy may be required. • Delayed resolution: PE usually normal within 2–4 weeks, with x-ray resolution as long as 8–18 weeks. • Lung abscess rare; may be associated with type 3. • Pleural effusion ~50%; usually sterile and absorbed spontaneously. • Empyema: <1% of treated cases; may have few cells early but progress to thick greenish pus; can cause extensive pleural scarring if not drained; may be complicated by brain abscess. • Pericarditis: Precordial pain and friction rub may be present, but consider in any seriously ill patient. • Arthritis, especially in children. • Paralytic ileus may occur in severely ill patients. • Impaired liver function: Abnormal LFTs and mild jaundice common.

Laboratory findings

• Gram's stain of sputum shows PMNs and lancet-shaped gram-positive organisms singly and in pairs. • Blood culture positive in 20–30%. • WBC usually 12–25,000 cells/mm^3; if normal or ↓, may have overwhelming infection with bacteremia. • Organisms may be seen in Wright's stained buffy coat; think of asplenia, multiple myeloma. • CXR: Usually homogeneous density, but may be >1 lobe or atypical with underlying pulmonary disease.

EXTRAPULMONARY PNEUMOCOCCAL INFECTION

Pneumococcal meningitis

• Second to meningococcus in adults and *Haemophilus influenzae* in children as cause of bacterial meningitis. • May be only site of infection or associated with otitis, mastoiditis, sinusitis, skull fracture with CSF leak, multiple myeloma, sickle cell disease. • CSF cloudy, ↑ protein, ↓ glucose, Gram's stain usually positive for bacteria. • CIE or latex agglutination positive in 80% of culture-positive patients. • 70% recover.

Pneumococcal endocarditis

• Usually complication of pneumonia or meningitis. • Clinical: Remittent fever, splenomegaly, metastatic infections. • Can infect normal valves, especially aortic with rapid development of heart failure, loud murmurs. • BC always positive without previous therapy.

Pneumococcal peritonitis

• Secondary to transient bacteremia; ↑ in young girls. • Associated with nephrotic syndrome, cirrhosis, liver cancer. • Ascitic fluid and BC positive.

TREATMENT

Pneumonia

• Sensitivity testing important only with new resistant strains. • 600,000 U penicillin G q 12 h until afebrile for 48–72 h. • Cephalosporins 1–2 g qd effective; use with caution if patient is allergic to penicillin. • With sensitive strains and uncomplicated disease, tetracycline 1–2 g qd, erythromycin 2.0 g qd, clindamycin 1.2 g qd.

Peritonitis: 2–4 million U penicillin qd.
Pneumococcal meningitis: 18–24 million U penicillin G IV qd; vancomycin (2 g qd) for resistant strains.
Pneumococcal endocarditis: 8–12 million U penicillin G IV qd; risk of valvular injury or myocardial abscesses which may require surgery.
Pneumococcal arthritis: Systemic antibiotics usually sufficient, but may require aspiration.
Empyema: All pleural effusions should be tapped diagnostically; chest tube is indicated if bacteria are present, pus, pH < 7.0, and/or pleural fluid glucose < 40 mg/dL.
Prevention: Vaccinate all patients over 55 and with heart disease; pulmonary, hepatic, or renal disease; diabetes; malignancies; patients with sickle cell disease > 2 years of age.

For more detailed discussion of this topic, see Austrian R: Pneumococcal Infections, Chap. 93, in HPIM-11, p. 533

---

35 STAPHYLOCOCCAL INFECTIONS

DISEASE SYNDROMES

SUPERFICIAL INFECTIONS

• Folliculitis. • Furuncles. • Hidradenitis suppurativa. • Carbuncles. • Impetigo, which cannot easily be distinguished from disease caused by group A streptococcus.

Treatment: Usually local heat, germicidal soaps; but for severe recurrent disease: dicloxacillin or cloxacillin 500 mg qid for 7–10 days.

TOXIC SHOCK SYNDROME

- Diagnostic criteria: high fever, diffuse "sunburn" rash that desquamates on palms and soles over 1–2 weeks, hypotension, involvement of three or more organ systems (GI, renal, hepatic, mucous membrane hyperemia, ↓ platelets, myalgia with ↑ CK, disorientation with normal CSF).
- Onset acute at start of menses.
- Non-menstrual-associated: cutaneous infections, focal tissue infections, postpartum and surgical wound infections (minimal signs of infection with onset typically on second day after surgery).
- Vaginal discharge: culture positive for *S. aureus* but blood cultures negative.
- Treatment: correct shock; treat renal failure, pulmonary insufficiency, DIC; drain focal collections; begin parenteral antibiotics.
- Up to 30% of women may have recurrences with subsequent menses.

BACTEREMIA AND ENDOCARDITIS

- A third of patients with bacteremia do not have identifiable focus; others have local infection, extravascular (skin, burns, cellulitis, osteomyelitis, arthritis) or intravascular (IV catheters, dialysis access sites, IV drug abuse) focus.
- Second most common cause of endocarditis and first among drug addicts.
- Nonaddicts: 30–60% involve normal mitral or aortic valves, often older patients with underlying disease; acute course with high fever, progressive anemia, frequent embolic and extracardiac complications.
- Addicts: tricuspid valve, septic pulmonary emboli.
- Diagnosis with up to three blood cultures; culture skin lesions, urine (positive in up to a third with bacteremia).
- Treatment: nafcillin 1.5 g q 4 h or oxacillin 2 g q 4 h; may add gentamicin (1.5 mg/kg then 1 mg/kg q 8 h) for 48–72 h; penicillin-sensitive strains: 4 million U q 4 h; penicillin-allergic or methicillin-resistant: vancomycin 0.5 g q 6 h.
- Duration of therapy: isolated bacteremia with normal heart valves and removable primary focus of infection—2 weeks; right-sided endocarditis in drug addicts—2 weeks of IV therapy and

4 weeks of oral dicloxacillin (1–1.5 g q 6 h); all others—4–6 weeks parenteral antibiotics; prosthetic valve endocarditis—penicillin or vancomycin + gentamicin and/or rifampin 600 mg qd × 6 weeks (surgery usually required).

- *S. epidermidis* most common isolate in primary nosocomial bacteremias, especially with IV catheters and prosthetic valves (40%); usually multiply antibiotic-resistant; treatment: vancomycin 0.5 g q 6 h for 6 weeks (plus gentamicin and/or rifampin with prosthetic valves).

OSTEOMYELITIS

- Especially children younger than 12 years; spine in adults; 50% preceding superficial staphylococcal infection.
- Acute in children; vertebral in adult is of slower onset, especially lumbar spine; increased bony fusion.
- Diagnosis: radionuclide scans may be abnormal first week; x-ray; needle aspiration or bone biopsy before therapy; sinus tract cultures not reliable in chronic osteomyelitis.
- Treatment: parenteral nafcillin or oxacillin for 4–6 weeks as for endocarditis (or cephalosporins, clindamycin, vancomycin for penicillin-allergic); surgery to remove devitalized bone, drain abscesses, relieve cord compression.

PNEUMONIA

- 1% of community-acquired, especially during influenza outbreaks.
- Older children and adults: usually preceded by influenza-like respiratory infection.
- Bronchopneumonia in cystic fibrosis; nosocomical infection in intubated or debilitated patients; obstructive pneumonia with bronchogenic cancer.
- Diagnosis: Gram's stain of sputum → many PMNs and gram-positive cocci; culture sputum and blood.
- Treatment: parenteral therapy as for endocarditis for 2 weeks unless complications.

URINARY TRACT INFECTION

- After *E. coli, S. saprophyticus* most common cause of nonobstructive UTI in sexually active women.
- Treatment: sensitive to ampicillin, trimethoprim, sulfonamides, nitrofurantoin; if relapse, look for renal calculi (produces urease).

For more detailed discussion of this topic, see Locksley RM: Staphylococcal Infections, Chap. 94, in HPIM-11, p. 537

GROUP A STREPTOCOCCAL INFECTIONS

Streptococcal pharyngitis

- Highest age 5–15 years; normally group A, occasionally C or G.
- Spread person-to-person, mostly by acutely ill.
- Incubation 2–4 days; abrupt sore throat, headache, malaise, fever; nausea, vomiting, abdominal pain in children.
- Physical exam: Temperature ≥ 101°F; diffuse erythema, edema, and lymphoid hyperplasia; tonsils enlarged and covered by off-white exudate; enlarged cervical nodes; fever usually abates within 1 week.
- Scarlet fever follows pharyngitis with lysogenic phage producing erythrogenic toxin in host without neutralizing antibody; rash develops within 2 days of sore throat: first neck, upper chest, and back, then over remainder of body, sparing palms and soles; rash diffuse, blanching erythema with 1- to 2-mm punctate elevations ("sandpaper" texture), increased along skin folds; erythema and petechiae of soft palate; lasts 4–6 days followed by desquamation.
- Complications: Acute otitis media and sinusitis, peritonsillar cellulitis, or abscess; pre-antibiotic-era meningitis, brain abscess, thrombosis of cerebral venous sinuses, bacteremia with metastatic infections; delayed nonsuppurative sequelae: acute rheumatic fever, acute glomerulonephritis.
- Diagnosis: Should culture or use direct antigen-detection kit; extremely rare in children 3 years old or less or in older adults; ASO (antistreptolysin O) titer confirms recent streptococcal infection in patients with rheumatic fever (ARF) or glomerulonephritis (AGN) but not useful with acute streptococcal infection.
- Treatment: To prevent ARF and AGN (if given within 9 days of onset): benzathine penicillin G 1.2 million units IM (600,000 U if <60 lbs) or penicillin VK 125–250 mg qid × 10 days; in the penicillin-allergic patient: erythromycin 250 mg qid × 10 days (resistance in Japan); higher doses of penicillin required if suppurative complications.

Streptococcal skin infections

- Erysipelas: Acute skin infection with marked involvement of cutaneous lymphatic vessels with group A streptococcus; especially infants, young children, and elderly on face; abrupt onset with fever, chills, malaise, headache, vomiting, spreading erythema → vesicles and bullae → crusts; central clearing; butterfly distribution; may have high fever and bacteremia.
- Pyoderma: Localized purulent streptococcal skin infections (impetigo); peak 2–6 years of age, especially lower legs; papules → vesicles with surrounding erythema → thick crusts over 4–6 days; diagnose by culture of base of lesion; treat with penicillin

as for pharyngitis; does not cause ARF but most commonly precedes AGN.
- Cellulitis: Acute inflammation of skin and subcutaneous tissues with pain, erythema, fever, and/or regional lymphadenopathy; margins not elevated or demarcated like erysipelas.

Lymphangitis and puerperal sepsis

- Red linear streaks from local trauma to enlarged regional lymph nodes with chills, fever, malaise (possible bacteremia).
- Puerperal sepsis follows abortion or childbirth with streptococcal invasion of endometrium and then lymphatics and bloodstream.

Pneumonia and empyema

- Uncommon; usually follows influenza, measles, pertussis, or varicella.
- May be epidemic, with abrupt fever, chills, myalgia, cough, hemoptysis, bronchopneumonia.
- Early and rapid accumulation of serosanguinous empyema fluid; 10–15% bacteremia.
- Treatment: 4–6 million units penicillin G IM or IV.

GROUP B STREPTOCOCCAL INFECTIONS

Perinatal infections

- Maternal chorioamnionitis, septic abortion, puerperal sepsis.
- One of two most frequent causes of neonatal sepsis and meningitis; early onset (within 10 days of birth) from maternal genital tract with lung involvement, 2 per 1000 live births, high mortality; late onset > 10 days from nosocomical transmission, meningitis, and bacteremia, lower mortality.

Adult infections

- Urinary tract infections in women and elderly men with prostatism.
- Suppurative gangrenous lesions in patients with adult-onset insulin-dependent diabetes and peripheral vascular insufficiency.
- Other: Endocarditis, pyogenic arthritis, pneumonia, empyema, meningitis, peritonitis.

OTHER STREPTOCOCCAL INFECTIONS

Group C

• Can cause pharyngitis, cervical adenitis, disseminated deep tissue infections. • Especially *S. equisimilis;* outbreak of *S. zooepidemicus* in unpasteurized milk.

Group G

• Bacteremia from cellulitis or decubitus ulcers with chronic lymphatic obstruction and venous insufficiency. • Often underlying malignancy, alcoholism, drug abuse.

Group D

• Urinary tract infections with structural abnormalities. • Infected decubitus ulcers, intraabdominal abscesses. • Enterococcal endocarditis: Must use high-dose penicillin or ampicillin plus aminoglycoside for synergism. • Nonenterococcal group D streptococcus (*S. bovis*) causes bacteremia or endocarditis, associated with colon cancer; penicillin-sensitive.

Viridans streptococci

• Most frequent cause of subacute bacterial endocarditis. • *S. milleri* may cause liver and brain abscesses, peritonitis, and empyema.

Anaerobic streptococci

• Found in abscess cavities with other bacteria. • Streptococcal myositis: Edema, crepitant myositis, pain, chains of group + cocci in seropurulent exudate. • Hemolytic streptococcal gangrene: Necrosis of subcutaneous and dermal tissues with spread along fascial planes following trauma or surgery. • Progressive synergistic gangrene: Ulcerated lesion about surgical incision surrounded by gangrenous skin. • Chronic burrowing ulcer: Deep soft-tissue infection which erodes through subcutaneous tissue to form ulcer. • Treatment: Drainage of abscesses, debridement of dead tissue, high-dose penicillin.

For more detailed discussion of this topic, see Bisno AB: Streptococcal Infections, Chap. 95, in HPIM-11, p. 543

---

37 ANAEROBIC INFECTIONS

TETANUS

Epidemiology and pathogenesis

- In U.S., almost exclusively in incompletely immunized; may follow surgery, skin testing, IM injections, burn wounds, chronic skin ulcers, otitis media, dental infections, abortion, pregnancy, or narcotic injection; 10–20% without history of injury or detectable lesion.
- Neonatal tetanus from infection of umbilical stump.

Clinical manifestations

- Incubation period 2–56 days; shorter with more severe disease.
- Initial symptoms: pain and stiffness in jaw, abdomen, or back; difficulty swallowing.
- 24–72 h later: rigidity, especially trismus, and reflex spasms; alert; low-grade fever; sweating; tachycardia.
- Physical exam: may precipitate spasms, hyperactive deep tendon reflexes; evaluate wounds, severity of trismus, potential respiratory compromise.
- Symptoms increase in severity 3–5 days; improvement by 10 days; complete recovery usually in 4 weeks.
- Complications: hypoxia; aspiration; venous thrombosis; vasomotor instability; hypertension; tachycardia, arrhythymias; pneumonia; vertebral fractures, acute peptic ulceration, paralytic ileus, constipation.

Diagnosis: Clinical; C. *tetani* recovered from wound in only 30%.

Treatment

- Drainage of infected wound.
- Quiet room; prevent aspiration, contractures.
- Antiserum as early as possible: human tetanus immune globulin 3–10,000 U IM; if only equine antiserum available, give 10,000 U after testing for hypersensitivity.
- Primary immunization once patient has recovered.
- Muscle relaxation: diazepam 40–120 mg qd.
- Tracheostomy if laryngospasm; ventilation.
- Penicillin G if treatment of wound necessary.

Prevention

- Immunization: children—DPT at 2, 4, 6, 18 months; adults—three doses Td (4–8 weeks, then 6 months to 1 year apart); boosters every 10 years.
- Wound prophylaxis: toxoid and antitoxin given simultaneously in separate syringes at separate sites.

BOTULISM

Etiology and pathogenesis: Ingestion of toxin produced by *Clostridium botulinum;* toxin A > B > E.

Food-borne botulism requires contamination with viable *C. botulinum* bacilli or spores and toxin production in anaerobic environment.
Wound botulism is caused by wound contaminated with soil containing toxin-producing *C. botulinum;* also associated with chronic drug abuse.
Clinical manifestations

- Symptoms usually 12–36 h after ingestion (extremes of 3 h to 14 days).
- Symptoms: bulbar dysfunction, symmetric paralysis of extremities (ascending or descending); weakness of respiratory muscles, constipation; urinary retention; ↓ salivation and lacrimation.
- Physical exam: alert; afebrile; ptosis, ↓ extraocular motion, sluggish pupils; symmetric flaccid weakness of palate, tongue, larynx, respiratory muscles, and extremities; paralytic ileus and bladder distention.

Laboratory findings: Examine blood, feces, gastric contents, and suspected food for toxin production.
Treatment
• Intubation or tracheostomy before respiratory failure. • Cathartics and enemas to remove unabsorbed toxin. • Trivalent ABE antitoxin following sensitivity testing to horse serum.

OTHER CLOSTRIDIAL INFECTIONS

FOOD POISONING

- *C. perfringens* second or third most common cause in U.S.
- Food sources: recooked meat, meat products, poultry.
- Symptoms develop 8–24 h after ingestion with epigastric pain, nausea, watery diarrhea.

ANTIBIOTIC-ASSOCIATED COLITIS Due to toxin-producing strains of *C. difficile.* May occur during or up to 4 weeks after all antibiotics except streptomycin or vancomycin (especially clindamycin, ampicillin, cephalosporins, aminoglycosides).
Clinical manifestations: Usually watery diarrhea, abdominal cramps and tenderness, fever, leukocytosis.
Laboratory findings: WBC may be ↑ to 50,000/mm^3; stool exam → WBCs.
Diagnosis: >95% positive stool toxin assay; characteristic pathology on sigmoidoscopy.
Treatment: mild—stop antibiotics; severe—vancomycin 125 mg PO qid × 7–10 days.

SUPPURATIVE TISSUE INFECTION

- *Clostridium* isolated from two-thirds of pts with intestinal perforation (esp. *C. ramnosum, C. perfringens, C. bifermentans).*
- *C. perfringens* frequent isolate from tuboovarian and pelvic abscesses (mild local disease); up to 20% of diseased gallbladders; up to 50% in emphysematous cholecystitis (gas in biliary radicles, esp. in diabetics); empyema.

Treatment: Usually requires broad-spectrum antibiotics for mixed infection.

LOCALIZED SKIN AND SOFT TISSUE INFECTION

• Localized, indolent infection without systemic toxicity, • Associated with cellulitis, perirectal abscesses, and diabetic foot ulcers. • Localized suppurative myositis in heroin addicts.

Treatment: Debridement; antibiotics only necessary with systemic sepsis.

SPREADING CELLULITIS

• Abrupt presentation with diffuse, spreading cellulitis and fasciitis but no myonecrosis or massive hemolysis. • Physical exam: subcutaneous crepitance with little localized pain. • Association with carcinoma of sigmoid or cecum.

Treatment: Incision of infected area; almost uniformly fatal within 48 h.

CLOSTRIDIAL MYONECROSIS Originates in deep, necrotic surgical or traumatic wounds.

Clinical manifestations: Sudden pain in wound → local swelling and edema → rapid toxemia, hypotension, renal failure, increased mental acuity.

Diagnosis: Wound smear showing positive rods; frozen section biopsy of muscle.

Treatment: Extensive debridement; penicillin G 20 million U qd; penicillin-allergic: check sensitivities to chloramphenicol (4 g qd), cefoxitin, carbenicillin, clindamycin, metronidazole, ? hyperbaric oxygen.

CLOSTRIDIAL SEPTICEMIA Differentiate from transient bacteremia when often with other bacteria; associated with GI, biliary, or uterine disease.

Etiology: Primarily following infection of uterus (esp. septic abortion), colon, or biliary tract.

Clinical manifestations: Sepsis; fever; chills 1–3 days after abortion with malaise, headache, severe myalgias, hemolysis, foul pelvic discharge; often no localizing signs; 50% hemolysis.

Treatment: Penicillin G 20 million U qd; drainage of infected sites.

MIXED ANAEROBIC INFECTIONS

ANAEROBIC INFECTIONS OF HEAD AND NECK

• Gingivitis. • Pharyngeal infections. • Facial infections (arise from diseases of mucous membranes, dental manipulations). • Sinusitis and otitis.

Complications: Contiguous spread → osteomyelitis of skull or mandible, brain abscesses, subdural empyema; caudad → mediastinitis; pleuropulmonary infections.

CENTRAL NERVOUS SYSTEM INFECTIONS

• Anaerobic bacteria in >85% of brain abscesses (peptostreptococci > fusobacteria > *Bacteroides*). • Direct extension of infection from sinuses, mastoids, or middle ear.

PLEUROPULMONARY INFECTIONS

- Anaerobic aspiration pneumonia: slow onset, low-grade fever, malaise, sputum; at risk—elderly, impaired consciousness; Gram stain of sputum → mixed bacterial flora; CXR—infiltrates in basilar segments of lower lobes.
- Necrotizing pneumonitis: numerous small abscesses involving several segments.
- Anaerobic lung abscesses: CXR—single or multiple cavities in dependent segments; oral anaerobes.
- Empyema: from long-standing anaerobic pulmonary infection.

INTRAABDOMINAL INFECTIONS

• Subphrenic abscess. • Liver abscess (50% have anaerobes).

PELVIC INFECTIONS Tuboovarian abscess, septic abortion, pelvic abscess, endometritis, postooperative wound infection.

SKIN AND SOFT TISSUE

- Synergistic gangrene: postoperative wound painful, red, and swollen for several days → erythema with central necrosis.
- Necrotizing fasciitis: rapidly spreading fascial infection by group A streptococcus or *Peptococcus* and *Bacteroides;* anaerobic cellulitis of scrotum, perineum, anterior abdominal wall—Fournier's gangrene.

BONE AND JOINT INFECTIONS Soft tissue infection adjacent to bone (maxilla and mandible); septic arthritis.

BACTEREMIA Transient bacteremia; may present like gram-negative sepsis.

Diagnosis: Consider with avascular sites, no culture isolates despite positive gram stain, failure to respond to antibiotics.

TREATMENT

- Drainage of abscesses; resection of dead tissue.
- Infections above diaphragm (*B. fragilis* unusual): 6–12 million U penicillin G qd × 4 weeks for lung abscess; if penicillin-resistant, clindamycin, chloramphenicol, cefoxitin.
- Colonic source (*B. fragilis*): clindamycin 600 mg IV q 8 h or metronidazole 500 mg IV q 8 h plus aminoglycoside.
- CNS: chloramphenicol 30–60 mg/kg qd, metronidazole, or penicillin.

For more detailed discussion of these topics, see Beaty HN: Tetanus, Chap. 99, p. 558; Beaty HN: Botulism, Chap. 100, p. 561; Kasper DL: Other Clostridial Infections, Chap. 101, p. 563; and Kasper DL: Infections due to Mixed Anaerobic Organisms, Chap. 102, p. 567, in HPIM-11

NOTES

38 DISEASES CAUSED BY OTHER GRAM-POSITIVE ORGANISMS

DIPHTHERIA

Epidemiology: *Corynebacterium diphtheriae;* in U.S. increased in Native Americans and in Pacific Northwest in indigent adults with symptomatic skin lesions—usually spread by droplet.

Clinical manifestations

- Incubation 1–7 days; temperature usually <101°F.
- Nasal pharyngeal: pain on swallowing, with thick, gray membrane over tonsils and pharynx; laryngeal: extension of membrane with airway occlusion.
- Cutaneous: invades wounds burns, or abrasions.

Complications

• Extension of membrane: airway obstruction and increased toxin absorption. • Toxic: myocarditis; peripheral neuritis.

Diagnosis

• Demonstration of organism (club-shaped gram-positive rod) by Gram stain or methylene blue; culture on Loeffler's medium. • Fluorescent-labeled antitoxin. • Toxin production.

Treatment

- Antitoxin after checking for hypersensitivity to horse serum; mild symptoms 10,000–20,000 units; moderate (pharyngeal membrane) 20,000–40,000; severe with laryngeal involvement 50,000–100,000 units IV.
- Acute and chronic carrier state: erythromycin 2 g qd × 7 days.
- Immunization (DPT): 3, 6, 12, 18 months, 6 years, and every 10 years with Td (tetanus toxoid and diphtheria).

LISTERIA MONOCYTOGENES

Epidemiology and pathogenesis

- Reservoir of most patients unclear, but there are food-borne outbreaks (coleslaw, milk, Mexican cheese).
- Increased in patients with lymphomas, diabetes, alcoholism, cardiovascular disease, or steroid or cytotoxic therapy.

Clinical manifestations: Sepsis in newborns; meningitis; bacteremia.

Diagnosis Culture.

Treatment

- Severe disease: penicillin G 240,000–320,000 U/kg qd in 6 doses + tobramycin 5–6 mg/kg qd in 3 doses; for 2 weeks in newborns, pregnant patients; 4 weeks in primary listeremia; 4–6 weeks in endocarditis and immunosuppressed patients.

- CNS infection: penicillin G 320,000–480,000 U/kg qd in 6 doses; *not* cephalosporins; in penicillin-allergic, cotrimoxazole 15 and 75 mg/kg qd in 3 doses for 14–21 days.

ANTHRAX

Epidemiology

- Outbreaks in Southern Europe, Middle East, Africa; in U.S. in workers who handle imported and unprocessed wool, hair, or hides.
- Infection by contact, inhalation, ingestion of contaminated meat, flies.

Clinical manifestations

- Cutaneous: 95% of cases in U.S.
- Inhalation: "Woolsorter's disease"—mediastinitis, hemoptysis, sudden dyspnea, cyanosis, stridor, shock; usually fatal within 24 h
- Meningeal: fulminant with hemorrhagic and/or purulent CSF.
- Intestinal: bloody diarrhea.

Diagnosis

• Gram stain of fluid usually positive unless previous antibiotics. • Cultures usually positive in 24 h. • Serology: indirect hemagglutination.

Treatment

• Cutaneous: penicillin procaine 600,000 U q 6 h until edema subsides then PO × 7–10 days. • Inhalation or meningeal: 20 million U penicillin IV qd (+300–400 mg hydrocortisone qd in meningeal). • Effective vaccine.

For more detailed discussion of these topics, see Harnisch JP: Diphtheria, Chap. 96, p. 550; Hoeprich PD: Infections Caused by *Listeria monocytogenes* and *Erysipelothrix rhusiopathiae*, Chap. 97, p. 554; and Kaye D, Petersdorf RG: Anthrax, Chap. 98, p. 556, in HPIM-11

39 MENINGOCOCCAL INFECTIONS

Epidemiology

• Person-to-person spread through nasopharyngeal secretions; attack rate highest ages 6 months to 1 year. • Disease caused by group B (50–55%) > C > W135 > Y > A (except in Alaska and Pacific Northwest). • Increased risks in household contacts, alcoholics, Alaskan natives, military recruits, patients with terminal complement component deficiencies.

Meningococcemia

• 30–50% have meningococcemia without meningitis. • Usually nonspecific prodrome of cough, headache, sore throat with sudden fever, chills, arthralgias, muscle pains; 75% have petechial rash on axillae, flanks, wrists, ankles. • Fulminant meningococcemia (Waterhouse-Friderichsen syndrome): 10–20% of patients with meningococcal infection, vasomotor collapse, large petechiae and purpuric lesions: high fatality. • Chronic meningococcemia: Intermittent fever, arthralgia, rash (maculopapular).

Meningitis

• Children 6 months to 10 years. • Usual URI symptoms with progression to fever, vomiting, headache, confusion (25% have abrupt onset). • Presumptive diagnosis with meningitis and petechial rash.

Other manifestations

• Purulent conjunctivitis or sinusitis. • Primary pneumonia. • Genital infections identical to gonococcus.

Complications

• After meningitis: Seizures or deafness acutely in 10–20% peripheral neuropathy, cranial nerve palsies usually clear within 2–4 months. • Arthritis: 2–10% with meningococcemia; often multiple joints involved while on therapy.

Diagnosis

• WBC usually 12–40,000, but may be normal to decreased. Meningitis: CSF with glucose < 35 mg/dL, 50% have + Gram's stain for bacteria, 100–40,000 PMNs. • Culture blood, spinal fluid, skin lesions. • Antigen in spinal fluid by latex agglutination or CIE (but not group B).

Treatment

• Adults: 12–24 million U penicillin G per day; children: 16 million U/m^2 per day for 7 days or 4–5 days past when afebrile. • Meningococcemia alone: 5–10 million U qd. Penicillin-allergic patients: Chloramphenicol 4–6 g qd.

Prevention

• Vaccine for outbreaks of A, C, Y, W135. • Prophylaxis of close contacts: Rifampin 600 mg bid (5–10 mg/kg) × 2 days.

For more detailed discussion of this topic, see Beaty NH: Meningococcal Infections. Chap. 103, in HPIM-11, p. 574

---

40 *HAEMOPHILUS* INFECTIONS

HAEMOPHILUS INFLUENZAE

Epidemiology

• Primarily affects children 6 to 48 months. • Increased risk: close contacts of primary cases, sickle cell disease, splenectomy, agammaglobulinemia, Hodgkin's, alcoholics. • 95% of systemic disease is type b.

Clinical manifestations

• Meningitis: most common bacterial cause at 9 months to 4 years. • Pneumonia: broncho- or lobar pneumonia (75% with empyema). • Bacteremia: especially 6–24 months; increased risk of sickle cell disease, splenectomy, Hodgkin's. • Cellulitis: cheek or periorbital area, rhinorrhea, fever, and/or ipsilateral otitis media; BC usually positive. • Epiglottis: mean 4 years old; *H. influenzae* b leading cause; 90% positive BC. • Pyarthrosis: ≤2 years old; single, large weight-bearing joints. • Other: second leading cause of childhood otitis media, sinusitis, chronic bronchitis, endocarditis, brain abscess.

Diagnosis

• 70% culture and Gram stain positive. • Antigen detection in serum, CSF, urine. • BC positive in up to 80%.

Treatment

- Chloramphenicol 100 mg/kg (up to 4 g qd) divided q 6 h and/or ampicillin 200–400 mg/kg qd (up to 6 g) given q 4 h with change to ampicillin if sensitive.
- For multiply resistant: moxolactam, ceftriaxone, ceftazadime.
- Outpatient: amoxicillin 50 mg/kg per day up to 2 g qd; if resistant, cefaclor, Septra.

Prevention

• Prophylaxis: rifampin 20 mg/kg (up to 600 mg) qd × 4 days for household contacts if other children <4 years old. • PRP vaccine for children 2–5 years old, 18 months if high risk.

BORDETELLA PERTUSSIS

Clinical manifestations: Occurs >50% in infants; incubation 6–20 days, with sneezing, fever, rhinorrhea, anorexia for 1–2 weeks → paroxysms of cough.
Diagnosis: Suggested by contact, "whooping cough," increased lymphocytes; culture; fluorescent antibody.
Treatment: Erythromycin if given early.
Prevention: Vaccine at 2, 4, 6, 18 months.

For more detailed discussion of this topic, see Feigin RD, Murphy FM: *Haemophilus* Infections, Chap. 109, in HPIM-11, p. 601

41 DISEASES CAUSED BY GRAM-NEGATIVE ORGANISMS

GRAM-NEGATIVE ENTERIC BACILLI

ESCHERICHIA COLI INFECTIONS

• UTI: causes >75%. • Peritoneal and biliary infections. • Bacteremia: most often from urinary tract, biliary, or intraperitoneal source. • Abscesses: especially at site of insulin administration in diabetics (with gas formation); in ischemic extremities, surgical wounds, perirectal phlegmons in leukemics.

Diagnosis: Cannot be differentiated on Gram stain; readily grows in culture.
Treatment: Uncomplicated infection (if sensitive)—ampicillin 2–4 g qd IV, IM, or PO; severe infections—ampicillin up to 12 g qd; cefazolin 1 g q 6–8 h, gentamicin or tobramycin 1.5 mg/kg then 1 mg/kg q 8 h; for meningitis, ceftriaxone 1–2 g q 12 h, cefotaxime 1–2 g q 4 h (adults).

KLEBSIELLA-ENTEROBACTER-SERRATIA INFECTIONS

• *Klebsiella:* complicated and obstructive UTI, biliary tract, peritoneal cavity, middle ear, mastoids, paranasal sinuses, meningitis, pneumonia (especially in alcoholics, diabetics, chronic pulmonary disease). • *Serratia* and *Enterobacter:* pneumonia, UTI; bacteremia (especially nosocomial).

Diagnosis: Gram's stain may be suggestive of *Klebsiella* with large capsule.
Treatment: *Klebsiella* usually sensitive to aminoglycosides and third generation cephalosporins; *Serratia* frequently multiply resistant, so sensitivity testing important; empiric therapy in ill patient—tobramycin or gentamicin (3–5 mg/kg/day or amikacin 15 mg/kg/day) plus cephalothin or cefazolin 4–12 g qd for 10–14 days.

PROTEUS, MORGANELLA, PROVIDENCIA INFECTIONS

• Cutaneous infections. • Ears and mastoid sinuses: very destructive; may extend to cause sinus thrombosis, meningitis, brain abscess, bacteremia. • Ocular infections: corneal ulcers, especially after trauma. • Peritonitis: isolated after perforation. • UTI: chronic bacteriuria, obstructive uropathy, renal stones. • Bacteremia: 75% from urinary tract; indistinguishable from other gram-negatives.

Diagnosis: Culture.
Treatment: *P. mirabilis* usually sensitive to penicillins; bacteriuria—ampicillin 0.5 g q 4–6 h; severe infection—6–12 g ampicillin IV + tobramycin or gentamicin 3–5 mg/kg/day.

PSEUDOMONAS

• Infections associated with local tissue damage (burns, wounds) or ↓ host resistance (cystic fibrosis, prematurity, leukemia). • Skin and subcutaneous tissues. • Osteomyelitis. • Ears, mastoids, paranasal sinuses: malignant otitis in diabetics. • Eye: corneal ulceration. • Urinary tract: obstructive uropathy and manipulation. • Respiratory tract: pneumonia infrequent. • Meningitis: following LPs, spinal anesthesia, head trauma. • Bacteremia: debilitated patients, premature infants, malignancies, after surgery of biliary or urinary tract. • Endocarditis: following open-heart surgery; IV drug abuse.

Treatment: Tobramycin and gentamicin 3–5 mg/kg/per day; amikacin if resistant (15 mg/kg/per day); ticarcillin or mezlocillin at 16–20 g qd.

BRUCELLOSIS

Epidemiology

- Four species: *B. melitensis* (goats), *B. suis* (hogs), *B. abortus* (cattle), *B. canis* (dogs).
- Exposure through infected tissues (slaughterhouse workers, butchers), milk, or milk products.

Clinical manifestations

- Acute brucellosis: incubation 7–21 days; usually insidious onset with low-grade fever, malaise, fatigue, sweats; 10–20% ↑ spleen.
- Localized: osteomyelitis of lumbosacral vertebrae; arthritis of knee; splenic abscesses; epididymoorchitis; endocarditis.
- Chronic: ill health for >1 year following onset.

Diagnosis: Positive culture of blood, lymph node, bone marrow; serology: IgG correlates with active infection; titers ⩾ 1:160 suggestive.

Treatment: Tetracycline 500 mg qid × 3–6 weeks + streptomycin 1 g q 12 h × 2 weeks or trimethoprim/sulfamethoxazole 480/2400 mg qd × 4 weeks.

TULAREMIA

Epidemiology: *Francisella tularensis* transmitted by contact with skin of rabbits, squirrels, muskrats, beavers, deer, cattle, or by tick bite; in U.S. by rabbit skin, bite of tick, or deer fly.

Clinical manifestations

• Incubation 2–5 days, then fever, chills, headache, myalgias. • Ulceroglandular: 75–85% from skin inoculation; papule → punched out ulcer with necrotic base; large, tender regional adenopathy. • Oculoglandular: purulent conjunctivitis with regional adenopathy. • Pulmonary: nonproductive cough, bilateral patchy infiltrates, high mortality. • Typhoidal: fever without skin lesions or adenopathy.

Diagnosis

• Serology: 4-fold rise over 2–3 weeks in agglutination titer; single titer ⩾ 1:160 suggestive. • Gram stain usually negative; culture (glucose-cysteine blood agar) requires special isolation.

Treatment: Streptomycin 7.5–10 mg/kg q 12 h IM × 7–10 days; if severe, 15 mg/kg q 12 h × 48–72 h or gentamicin 1.7 mg/kg q 8 h; fever responds within 2 days.

PLAGUE

Epidemiology: Humans infected with *Yersinia pestis* by bite of rodent flea; concentrated in southwestern U.S.
Clinical manifestations: Bubonic—painful, enlarged lymph nodes, fever, headache, prostration 2–7 days after flea bite; may proceed to sepsis; pneumonia with multilobar involvement.
Diagnosis: Laboratory: WBC ↑ 15,000–20,000 (up to 100,000); ↑ SGOT; DIC; smear of aspirate of bubo on Wayson's or Giemsa's stain → bipolar, "safety pin" forms; culture usually positive but may require 48–72 h.
Treatment: streptomycin 7.5–15 mg/kg IM q 12 h and/or tetracycline 5–10 mg/kg q 6 h IV for 3–4 days after afebrile; treat contacts with tetracycline 250 mg qid.

For more detailed discussion of these topics, see Schaberg DR, Turck M: Diseases Caused by Gram-Negative Enteric Bacilli, Chap. 105, p. 583; Sanford JP: Meloidosis and Glanders, Chap. 106, p. 589; Kaye D, Petersdorf RG: Brucellosis, Chap. 112, p. 610; Kaye D: Tularemia, Chap. 113, p. 613; Palmer DL: Plague and Other *Yersinia* Infections, Chap. 114, p. 615; Plorde JJ: Bartonellosis, Chap. 116, p. 620; and Corey L: Cat-Scratch Disease, Chap. 118, p. 623, in HPIM-11

---

42 TUBERCULOSIS AND OTHER MYCOBACTERIAL INFECTIONS

TUBERCULOSIS

CLINICAL MANIFESTATIONS

- Primary TBC: Usually asymptomatic; lower or midlung zone pneumonitis with enlarged hilar lymph nodes.
- Reactivation: Chronic wasting disease with weight loss and low-grade fever.
- Pulmonary TBC: Apical posterior segments of upper lobes and superior segments of lower lobes; usually insidious onset; chronic cough with scant, nonpurulent sputum; hemoptysis with cavitary disease.
- Pleurisy with effusion: Abrupt pleuritic pain following formation of effusion next to peripheral primary lesion; usually in young patients but in U.S. half > 35 years old and have simultaneous pulmonary TBC; fluid; >3.0 g/dL protein, ↑ lymphocytes; a third are PPD-negative; good response to treatment; empyema requires surgical drainage.
- Pericarditis: Usually from drainage of infected lymph node or extension of pleurisy; may develop tamponade or late chronic constrictive pericarditis.
- Peritonitis: Hematogenous seeding, abdominal lymphatic or GU source; insidious onset; diagnose by culture of paracentesis fluid or biopsy.
- Laryngeal and endobronchial: Usually with advanced pulmonary disease; laryngitis → hoarseness, bronchitis → cough and minor hemoptysis; highly infectious; respond well to therapy.
- Adenitis: Scrofula: chronic cervical adenitis, just below mandible, rubbery, nontender; diagnose by surgical biopsy for culture and histology, with therapy at or immediately before surgery to prevent fistulas; in children < 5 years old, usually *M. scrofulaceum* and *M. intracellulare*.
- Skeletal: Pott's: infection of midthoracic spine with anterior erosion of vertebral bodies; may be large abscesses; responds to chemotherapy alone unless neurologic compromise.
- Genitourinary: Renal TBC usually as microscopic pyuria and hematuria with sterile urine cultures; may cause cavitation of renal parenchyma and ureteral stricture; females: salpingitis and sterility; males: prostate and seminal vesicles.
- Meningeal: Meningeal and cranial nerve signs: CSF: ↑ protein, ↓ glucose, lymphocytosis.
- Ocular: Chorioretinitis, uveitis; choroid tubercles in miliary TBC.
- Gastrointestinal: Ileitis in extensive cavitary disease and swallowed organisms with chronic diarrhea and fistulas.
- Adrenal: Cortical involvement may cause insufficiency.
- Cutaneous: Lupus vulgaris.

- Miliary: fever, anemia, splenomegaly; 4–6 weeks into illness: fine nodules on CXR; transbronchial, liver, and bone marrow biopsy positive in two-thirds; more fulminant in previously diseased individual with diffuse pulmonary infiltrates and positive sputum; PPD often negative.

DIAGNOSIS

- Detect in sputum, body fluids, or tissues by acid-fast stain or fluorescence with auramine-rhodamine (not specific for *M. tuberculosis*).
- Primary isolation takes 4–8 weeks.
- CXR: Healed first-degree lesion with calcified hilar node and peripheral lesion—Ghon's complex; multinodular infiltrates and/or cavitation in apical posterior segments of upper lobes.
- Skin testing: Positive reaction >10 mm induration to PPD-S; half of patients with miliary TBC and a third with new pleurisy are PPD-negative.

TREATMENT

- Symptomatic improvement in 2–3 weeks; sputum conversion usually within 2 months.
- Renal failure: isoniazid and ethambutol 2–3 times per week or after each dialysis; rifampin dose unchanged.
- Suspect drug resistance from Haiti, Southeast Asia, Latin America, and begin therapy with isoniazid, rifampin, and ethambutol.
- Prophylaxis: 1 year of isoniazid 300 mg qd for all patients with +PPD <35 years old and with any +PPD in patients with AIDS, Hodgkin's, chronic steroids, renal failure, and abnormal CXR in untreated older patient.

OTHER MYCOBACTERIAL INFECTIONS

M. ulcerans: Cause of Buruli ulcer, small painless nodule → extensive granulomatous ulceration on extremities; occurs in Australia and Africa.

M. marinum: Infection from exposure to freshwater or saltwater fish; nodule with lymphatic spread or ulcer; sensitive to rifampin, ethambutol, and/or tetracycline, trimethoprim-sulfamethoxazole; must be cultured at 30–32°C.

M. kansasii: Pigment with light exposure, grows at 37°C, can be identified on initial stains by prominent transverse banding; pulmonary disease similar to tuberculosis but milder symptoms; disseminated disease with pancytopenia, hairy-cell leukemia, malignancies, transplants; treat with rifampin and ethambutol or isoniazid.

M. scrofulaceum: Lymphadenitis in children with few systemic symptoms; treat surgically.

M. avium-intracellulare: Pulmonary disease like TBC, risk factors are underlying pulmonary disease, age; lymphadenitis in children; disseminated disease with fever, anemia, leukocytosis, hepatosplenomegaly. Overwhelming infection with no cellular response in

AIDS patients; may cause severe diarrhea. Treatment: Poor; 3–6 drugs and/or clofazamine, ansamycin.

***M. fortuitum* and *M. chelonei*:** Grow within 1–5 weeks on most media. *M. fortuitum:* Posttraumatic and postoperative skin and soft-tissue infection. *M. chelonei:* Pulmonary infections and disseminated disease. Often resistant; sensitivity testing more reliable: amikacin, cefoxitin, doxycyline, gentamicin, erythromycin, sulfonamides.

For more detailed discussion of this topic, see Daniel TM: Tuberculosis, Chap. 119 in HPIM-11, p. 625 and Freedman SD: Other Mycobacterial Infections, Chap. 121, in HPIM-11, p. 637

---

43 INFLUENZA AND OTHER VIRAL RESPIRATORY DISEASES

INFLUENZA

Epidemiology

• Major outbreaks from "antigenic shifts": reassortment of genomic segments with expression of new neuraminidase (N) or hemagglutination (H) of influenza A. • Influenza B less variation, with outbreaks in schools and military camps.

Clinical manifestations

• Abrupt onset of headache, fevers, chills, cough, sore throat, myalgias. • Acute illness usually resolves over 2–5 days.

Complications

• Primary influenza pneumonia: Persistent fever, dyspnea, scanty sputum; CXR: diffuse interstitial infiltrates; ↑ with cardiac disease, especially mitral stenosis. • Secondary bacterial pneumonia: Improvement 2–3 days after acute influenza, then fever, productive cough; *Streptococcus pneumoniae, S. aureus, H. influenzae.* • Reye's syndrome: Onset of nausea and vomiting, CNS symptoms (lethargy, delirium, seizures); ↑ SGOT, SGPT, and ammonia, especially after influenza B; normal CSF; association with aspirin therapy. • Myositis, rhabdomyolysis: Marked muscle tenderness with ↑ CPK and aldolase.

Diagnosis

• Isolation of virus from throat swabs, nasopharyngeal washes, or sputum in tissue culture within 48–72 h. • Serology: Fourfold rise in hemagglutination, complement fixation over 10–14 days.

Treatment/prophylaxis

• Symptomatic therapy but no salicylates for patients younger than 16 years of age. • Amantadine for influenza A will decrease systemic symptoms if started within 48 hours—200 mg qd for 3–5 days; rimantadine has fewer CNS side effects (jitteriness, anxiety, insomnia). • Inactivated influenza vaccine for A and B yearly, especially for patients with chronic cardiovascular or pulmonary disease, those older than 65 years, medical personnel; amantadine can be given simultaneously during outbreaks until vaccine is effective (2 weeks).

OTHER VIRAL RESPIRATORY INFECTIONS

RHINOVIRUS Epidemiology: Major cause of common cold; seasonal peaks in fall and spring; spread by contact with infected secretions.

Clinical manifestations: Incubation 1–2 days, then rhinorrhea, sneezing, nasal congestion, sore throat; systemic symptoms unusual; in children may cause bronchitis, bronchiolitis, bronchopneumonia; exacerbation of asthma and chronic obstructive pulmonary disease.

CORONAVIRUS Epidemiology: 10–20% of colds, especially late fall, early winter, spring.
Clinical manifestations: Incubation 3 days, duration 6–7 days.

RESPIRATORY SYNCYTIAL VIRUS Epidemiology: Major respiratory pathogen of young children, peak 2–3 months; lower respiratory disease in young infants (20–25% of hospital admissions for pneumonia); nosocomial pathogen.
Clinical manifestations: Infants: rhinorrhea, low-grade fever and cough → lower respiratory tract involvement in 25–40%, especially severe with congenital cardiac disease; adults: common cold with moderate systemic symptoms.
Diagnosis: Isolation from respiratory secretions; rapid diagnosis by immunofluorescence of nasal scrapings; serology (CSF) useful if >4 months old.
Treatment: Aerosolized ribavirin in hospitalized infants.

PARAINFLUENZA VIRUS Epidemiology: Major cause of lower respiratory illness, especially croup, in children.
Clinical manifestations: Children: acute fever, coryza, sore throat, cough; may progress to barking cough and frank stridor; older children and adults: common cold.
Diagnosis: Viral cultures.

ADENOVIRUS Epidemiology: Children, military recruits; spread through aerosols, inoculation of conjunctival sac, or fecal-oral.
Clinical manifestations: Acute URI with rhinitis; pharyngoconjunctival fever: bilateral conjunctivitis, low-grade fever, rhinitis, sore throat, cervical adenopathy; acute respiratory disease (ARD) in military recruits with fever, cough, coryza; acute diarrheal illness in young children; hemorrhagic cystitis; epidemic keratoconjunctivitis.
Diagnosis: Culture, serology.
Treatment: Live unattenuated vaccine against types 4 and 7; stimulates antibodies against subsequent ARD.

For more detailed discussion of this topic, see Dolin R: Influenza, Chap. 130, in HPIM-11, p. 672, and Common Viral Respiratory Infections, Chap. 131, in HPIM-11, p. 677

---

44 RUBEOLA, RUBELLA, CHICKENPOX, AND OTHER VIRAL EXANTHEMS

MEASLES (RUBEOLA)

Epidemiology: Transmitted by droplets of nasopharyngeal secretions; highly contagious; increased outbreaks in teenagers and young adults.
Manifestations: Incubation approximately 10 days; then malaise, irritability, high fever, conjunctivitis, severe cough, coryza; 3–4 days after prodromal symptoms—Koplik's spots and rash: forehead → face → trunk.
Complications: Croup, bronchitis, bronchiolitis, interstitial giant cell pneumonia (immunocompromised children); conjunctivitis; myocarditis; acute glomerulonephritis; bacterial pneumonia; encephalomyelitis: 1 in 1000 patients, usually 4–7 days after rash (high fever, drowsiness, coma, fatal in 10%); late complication—subacute sclerosing panencephalitis.
Diagnosis: Leukopenia during prodrome; <2000 lymphocytes/mm^3 is poor prognostic sign; multinucleated giant cells in secretions; viral culture; serology.
Prophylaxis: Passive immunization with 0.5 mL/kg γ-globulin (to 15 mL) for children <3 years old, pregnant women, patients with TBC, immunocompromised; live attentuated vaccine at 15 months.

RUBELLA (GERMAN MEASLES)

Clinical Manifestations

- Incubation 14–21 days; prodrome of malaise, headache, fever, mild conjunctivitis.
- Maculopapular rash begins on forehead and face → trunk and extremities; enlarged lymph nodes, especially postauricular and suboccipital; arthralgias.
- Congenital: patent ductus, interventricular septal defect, pulmonic stenosis, corneal clouding, cataracts, chorioretinitis; microcephaly, mental retardation, deafness.

Diagnosis: Viral cultures; serology; hemagglutinating antibodies by second day of rash.
Prevention: Live attenuated vaccine should not be given to a woman who may become pregnant within 3 months; contraindicated in immunodepressed.

VARICELLA-ZOSTER

CHICKENPOX

- Incubation 10–21 days; 90% attack rate among susceptibles.
- Prodrome of fever and lassitude → maculopapules, vesicles, and scabs in varying stages of evolution; first on trunk and face.

Complications: Bacterial superinfection (skin); pneumonitis in up to 20% of adults; myocarditis; corneal lesions; arthritis; acute glomerulonephritis, hepatitis.

HERPES ZOSTER

• Reactivation of latent virus from dorsal root ganglia. • Pain within dermatome for 48–72 h → erythematous rash → vesicular lesions.

Complications: Meningoencephalitis; granulomatous angiitis with contralateral hemiplegia; 40% cutaneous dissemination with lymphoma.
Diagnosis: Tzanck smear—multinucleated giant cells at base of lesions; viral culture; serology.
Prophylaxis: Varicella-zoster immune globulin (VZIG) to immunodeficient patients <15 years old.
Treatment: Zoster ophthalmicus—analgesics, atropine, topical antivirals (IUDR, ara-A, acyclovir); immunocompromised—acyclovir 15 mg/kg qd over 12 h.

POXVIRUSES

SMALLPOX (VARIOLA)

Epidemiology: Last case in 1977; spread through airborne transmission.
Clinical manifestations: Incubation 14–17 days with prodrome of fever, headache, myalgia, transient erythematous eruption → painful ulcers on buccal mucosa and papules on extremities → hemorrhagic vesicles; infectious until scabs fall off (3 weeks).
Diagnosis: EM of vesicle fluid for viral particles or agar precipitation of antigen from vesicles; cell culture.

VACCINIA Virus used to induce immunity to smallpox; only indicated for laboratory workers involved with smallpox (*not* to treat HSV, warts).
Complications: Vaccinia gangrenosum (destruction of large areas of skin), eczema vaccination (widespread infection in patient with eczema), generalized vaccinia.

For more detailed discussion of these topics, see Ray CG: Measles (Rubeola), Chap. 132, p. 682; Ray CG: Rubella ("German Measles") and Other Viral Exanthems, Chap. 133, p. 684; Ray CG: Smallpox, Vaccinia, and Other Poxviruses, Chap. 134, p. 686; and Whitley RJ: Varicella-Zoster Virus Infections, Chap. 135, p. 689, in HPIM-11

---

45 MUMPS

Epidemiology

• Paramyxovirus; only reservoir is in humans. • Transmitted by infected salivary secretions or urine for 6 days prior to parotitis to up to 2 weeks later. • Incubation 15–21 days; peak ages 5–9 years.

Clinical manifestations

- Salivary adenitis: usually sudden parotitis with marked pain; skin over gland not warm or red (vs. bacterial parotitis); fever 100–103°F, malaise, headache, anorexia.
- Epididymoorchitis: 20–35% of postpubertal males; usually 7–10 days after parotitis with recrudescence of malaise, chills, fevers; half followed by testicular atrophy; sterility if bilateral.
- Pancreatitis: abdominal pain and tenderness rarely complicated by shock or pseudocyst; may see increased amylase with parotitis alone (but increased lipase only with pancreatitis).
- CNS: half show increased cells in CSF, usually 3–10 days after onset of parotitis; rare—true encephalitis, paralytic polio-like syndrome, transverse myelitis, cerebellar ataxia.
- Other: subacute thyroiditis, dacryoadenitis, optic neuritis, iritis, conjunctivitis, myocarditis, hepatitis, thrombocytopenic purpura, interstitial pneumonia, migratory polyarthritis (esp. males ages 20–30).

Diagnosis

- Laboratory findings: relative lymphocytosis in uncomplicated parotitis; marked leukocytosis with orchitis; increased amylase; CSF—1000–2000 WBCs with PMNs early (higher than aseptic meningitis with polio-, coxsackie-, and echoviruses).
- Culture from blood, throat swabs, CSF, urine; in tissue culture, immunofluorescence positive in 2–3 days.
- Serology: fourfold increases in titer by ELISA, CF (S antigen early, V later).

Treatment

- Prednisone 60 mg qd tapered over 7–10 days may give symptomatic relief in orchitis.
- Prevention: Live attenuated vaccine after 1 year of age; contraindicated if hypersensitivity reaction, febrile illness, malignancy, pregnancy.

For more detailed discussion of this topic, see Ray CG: Mumps, Chap. 141, in HPIM-11, p. 709

46 ENTEROVIRUSES AND REOVIRUSES

Characteristics

• Picornavirus: small, single-stranded RNA; can survive in sewage and chlorinated water with organic debris. • Asymptomatic infection common; epidemics in summer and fall. • Fecal-oral transmission; incubation 2–10 days. • Two-thirds of isolates from children <9 years old.

Diagnosis: Virus isolation from throat, stool, body fluids; CSF positive 10–85% (except polio), but may shed in stool for 4 months.

POLIOVIRUS

Clinical manifestations

- 90% subclinical or mild; abortive poliomyelitis—nonspecific febrile illness for 2–3 days.
- Aseptic meningitis: usually complete recovery.
- Paralytic poliomyelitis: fever recurs 5–10 days later with meningeal irritation, asymmetric flaccid paralysis, absent DTRs, normal sensation; 6–25% bulbar; recovery continues for up to 6 months.

Prevention

- OPV (oral poliovaccine): live attenuated virus; 2, 4, 12 months of age; advantages—ease of administration, secondary immunization of nonimmune contacts; risk of paralytic polio (1 in 3.7 million doses).
- IPV: inactivated; 4 doses (3 doses 4–8 weeks apart, then 1 dose 6–12 months later).

COXSACKIE AND ECHOVIRUSES

ASEPTIC MENINGITIS

- Symptoms: fever, headache, stiff neck, confusion.
- Laboratory findings: <500 WBC in CSF (may be ↑ PMNs early), protein slightly ↑, normal glucose.
- CSF usually culture-positive early.
- >90% recover completely.

OTHER

- Generalized disease of the newborn: overwhelming enteroviral infection.
- Myocarditis and pericarditis: 50% coxsackievirus B.
- Exanthems: coxsackievirus A16 hand-foot-mouth disease.
- Herpangina: acute fever, sore throat, small vesicles posterior half of palate; coxsackievirus A.
- Epidemic myalgia: sudden fever, upper abdominal pain; coxsackievirus B.

REOVIRUS

Characteristics: Double-stranded RNA; sporadic upper respiratory infections, exanthems, pneumonia, hepatitis, encephalitis.

For more detailed discussion of this topic, see Ray CG: Enteroviruses and Reoviruses, Chap. 139, in HPIM-11, p. 703

---

47 HERPES SIMPLEX VIRUSES

CLINICAL DISEASE

ORAL-FACIAL INFECTIONS

- Primary infection: pharyngitis and gingivostomatitis with fever, malaise, myalgias lasting 3–14 days.
- Reactivation: intraoral or external facial lesions.
- Immunosuppressed patients: can develop severe mucositis; with atopic eczema, severe oral-facial infections (eczema herpeticum) with dissemination to visceral organs; associated with erythema multiforme.

GENITAL INFECTIONS

- Primary: fever, headache, malaise, myalgias with local pain, itching, dysuria, tender inguinal adenopathy; 80% cervical involvement.
- Recurrences: 80% with HSV-2 infection will have recurrence within 1 year vs. 55% with HSV-1 infection.
- Rectal and perianal: especially homosexual men; anorectal pain, discharge, tenesmus, constipation; autonomic dysfunction with sacral paresthesias, impotence, urinary retention.

HERPETIC WHITLOW Infection of finger with abrupt edema, erythema, vesicular or pustular lesions; may be indistinguishable from pyogenic infections, but surgery may exacerbate.

EYE INFECTIONS

- Most frequent cause of corneal blindness in U.S.
- Keratitis: acute-onset pain, blurring of vision, chemosis, conjunctivitis, dendritic lesions of cornea.

ENCEPHALITIS

- Most common cause of acute, sporadic viral encephalitis in U.S.; >95% HSV-1.
- Symptoms: acute onset of fever and focal temporal lobe symptoms.
- Diagnosis: brain biopsy.

PERIPHERAL NERVOUS SYSTEM

- Autonomic nervous system dysfunction with numbness, tingling of buttock, urinary retention, constipation resolving over days to weeks.
- Transverse myelitis with symmetrical paralysis of lower extremities or Guillain-Barré syndrome.
- Bell's palsy following reactivation of HSV-1.

VISCERAL INFECTIONS

- Esophagitis: dysphagia, substernal pain, weight loss; especially distal esophagus; diagnose by culture and cytologic exam of secretions from endoscopy.

- HSV pneumonitis: in severely immunosuppressed patients; extension of herpetic tracheobronchitis → focal necrotizing pneumonitis; hematogenous dissemination → bilateral interstitial pneumonitis; mortality >80%.
- Hepatitis: immunosuppressed; fever; increased bilirubin, SGOT.

NEONATAL INFECTION

- 6–7 weeks of age highest rate of visceral or CNS infection.
- 70% HSV-2 from infected genital secretions at delivery.

DIAGNOSIS

Rapid diagnosis: Demonstration of giant cells or intranuclear inclusions on Wright, Giemsa (Tzanck prep), or Pap stain of scrapings of base of lesions (could also be varicella-zoster). Culture usually positive in 48–96 h; serology useful only during primary infection.

THERAPY

Mucocutaneous HSV infections

Immunosuppressed patients

Acute symptomatic first or recurrent episodes: IV acyclovir (5 mg/kg every 8 h) or oral acyclovir (200 mg PO 5 times per day for 7 to 10 days) relieves pain and speeds healing. With localized external lesions 5% topical acyclovir ointment applied 4 to 6 times daily may be beneficial.

Suppression of reactivation disease: IV (5 mg/kg every 8 h) or oral acyclovir (400 mg PO 4 to 5 times per day) will when taken daily prevent recurrences during high-risk period, e.g., immediate posttransplantation period.

Immunocompetent patients

Genital herpes

First episodes: oral acyclovir (200 mg PO 5 times per day for 10 to 14 days) is the treatment of choice. IV acyclovir (5 mg/kg every 8 h for 5 days) is given for severe disease or neurologic complications such as aseptic meningitis. Topical 5% ointment or cream applied 4 to 6 times daily for 7 to 10 days may be beneficial in patients without cervical, urethral, or pharyngeal involvement.

Symptomatic recurrent genital herpes: Oral acyclovir (200 mg PO 5 times per day for 5 days) has modest benefit in shortening lesions and viral excretion time. Routine use for all episodes not recommended.

Suppression of recurrent genital herpes: Daily oral acyclovir 200-mg capsules, 2 to 3 times daily will prevent reactivation of symptomatic recurrences; use at present limited to 6-month course in frequent recurrers.

Oral-labial HSV

First episode: Oral acyclovir has not been studied yet.

Recurrent episodes: Topical acyclovir ointment is of no clinical benefit. Oral acyclovir is not routinely recommended.

Herpetic whitlow: Studies of antiviral chemotherapy have not yet been performed.

HSV proctitis: Oral acyclovir (400 mg PO 5 times per day) is useful in shortening course of infection. In immunosuppressed patients or in severe infection, IV acyclovir 5 mg/kg every 8 h may be useful.

Herpetic eye infections

Acute keratitis: Topical trifluorothymidine, vidarabine, idoxuridine, acyclovir, and interferon are all beneficial. Debridement may be required; topical steroids may worsen disease.

CNS HSV infection
HSV encephalitis: intravenous acyclovir 10 mg/kg 8 h (30 mg/kg per day) for 10 days or vidarabine (15 mg/kg per day) decrease mortality; acyclovir is the preferred agent.
HSV aseptic meningitis: No studies of systemic antiviral chemotherapy. If therapy is to be given IV, acyclovir at 15 to 30 mg/kg per day should be utilized.
Autonomic radiculopathy: No studies are available.
Neonatal HSV infection: Intravenous vidarabine (30 mg/kg per day) or acyclovir (30 mg/kg per day). Neonates appear to tolerate this high dose of vidarabine.
Visceral HSV infections
HSV esophagitis: Systemic acyclovir (15 mg/kg per day) or vidarabine (15 mg/kg per day) should be considered.
HSV pneumonitis: No controlled studies: systemic acyclovir (15 mg/kg per day) or vidarabine (15 mg/kg per day) should be considered.
Disseminated HSV: No controlled studies, intravenous acyclovir or vidarabine should be attempted. No definite evidence that therapy will decrease mortality.
Erythema multiforme associated with HSV: Anecdotal observations suggest oral acyclovir capsules 2 to 3 times daily will suppress EM.

Reproduced from Corey L: HPIM-11, p. 696.

For more detailed discussion of this topic, see Corey L: Herpes Simplex Viruses, Chap. 136, in HPIM-11, p. 692

48 CYTOMEGALOVIRUS AND EPSTEIN-BARR VIRUS INFECTIONS

CYTOMEGALOVIRUS (CMV) INFECTION

Epidemiology and pathogenesis

• 1% of newborns in U.S. infected. • Spread by repeated or prolonged intimate contact: day-care centers, venereal transmission; 2–10% transmission per unit of blood with viable WBCs transfused. • Clinical disease in fetus or newborn from primary maternal infection. • Virus persists indefinitely in tissues of host and may be reactivated during immunosuppression.

Clinical manifestations

- Congenital CMV infection: cytomegalic inclusion disease in ~5% infected fetuses of mothers with primary infections; petechiae, hepatosplenomegaly, jaundice; 30–50% have microcephaly and/or cerebral calcifications; 20–30% mortality with severe disease; most congenital infections clinically inapparent at birth.
- Perinatal: acquired at delivery from infected birth canal or contact with maternal milk; rare cause of protracted interstitial pneumonia in premature infants.
- CMV mononucleosis: incubation 20–60 days; lasts 2–6 weeks; prolonged high fevers, profound fatigue, malaise, myalgias, headache, splenomegaly (exudative pharyngitis and cervical adenopathy rare, unlike EBV); lymphocytosis with >10% atypicals; moderate ↑ SGOT, alkaline phosphatase.
- Immunocompromised host: maximum risk 1–4 months after organ transplant, causing fever, leukopenia, hepatitis, pneumonia, colitis, retinitis; pneumonia in 20% of bone marrow recipients; very frequent in patients with AIDS.

Diagnosis

- Culture: may be positive in days with high titer (congenital infection or AIDS) or several weeks (CMV mononucleosis); urine or saliva may be culture positive for months to years.
- Serology: antibody rises may not be detectable for up to 4 weeks after primary infection.

EPSTEIN-BARR VIRUS INFECTIONS

Epidemiology and pathogenesis

• Transmitted by saliva (rarely by blood transfusions). • Shed from oropharynx for up to 18 months after primary infection; can be isolated from 25–50% of oropharyngeal washings from renal transplant patients and virtually all patients with AIDS. • Infected B lymphocytes polyclonally stimulated to produce immunoglobulin.

Clinical manifestations

- Symptoms: incubation 4–8 weeks; malaise, anorexia, chills, then pharyngitis, fever, and lymphadenopathy.
- Physical exam: >90% febrile; diffuse pharyngitis; cervical adenopathy; 50% splenomegaly.
- Clinical course: pharyngitis persists 7–10 days; fever 7 to 14 days: malaise may persist more than 3 to 4 weeks.
- Complications: hematologic—autoimmune hemolytic anemia, thrombocytopenia, granulocytopenia; splenic rupture during second or third week of illness; neurologic—cranial nerve palsies, encephalitis; hepatitis; cardiac—pericarditis, myocarditis rare; may have overwhelming infection with X-linked lymphoproliferative syndrome.

Diagnosis

- Heterophil antibodies: antibodies to sheep red blood cells removed by absorption with beef red blood cells; 10–15% may be negative in first week; may be positive up to 9 months after onset of illness.
- Atypical lymphocytosis: activated T lymphocytes.
- Specific antibodies: IgM to VCA (viral capsid antigen) diagnostic of primary infection (but only in reference lab); IgG-VCA positive for life.

Management: Corticosteroids for airway obstruction or severe hemolytic anemia or thrombocytopenia.

EBV-associated Malignancy

• Burkitt's lymphoma, anaplastic nasopharyngeal cancer. • B-cell lymphomas, especially in immunosuppressed (organ transplant, ataxia telangectasia, AIDS.)

For more detailed discussion of these topics, see Hirsch MS: Cytomegalovirus Infection, Chap. 137, p. 697; and Schooley RT: Epstein-Barr Virus Infections, Including Infectious Mononucleosis, Chap. 138, p. 699, in HPIM-11

49 VIRAL ENCEPHALITIS, RABIES, AND DENGUE

VIRAL ENCEPHALITIS

"ARBOVIRUS INFECTIONS" Transmitted by mosquitoes, so spread in late spring through early fall.
Clinical manifestations: Differ by age; <1 year old—sudden fever and convulsions, rigidity of extremities, abnormal reflexes; 5–14 years old—headache, fever, drowsiness, nausea, vomiting, photophobia, nuchal rigidity; adults—abrupt fever, nausea with vomiting, severe headache, confusion; may have tremors, cranial nerve abnormalities, abnormal reflexes (suck and snout).
Laboratory findings: Slight to moderate ↑ WBC; CSF—100–1000 WBC, ↑ PMNs early, slightly ↑ protein, glucose normal.

CALIFORNIA ENCEPHALITIDES **Epidemiology:** LaCrosse encephalitis second only to enteroviruses causing acute CNS disease in Midwest, North Central states.
Clinical manifestations: Mild form—2–3 days of fever, headache, malaise with meningeal signs decreasing over 7–8 days; severe form—abrupt fever, headache, vomiting with seizures, focal neurologic signs.
Laboratory findings: WBC 7000–30,000; CSF 10–500 WBC/mm^3, protein < 100 mg/dL, normal glucose; EEGs abnormal in 80%.
Diagnosis: Serum and CSF tested for IgM antibodies for LaCrosse virus.
Treatment: Parenteral diazepam most effective for seizures; with severe disease, should be discharged on phenobarbital for 6–12 months.
Prognosis: <2% fatality; but a third with neurologic findings.

EASTERN EQUINE ENCEPHALITIS **Epidemiology:** Eastern coast of Americas; affects mainly children and adults >55 years; 25:1 inapparent infection to overt encephalitis.
Clinical manifestations: CSF may have >1000 WBC/mm^3.
Diagnosis: Detection of specific IgM in CSF or serum.
Prognosis: Mortality in clinical infection >50%.

ST. LOUIS ENCEPHALITIS (SLE) **Epidemiology:** In West, mixed outbreaks of western equine encephalitis and SLE in rural areas; urban epidemics primarily in older patients.
Clinical manifestations: Most often inapparent; three-quarters with symptoms have encephalitis; others with aseptic meningitis.
Diagnosis: 40% positive hemagglutination inhibition at onset of illness.
Prognosis: 20% case fatality ratio.

WESTERN EQUINE ENCEPHALITIS **Epidemiology:** Entire U.S., especially central valley of California; a quarter of patients <1 year old; highest attack rates >55 years old.

Prognosis: Severe sequelae if <3 months old (>60%), but <5% of adults.

RABIES

Epidemiology

- In U.S. human cases from skunks, bats, raccoons, or domestic animal bites outside of country.
- Highest prevalence: S.E. Asia, Philippines, Africa, Indian subcontinent.
- Human-to-human transmission through corneal transplants.

Clinical manifestations

- Prodrome: 1–4 days of fever, headache, malaise, myalgias, anorexia, sore throat; 50–80% have paresthesias and/or fasciculations at site of inoculation.
- Encephalitis: excessive motor activity, excitation, agitation, hallucinations, muscle spasms, seizures, focal paralysis, hyperesthesia, fever, autonomic dysfunction (dilated, irregular pupils, ↑ lacrimation and salivation).
- Brainstem dysfunction: cranial nerve palsies, 50% hydrophobia (involuntary contraction of respiratory muscles with swallowing liquids); prominence of early brainstem dysfunction distinguishes from other encephalitides.
- Late complications: median survival 4 days; with respiratory support develop syndrome of inappropriate secretion of antidiuretic hormone, diabetes insipidus, cardiac arrhythmias; three nonfatal cases to date.

Diagnosis

- Isolation of virus from saliva or brain by mouse inoculation.
- Serology: 4-fold rise in neutralizing antibody or CSF antibody titers >1:64 (if received rabies vaccine).
- Antigen detection: fluorescent antibody staining of corneal impression smears; skin or brain biopsies.

Prevention and Treatment

- Indications for postexposure prophylaxis: physical contact with saliva, exposure to escaped wild animal at risk (bats, skunks, coyotes, foxes, raccoons), or positive fluorescent antibody test of brain of captured animal.
- Local wound therapy: vigorous cleansing with soap and water.
- Passive immunization: human rabies immune globulin (RIG), 20 U/kg (half locally in wound, half IM) or equine globulin 40 U/kg.
- Active immunization: human diploid cell vaccine (HDCV) 1 mL IM on days 0, 3, 7, 14, 28.
- Preexposure prophylaxis: at risk—veterinarians, spelunkers, laboratory workers, animal handlers—HDCV 1 mL IM on days 0, 7, 21; check for neutralizing antibody titer ≥1:5; and/or booster every 2 years.

DENGUE

Epidemiology

- Major areas: tropical Asia, especially <1 year old; Caribbean.
- Dengue hemorrhagic fever (DHF) almost exclusively in previously immune.

Clinical manifestations

- Prodrome of fever, cough, pharyngitis, headache, vomiting, abdominal pain, high fevers, myalgias, and bone pain.
- DHF: abrupt deterioration with hypotension, petechiae.

Diagnosis

- DHF: fever (acute onset, continuous for 2–7 days); hemorrhagic manifestations (petechiae, purpura, epistaxis); thrombocytopenia; hemoconcentration (20% have ↑ Hct).
- Dengue shock syndrome: hypotension, pulse pressure ≤ 20 mmHg.

Treatment: Fluid replacement; questionable role of heparin with DIC.

For more detailed discussion of these topics, see Corey L: Rabies and Other Rhabdoviruses, Chap. 142, p. 712; and Sanford JP: Arbovirus Infections, Chap. 143, p. 717, in HPIM-11

50 FUNGAL AND RELATED INFECTIONS

CRYPTOCOCCOSIS

Etiology/pathogenesis: Infection by inhalation of *Cryptococcus neoformans;* 50% underlying lymphoma, sarcoid, steroid therapy, AIDS.

Clinical manifestations

- Meningoencephalitis: fever and nuchal rigidity often absent; 50% with papilledema, 25% with cranial nerve palsies.
- Pulmonary: 40% with chest pain, 20% with cough, ≥1 well-circumscribed dense infiltrate.

Diagnosis

- CSF: 50% india ink +, glucose ↓, protein ↑; 20–600 WBC/mm^3; 90% cryptococcal antigen +.
- Pulmonary: sputum culture + in 10%; serum antigens + in 33%; requires biopsy for Dx.

Treatment: Amphotericin B 0.3 mg/kg per day + flucytosine 150 mg/kg per day × 6 weeks.

BLASTOMYCOSIS

Etiology/pathogenesis: Inhalation of *Blastomyces dermatitidis;* Southeastern, central mid-Atlantic states.

Clinical manifestations

- Acute self-limited pneumonia.
- Chronic: progressive fever, cough, weight loss, skin lesions (pimple → verrucous, crusted, or ulcerated lesion); two-thirds have abnormal CXR; osteolytic lesions.

Diagnosis: Wet smear and/or culture.
Treatment: Progressive disease or meningitis: amphotericin B, total 2.0–2.5 g; indolent disease: ketoconazole 400 mg qd.

HISTOPLASMOSIS

Etiology/pathogenesis: Inhalation of *Histoplasma capsulatum;* in U.S., southeastern, mid-Atlantic, central states.

Clinical manifestations

- Acute pulmonary disease: most asymptomatic or mild; hilar adenopathy; erythema nodosum.
- Chronic pulmonary disease: weight loss; CXR—fibronodular apical infiltrates; 33% stabilize or improve spontaneously.
- Acute disseminated disease: fever, hepatosplenomegaly, lymphadenopathy, jaundice, anemia, leukopenia; 25% have indurated ulcers of mouth; 50% of CXRs show discrete nodules or miliary pattern.
- Ocular: uveitis.

Diagnosis

- Serology: CF > 1:32 suggestive but not diagnostic; may cross-react with blastomycosis.
- Culture (+ in 2–6 weeks) or histology.

Treatment: Same as for blastomycosis.

COCCIDIOIDOMYCOSIS

Etiology/pathogenesis: Infection from inhalation of arthrospores of *Coccidioides immitis;* California, Arizona, W. Texas, New Mexico.

Clinical manifestations

- Symptomatic pulmonary infection: CXR–infiltrate, hilar adenopathy, or pleural effusion; may have mild eosinophilia.
- Chronic progressive pulmonary infection.
- Dissemination: persistence of fever, malaise, hilar or paratracheal adenopathy.

Diagnosis

- Wet smear and culture (biohazard).
- Serology: seroconversion may not occur for up to 8 weeks following onset of primary pulmonary disease, + CF in CSF diagnostic of infection.
- Skin test: converts between third and twenty-first day.

Treatment

- Seriously ill—amphotericin B 0.5–0.7 mg/kg qd × 10–12 weeks; meningitis—long-term intrathecal amphotericin.
- Nonmeningeal disease—ketoconazole 200–400 mg qd × 1 year.

CANDIDIASIS

Etiology/pathogenesis: Increased risk: skin maceration, pregnancy, diabetes, AIDS, hematologic malignancy, antibiotic or steroid therapy.

Clinical manifestations

- Oral thrush.
- Cutaneous candidiasis: red, macerated intertriginous areas.
- Chronic mucocutaneous candidiasis: circumscribed hyperkeratotic skin lesions, dystrophic nails, partial alopecia, oral and vaginal thrush; associated hypofunction of parathyroid, adrenal, or thyroid glands, T-cell function defects.
- Gastrointestinal: ulcerations of distal esophagus.
- Hematogenous: fever; retinal abscesses; pulmonary nodular infiltrate; endocarditis.

Diagnosis: Demonstration of pseudohyphae on wet smear, culture, histology.

Treatment

- Cutaneous: nystatin, ciclopirox, imidazole creams.
- Oral: clotrimazole troches, nystatin suspension.

- Esophageal: ketoconazole 200–400 mg qd; severe—amphotericin B 0.3 mg/kg per day × 5–10 days.
- Bladder: irrigation with amphotericin B 50 μg/mL × 5 days.
- Disseminated: amphotericin B 0.4–0.5 mg/kg × several weeks ± flucytosine 100–150 mg/kg per day.

ASPERGILLOSIS

Etiology/pathogenesis: Inhalation of spores in immunosuppressed patients: < 500 PMNs, high-dose steroids, cytotoxic drugs.

Clinical manifestations

- Allergic bronchial aspergillosis: preexisting asthma, eosinophilia, IgE Ab to *Aspergillus,* fleeting pulmonary infiltrates.
- Endobronchial pulmonary aspergillosis: chronic productive cough, hemoptysis, chronic lung disease.
- Aspergilloma: ball of hyphae within lung cyst or cavity.
- Invasive: acute pneumonia in immunosuppressed.
- Sinusitis: chronic in nonimmunosuppressed.

Diagnosis

• Repeated isolation from sputum suggestive of colonization or infection. • Fungus ball on CXR. • Histopathology and cultures (BC rarely +).

Treatment: Lobectomy for severe hemoptysis with fungus ball. Invasive: amphotericin B can arrest or cure.

MUCORMYCOSIS

Etiology/pathogenesis: Infection by *Rhizopus* or *Mucor* in patients with poorly controlled diabetes (paranasal sinuses and nose); hematologic malignancy or organ transplantation (lung); uremia, severe malnutrition, diarrhea (gastrointestinal).
Diagnosis: Biopsy and histology of nonseptate hyphae; culture difficult.
Treatment: Regulation of diabetes; decrease immunosuppressive drugs; extensive debridement + amphotericin B at least 10–12 weeks: cure in ~50%.

SPOROTRICHOSIS

Etiology/pathogenesis: Inoculation of *Sporothrix schenckii* into subcutaneous tissue by minor trauma; increased risk: nursery workers, florists, gardeners.
Clinical manifestations: Painless red papule at site of inoculation with proximal extension along lymphatic channels.
Diagnosis: Culture of pus, joint fluid, sputum, or skin biopsy.

Treatment

- Cutaneous: saturated potassium iodide in increasing doses up to 4.5–9 mL/per day for 1 month after complete resolution.
- Extracutaneous: amphotericin B.

ACTINOMYCOSIS

Etiology/pathogenesis: Infection by break in mucosa or aspiration of *Actinomyces,* anaerobic higher gram-positive branching bacteria.
Clinical manifestations: cervicofacial; thoracic; abdominal; pelvic: increased with IUD.
Diagnosis: Culture and histologic section (not acid-fast).

Treatment

- Mild cervicofacial: oral tetracycline; penicillin V, or erythromycin 500 mg qid × 2–4 months.
- Thoracic and abdominal: IV penicillin G 2–6 million U qd × 6 weeks, then PO penicillin or tetracycline for 6–12 months; drainage of necrotic tissue and abscesses.

NOCARDIOSIS

Etiology/pathogenesis: Infection through inhalation or local trauma by *N. asteroides* (nocardiosis); increased risk: steroids, cancer, pulmonary alveolar proteinosis, chronic granulomatous disease.

Clinical manifestations

- Pneumonia: fever and productive cough; infiltrate → cavitation.
- CNS: multiple abscesses; if abscess ruptures into ventricle → purulent meningitis.

Diagnosis: Branching, weakly acid-fast organisms in histologic sections or smear of pus or sputum.

Treatment

- Surgical drainage of abscesses or empyemas.
- Sulfisoxazole PO or IV 100 mg/kg per day then to peak blood concentration of 10–15 mg/dL or trimethoprim-sulfamethoxazole PO or IV as 50 mg/kg per day of sulfamethoxazole in 2 doses per day × 6–12 months.

For more detailed discussion of these topics, see Bennett JE: Fungal Infections, Chap. 146, p. 736; and Bennett JE: Actinomycosis and Nocardiosis, Chap. 147, p. 745, in HPIM-11

---

51 RICKETTSIAL INFECTIONS

ROCKY MOUNTAIN SPOTTED FEVER (RMSF)

Epidemiology: Transmission of *Rickettsia rickettsii* by bite of infected tick; >50% of cases from south Atlantic and south central states.

Clinical manifestations

- Incubation 3–12 days: abrupt onset of severe headache, rigors, prostration, generalized myalgia, fevers to 103–104°F; occasionally only low-grade fever, anorexia, lethargy.
- Rash: pink macular lesions on extremities, including palms and soles on fourth day of fever → maculopapular → petechial → ecchymoses.
- Severe infection: shock with gangrene of extremities, buttocks, earlobes, nose.
- Neurologic manifestations: headache, restlessness, stiff back, insomnia; CSF normal.
- Course: in mild cases, all symptoms may abate within 2 weeks without therapy; deaths usually in second week.

Diagnosis

- Serology: Weil-Felix OX-19 > 1:40, OX-2 > 1:20 by tenth day; 4-fold rise in CF.
- Immunofluorescence of skin lesions may be positive by fourth day.

Treatment: Chloramphenicol 50 mg/kg or tetracycline 25 mg/kg loading, then divided q 6 h until afebrile 24 h.

MURINE (ENDEMIC) TYPHUS FEVER

Epidemiology: Infection by bite of rat flea with *Rickettsia typhi;* predominantly urban, late summer; prevalent in southeastern and Gulf Coast states.

Clinical manifestations

- Incubation 8–16 days: headache, backache, arthralgia, nausea, shaking chills; severe frontal headache, fever, nonproductive cough; fever usually lasts 12 days.
- Rash: early lesions in axilla and inner aspect of arm → sudden generalized red, discrete macular rash of upper abdomen, shoulders, chest, arms, thighs → maculopapular; little involvement of extremities.
- Neurologic manifestations: severe frontal headache.
- Course: rapid recovery after defervesence; fatalities unusual.

Diagnosis: Fourfold rise in specific CF by third week; Weil-Felix OX-19 > 160 by tenth day.
Treatment: As for RMSF, but parenteral antibiotics rarely necessary.

EPIDEMIC (LOUSE-BORNE) TYPHUS FEVER

Epidemiology: Infection by exposure to feces of body louse with *Rickettsia prowazekii;* new epidemics from patients with recrudescent typhus (Brill-Zinsser disease) or flying squirrels.

Clinical manifestations

- Incubation 7 days: abrupt headache, chills, fever, malaise; symptoms more severe than murine typhus.
- Rash: macular in axillary folds, trunk, and extremities.
- Neurologic: headache, general spasticity to extreme agitation, stupor, coma.
- Complications: azotemia, thrombosis, cutaneous gangrene.
- Brill-Zinsser disease: recrudescent episode years after initial attack with good recovery.

Diagnosis: Rise in specific CF serology, positive OX-19; in Brill-Zinsser, specific IgG rise as early as fourth day.
Treatment: As for RMSF, usually afebrile after second day.

Q FEVER

Epidemiology: Inhalation of dust or drinking milk contaminated with *Coxiella burnetti.*
Clinical manifestations

- Incubation ~19 days: headache, chills, fever, malaise, myalgia, anorexia; dry cough and chest pain after 5 days; fever may persist 4 weeks if untreated.
- Hepatitis: a third develop protracted disease; granulomas on biopsy.
- Endocarditis: subacute endocarditis with negative BC.

Diagnosis: High CF titer to phase I antigen.
Treatment: Tetracycline or chloramphenicol for at least 2 weeks; endocarditis may require therapy for 2–5 years plus surgery.

For more detailed discussion of this topic, see Woodward TE: Rickettsial Diseases, Chap. 148, in HPIM-11, p. 747

52 *MYCOPLASMA* INFECTIONS

MYCOPLASMA PNEUMONIAE

Epidemiology: 50% of pneumonia in college students; antibody only protective several years.

Clinical manifestations

- Pharyngitis, tracheobronchitis, bullous myringitis, pneumonia.
- Almost all have cough; fever may persist 1–2 weeks if untreated, with prolonged malaise and weakness.
- Rare complications: meningoencephalitis, polyneuritis, monarticular arthritis, Stevens-Johnson syndrome, pericarditis, myocarditis, hepatitis, DIC, hemolytic anemia.

Diagnosis

- Laboratory: 25% WBC 10,000–15,000; ESR > 40 in two-thirds.
- Fourfold rise in CF.
- Cold agglutinins: development of IgM to I antigen on type O RBC; positive in half in first week of illness to 6 weeks.

Treatment: Erythromycin 500 mg tid or tetracycline 250 mg qid × 10–14 days if mild, 21 days if severe.

For more detailed discussion of this topic, see Clyde WA, Jr.: *Mycoplasma* Infections, Chap. 149, in HPIM-11, p. 757

53 CHLAMYDIAL INFECTIONS

C. TRACHOMATIS GENITAL INFECTIONS

Epidemiology: Most common sexually transmitted disease in U.S.; caused by serovars D through K; peak incidence late teens, early twenties.

Clinical manifestations

- Nongonococcal (NGU) and postgonococcal urethritis (PGU).
- Epididymitis: major cause in men under 35.
- Reiter's syndrome: up to 70% of men with untreated nondiarrheal Reiter's with urethritis positive for *chlamydia*.
- Proctitis: symptoms—mild rectal pain, mucus discharge; lymphogranuloma venereum (LGV) more severe.
- Mucopurulent cervicitis.
- Pelvic inflammatory disease (PID).
- Urethral syndrome: most common isolate from young women with acute dysuria, frequency, and pyuria with urine cultures negative for bacteria.

Diagnosis

- Antigen detection: direct immunofluorescence of infected secretions, ELISA.
- Culture: difficult to grow in tissue culture except for LGV stains.
- Serology: fourfold increase in CF or microimmunofluorescence useful in LGV, infant pneumonia, or perihepatitis.

Treatment

- NGU: tetracycline 500 mg qid, doxycycline 100 mg bid, or erythromycin 500 mg qid × 7 days.
- Cervical: tetracycline 500 mg qid × 14 days; erythromycin if pregnant.
- Should treat all patients with gonorrhea and sexual partners for *chlamydia*.

LYMPHOGRANULOMA VENEREUM (LGV)

Epidemiology: Sexually transmitted disease by strains L_1, L_2, or L_3; occasional nonsexual transmission.

Clinical manifestations

- Primarily genital lesion: in heterosexuals 3 days to 3 weeks after exposure; small painless vesicle or nonindurated ulcer.
- Primary rectal infection: women and homosexual men; proctitis.
- Inguinal syndrome: painful inguinal lymphadenopathy 2–6 weeks after exposure; two-thirds unilateral; may progress to matted nodes and fistulas.
- Constitutional symptoms: fever, chills, headache, meningismus, anorexia, arthralgias, myalgias.
- Complications: perirectal abscess, fistulas, strictures.

Diagnosis

• Laboratory findings: elevated WBC, ESR; may have elevated LFTs. • Culture of bubo aspirate and rectum. • Serology: CF titer ≥ 1:64 suggestive.

Treatment: Tetracycline 500 mg qid or sulfonamide 4 g qd × 3 weeks; aspirate all buboes.

TRACHOMA AND ADULT INCLUSION CONJUNCTIVITIS

Epidemiology

- Trachoma: serovars A, B, and C; eye-to-eye spread in endemic areas.
- Inclusion conjunctivitis: sexually transmitted through infected genital secretions.

Clinical manifestations

- Endemic trachoma: conjunctivitis with small lymphoid follicles (usually < 2 years old); cornea with leukocytic infiltration and superficial vascularization (pannus) → conjunctival scarring → inturned eyelashes → bacterial corneal ulcer → blindness.
- Genital strains: acute unilateral follicular conjunctivitis and periauricular lymphadenopathy in sexually active young adults.

Diagnosis

- Clinical diagnosis of classical trachoma if two of following present: (1) lymphoid follicles on upper tarsal conjunctiva, (2) conjunctival scarring, (3) vascular pannus, (4) limbal follicles.
- Giemsa- or immunofluorescent-stained smears of conjunctiva; culture; antibody not diagnostic.

Treatment: Topical tetracycline or erythromycin for 21–60 days or oral erythromycin for 3 weeks.

PSITTACOSIS

Epidemiology: Respiratory transmission of *C. psittaci* from any avian species, especially psittacine.
Clinical manifestations: Incubation 7–14 days: fever, chills, headache, dry cough, myalgias; splenomegaly 10–70%.

Diagnosis

- Laboratory findings: usually patchy infiltrate on CXR; WBC normal or elevated; LFTs usually normal.
- Diagnose by culture or serology (but may cross-react with *C. trachomatis*).

Treatment: Tetracycline 500 mg qid for at least 7 days after defervescence.

For more detailed discussion of this topic, see Stamm WE, Holmes KK: Chlamydial Infections, Chap. 150, in HPIM-11, p. 759

54 PARASITIC DISEASES

AMEBIASIS

Epidemiology: Infection caused by ingestion of cyst of *E. histolytica;* risk: poor hygiene (poverty, poor sanitation, mental retardation), homosexuals.

Clinical manifestations

- Intestinal: intermittent diarrhea with watery stools and/or mucus and blood.
- Hepatic: insidious or abrupt onset with fever, sweats, weight loss, RUQ pain, nausea, ↑ WBCs; ↑ SGOT and bilirubin with more severe disease.
- Pleuropulmonary: direct extension into right pleural cavity and lung in 10–20% with liver abscess.
- Other extraintestinal: pericarditis, peritonitis.

Diagnosis

- Identification: cysts in formed stools; motile trophozoites in liquid stools.
- Serology: + in >90% of patients with hepatic abscess and most with colitis.
- Liver abscess: liver scan, ultrasound, or CT very sensitive (must differentiate from pyogenic abscess or hydatid cyst).

Treatment

- Asymptomatic carrier: iodoquinol 650 mg tid × 20 days or dilanoxide furoate (from CDC) 500 mg tid × 10 days. Intestinal disease: mild to moderate—metronidazole 750 mg tid × 5–10 days + luminal agent; severe—metronidazole + dehydroemetine 1.0–1.5 mg/kg IM daily × 5 days.
- Extraintestinal: metronidazole + luminal agent or chloroquine phosphate 1 g qd × 2, then 500 mg qd × 4 weeks + dehydroemetine for 10 days or emetine 1 mg/kg IM qd × 10 days; aspirate if imminent rupture, failure to respond to medical therapy in 72 h.

MALARIA

Epidemiology

- Four species: *Plasmodium vivax, P. ovale, P. malariae, P. falciparum;* transmitted by bite of female anopheles mosquito.
- Infection starts with attachment to specific receptor on red blood cell surface; most W. Africans resistant to *P. vivax*.
- Drug-resistant *P. falciparum* in areas of S. Asia, W. Pacific, Central America, S. America, Africa, India.
- Parasitemia limited in sickle cell trait, thalassemia, G6PD deficiency.

TABLE 54-1 **Treatment of acute malaria**

Infection	Drug	Dosage
Chloroquine-resistant *P. falciparum*	Quinine sulftate	650 mg PO tid × 10–14 days
	or quinine dihydrochloride (from CDC)	600 mg in 300 mL normal saline (NS) IV over 1 h, repeat in 6–8 h
	or quinidine gluconate	800 mg in 300 mL NS IV over 1 h, repeat in 6–8h
	plus pyrimethamine	25 mg PO bid × 3 days
	plus sulfadiazine	500 mg PO bid × 5 days
	or quinine as above	
	plus tetracycline	250 mg qid × 7 days
	or quinine	
	plus clindamycin	900 mg tid × 3 days
P. malariae and chloroquine-sensitive *P. falciparum*	Chloroquine	1 g (600 mg base) PO, then 500 mg in 6 h, then 500 mg qd × 2 days
	or chloroquine hydrochloride	250 mg (200 mg base) IM or IV q 6 h
P. vivax, P. ovale	Same as *P. malariae plus* primaquine phosphate	26.3 mg (15 mg base) PO qd × 14 days (rule out G6PD deficiency)

Modified from Plorde JJ, White NJ: HPIM-11, p. 782.

Clinical manifestations

- *P. vivax* or *P. ovale:* incubation 10–14 days; prodrome of myalgia, headache, chills before paroxysm of rigor, sudden fever, then defervesence; occur every other day with synchronized infection.
- *P. malariae:* paroxysms every third day; mildest and most chronic; immune-complex nephropathy.
- *P. falciparum:* onset insidious with irregular fever; splenomegaly, headache, confusion, hypotension, edema; GI symptoms common; encephalopathy, abnormal renal function.
- Complications of *P. falciparum:* acute pulmonary insufficiency third or fourth day of therapy; blackwater fever—massive intravascular hemolysis → hemoglobinuria → acute renal failure.

Diagnosis: Laboratory findings: WBC normal or ↓, ↑ ESR; thin or thick blood smears on Wright or Giemsa stain; *P. vivax*—immature (enlarged) RBCs, diffuse red dots (Schuffner's dots); *P. ovale*—RBC often oval; *P. malariae*—"band" forms; *P. falciparum*—small rings, often two chromatin dots, banana-shaped gametocyte.

TREATMENT

- See Table 54-1.
- Severe falciparum malaria: exchange transfusion if >10% parasitemia; dexamethasone, mannitol, and heparin should be avoided.
- Prophylaxis (see Table 54-2).

TABLE 54-2 **Prophylaxis for malaria**

Purpose	Drug	Dosage
Suppression in areas without chloroquine resistance	Chloroquine phosphate	500 mg (300 mg base) PO weekly for 6 weeks after return
	or amodiaquine dihydrochloride	520 mg (400 mg base) PO weekly + 6 weeks after return
Areas with chloroquine resistance		
>3 weeks	Chloroquine as above	
	plus Fansidar	25 mg pyrimethamine/500 mg sulfadoxine weekly + 6 weeks after return
	or mefloquine	250 mg weekly + 6 weeks after return
<3 weeks	Chloroquine as above	
	Fansidar	Take along therapeutic dose—3 tablets
Prevent relapse of *P. vivax* and *P. ovale*	Primaquine phosphate	26.3 mg (15 mg base) PO qd × 14 days or 45 mg base weekly × 8 during last 2 weeks of suppressive therapy

Modified from Plorde JJ, White NJ: HPIM-11, p. 784.

TOXOPLASMOSIS

Clinical manifestations

- Lymphadenopathy: acute acquired infection in immunocompetent host; also confusion, malaise, stiff neck, sore throat, macular rash sparing palms and soles, hepatosplenomegaly, reactive lymphocytes can occur.
- Ocular involvement: 35% of all chorioretinitis; usually reactivation of congenital disease; systemic symptoms rare.
- Immunocompromised: increased with immunosuppression for lymphoproliferative disorders, hematologic malignancy, organ transplants; >50% CNS involvement, CSF—slight increase in mononuclear cells and protein, normal glucose.
- Encephalitis and AIDS: chills, fever, headache, seizures, decreased mental status, neurologic findings; usually no increased antibody titers, CSF normal or ↑ WBCs and protein, ↓ glucose; CT—diffuse encephalitis and/or mass lesion(s).

Diagnosis

• Tissue culture; intraperitoneal in mice. • Histology: demonstration of tachyzoites in tissue sections. • Serology: Sabin-Feldman dye test and IFA measure IgG; ocular toxo usually with low positive titers; acute disease in pregnant women— ↑ IgM.

Therapy: Pyrimethamine—loading 100–200 mg in two doses × 2 days then 1 mg/kg up to 25 mg qd (50 mg in immunodeficient) + folinic acid 5–20 mg qd + sulfadiazine 50–75 mg/kg, then 75–

100 mg/kg qd in 4 divided doses for 4–6 weeks with active chorioretinitis or 4–6 weeks after resolution of active disease in immunocompromised patient.

PNEUMOCYSTIS CARINII PNEUMONIA

Epidemiology/pathogenesis: Airborne transmission of protozoa; most pneumonia reactivation. Increased risk: premature, malnourished infants; children with primary immunodeficiency diseases; immunosuppressive therapy (especially corticosteroids) for cancer, organ transplantation; AIDS.
Clinical manifestations: Pneumonia.
Diagnosis: Histopathologic staining by methenamine silver of sputum (rare), transtracheal aspiration, bronchoalveolar lavage and/or transbronchial biopsy, open lung biopsy.

Treatment

- Trimethoprim/sulfamethoxazole 20/100 mg/kg per day PO or IV in four doses × 14 days; 60–80% AIDS patients develop rash, fever, leukopenia.
- Pentamidine: 4 mg/kg per day × 14 days IM or slow IV infusion; 50% develop hypoglycemia, hyperglycemia, hypocalcemia, azotemia, hepatic dysfunction.

GIARDIASIS

Epidemiology/pathogenesis

- Ingestion of cysts of protozoa, *Giardia lamblia.*
- Most frequent cause of outbreaks of waterborne diarrhea in U.S.
- Increased risk: contaminated water supplies, male homosexuals, children in day-care centers; Ig deficiencies, achlorhydria.

Clinical manifestations: Diarrhea 1–3 weeks.
Diagnosis: Identification of cyst in feces or trophozoite in diarrheal stool, duodenal secretions (Enterotest), or jejunal biopsies.

Treatment

- Quinacrine 100 mg tid × 5 days; 70–95% effective; may produce GI disturbances.
- Metronidazole 2 g qd × 3 days or 750 mg tid × 5 days; fewer side effects; should not be used in pregnancy.

CRYPTOSPORIDIOSIS

Epidemiology: Fecal-oral transmission of oocysts; increased risk—homosexuals, day-care centers, immunosuppression, ↓ Ig.
Clinical manifestations: abdominal cramps.
Diagnosis: Demonstration of oocysts in stool.
Treatment: Self-limited in immunocompetent patients; no proven therapy in immunosuppressed patients.

ISOSPORIASIS

Epidemiology: Ingestion of cysts of *Isospora belli;* increased in children in tropical areas and male homosexuals.
Clinical manifestations: Abdominal cramps, diarrhea.
Diagnosis: 50% with increased eosinophils; acid-fast oocysts in stool, duodenal aspirates, jejunal biopsies.
Treatment: Trimethoprim/sulfamethoxazole 160/800 mg qid × 10 days, then bid × 3 weeks.

TRICHINOSIS

Epidemiology/pathogenesis: Ingestion of meat containing encysted larvae of *Trichinella spiralis,* especially pork or walrus; prevalent in Europe, New England, Louisiana, Hawaii, Alaska.

Clinical manifestations

- Asymptomatic → severe disease.
- Intestinal phase: diarrhea, abdominal pain, nausea, fever.
- Muscular invasion: fever, periorbital edema, conjunctivitis, subconjunctival hemorrhages, muscle pain and tenderness, subungual hemorrhages.
- Lung: hemoptysis, consolidation on CXR.
- CNS: polyneuritis, meningitis, encephalitis, normal CSF.
- Cardiac: persistent tachycardia, CHF; 20% ST-T wave abnormalities.

Diagnosis: Eosinophilia; serology; demonstration of larvae in muscle biopsy.

Treatment: Thiabendazole 25 mg/kg bid × 5–7 days; prednisone 20–60 mg qd if myocardial, CNS, or allergic.

SCHISTOSOMIASIS

Epidemiology/pathogenesis

- Infection after contact with water containing infective stage (cercariae) → migrate to lungs → portal veins where mature to adult schistosomes; pathology due to granulomatous reaction to eggs, dependent on duration and intensity of exposure.
- *S. mansoni:* S. America (Brazil, Venezuela, Surinam), Caribbean Islands, Africa, Middle East.
- *S. japonicum:* China, Philippines.
- *S. haematobium:* Africa, Middle East.

Clinical manifestations

- Acute schistosomiasis: *S. mansoni* and *japonicum;* intense itching; 2–6 weeks later fever, chills, headache, angioedema, weakness, abdominal pain, diarrhea; may last 2–3 months.
- Liver fibrosis: *S. mansoni* and *S. japonicum.*
- Glomerulonephritis and pulmonary hypertension.
- Urinary tract: *S. haematobium;* dysuria and hematuria, anatomic obstruction, hydroureter, hydronephrosis, renal failure rare.

Diagnosis: Acute schistosomiasis: eosinophilia >50%, positive serology; identification of ova in stool (*S. mansoni, S. japonicum*) or urine (*S. haematobium*); serology.
Treatment: Prazequantel 40 mg/kg single dose or 20 mg/kg × 2 4 h apart.

INTESTINAL NEMATODES

ENTEROBIASIS (PIN WORM) Epidemiology: Ingestion of eggs of *Enterobius vermicularis;* most common helminthic infection.
Clinical manifestations: Pruritus ani at night.
Diagnosis: Identification of ova in perianal area using tape over end of tongue blade.
Treatment: Mebendazole 100 mg bid × 3 days.

TRICHURIASIS (WHIPWORM) Epidemiology: Ingestion of eggs of *Trichuris trichuria;* especially in tropics and southeastern U.S.; most common helminthic infection in Americans returning from tropics.
Clinical manifestations: Symptoms only with heavy infection, especially in children—nausea, abdominal pain, diarrhea.
Diagnosis: Identification of eggs in feces.
Treatment: Mebendazole 100 mg bid × 3 days.

ASCARIASIS Epidemiology: Ingestion of embryonated eggs of *Ascaris lumbricoides* from contaminated food or soil; larvae migrate through intestinal wall → lungs → swallowed → jejunum.
Clinical manifestations: Fever, cough, dyspnea, ↑ eosinophils, migratory pulmonary infiltrates, abdominal pain with heavy infection, malabsorption.
Diagnosis: Ova in feces; passage of adult worm.
Treatment: Mebendazole 100 mg bid × 3 days.

HOOKWORM DISEASE Epidemiology: Infection through skin penetration of filariform larvae of *Ancyclostoma duodenale* or *Necator americanus;* migrate through lungs to intestine.
Clinical manifestations: If severe, iron-deficiency anemia and hypoalbuminemia.
Diagnosis: Identification of ova in feces.
Treatment: Mebendazole as for ascariasis.

STRONGYLOIDIASIS Epidemiology: Infection by penetration of skin by larva of *Strongyloides stercoralis;* after migration through lung, adults mature in small intestine; may develop autoinfection where larvae invade intestinal mucosa or perianal skin without going through soil phase.
Clinical manifestations: Transitory skin eruptions with blotchy erythema, urticaria, cough, dyspnea, bronchospasm, epigastric pain, tenderness, nausea; debilitated and immunodepressed patients—widespread dissemination of larvae to extraintestinal organs.
Diagnosis: Identification of larvae in fresh fecal specimens, duodenal aspirates, or jejunal biopsies; ↑ eosinophils except in very severe cases.

Treatment: Thiabendazole 25 mg/kg bid × 2–3 days (7 days with disseminated infection).

TREMATODES OR FLUKES (see HPIM-11, Chap. 167)

CESTODE (TAPEWORM) INFECTIONS (see HPIM-11, Chap. 168)

For more detailed discussion of these topics, see Plorde JJ: Amebiasis, Chap. 153, p. 773; Plorde JJ, White NJ: Malaria, Chap. 154, p. 778; Locksley RM, Plorde JJ: Leishmaniasis, Chap. 155, p. 785; Plorde JJ: Trypanosomiasis, Chap. 156 p. 787; McLeod R, Remington JS: Toxoplasmosis, Chap. 157, p. 791; Walzer PD: *Pneumocystis carinii* Pneumonia, Chap. 158, p. 797; Plorde JJ: Babesiosis, Chap. 159, p. 799; Plorde JJ: Giardiasis, Chap. 160, p. 800; Plorde JJ: Cryptosporidiosis and Other Protozoan Infections, Chap. 161, p. 801; Plorde JJ: Trichinosis, Chap. 162, p. 805; Plorde JJ: Filariasis, Chap. 163, p. 807; Nash TE: Schistosomiasis, Chap. 164, p. 810; Plorde JJ: Tissue Nematodes, Chap. 165, p. 814; Plorde JJ: Intestinal Nematodes, Chap. 166, p. 816; Plorde JJ: Other Trematodes or Flukes, Chap. 167, p. 822; and Ramsey PG, Plorde JJ: Cestode (Tapeworm) Infections, Chap. 168, p. 825, in HPIM-11

---

55 OTHER INFECTIONS OF CLINICAL IMPORTANCE

LEGIONELLA INFECTIONS

Etiology/epidemiology

- Aerobic gram-negative rods with complex growth requirements; thrive in hot water distribution systems of buildings, causing common-source outbreaks.
- Infection by respiratory inhalation; incubation 2–10 days.
- Increased risk with smoking, chronic renal failure, malignancy, immunosuppression.

Clinical manifestations

- Malaise, headache, nonproductive cough → cough productive of mucoid sputum, pleuritic chest pain, myalgia; ~25% GI symptoms.
- May require 4–5 days to show clinical response despite antibiotics.
- Complications: 10–15% respiratory failure; hypotension, shock.

Diagnosis

Laboratory findings: normal to ↑ WBCs (20% > 20,000), ↑ ESR, mild proteinuria. CXR: 65% unilateral pulmonary parenchymal infiltrates → bilateral; a third show pleural effusions. Culture requires selective media. Immunofluorescent staining of specimens: less sensitive than culture. Serology.
Treatment: Erythromycin 0.5–1 g q 6 h IV or PO × 14 days.

LEPROSY

Etiology/epidemiology: Chronic granulomatous infection with *Mycobacterium leprae*; human-to-human transmission, probably from nasal secretions of untreated lepromatous patients.

Clinical manifestations

- Early leprosy: one or more hypopigmented or hyperpigmented mascules or plaques, often anesthetic.
- Tuberculoid: early—hypopigmented macule; nerve involvement early; ulnar, peroneal, and greater auricular nerves may be palpable → muscle atrophy; contractures; trauma; corneal ulcerations.
- Lepromatous: hypopigmented macules, nodules, plaques, papules, especially face, ears, wrists, buttocks, knees; loss of lateral eyebrows; early nasal symptoms → nasal obstruction, laryngitis, hoarseness.
- Borderline: borderline tuberculoid—increased skin lesions and involvement of multiple peripheral nerves; borderline lepromatous—heterogeneous and symmetric skin lesions.
- Reactional states: erythema nodosum leprosum (ENL) in lepromatous; reversal reaction.

- Complications: most frequent cause of crippling of hand in world; trauma and secondary chronic infections → loss of digits; blindness.

Diagnosis: Demonstration of acid-fast bacilli in skin smears, skin or nerve biopsies, but may be negative in tuberculoid; 10–40% of lepromatous false positive VDRL.

Treatment

- Tuberculoid, borderline tuberculoid: dapsone 50–100 mg qd + rifampin 600 mg qd × 6–12 months, then dapsone alone × 18 months.
- Borderline, borderline lepromatous: dapsone + rifampin for minimum of 2 years if dapsone-sensitive.
- Lepromatous: dapsone + rifampin + clofazamine 50–200 mg qd indefinitely.

LEPTOSPIROSIS

Epidemiology: Infection by contact with urine or tissue of infected animal through abrasions or mucous membranes; two-thirds by incidental exposure to contaminated water.

Clinical manifestations

- Incubation average of 10 days; leptospiremic phase—abrupt headache, severe myalgias, chills, high fevers, conjunctival suffusion, pharyngeal infection, cutaneous hemorrhages, maculopapular rashes on trunk; lasts 4–9 days.
- "Immune phase": appearance of IgM; fever and/or meningismus (50–90% pleocytosis in CSF).
- Weil's syndrome: severe leptospirosis with jaundice, azotemia.
- Aseptic meningitis.
- Myocarditis.

Diagnosis

- Laboratory findings: >70% PMN; increased to >70,000 WBCs; platelets may be <30,000; half show increased CK in first phase; mild proteinuria.
- Cultured from blood or CSF during first phase or urine during second on semisolid medium (Fletcher's).
- Serology: fourfold rise in agglutination; 6–12th day of illness.

Treatment: Only useful within 4 days of onset; doxycycline 100 mg bid × 7 days or penicillin G; Jarisch-Herxheimer reaction.

LYME DISEASE

Epidemiology: Infection with spirochete *Borrelia burgdorferi*, through bite of ixodid tick; greatest incidence in Northeast and Midwest (Wisconsin, Minnesota).

Clinical manifestations

- Stage 1: 3–32 days; erythema chronicum migrans + severe headache, mild neck stiffness, fever, chills, malaise.

- Stage 2: several weeks to months; 15% frank neurologic abnormalities—meningitis, cranial neuritis, mononeuritis multiplex, chorea; CSF—~100 lymphs, ↑ protein, normal to ↓ glucose; 8% cardiac—AV block, acute myocarditis, usually lasts a few weeks.
- Stage 3: weeks–2 years after onset, 60% arthritis—lasts weeks to months with recurrences.

Diagnosis

• Serology: ↑ IgG after 2–3 weeks; may cross-react with *T. pallidum*. • Culture: may be positive early in disease from blood, skin, CSF but difficult.

Treatment

• Early: tetracycline 250 mg qid, penicillin V 500 mg qid, erythromycin 250 mg qid × 10–20 days. • Meningitis, neuropathies, AV block: 20 million U penicillin G per day × 10 days.

For more detailed discussion of these topics, see Beaty HN, Pasculle AW: *Legionella* Infections, Chap. 117, p. 620; Miller RA: Leprosy (Hansen's Disease), Chap. 120, p. 633; Sanford JP: Leptospirosis, Chap. 124, p. 652; Hirschmann JV: Rat-Bite Fever (*Streptobacillus moniliformis* and *Spirillum minus* Infections), Chap. 125, p. 655; and Steere AC: Lyme Disease, Chap. 127, p. 657, in HPIM-11

SECTION III
CARDIOVASCULAR DISEASE

56 PHYSICAL EXAMINATION OF THE HEART

General examination of a patient with suspected heart disease should include vital signs (respiratory rate, pulse, blood pressure), skin color, clubbing, edema, evidence of decreased perfusion (cool and sweaty skin), and hypertensive changes in optic fundi. Important findings on cardiovascular examination include:

CAROTID ARTERY PULSE

1 *Pulsus parvus:* Weak upstroke due to decreased stroke volume (hypovolemia, LV failure, aortic or mitral stenosis).

2 *Pulsus tardus:* Delayed upstroke (aortic stenosis).

3 *Bounding pulse:* Hyperkinetic circulation, aortic regurgitation, patent ductus arteriosus, marked vasodilatation.

4 *Pulsus bisferiens:* Double systolic pulsation in aortic regurgitation, hypertrophic cardiomyopathy.

5 *Pulsus alternans:* Regular alteration in pulse pressure amplitude (severe LV dysfunction).

6 *Pulsus paradoxus:* Exaggerated inspiratory fall (>10 mmHg) in systolic BP (pericardial tamponade, obstructive lung disease).

JUGULAR VENOUS PULSATION (JVP) (Fig. 56-1) Jugular venous distention develops in right-sided heart failure, constrictive pericarditis, pericardial tamponade, obstruction of superior vena cava. JVP normally *falls* with inspiration, but may *rise* (Kussmaul's sign) in constrictive pericarditis. Abnormalities in examination include:

1 *Large "a" wave:* Tricuspid stenosis, pulmonic stenosis, AV dissociation (right atrium contracts against closed tricuspid valve).

2 *Large "v" wave:* Tricuspid regurgitation, atrial septal defect.

3 *Steep "y" descent:* Constrictive pericarditis.

4 *Slow "y" descent:* Tricuspid stenosis.

PRECORDIAL PALPATION Cardiac apical impulse is normally localized in the fifth intercostal space, midclavicular line. Abnormalities include:

1 *Forceful apical thrust:* Left ventricular hypertrophy.

2 *Lateral and downward displacement of apex impulse:* Left ventricular dilatation.

3 *Prominent presystolic impulse:* Hypertension, aortic stenosis, hypertrophic cardiomyopathy.

4 *Double systolic apical impulse:* Hypertrophic cardiomyopathy.
5 *Sustained "lift" at lower left sternal border:* Right ventricular hypertrophy.
6 *Dyskinetic (outward bulge) impulse:* Ventricular aneurysm, large dyskinetic area post MI, cardiomyopathy.

AUSCULTATION

HEART SOUNDS **S_1:** *Loud:* Mitral stenosis, short PR interval, hyperkinetic heart, thin chest wall; *Soft:* Long PR interval, heart failure, mitral regurgitation, thick chest wall, pulmonary emphysema.

S_2: Normally A_2 precedes P_2 and splitting increases with inspiration; abnormalities include:

- *Widened* splitting: right bundle branch block, pulmonic stenosis, mitral regurgitation.
- *Fixed* splitting (no respiratory change in splitting); atrial septal defect.
- *Narrow* splitting: pulmonary hypertension.
- *Paradoxical* splitting (splitting *narrows* with inspiration): Aortic stenosis, left bundle branch block, CHF.
- *Loud* A_2: systemic hypertension.
- *Soft* A_2: Aortic stenosis (AS).
- *Loud* P_2: Pulmonary arterial hypertension.
- *Soft* P_2: Pulmonic stenosis (PS).

S_3: Low-pitched, heard best with bell of stethoscope at apex, following S_2; normal in children; after age 30–35, indicates LV failure or volume overload.

FIG. 56-1. *Normal jugular venous pressure recording.*

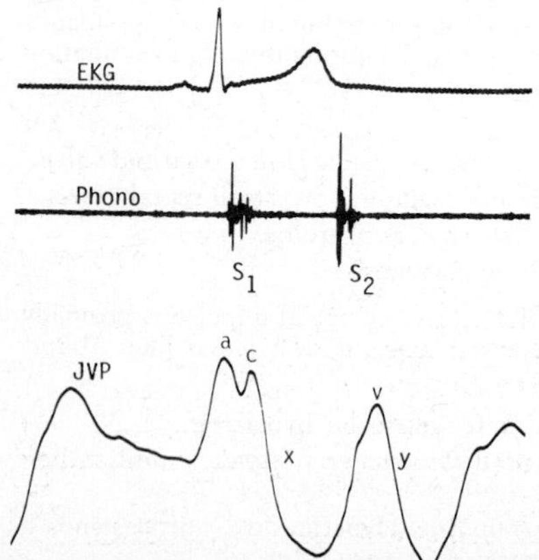

TABLE 56-1

Lesion	Type of murmur	Maneuver: Valsalva	Hand grip	Squat	Stand
Aortic stenosis	Crescendo-decrescendo	↓	↓	↑	↓
Mitral regurgitation	Holosystolic	↓	↑	↑	↓
Ventricular septal defect	Holosystolic	↓	↑	↑	↓
Mitral valve prolapse	Late systolic (follows click)	↑	↓	↓	↑
Hypertrophic obstructive cardiomyopathy	Harsh, diamond-shaped at left sternal border; holosystolic at apex	↑	↓	↓	↑

S_4: Low-pitched, heard best with bell at apex, preceding S_1; reflects atrial contraction into a noncompliant ventricle; found in AS, hypertension, hypertrophic cardiomyopathy, and CAD.
Opening snap (OS): High-pitched; follows S_2 (by 0.06–0.12 s), heard at lower left sternal border and apex in mitral stenosis (MS); the more severe the MS, the shorter the OS–S_2 interval.
Ejection clicks: High-pitched sounds following S_1; observed in dilatation of aortic root or pulmonary artery, congenital AS (loudest at apex) or PS (upper left sternal border); the latter *decreases* with inspiration.
Midsystolic clicks: At lower left sternal border and apex, often followed by late systolic murmur in mitral valve prolapse.

HEART MURMURS **Systolic murmurs:** May be "crescendo-decrescendo" ejection type, pansystolic, or late systolic; right-sided murmurs (e.g., tricuspid regurgitation) typically increased with inspiration. A number of simple maneuvers produce characteristic changes depending on etiology of murmur (Table 56-1).
Diastolic murmurs:

1 *Early diastolic murmurs:* Begin immediately after S_2, are high-pitched, and usually are caused by aortic or pulmonary regurgitation.

2 *Mid-to-late diastolic murmurs:* Low-pitched, heard best with bell of stethoscope; observed in MS or TS (Chap. 62); less commonly due to abnormally increased transvalvular flow as in atrial myxoma.

3 *Continuous murmurs:* Present in systole and diastole (envelops S_2); found in patent ductus arteriosus and sometimes in coarctation of aorta; less common causes are systemic or coronary AV fistula, aortic septal defect, ruptured aneurysm of sinus of Valsalva.

For more detailed discussion of this topic, see O'Rourke RA, Braunwald E: Physical Examination of the Heart, Chap. 177, in HPIM-11, p. 865

57 ELECTROCARDIOGRAPHY AND ECHOCARDIOGRAPHY

STANDARD APPROACH TO THE ECG

Normally, standardization is 1.0 mV per 10 mm, and paper speed is 25 mm/s (each horizontal small box = 0.04 s).

HEART RATE Beats/min = 300 divided by the number of *large* boxes (each 5 mm apart) between consecutive QRS complexes. For faster heart rates, divide 1500 by number of *small* boxes (1 mm apart) between each QRS.

RHYTHM *Sinus rhythm* is present if every P wave is followed by a QRS, PR interval ≥ 0.12 s, every QRS is preceded by a P wave, and the P wave is upright in leads I, II, and III. Abnormal rhythms are discussed in Chap. 60.

MEAN AXIS If QRS is primarily positive in limb leads I and II, then axis is *normal.* Otherwise, find limb lead in which QRS is most isoelectric (R = S). The mean axis is perpendicular to that lead (Fig. 57-1). If the QRS complex is *positive* in that perpendicular lead, then mean axis is in the direction of that lead; if *negative,* then mean axis points directly away from that lead.

Left-axis deviation (< −30°) occurs in diffuse left ventricular disease, inferior MI; also in left anterior hemiblock (small r, deep S in leads II, III, aVF).

Right-axis deviation (>90°) occurs in right ventricular hypertrophy (R > S in V_1) and left posterior hemiblock (small Q and tall R in leads II, III, and aVF). Mild right-axis deviation is seen in thin, healthy individuals (up to 110°).

INTERVALS (normal values in parentheses)
PR (0.12–0.20 s):

- *Short:* (1) preexcitation syndrome (look for slurred QRS upstroke due to "delta" wave), (2) nodal rhythm (inverted P in aVF).
- *Long:* first-degree AV block (Chap. 60).

QRS (0.06–0.10 s).

- *Widened:* (1) ventricular premature beats, (2) bundle-branch blocks: *right* (RsR′ in V_1, deep S in V_6) and *left* (RR′ in V_6) (see Fig. 57-2), (3) toxic levels of certain drugs (e.g., quinidine), (4) severe hypokalemia.

QT (≤0.43 s; <50% of RR interval):

- *Prolonged* congenital: hypokalemia, hypocalcemia, drugs (quinidine, procainamide, tricyclics).

HYPERTROPHY

- *Right atrium:* P wave ≥ 2.5 mm in lead II.
- *Left atrium:* P biphasic (positive, then negative) in V_1, with terminal negative force wider than 0.04 s.

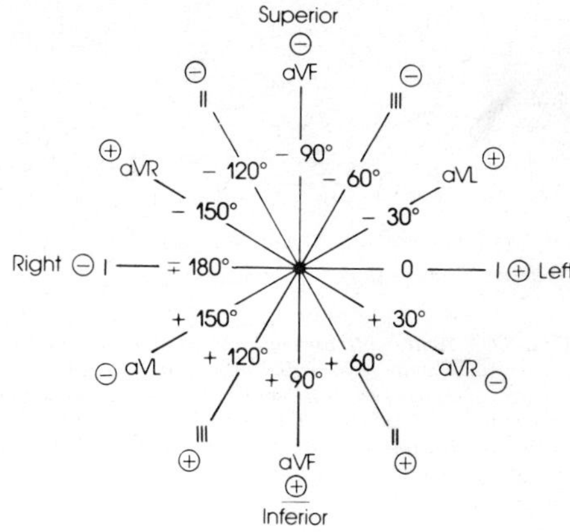

FIG. 57-1 *Electrocardiographic lead systems: The hexaxial frontal plane reference system to estimate electrical axis. Determine leads in which QRS deflections are maximum and minimum. For example, a maximum positive QRS in I which is isoelectric in aVF is oriented to 0°. Normal axis ranges from −30° to +90°. An axis >+90° is right axis deviation and <30° is left axis deviation. Normal ranges are described in the text, and applications are derived in Figs. 178-5 and 178-6 in HPIM-11. (Reproduced from Myerburg RJ: HPIM-11, p. 872.)*

FIG. 57-2 *Intraventricular conduction abnormalities. Illustrated are right bundle branch block (RBBB); left bundle branch block (LBBB); left anterior hemiblock (LAH); right bundle branch block with left anterior hemiblock (RBBB + LAH); and right bundle branch block with left posterior hemiblock (RBBB + LPH). (Reproduced from Myerburg RJ: HPIM-11, p 879.)*

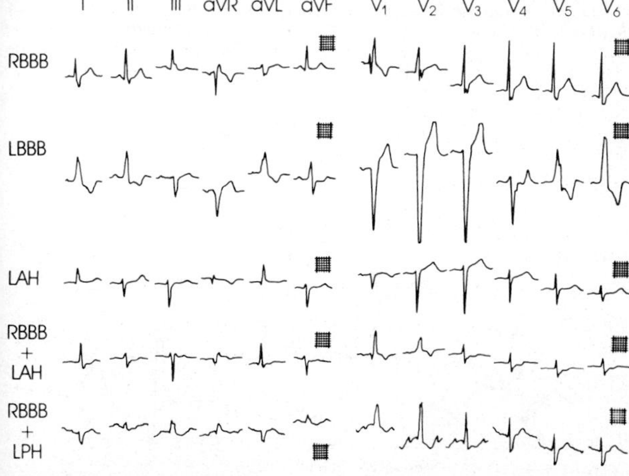

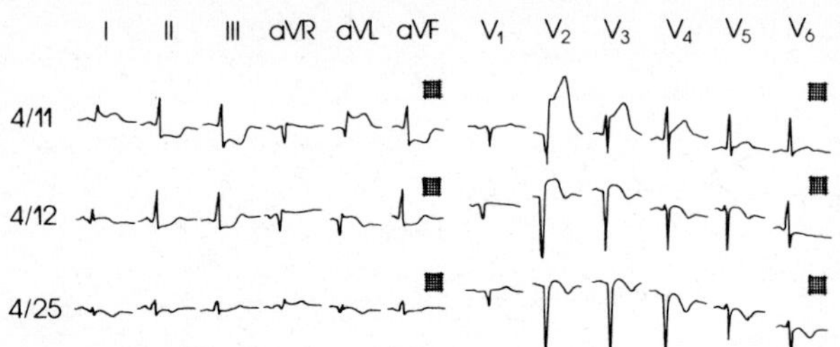

FIG. 57-3 *Acute anterior wall myocardial infarction. On 4/11, changes of a very early acute myocardial infarction in leads I, aVL, V_2, and V_3, with reciprocal changes in II, III, and aVF. On 4/12, ST segments remain elevated in the anterior leads, but T waves are inverted. On 4/25, a completed large anterior myocardial infarction is recorded—Q in I, aVL, V_1 to V_4. (Reproduced from Myerburg RJ: HPIM-11, p 878.)*

- *Right ventricle:* R > S in V_1 and R in V_1 > 5 mm; deep S in V_6; right-axis deviation.
- *Left ventricle:* S in V_1 plus R in V_5 or $V_6 \geq 35$ mm or R in aVL > 11 mm.

INFARCTION (Fig. 57-3 and 57-4) *Q-wave MI:* Pathologic Q waves (≥0.04 s and ≥25% of total QRS height) in leads shown in Table 57-1; acute *non-Q-wave MI* shows ST-T changes in these leads without Q wave development:

FIG. 57-4 *Acute inferior wall myocardial infarction. The ECG of 11/29 shows minor nonspecific ST-segment and T-wave changes. On 12/5 an acute myocardial infarction occurred. There are pathologic Q waves (1), ST-segment elevation (2), and terminal T-wave inversion (3) in leads II, III and aVF indicating the location of the infarct on the inferior wall. Reciprocal changes in aVL (small arrow). Increasing R-wave voltage with ST depression and increased voltage of the T wave in V_2 is characteristic of true posterior wall extension of the inferior infarction. (Reproduced from Myerburg RJ: HPIM-11, p 878.)*

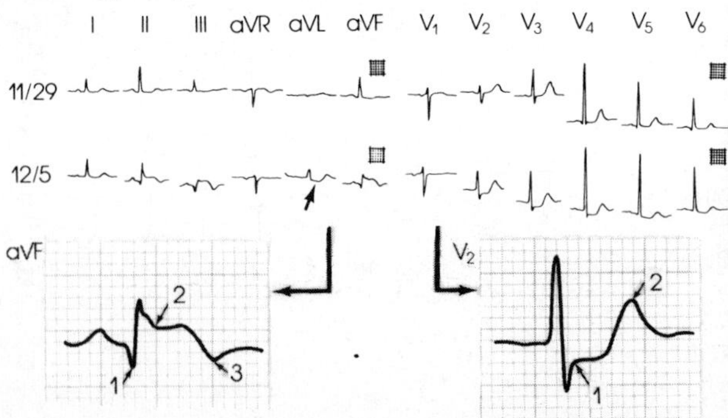

TABLE 57-1

Leads	Site of infarction
V_1–V_2	Anteroseptal
V_3–V_4	Apical
I, aVL, V_5–V_6	Anterolateral
II, III, aVF	Inferior
V_1–V_2 (tall R, *not* deep Q)	True posterior

ST-T WAVES

- *ST elevation:* Acute MI, coronary spasm, pericarditis (concave upward), LV aneurysm.
- *ST depression:* Digitalis effect, strain (due to ventricular hypertrophy), ischemia, or nontransmural MI.
- *Tall peaked T:* Hyperkalemia; acute MI ("hyperacute T").
- *Inverted T:* Non-Q-wave MI, ventricular "strain" pattern, drug effect (e.g., digitalis), hypokalemia, hypocalcemia, increased intracranial pressure (e.g., subarachnoid bleed).

INDICATIONS FOR ECHOCARDIOGRAPHY (Fig. 57-5)

VALVULAR STENOSIS Both native and artificial valvular stenosis can be evaluated, and severity can be determined by Doppler [peak gradient = 4 × (peak velocity)^2].

VALVULAR REGURGITATION Structural lesions (e.g., flail leaflet, vegetation) resulting in regurgitation may be identified. Echo can demonstrate whether ventricular function is normal; Doppler can identify and estimate severity of regurgitation through each valve.

VENTRICULAR PERFORMANCE Global and regional wall-motion abnormalities of both ventricles can be assessed; ventricular hypertrophy/infiltration may be visualized; evidence of pulmonary hypertension may be obtained.

CARDIAC SOURCE OF EMBOLISM May visualize atrial or ventricular thrombus, intracardiac tumors, and valvular vegetations. Yield of identifying cardiac source of embolism is *low* in absence of cardiac history or physical findings.

ENDOCARDITIS Vegetation visualized in more than half of patients, but management is generally based on clinical, not echo, findings. Complications of endocarditis (e.g., valvular regurgitation) may be evaluated.

CONGENITAL HEART DISEASE Echo, Doppler, and contrast echo (rapid IV injection of saline) are noninvasive procedures of choice in identifying congenital lesions.

AORTIC ROOT Aneurysm and dissection of the aorta may be evaluated and complications (aortic regurgitation, tamponade) assessed (Chap. 69).

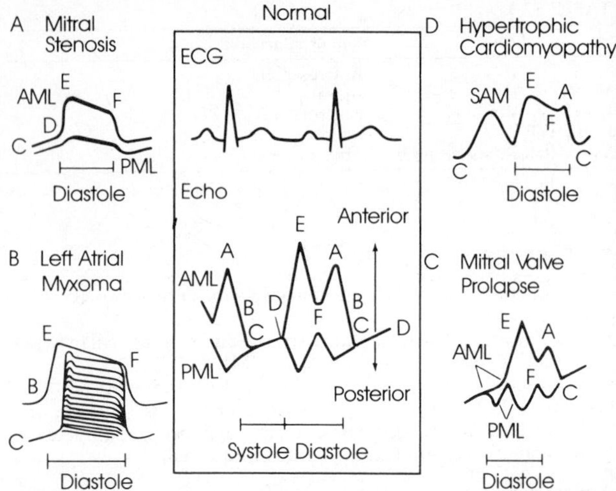

FIG. 57-5 *A schematic presentation of the normal M-mode echocardiographic (ECHO) recording of anterior (AML) and posterior mitral leaflet (PML) motion is shown in the center with the simultaneous ECG. Abnormal mitral echocardiograms which occur in (A) mitral stenosis, (B) left atrial myxoma, (C) mitral valve prolapse, and (D) obstructive hypertrophic cardiomyopathy are also depicted. In the ECHO, the A point represents the end of anterior movement resulting from left atrial contraction, the CD segment represents the closed position of both mitral leaflets during ventricular systole, and panel E ends the anterior movement as the leaflet opens. The slope EF results from posterior motion of the AML during rapid ventricular filling. In obstructive hypertrophic cardiomyopathy, SAM represents systolic anterior movement. (Reproduced from Wynne J, O'Rourke RA, Braunwald E: HPIM-10, p. 1333.)*

HYPERTROPHIC CARDIOMYOPATHY, MITRAL VALVE PROLAPSE, PERICARDIAC EFFUSION Echo is the diagnostic technique of choice for identifying these conditions.

For more detailed discussion of this topic, see Myerburg RJ: Electrocardiography, Chap. 178, in HPIM-11, p 872, and Come PC, Wynne J, Braunwald E: Noninvasive Methods of Cardiac Examination, Chap. 179, in HPIM-11, p. 881

---

58 CONGESTIVE HEART FAILURE

DEFINITION Heart is unable to pump the blood required by metabolizing tissues or can do so only from an abnormally elevated filling pressure. It is important to identify the *underlying* nature of the cardiac disease, and the factors which precipitate acute CHF.

UNDERLYING CARDIAC DISEASE Includes states which depress ventricular function (coronary artery disease, hypertension, dilated cardiomyopathy, valvular disease, congenital heart disease) and states which restrict ventricular filling (mitral stenosis, restrictive cardiomyopathy, pericardial disease).

ACUTE PRECIPITATING FACTORS Include (1) increased Na intake, (2) noncompliance with anti-CHF medications, (3) acute MI (may be silent), (4) exacerbation of hypertension, (5) acute arrhythmias, (6) infections and/or fever, (7) pulmonary embolism, (8) anemia, (9) thyrotoxicosis, (10) pregnancy, (11) acute myocarditis or infective endocarditis.

SYMPTOMS Due to inadequate perfusion of peripheral tissues (fatigue, dyspnea) and elevated intracardiac filling pressures (orthopnea, paroxysmal nocturnal dyspnea, peripheral edema).

PHYSICAL EXAMINATION Jugular venous distention, S_3, pulmonary congestion (rales, dullness over pleural effusion, peripheral edema, hepatomegaly and ascites).

LABORATORY CXR can reveal cardiomegaly, pulmonary vascular redistribution, Kerley B lines, pleural effusions. Left ventricular contraction can be assessed by *echocardiography* or *radionuclide ventriculography.* In addition, echo can identify underlying valvular, pericardial, or congenital heart disease, as well as regional wall-motion abnormalities typical of coronary artery disease.

CONDITIONS WHICH MIMIC CHF **Pulmonary disease:** Chronic bronchitis, emphysemas, and asthma (see Chaps. 73 and 75); look for sputum production and abnormalities on CXR and pulmonary function tests.
Other causes of peripheral edema: Liver disease, varicose veins, and cyclic edema, none of which results in jugular venous distention. Edema due to renal dysfunction is accompanied by elevated serum creatinine and abnormal urinalysis. (See Chap. 13.)

THERAPY Aimed at symptomatic relief, removal of precipitating factors, and control of underlying cardiac disease:

1 Reduction of physical activity and dietary restriction of NaCl (<2 g/day).

2 *Diuretic* (see Tables 13-1 and 13-2), e.g., furosemide 40–120 mg/day PO (given IV to sicker, hospitalized patients). Aim to diurese no more than 1–2 kg per day. Body weight, electrolytes,

BUN, and creatinine should be carefully followed. Hypokalemia must be avoided with K supplements or K-sparing diuretics, particularly in patients taking digitalis glycosides.

3 *Digoxin* (0.125–0.25 mg/day PO after 1-mg loading dose over 24 hours). Useful in CHF due to systolic dysfunction and in atrial fibrillation (AF) with rapid ventricular rate, but *not* for pericardial disease, restrictive cardiomyopathy, or mitral stenosis (unless AF is present). Dosage should be reduced in patients with renal failure. Digoxin is *contraindicated* in hypertrophic cardiomyopathy and in patients with AV conduction blocks.

Digitalis toxicity may be precipitated by hypokalemia, hypoxemia, hypercalcemia, hypomagnesemia, hypothyroidism, or myocardial ischemia. *Note:* The addition of quinidine will increase the digoxin level; therefore, digoxin dose should be halved.

Early signs of digitalis toxicity include anorexia, nausea, and lethargy. *Cardiac toxicity* includes ventricular extrasystoles, ventricular tachycardia, and fibrillation; atrial tachycardia with block; sinus arrest and sinoatrial block; all degrees of AV block. *Chronic* digitalis intoxication may cause cachexia, gynecomastia, yellow vision, or confusion. At first sign of digitalis toxicity, discontinue the drug; maintain serum K concentration in 4.0–5.0 meq/L range. Bradyarrhythmias and AV block may respond to atropine (0.6 mg IV); otherwise a temporary pacemaker may be required. Treatment of choice for digitalis-induced ventricular arrhythmias is lidocaine and phenytoin (Chap. 60). Antidigoxin antibodies are available for massive overdose.

4 *Vasodilators* (Table 58-1) should be added if symptoms persist despite regimen of digitalis and diuretics. *Venous* dilators (e.g., nitrates) reduce pulmonary congestion; *arterial* dilators (e.g., hydralazine) augment forward stroke volume. Converting-enzyme inhibitors are mixed (venous and arterial) dilators and are particularly useful. Vasodilators may result in serious hypotension in patients who are overdiuresed; therefore, start at lowest dosage, and patient should remain supine for 2 hours after initial dose.

5 *IV sympathomimetic amines* May be administered to hospitalized patients for refractory symptoms or acute exacerbation of

TABLE 58-1 **Vasodilators for treatment of congestive heart failure**

Drug	Site of action (veins or arteries)	Usual dosage
IV agents:		
Nitroprusside	V = A	0.5–5 μg/kg/min
Nitroglycerin	V > A	10–200 μg/min
Oral agents:		
Captopril	V = A	6.25–25 mg tid
Hydralazine	A	50–200 mg tid
Nitrates	V	
(e.g., isosorbide dinitrate)		20–80 mg qid
Prazosin	V = A	1–5 mg qid

Note: Arteriolar dilator may be combined with venous dilator (e.g., hydralazine plus nitrate).

CHF. They are *contraindicated* in hypertrophic cardiomyopathy (Chap. 68). *Dobutamine* (2.5–10 μ/kg/min) augments cardiac output without significant peripheral vasoconstriction or tachycardia. *Dopamine* at low dosage (1–5 μg/kg/min) facilitates diuresis; at higher dosage (5–10 μg/kg/min) positive inotropic effects predominate; peripheral vasoconstriction is greatest at dosage > 10 μg/kg/min). *Amrinone* is a nonsympathetic positive inotrope and vasodilator. Vasodilators and inotropic agents may be used together for additive effect.

Patients with severe refractory CHF with less than 6 months expected survival who meet stringent criteria may be candidates for cardiac transplantation.

PULMONARY EDEMA

Pulmonary edema of cardiac origin presents with severe dyspnea and clinical (tachypnea, rales, S_3) and radiologic signs (pulmonary vascular redistribution, perihilar "butterfly" appearance) of pulmonary congestion. Immediate therapy: (1) administer O_2 by mask or nasal cannula to achieve $P_{O_2} > 60$ mmHg; (2) sit patient upright to reduce venous return; (3) IV furosemide (20–160 mg IV); use lower dose if patient does not take diuretic chronically; (4) morphine 2–5 mg IV prn; assess frequently for hypotension or respiratory depression; naloxone should be available to reverse effects of morphine, if necessary; (5) afterload reduction (IV nitroprusside) if systolic BP >100 mmHg.

Additional therapy may be required: (1) phlebotomy (removal of 250 mL to decrease venous return); (2) aminophylline reduces bronchospasm and augments myocardial contractility and diuresis; can be used as initial therapy (in place of morphine) if not clear whether dyspnea is due to pulmonary edema or severe obstructive lung disease before CXR is obtained; (3) digoxin, especially if supraventricular arrhythmia is present; (4) intubation may be needed for persistent hypoxemia or hypercapnia.

A precipitating cause of pulmonary edema should always be sought, especially acute arrhythmias or infection.

For more detailed discussion of this topic, see Braunwald E: Heart Failure, Chap. 182, in HPIM-11, p. 905, and Ingram RH Jr, Braunwald E: Dyspnea and Pulmonary Edema, Chap. 26 in HPIM-11, p. 141

---

59 HYPERTENSION

DEFINITION Chronic elevation in BP > 140/90; etiology unknown in 90–95% of patients ("essential hypertension"). Always consider a secondary correctable form of hypertension, especially in patients under age 30 or those who become hypertensive after 55.

SECONDARY HYPERTENSION

RENAL ARTERY STENOSIS Due either to atherosclerosis (older men) or fibromuscular dysplasia (young women). Presents with sudden onset of hypertension, refractory to usual antihypertensive therapy. Abdominal bruit often audible; mild hypokalemia due to activation of the renin-angiotensin-aldosterone system may be present.

RENAL PARENCHYMAL DISEASE Elevated serum creatinine and/or abnormal urinalysis, containing protein, cells, or casts.

COARCTATION OF AORTA Presents in children or young adults; constriction is usually present in aorta at origin of left subclavian artery. Exam shows diminished, delayed femoral pulsations; late systolic murmur loudest over the midback. CXR shows indentation of the aorta at the level of the coarctation and rib notching (due to development of collateral arterial flow).

PHEOCHROMOCYTOMA Catecholamine-secreting tumor of the adrenal gland; presents with paroxysms of headache, sweating, and palpitations. Elevated urinary catecholamine metabolites (see below).

HYPERALDOSTERONISM Due to aldosterone-secreting adenoma or bilateral adrenal hyperplasia. Should be suspected when hypokalemia is present in a hypertensive patient off diuretics.

OTHER CAUSES Oral contraceptive usage, Cushing's and adrenogenital syndromes (Chap. 137), thyroid disease (Chap. 136), hyperparathyroidism (Chap. 143), and acromegaly (Chap. 134).

APPROACH TO PATIENT

HISTORY Most patients are asymptomatic. Severe hypertension may lead to headache, epistaxis, or blurred vision.
Clues to specific secondary forms of hypertension: Use of birth control pills or glucocorticoids; paroxysms of headache, sweating, or tachycardia (pheochromocytoma); history of renal disease or abdominal traumas (renal hypertension).

PHYSICAL EXAM Measure BP with appropriately sized cuff (large cuff for large arm). Measure BP in both arms as well as a leg (to evaluate for coarctation). Signs of hypertension include retinal arteriolar changes (narrowing/nicking); left ventricular lift, loud A_2, S_4. Clues to secondary forms of hypertension include cushinoid appearance (Chap. 137), thyromegaly, abdominal bruit (renal artery stenosis), delayed femoral pulses (coarctation of aorta).

SCREENING TESTS FOR SECONDARY HYPERTENSION Should be carried out on all patients with documented hypertension: (1) serum creatinine, BUN, and urinalysis (renal parenchymal disease); (2) serum K measured off diuretics (hypokalemia prompts workup for hyperaldosteronism or renal artery stenosis); (3) CXR (rib notching or indentation of distal aortic arch in coarctation of the aorta); (4) ECG (left ventricular hypertrophy suggests chronicity of hypertension), (5) other useful screening blood tests include CBC, glucose, cholesterol, triglycerides, CA, uric acid.

FURTHER WORKUP Indicated for specific diagnoses if screening tests are abnormal or BP is refractory to antihypertensive therapy: (1) renal artery stenosis: digital subtraction angiography, IVP, renal arteriography, and measurement of renal vein renin; (2) Cushing's syndrome: dexamethasone suppression test (Chap. 137); (3) pheochromocytoma: 24- urine collection for catecholamines, metanephrines, and vanillymandelic acid; (4) primary hyperaldosteronism: depressed plasma renin activity and hypersecretion of aldosterone, both of which fail to change with volume expansion; (5) renal parenchymal disease: see Section V.

DRUG THERAPY OF ESSENTIAL HYPERTENSION

Initial therapy consists of a diuretic or beta blocker alone or in combination.

DIURETICS Begin with hydrochlorthiazide 25–100 mg qd or equivalent. Side effects: hypokalemia, hyperglycemia, hyperuricemia. Hypokalemia may be minimized by K supplements or a K-sparing diuretic (e.g., spironolactone) (see Table 13-1). Use lowest effective dosage, particularly in elderly who may become volume-depleted. Monitoring of serum K is particularly important in patients on digitalis glycosides.

BETA BLOCKERS (Table 59-1) Particularly effective in young patients with "hyperkinetic" circulation. Relative contraindications: bronchospasm, CHF, A-V block, bradycardia, and "brittle" insulin-dependent diabetes.

If BP is not adequately controlled with diuretics/beta blockers, add a *converting-enzyme inhibitor* (captopril 12.5–50 mg bid or enalapril 5–40 mg qd); discontinue K supplements and K-sparing diuretics when using these drugs. Side effects include rash and, rarely, proteinuria or neutropenia.

If BP proves refractory to preceding regimen, work up for secondary forms of hypertension, especially renal artery stenosis and pheochromocytoma and consider other antihypertensive drugs (see HPIM-11, p. 1032 for detailed list of antihypertensives).

TABLE 59-1 **Beta blockers***

Drug	Usual dosage (PO)	Features
Propranolol (Inderal)	10–120 mg q 6–12 h	
Metoprolol (Lopressor)	25–150 mg q 12 h	$Beta_1$ selective
Nadolol (Corgard)	20–120 mg q 24 h	Once-a-day dosage
Atenolol (Tenormin)	25–100 mg q 24 h	$Beta_1$ selective; once-a-day dosage
Timolol (Blocadren)	10–30 mg q 12 h	
Pindolol (Visken)	10–30 mg q 12 h	Partial beta-agonist activity
Labetolol (Trandate, Normodyne)	100–600 mg 12 h	Both alpha and beta blocker

**Side effects:* Bradycardia (less common with pindolol), GI side effects, left ventricular dysfunction, bronchospasm (less common with atenolol and metoprolol), exacerbation of diabetes or impaired response to insulin-induced hypoglycemia, impotence.

SPECIAL CIRCUMSTANCES

PREGNANCY Safest antihypertensives include methyldopa (250–1000 mg PO bid-tid), hydralazine (10–150 mg PO bid-tid), and a beta blocker (Table 59-1).

RENAL FAILURE Standard thiazide diuretics may not be effective. Consider metolazone, furosemide, or bumetanide alone or in combination.

MALIGNANT HYPERTENSION Diastolic BP > 120 mmHg is a medical emergency. IV therapy is mandatory if there is evidence of cardiac decompensation (CHF, angina), encephalopathy (headache, seizures, visual disturbances), or deteriorating renal function. Drugs to treat hypertensive crisis are listed in Table 59-2. Replace with PO antihypertensive as patient becomes asymptomatic and diastolic BP improves.

TABLE 59-2 **Treatment of malignant hypertension and hypertensive crisis**

Drug	Dosage (IV)	Side effects
Diazoxide	150–300 mg	Na^+ retention,* hyperglycemia
Nitroprusside†	0.5–8.0 μg/kg/min	Hypotension; after 24 h watch for tinnitus, blurred vision, altered mental status
Trimethaphan†	1–10 μg/min	Urinary retention

*Administer furosemide 20–80 mg IV to prevent Na^+ retention.
†Intraarterial BP monitoring is recommended to avoid rapid fluctuations in BP.

For more detailed discussion of this topic, see Williams GH, Braunwald E: Hypertensive Vascular Disease, Chap. 196, in HPIM-11, p. 1024

NOTES

60 ARRHYTHMIAS AND SUDDEN DEATH

Arrhythmias may appear in the presence or absence of structural heart disease; they are more serious in the former. Conditions which provoke arrhythmias include (1) coronary artery disease, (2) CHF, (3) hypoxemia, (4) hypercapnia, (5) hypotension, (6) electrolyte disturbances (especially involving K, Ca, and Mg), (7) drug toxicity (digoxin, antiarrhythmic agents which prolong QT interval), (8) caffeine, (9) ethanol.

DIAGNOSIS Examine ECG for evidence of ischemic changes (Chap. 57), prolonged QT interval, and characteristics of Wolff-Parkinson-White (WPW) syndrome (see below). See Table 60-1 for diagnosis of tachyarrhythmias; always identify atrial activity and relationship between P waves and QRS complexes. Aids in the diagnosis include the following:

- Obtain long rhythm strip of leads II, aVF, or V_1. Double the ECG voltage and increase paper speed to 50 mm/s to identify P waves.
- Place accessory ECG leads (right-sided chest, esophageal, right-atrial) to identify P waves. Record ECG during carotid sinus massage (Table 60-1) for 5 s. *Note:* Do not massage both carotids simultaneously.

Tachyarrhythmias with wide QRS complex beats may represent ventricular tachycardia or supraventricular tachycardia with aberrant conduction. Factors favoring *ventricular tachycardia* include (1) AV dissociation, (2) QRS > 0.14 s, (3) LAD, (4) no response to carotid sinus massage, (5) morphology of QRS is similar to that of previous ventricular premature beats.

GUIDELINES FOR TREATMENT OF TACHYARRHYTHMIAS (Tables 60-1 and 60-2) Precipitating causes (listed above) should be corrected. If pt is hemodynamically compromised (angina, hypotension, CHF), proceed to immediate cardioversion. *Note:* Do not cardiovert sinus tachycardia or if digitalis toxicity is suspected. Initiate drugs as indicated in the tables; follow drug levels and ECG intervals (especially QRS and QT). Reduce dosage for pts with hepatic or renal dysfunction as indicated in Table 60-2. Drug efficacy is confirmed by ECG monitoring (or Holter), stress testing, and in special circumstances, invasive electrophysiologic study.

PREEXCITATION SYNDROME (WPW) Conduction occurs through an accessory pathway between atria and ventricles. Baseline ECG typically shows a short PR interval and slurred upstroke of the QRS ("delta" wave) (Fig. 60-1*N*). Associated tachyarrhythmias are of two types:

- *Narrow QRS complex tachycardia* (antegrade conduction through AV node): usually paroxysmal supraventricular tachycardia. Treat cautiously with IV verapamil, digoxin, or propranolol (Table 60-2).

TABLE 60-1 **Clinical and electrocardiographic features of common arrhythmias**

Rhythm	Example (Fig. 60-1)	Atrial rate	Features	Carotid sinus massage	Precipitating conditions	Initial treatment
Narrow QRS complex:						
Atrial premature beats	*A*	—	P wave abnormal; QRS width normal	—	Can be normal; or due to anxiety, CHF, hypoxia, caffeine, abnormal electrolytes (K^+, Ca^{2+}, Mg^{2+})	Remove precipitating cause; if symptomatic: beta blocker or group IA drug*
Sinus tachycardia	*B*	100–160	Normal P wave	Rate gradually slows	Fever, dehydration, pain, CHF, hyperthyroidism, COPD	Remove precipitating cause; if symptomatic: beta blocker
Paroxysmal SVT	*C*	140–250	P wave "peaked" or inverted in leads II, III, aVF	Abruptly converts to sinus rhythm (or no effect)	Healthy individuals; preexcitation syndromes (see text)	Vagal maneuvers; if unsuccessful: verapamil, beta blocker, group IA drug, cardioversion (150 J)
Paroxysmal atrial tachycardia with block	*D*	130–250	Upright "peaked" P; 2:1, 3:1, 4:1, block	No effect on atrial rate; block may ↑	Digitalis toxicity	Hold digoxin, correct [K^+]; phenytoin (250 mg IV over 5 min)

(*continued*)

TABLE 60-1 **Clinical and electrocardiographic features of common arrhythmias (*continued*)**

Rhythm	Example (Fig. 60-1)	Atrial rate	Features	Carotid sinus massage	Precipitating conditions	Initial treatment
Atrial flutter	*E*	250–350	"Sawtooth" flutter waves; 2:1, 4:1 block	↑ Block; ventricular rate	Mitral valve disease, hypertension, pulmonary embolism, pericarditis, post-cardiac surgery, hyperthyroidism, obstructive lung disease, EtOH, idiopathic (atrial flutter and atrial fibrillation)	1. Slow the ventricular rate: digoxin, beta blocker, or verapamil 2. Convert to NSR (after anticoagulation if chronic) with quinidine† or procainamide; may require electrical cardioversion (flutter: 50 J; fib: 100–200 J). Atrial flutter may respond to rapid atrial pacing (atrial flutter and atrial fibrillation)
Atrial fibrillation	*F*	>350	No discrete P; irregularly spaced QRS	Ventricular rate ↓		
Multifocal atrial tachycardia		100–220	More than 3 different P wave shapes with varying P-P intervals	No effect	Severe respiratory insufficiency	Treat underlying lung disease; verapamil may be used to slow ventricular rate

Wide QRS complex:					
Ventricular premature beats	*G*	Fully compensatory pause between normal beats	No effect	Coronary artery disease, myocardial infarction, CHF, hypoxia, hypokalemia, digitalis toxicity, prolonged QT interval (congenital or drugs: quinidine and other antiarrhythmics, tricyclics, phenothiazines)	May not require therapy;‡ use same drugs as ventricular tachycardia
Ventricular tachycardia	*H*	QRS rate 100–250; slightly irregular rate	No effect		If unstable: electrical conversion (100 J); otherwise: Acute (IV): lidocaine, procainamide, bretylium; chronic (PO) prevention: group IA, IB, IC, III drugs*
Ventricular fibrillation	*I*	Erratic electrical activity only	No effect		Immediate defibrillation (200–400 J)
Torsades de pointes		Ventricular tachycardia with sinusoidal oscillations of QRS height	No effect	Prolonged QT interval (congenital or drugs: quinidine and other antiarrhythmics, tricyclics, phenothiazines)	Lidocaine; isoproterenol (unless CAD present); overdrive pacing; magnesium; bretylium. Drugs that prolong QT interval (e.g., quinidine) are contraindicated.
Supraventricular tachycardias with aberrant ventricular conduction		P wave typical of the supraventricular rhythm; wide QRS complex due to conduction through refractory pathways		Etiologies of the respective supraventricular rhythms listed above; atrial fibrillation with rapid, wide QRS may be due to preexcitation (WPW)	Same as treatment of respective supraventricular rhythm; if ventricular rate rapid (>200), treat as WPW (see text)

*Antiarrhythmic drug groups listed in Table 60-2.
†Decrease digoxin dose when starting quinidine.
‡Indications for treating VPCs listed in Chap. 64.
Note: J = joules.

TABLE 60-2 **Antiarrhythmic drugs**

Drug	Loading dose	Maintenance dose	Side effects	Excretion
Group IA:				
Quinidine sulfate		PO: 200–400 mg q 6 h	Diarrhea, tinnitus, QT prolongation, hypotension, anemia, thrombocytopenia	Hepatic
Quinidine gluconate		PO: 324–628 mg q 8 h		Hepatic
Procainamide	IV: 500–1000 mg	IV: 2–5 mg/min PO: 500–1000 mg q 4 h	Nausea, lupus-like syndrome, agranulocytosis, QT prolongation	Renal and hepatic
Sustained-release:		PO: 500–1250 mg q 6 h		
Disopyramide		PO: 100–300 mg q 6–8 h	Myocardial depression, AV block, QT prolongation, anticholinergic effects	Renal
Group IB:				
Lidocaine	IV: 20–50 mg/min to 1.4 mg/kg; repeat after 5 min	IV: 1–4 mg/min	Confusion, seizures, respiratory arrest	Hepatic
Tocainide		PO: 400–600 q 8 h	Nausea, confusion, tremors, lupus-like reaction	Hepatic and renal
Group IC:				
Flecainide		PO: 100–200 q 12 h	Nausea, exacerbation of ventricular arrhythmia, prolongation of PR and QRS intervals	Renal

Group II:				
Propranolol	IV: 0.5–1 mg/min to 0.15–0.2 mg/kg	PO: 10–200 mg q 6 h	CHF, bradycardia, AV block, bronchospasm	Hepatic
Group III:				
Amiodarone	PO: 800–1400 mg qd × 1–2 weeks	PO: 200–600 mg qd	Thyroid abnormalities, pulmonary fibrosis, hepatitis, corneal microdeposits, bluish skin, QT prolongation	—
Bretylium	IV: 5–10 mg/kg	IV: 0.5–2.0 mg/min	Hypertension, orthostatic hypotension, nausea, parotid pain	Renal
Group IV:				
Verapamil	IV: 2.5–10 mg	PO: 80–120 mg tid-qid	AV block, CHF, hypotension, constipation	Hepatic
Other				
Digoxin	IV, PO: 0.75–1.5 mg over 24 hours	IV, PO: 0.125–0.25 mg qd	Nausea, AV block, ventricular and supraventricular arrhythmias	Renal

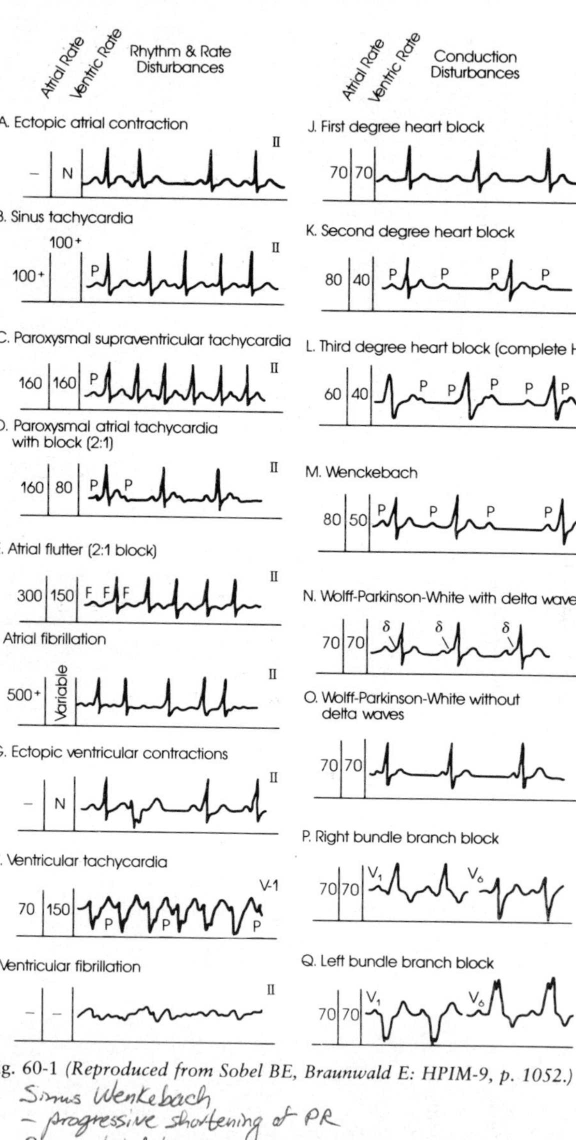

Fig. 60-1 *(Reproduced from Sobel BE, Braunwald E: HPIM-9, p. 1052.)*

Sinus Wenkebach
- progressive shortening of PR
Sino-atrial block vs. Sinus pause
- next P-QRS comes on time vs. randomly c̄ pauses

- *Wide QRS complex tachycardia* (antegrade conduction through accessory pathway): often associated with AF with a very *rapid* (>250/min) ventricular rate (which may degenerate into VF). If hemodynamically compromised, immediate cardioversion is indicated; otherwise, treat with IV lidocaine or procainamide, *not* digoxin or verapamil.

AV BLOCK

FIRST DEGREE (Fig. 60-1*J*) Prolonged, constant PR interval (>0.20 s). May be normal or secondary to increased vagal tone or digitalis; no treatment required.

SECOND DEGREE Mobitz I (Wenkebach) (Fig. 60-1*M*): Narrow QRS, progressive increase in PR interval until a ventricular beat is dropped, then sequence is repeated. Seen with digitalis toxicity, increased vagal tone, inferior MI. Usually transient, no therapy required; if symptomatic, use atropine (0.6 mg IV, repeated × 3–4) or temporary pacemaker.

Mobitz II (Fig. 60-1*K*): Fixed PR interval with occasional dropped beats, in 2:1, 3:1, or 4:1 pattern; the QRS complex is usually wide. Seen with MI or degenerative conduction system disease; a dangerous rhythm—may progress suddenly to complete AV block; pacemaker is indicated.

Third degree (complete AV block) (Fig. 60-1*L*) Atrial activity is not transmitted to ventricles; atria and ventricles contract independently. Seen with MI, digitalis toxicity, or degenerative conduction system disease. Permanent pacemaker is indicated, except when associated transiently with inferior MI or in asymptomatic congenital heart block.

SUDDEN DEATH

Unexpected collapse and death may result from (1) ventricular tachycardia, VF (usually associated with severe coronary artery disease, sometimes with acute MI); (2) pronounced bradyarrhythmia or AV conduction block; (3) sudden marked drop in cardiac output (massive PE, cardiac tamponade, critical aortic stenosis); (4) sudden drop in circulating volume (ruptured aneurysm, aortic dissection); (5) catastrophic CNS event. Immediate institution of cardiopulmonary resuscitation and rapid transportation to a medical facility are mandatory. Prognosis following initial resuscitation is dependent on identification of underlying cause and aggressive treatment.

For more detailed discussion of this topic, see Sobel BE, Braunwald E: Sudden Cardiovascular Collapse and Death, Chap. 30, in HPIM-11, p 158, and Josephson ME, Buxton AE, Marchlinski FE: The Bradyarrhythmias, Chap. 183, and Tachyarrhythmias, Chap. 184, in HPIM-11, pp 916 and 923.

61 CONGENITAL HEART DISEASE IN THE ADULT

ATRIAL SEPTAL DEFECT (ASD)

HISTORY Usually asymptomatic until third or fourth decades, when exertional dyspnea, fatigue, and palpitations may develop. Symptoms often associated with pulmonary hypertension (see below).

PHYSICAL EXAM Parasternal RV lift, wide fixed splitting of S_2, systolic flow murmur along sternal border, diastolic flow rumble across tricuspid valve, prominent jugular venous *v* wave.

LABORATORY **ECG:** Incomplete RBBB. LAD common with ostium primum (lower septal) defect.
CXR: Increased pulmonary vascular markings, prominence of RV and main pulmonary artery (LA enlargement *not* usually present).
Echocardiogram: RA and RV enlargement; Doppler shows abnormal turbulent transatrial flow.
Radionuclide angiogram: Noninvasively estimates ratio of pulmonary flow to systemic flow (PF:SF).

TREATMENT Dyspnea and palpitations may respond to digitalis and mild diuretic (e.g., hydrochlorthiazide 50 mg/day). An ASD with PF:SF > 1.5:1.0 should be surgically repaired. Surgery is contraindicated with significant pulmonary hypertension and PF:SF < 1.2:1.0.

VENTRICULAR SEPTAL DEFECT (VSD)

Congenital VSDs may close spontaneously during childhood. Symptoms relate to size of the defect and pulmonary vascular resistance.

HISTORY CHF in infancy. Adults may be asymptomatic or develop fatigue and reduced exercise tolerance.

PHYSICAL EXAM Systolic thrill and holosystolic murmur at lower left sternal border, loud P_2, S_3; flow murmur across mitral valve.
ECG: Normal with small defects. Large shunts result in LA and LV enlargement.
CXR: Enlargement of main pulmonary artery, LA and LV, with increased pulmonary vascular markings.
Echocardiogram: LA and LV enlargement; defect may be visualized; Doppler shows high-velocity flow in RV outflow tract, near the defect.

TREATMENT Fatigue and mild dyspnea are treated with digitalis, mild diuretics, and afterload reduction (Chap. 58). Surgical closure is indicated if PF:SF > 1.5:1. Antibiotic prophylaxis for endocarditis is essential.

PATENT DUCTUS ARTERIOSUS (PDA)

Abnormal communication between the descending aorta and pulmonary artery; associated with birth at high altitudes and maternal rubella.

HISTORY Asymptomatic or dyspnea on exertion and fatigue.

PHYSICAL EXAM Hyperactive LV impulse; loud systolic-diastolic "machinery" murmur at upper left sternal border. If pulmonary hypertension develops, diastolic component of the murmur may disappear.
ECG: LV hypertrophy is common; RV hypertrophy with pulmonary hypertension.
CXR: Increased pulmonary vascular markings; enlarged main pulmonary artery, ascending aorta, LV; occasional calcification of ductus.
Echocardiography: Hyperdynamic, enlarged LV; the PDA can often be visualized on 2-dimensional echo; Doppler demonstrates abnormal flow contained within it.

TREATMENT In absence of pulmonary hypertension, PDA should be ligated to prevent infective endocarditis, LV dysfunction, and pulmonary hypertension.

PROGRESSION TO PULMONARY HYPERTENSION (PHT)

Patients with significant, uncorrected ASD, VSD, or PDA may develop progressive, irreversible PHT with shunting of desaturated blood into the arterial circulation (right-to-left shunting). Fatigue, light-headedness, and chest pain due to RV ischemia are common, accompanied by cyanosis, clubbing of digits, loud P_2, murmur of pulmonary valve regurgitation, and signs of RV failure. ECG and echocardiogram show RV hypertrophy. Surgical correction of congenital defects contraindicated with severe PHT and right-to-left shunting.

PULMONIC STENOSIS (PS)

A transpulmonary valve gradient less than 50 mmHg rarely causes symptoms, and progression tends not to occur. Higher gradients result in dyspnea, fatigue, light-headedness, chest pain (RV ischemia).

PHYSICAL EXAM Shows jugular venous distention with prominent *a* wave, RV parasternal impulse, wide splitting of S_2 with soft P_2, ejection click followed by "diamond-shaped" systolic murmur at upper left sternal border, S_4.
ECG: RV and RA enlargement in advanced PS.
CXR: Often shows poststenotic dilatation of the pulmonary artery and RV enlargement.
Echocardiography: RV hypertrophy and "doming" of the pulmonic valve. Doppler accurately measures transvalvular gradient.

TREATMENT Prophylaxis for infective endocarditis is mandatory. Moderate or severe stenosis (gradient $>$ 50 mmHg) requires surgical (or balloon) valvuloplasty.

COARCTATION OF THE AORTA

Aortic constriction just distal to the origin of the left subclavian artery is a surgically correctable form of hypertension (Chap. 59). Usually asymptomatic, but it may cause headache, fatigue, or claudication of lower extremities.

PHYSICAL EXAM Hypertension in upper extremities; delayed femoral pulses with decreased pressure in lower extremities. Pulsatile collateral arteries can be palpated in the intercostal spaces. Systolic (and sometimes diastolic) murmur is best heard over the mid-upper back.
ECG: LV hypertrophy.
CXR: Notching of the ribs due to collateral arteries; "figure 3" appearance of distal aortic arch.

TREATMENT Surgical correction, although hypertension may persist. Antibiotic prophylaxis against endocarditis is required even after correction.

For more detailed discussion of this topic, see Friedman WF: Congenital Heart Disease, Chap. 185, HPIM-11, p. 938

---

62 VALVULAR HEART DISEASE

MITRAL STENOSIS (MS)

ETIOLOGY Most commonly rheumatic, although history of acute rheumatic fever is not uncommon; congenital MS is an uncommon cause, observed primarily in infants.

HISTORY Symptoms most commonly begin in the fourth decade, but MS often causes severe disability by age 20 in economically deprived areas. Principal symptoms are dyspnea and pulmonary edema precipitated by exertion, excitement, fever, anemia, paroxysmal tachycardia, pregnancy, sexual intercourse, etc.

PHYSICAL EXAM Peripheral and facial cyanosis in severe MS. Right ventricular lift; palpable S_1; opening snap (OS) follows A_2 by 0.06 to 0.12 s; OS–A_2 interval inversely proportional to severity of obstruction. Diastolic rumbling murmur with presystolic accentuation in sinus rhythm. Duration of murmur correlates with severity of obstruction.

COMPLICATIONS Hemoptysis, pulmonary embolism, pulmonary infection, systemic embolization; endocarditis is *uncommon* in pure MS.

LABORATORY **ECG:** Typically shows atrial fibrillation (AF) or left atrial (LA) enlargement when sinus rhythm is present. Right-axis deviation and RV hypertrophy in the presence of pulmonary hypertension.
CXR: Shows LA and RV enlargement and Kerley B lines.
Echocardiogram: Most useful noninvasive test; shows inadequate separation, calcification and thickening of valve leaflets, and LA enlargement. Doppler echocardiogram allows estimation of transvalvular gradient.

TREATMENT Pts should receive rheumatic fever and subacute infective endocarditis prophylaxis. In the presence of dyspnea, medical therapy for heart failure: digitalis to slow ventricular rate in AF, diuretics, and sodium restriction. Anticoagulants for pts with AF and/or history of systemic and pulmonic emboli. Open mitral valvuloplasty in the presence of symptoms and mitral orifice $\leq$ approximately 1.2 cm^2.

MITRAL REGURGITATION (MR)

ETIOLOGY Rheumatic heart disease in approximately 50%. Other causes: mitral valve prolapse, ischemic heart disease with papillary muscle dysfunction, LV dilatation of any cause, mitral annular calcification, hypertrophic cardiomyopathy, infective endocarditis, congenital.

CLINICAL MANIFESTATIONS Fatigue, weakness, and exertional dyspnea. Physical examination: sharp upstroke of arterial pulse, LV lift, S_1 diminished: wide splitting of S_2; S_3; loud holosystolic murmur often followed by brief early diastolic murmur.

ECHOCARDIOGRAM Enlarged LA, hyperdynamic LV; Doppler echocardiogram helpful in diagnosing and assessing severity of MR.

TREATMENT As for heart failure (see Chap. 58). Surgical treatment, most commonly valve replacement, is indicated in the presence of symptoms and impairment of LV function. Operation should be carried out *before* development of severe chronic heart failure.

MITRAL VALVE PROLAPSE (MVP)

ETIOLOGY Most commonly idiopathic; ?familial; often accompanies rheumatic fever, ischemic heart disease, ASD, Marfan's syndrome.

PATHOLOGY Redundant mitral valve tissue with myxedematous degeneration and elongated chordae tendineae.

CLINICAL MANIFESTATIONS More common in females. Most pts are asymptomatic and remain so. Most common symptoms are atypical chest pain and a variety of supraventricular and ventricular arrhythmias. Most common complication is severe MR resulting in LV failure. Rarely, systemic emboli from platelet-fibrin deposits on valve. Sudden death is a *very rare* complication.

PHYSICAL EXAM Mid or late systolic click(s) followed by late systolic murmur; exaggeration by Valsalva maneuver, reduced by squatting and isometric exercise (Chap. 56).
Echocardiogram: Shows posterior displacement of posterior (occasionally anterior) mitral leaflet late in systole.

TREATMENT Asymptomatic pts should be reassured but require prophylaxis for infective endocarditis. Valve replacement for pts with severe mitral regurgitation; anticoagulants for pts with history of embolization.

AORTIC STENOSIS (AS)

ETIOLOGY: Often congenital; rheumatic AS is usually associated with mitral valve disease. Idiopathic, calcific AS is a degenerative disorder common in the elderly and usually mild.

SYMPTOMS: Dyspnea, angina, and syncope are cardinal symptoms; they occur late, after years of obstruction.

PHYSICAL EXAM Weak and delayed arterial pulses with carotid thrill. Double apical impulse; A_2 soft or absent; S_4 common. Diamond-shaped systolic murmur $\geq$ grade 3/6, often with systolic thrill.

LABORATORY ECG and CXR: Often show LV hypertrophy, but not useful for predicting gradient.
Echocardiogram: Shows thickening of LV wall, calcification and thickening of aortic valve cusps. Dilatation and reduced shortening of LV indicate poor prognosis. Doppler echogram useful for predicting gradient.

TREATMENT Avoid strenuous activity in asymptomatic phase. Treat heart failure in standard fashion (see Chap. 58), but *avoid afterload reduction*. Valve replacement is indicated in adults with symptoms resulting from AS and hemodynamic evidence of severe obstruction. Operation should be carried out *before* frank failure has developed.

AORTIC REGURGITATION (AR)

ETIOLOGY Rheumatic in 70%; may also be due to infective endocarditis, syphilis, or aortic dilatation due to cystic medionecrosis; three-fourths of pts are males.

CLINICAL MANIFESTATIONS Exertional dyspnea and awareness of heart beat, angina pectoris, and signs of LV failure. Wide pulse pressure, waterhammer pulse, capillary pulsations (Quincke's sign), A_2 soft or absent, S_3 common. Blowing, decrescendo diastolic murmur along left sternal border (along right sternal border with aortic dilatation). May be accompanied by systolic murmur.

LABORATORY **ECG and CRX:** Show LV enlargement. **Echocardiogram:** Shows increased excursion of posterior LV wall, LA enlargement, LV enlargement, high-frequency fluttering of mitral valve. Doppler studies useful in detection and quantification of AR.

TREATMENT Standard therapy for LV failure (see Chap. 58). Surgical valve replacement should be carried out in patients with severe AR soon after development of symptoms or in asymptomatic patients with LV dysfunction on radionuclide ventriculogram, angiogram, or echocardiogram.

TRICUSPID STENOSIS (TS)

ETIOLOGY Usually rheumatic; most common in females; almost invariably associated with MS.

CLINICAL MANIFESTATIONS Hepatomegaly, ascites, edema, jaundice, jugular venous distention with slow *y* descent (Chap. 56). Diastolic rumbling murmur along left sternal border increased by inspiration with loud presystolic component. Right atrial and superior vena caval enlargement on x-ray.

TREATMENT In severe TS, surgical relief is indicated and usually requires valve replacement.

TRICUSPID REGURGITATION (TR)

ETIOLOGY Usually functional and secondary to marked RV dilatation of any cause and often associated with pulmonary hypertension.

CLINICAL MANIFESTATIONS Severe RV failure, with edema, hepatomegaly, and prominent *v* waves in jugular venous pulse with rapid *y* descent (Chap. 56). Systolic murmur along sternal edge is increased by inspiration.

TREATMENT Intensive diuretic therapy. In severe cases (in absence of severe pulmonary hypertension), surgical treatment consists of tricuspid annuloplasty or valve replacement.

For more detailed discussion of this topic, see Braunwald E: Valvular Heart Disease, Chap. 187, in HPIM-11, p. 956

---

63 INFECTIVE ENDOCARDITIS

ETIOLOGY See Table 63-1

MANIFESTATIONS

1 *Subacute infective endocarditis:* symptoms—insidious onset of weakness, fatigue, fever, night sweats, painful fingers, toes, or skin lesions; physical exam ± petechiae (mouth, conjunctiva), linear hemorrhages under nails; erythematous or purple tender nodules on palms, soles, or fingers (Osler's nodes); changes in cardiac mumur, splenomegaly; arthralgias; emboli.

TABLE 63-1

Predisposing condition	Organism	Comment
Dental manipulations	Viridans streptococci	
Parenteral drug addicts	*S. aureus* Group A streptococcus Gram-negative rods *Candida* spp.	Septic phlebitis and right-sided endocarditis are common.
Prosthetic valve recipients:		
< 2 months after surgery	*S. epidermidis* Diphtheroids Gram-negative rods *Candida* spp. Enterococcus *S. aureus*	Early-onset infections tend to be resistant to prophylactic antimicrobials administered at surgery.
> 2 months after surgery	*Streptococcus* spp. *S. epidermidis* Diphtheroids Enterococcus *S. aureus*	Some low-virulence infections implanted at surgery are slow to develop.
Urinary tract infections	Enterococcus Gram-negative rods	Associated in older males with prostatism and in women with genitourinary tract infections.
Catheter-related phlebitis	*S. aureus* *S. epidermidis* *Candida* spp. Gram-negative rods	An increasingly common source of endocarditis in hospitalized patients.
Alcoholism	Pneumococcus	May be associated with simultaneous pneumonia and meningitis.
Colon cancer	*Streptococcus bovis*	

Reproduced from Pelletier LL Jr., Petersdorf RG: HPIM-11, p. 972.

2 *Acute endocarditis:* fever, chills, numerous petechiae, emboli, retinal hemorrhages with pale centers (Roth's spots), nontender subcutaneous maculopapular lesions of pulp of fingers (Janeway's spots).

3 *Right-sided:* high fevers, pleuritic chest pain, dyspnea, malaise over several weeks; increased risk—parenteral drug addicts, infected venous catheters or pacing wires.

4 *Prosthetic:* symptoms indistinguishable from native valve endocarditis but increased valve ring infection, myocardial abscess, conduction disturbances, valve stenosis secondary to vegetations or new regurgitant murmur from valve dehiscence.

LABORATORY FINDINGS

- ↑ WBC usually, normochromic normocytic anemia in subacute, ↑ ESR, proteinuria, ↓ CH_{50} or C3
- Echo: cannot differentiate active from healed lesions
- Blood cultures: 3–5 sets of venous blood (arterial not necessary)

PROPHYLAXIS

- At risk: congenital or acquired valvular disease, prosthetic valves, ventriculoseptal patches, prior history of endocarditis; lower risk—mitral valve prolapse with regurgitation, asymmetrical septral hypertrophy, tricuspid or pulmonary valve lesions.
- Upper respiratory tract: dental manipulation, oral surgery, tonsillectomy, adenoidectomy, bronchoscopy—1.2 million U procaine penicillin + 1.0 g streptomycin IM 30 minutes before surgery, then penicillin V 0.5 g q 6 h × 4; penicillin-allergic—vancomycin 1.0 g IV over 30 minutes or 1.0 g erythromycin PO, then erythromycin 0.5 g q 6 h × 4.
- GI and GU tract: bladder catheterization; cystoscopy, prostatectomy, obstetrical or gynecologic manipulation of infected tissues, colon surgery (not endoscopy or proctoscopy without biopsies, BE, pelvic exam)—ampicillin 1 g + gentamicin 1.0 mg/kg IM or IV 30–60 minutes before, then q 8 h × 2; penicillin-allergic—vancomycin 1 g + gentamycin 1.0 mg/kg IV and in 12 h.

TREATMENT See Table 63-2.

TABLE 63-2

S. viridans and nonenterococcal group D streptococci (penicillin G MIC < 0.1 μg/mL)	Penicillin G 10–20 million U per day IV in divided doses every 4–6 h × 4 weeks Penicillin G 10–20 million U per day IV with streptomycin 7.5 mg/kg IV or IM every 12 h or gentamicin 1 mg/kg IV every 8 h × 2 weeks Penicillin G 10–20 million U per day IV × 2 weeks, followed by amoxacillin 1 g PO every 6 h × 2 weeks Cefazolin 2 g IV every 6–8 h × 4 weeks if allergic to pencillin Vancomycin 15 mg/kg IV every 12 h × 4 weeks if allergic to penicillin
Enterococcus or relatively penicillin-resistant viridans streptococci (penicillin G MIC > 0.1 μg/mL)	Penicillin G 15–24 million U per day IV in divided doses every 4–6 h with gentamicin 1 mg/kg IV every 8 h × 4–6 weeks Ampicillin 2 g IV every 6 h possible substitute for penicillin G Streptomycin 7.5 mg/kg IV or IM possible substitute for gentamicin if the MIC for streptomycin is < 2000 μg/mL Vancomycin 15 mg/kg IV every 12 h with gentamicin 1 mg/kg IV every 8 h × 4–6 weeks, if allergic to penicillin
Pneumococcus or group A streptococcus	Penicillin G 6–12 million U per day IV in divided doses every 4–6 h × 4 weeks Cefazolin 2 g IV every 6–8 h × 4 weeks if allergic to penicillin
Methicillin-susceptible *S. aureus* or *S. epidermidis*	Nafcillin 2 g IV every 4 h × 4–6 weeks or longer Cefazolin 2 g IV every 6 h × 4–6 weeks or longer, if allergic to penicillin Vancomycin 15 mg/kg IV every 12 h × 4–6 weeks or longer, if allergic to pencillin
Methicillin-resistant *S. aureus*, *S. epidermidis*, or *Corynebacterium* spp.	Vancomycin 15 mg/kg IV every 12 h × 4–6 weeks or longer Vancomycin in combination with rifampin 900–1200 mg PO once daily for 4–6 weeks or longer with gentamicin 1 mg/kg IV every 8 h × 2 weeks

Reproduced from Pelletier LL Jr., Petersdorf RG: HPIM-11, p. 974.

For more detailed discussion of this topic, see Pelletier LL Jr., Petersdorf RG: Infective Endocarditis, Chap. 188 in HPIM-11, p. 970

ACUTE MYOCARDIAL INFARCTION (AMI)

Early recognition and immediate treatment of AMI are essential; diagnosis is based on characteristic history, ECG, and evolution of cardiac enzymes.

SYMPTOMS Chest pain similar to angina (Chap. 2), but more intense and persistent (>30 min); but fully relieved by rest or nitroglycerin, often accompanied by nausea, sweating, apprehension. However, 25% of MIs are clinically silent.

PHYSICAL EXAM Pallor, diaphoresis, tachycardia, S_4, dyskinetic cardiac impulse may be present. If CHF exists, there is jugular venous distention, rales, S_3.

ECG **Q-wave MI:** ST elevation, followed by T-wave inversion, then Q-wave development (Chap. 57) over several hours.
Non-Q-Wave MI: ST depression followed by persistent ST-T wave changes *without* Q-wave development. Comparison with old ECG helpful.

CARDIAC ENZYMES Time course is important for diagnosis; creatine phosphokinase (*CK*) level should be checked every 8 h for first day: CK rises within 6–8 h, peaks at 24 h, returns to normal by 36–48 h. CK-MB isoenzyme is more specific for MI. Total CK (but not CK-MB) rises after IM injection or electrical cardioversion. *SGOT* levels rise within 8–12 h, peak at 18–36 h, and return to normal by 4 days. *LDH* peaks at day 3–4 and is normal within 14 days; LDH_1 isoenzyme is more specific for MI than total LDH.

NONINVASIVE IMAGING TECHNIQUES Useful when diagnosis of MI is not clear. *^{99m}Tc-pyrophosphate* scan shows "hot spot" 2–5 days after MI (less reliable for nontransmural MI); false-positives seen with ventricular aneurysm and pericarditis and after cardioversion. *Thallium 201 scan* after MI shows "cold spot" within a few hours, but cannot distinguish from old infarction. *Echocardiogram* or *radionuclide ventriculogram* are used to characterize wall-motion abnormalities after AMI. Echo is also useful in detecting RV infarction, LV aneurysm, LV dyskinesis, and LV thrombus.

STANDARD INITIAL THERAPY

GOALS Relieve pain, minimize mass of infarcted tissue, prevent/treat arrhythmias and mechanical complications:

1 Hospitalize in coronary care unit
2 Continuous ECG monitoring for arrhythmias
3 IV line for emergency treatment of arrhythmia
4 Control of pain: (a) morphine sulfate 2–4 mg IV prn (watch for hypotension, respiratory depression); (b) nitroglycerin 0.3 mg SL if systolic BP > 100; for refractory pain: IV nitroglycerin (begin at 10 μg/min)

5 Oxygen 2–4 L/min by nasal cannula (maintain $P_{O_2} > 70$ mmHg)
6 Mild sedation (diazepam 5 mg PO qid)
7 Stool softeners
8 Low-dose heparin (5000 U SC q 12 h); use full-dose IV heparin if severe CHF is present or ventricular thrombus is demonstrated by echocardiogram

ACUTE REPERFUSION IV streptokinase (1.5 million units) or tissue plasminogen activator (100 mg) may be given within 4 h of chest pain onset. Little benefit with later administration. Complications include bleeding and reperfusion arrhythmias. Residual high-grade stenosis may be treated with balloon angioplasty (PTCA).

VENTRICULAR ARRHYTHMIAS Isolated ventricular premature beats (VPBs) occur frequently. Precipitating factors should be corrected (hypoxemia, acidosis, hypokalemia, hypercalcemia, hypomagnesemia, CHF, arrhythmogenic drugs). For prophylaxis against serious ventricular arrhythmia, consider prophylactic IV lidocaine (Chap. 60); infusion rate should be lower in patients with CHF and liver disease, and in the elderly.

More definitive indications for lidocaine: (1) more than 5 isolated VPBs per minute, (2) ventricular couplets or runs of ventricular tachycardia, (3) "R-on-T" VPBs. If lidocaine fails to suppress ventricular ectopy, add IV procainamide, a beta blocker, or bretylium (Chap. 60). Ventricular tachycardia with hemodynamic instability requires immediate cardioversion (Chap. 60).

VENTRICULAR FIBRILLATION VF requires immediate defibrillation (200–400 W·s). If unsuccessful, initiate CPR, administer $NaHCO_3$ and repeat defibrillation at 400 W·s. Ventricular arrhythmias which appear several days or weeks following MI warrant chronic oral antiarrhythmic therapy (Chap. 60) and possibly invasive electrophysiologic study.

ACCELERATED IDIOVENTRICULAR RHYTHM Wide QRS complex, regular rhythm, rate 60–100 beats/min is common and usually benign; if it causes hypotension, treat with atropine 0.6 mg IV. *Sinus tachycardia* may result from CHF, hypoxemia, pain, fever, pericarditis, hypovolemia, administered drugs. If no cause identified, may treat with beta blocker (Table 59-1). For persistent sinus tachycardia (>120), use Swan-Ganz catheter to differentiate CHF from decreased intravascular volume.

BRADYARRHYTHMIAS AND AV BLOCK (Chap. 60) In *inferior MI,* usually represent heightened vagal tone or discrete AV nodal ischemia. If hemodynamically compromised (CHF, hypotension, emergence of ventricular arrhythmias), treat with atropine 0.5 mg IV q 5 min (up to 2 mg). If no response, use temporary pacemaker. Isoproterenol should be avoided. In *anterior MI,* AV conduction defects usually reflect extensive tissue necrosis. Temporary pacemaker indicated for (1) Mobitz type II block (Chap. 60), (2) complete heart block, (3) new bifascicular block (LBBB, RBBB + left anterior hemiblock, RBBB + left posterior hemiblock), (4) any bradyarrhythmia associated with hypotension or CHF.

CONGESTIVE HEART FAILURE Results from systolic "pump" dysfunction or increased LV "stiffness."
Symptoms: Dyspnea, orthopnea, tachycardia.
Examination: Jugular venous distention, S_3, rales.
Therapy (Chap. 58): Includes diuretics, vasodilators (especially PO, topical, or IV nitrates), and inhaled oxygen; digitalis is usually of little benefit in AMI unless treating supraventricular arrhythmia. If hypotension accompanies CHF, place Swan-Ganz catheter to determine pulmonary capillary wedge pressure (PCW) (see Table 64-1 and Fig. 64-1).

CARDIOGENIC SHOCK Severe LV failure with hypotension (BP <80 mmHg) and elevated PCW, accompanied by oliguria and metabolic acidosis.
Treatment (see Chap. 58): Swan-Ganz catheter and intraarterial BP monitoring are essential; aim for mean PCW of 18–20 mmHg with adjustment of volume (diuretics or infusion) as needed. Intraaortic balloon counterpulsation may be necessary to maintain BP and reduce LV filling pressures. Administer high concentration of O_2 by mask; if pulmonary edema coexists, intubation and mechanical ventilation are indicated. Acute mechanical complications (see below) should be sought and promptly treated.

Hypotension also may result from *RV MI,* which should be suspected in the setting of inferior or posterior MI, if jugular venous distention and elevation of right-heart pressures predominate (rales are typically absent and PCW may be normal); *treatment* consists of volume infusion, gauged by PCW and arterial pressures. Noncardiac causes of hypotension should be considered: hypovolemia, acute arrhythmia, or sepsis.

ACUTE MECHANICAL COMPLICATIONS Ventricular septal rupture and acute mitral regurgitation due to papillary muscle ischemia/infarct develop during the first week following MI and are characterized by sudden onset of CHF and new systolic murmur. PCW tracings may show large *v* waves in either condition, but an oxygen "step-up" as catheter is advanced from RA to RV suggests septal rupture. Acute medical therapy of these conditions includes vasodilator therapy (IV nitroprusside: begin at 10 μg/min and titrate to maintain systolic BP ≃ 100 mmHg); intraaortic balloon pump may be required to maintain cardiac output. Surgical correction is postponed for 4–6 weeks after AMI if pt is stable; surgery should not be deferred if pt is unstable. Acute ventricular free-wall rupture presents with sudden loss of BP, pulse, and

TABLE 64-1 **Indications for Swan-Ganz catheter in acute myocardial infarction**

1. Moderate to severe CHF
2. Hypotension not corrected by volume infusion
3. Unexplained sinus tachycardia or tachypnea
4. Suspected acute mitral regurgitation or ventricular septal rupture
5. To manage IV vasodilator therapy

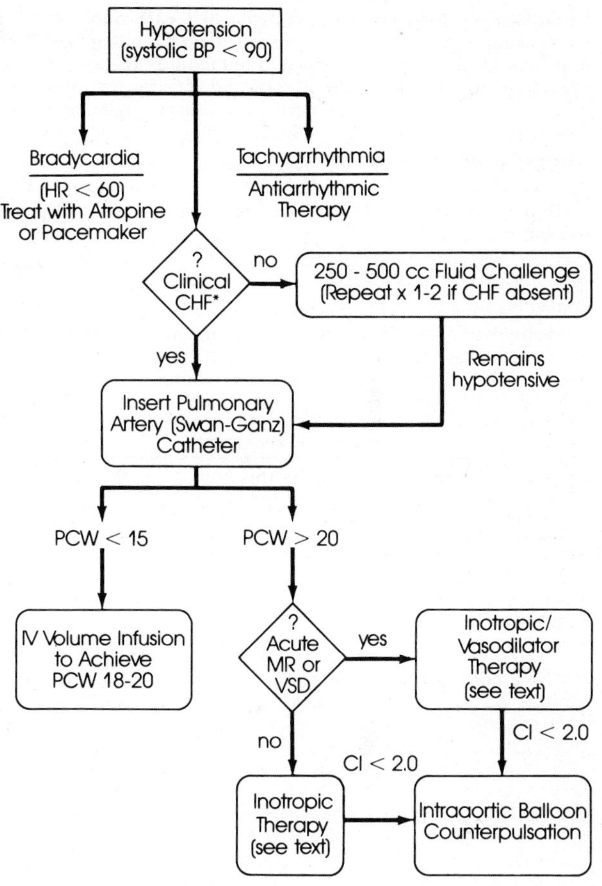

FIG. 64-1 *Approach to hypotension in acute myocardial infarction.*

consciousness, while ECG shows an intact rhythm; emergent surgical repair is crucial, and mortality is high.

PERICARDITIS Characterized by *pleuritic, positional* pain and pericardial rub (Chap. 67); must be distinguished from recurrent angina. Often responds to aspirin 650 mg PO qid. Anticoagulants should be withheld when pericarditis is suspected.

RECURRENT ANGINA Usually associated with transient ST-T wave changes; antianginal treatment should be maximized with oral beta blockers, nitrates, calcium antagonists (Chap. 65). For refractory angina, add IV nitroglycerin and, if necessary, intraaortic balloon counterpulsation followed by coronary angiography and consideration of angioplasty or bypass surgery.

DRESSLER'S SYNDROME Syndrome or fever, pleuritic chest pain, pericardial effusion which may develop 2–6 weeks following AMI; pain and ECG characteristic of pericarditis; usually responds to aspirin or NSAIDs.

SECONDARY PREVENTION

Exercise testing should be performed at, or soon after discharge. A positive test (Chap. 65) suggests need for cardiac catheterization to evaluate myocardium at risk of recurrent infarction. Beta blockers should be prescribed routinely commencing 7–14 days following AMI (Table 59-1), unless contraindication present (asthma, CHF, bradycardia, "brittle" diabetes).

For more detailed discussion of this topic, see Pasternak RC, Braunwald E, and Alpert JS: Acute Myocardial Infarction, Chap. 190, in HPIM-11, p. 982

---

65 CHRONIC CORONARY ARTERY DISEASE

Angina pectoris, the most common clinical manifestation of CAD, results from an imbalance between myocardial O_2 supply and demand, most commonly resulting from atherosclerotic coronary artery obstruction. Other conditions which upset this balance and result in angina include aortic stenosis (Chap. 62), hypertrophic cardiomyopathy (Chap. 68), and coronary artery spasm (see below).

SYMPTOMS Angina is typically associated with exertion or emotional upset; relieved quickly by rest or nitroglycerin (TNG) (see Chap. 2). Major risk factors are cigarette smoking, hypertension, hypercholesterolemia (↑ LDL fraction), diabetes, and family history.

PHYSICAL EXAM Often normal: arterial bruits or retinal vascular abnormalities suggest generalized atherosclerosis; S_4 is common. During acute anginal episode other signs may appear: loud S_3 or S_4, diaphoresis, rales, and a transient murmur of mitral regurgitation.

ECG May be normal between anginal episodes or show previous infarction (Chap. 57). During angina, ST- and T-wave abnormalities typically appear (ST-segment depression reflects subendocardial ischemia; ST-segment elevation may reflect acute infarction or transient coronary artery spasm). Ventricular arrhythmias frequently accompany acute ischemia.

STRESS TESTING Enhances diagnosis of CAD. Exercise is performed on treadmill or bicycle until target heart rate is achieved or pt becomes symptomatic (chest pain, light-headedness, hypotension, marked dyspnea, ventricular tachycardia) or develops diagnostic ST-segment changes. Useful information includes duration of exercise achieved; peak heart rate and BP; depth, morphology, and persistence of ST-segment depression; and whether and at which level of exercise pain, hypotension, or ventricular arrhythmias develop. *Thallium 201* imaging increases sensitivity and specificity and is particularly useful if baseline ECG abnormalities prevent interpretation of test (e.g., LBBB). *Note*: Exercise testing should not be performed in pts with unstable angina or aortic stenosis.

Some pts do not experience chest pain during ischemic episodes with exertion ("silent ischemia"), but are identified by transient ST-T wave abnormalities during stress testing or Holter monitoring.

CORONARY ARTERIOGRAPHY The definitive test for assessing severity of CAD; major indications are (1) angina refractory to medical therapy, (2) markedly positive exercise test (≥2-mm ST-segment depression, or hypotension with exercise) suggestive of left main or three-vessel disease, (3) to assess for coronary artery spasm, (4) to evaluate pts with perplexing chest pain in whom noninvasive tests are not diagnostic.

TABLE 65-1 **Examples of long-acting nitrate preparations**

Drug	Dosage
Isosorbide dinitrate	
Oral	10–60 mg tid-qid
Sublingual	5–20 mg q 3 h
Long-acting oral tembid*	40–80 mg PO bid-qid
Nitroglycerin skin ointment*	0.5–2.0 in qid
Transdermal nitroglycerin patch	5–25 mg per day

* Particularly useful at bedtime to prevent nocturnal angina during sleep.

MANAGEMENT

GENERAL

- Identify and treat risk factors; mandatory cessation of smoking.
- Correct exacerbating factors contributing to angina: hypertension, marked obesity, CHF, anemia, hyperthyroidism.
- Reassurance and pt education.

DRUG THERAPY Sublingual nitroglycerin (TNG 0.3–0.6 mg); may be repeated at 5-min.-intervals; warn pts of possible headache or light-headedness; teach prophylactic use of TNG prior to activity that evokes angina. If chest pain persists for more than 20 min despite 2–3 TNG, pt should report promptly to nearest medical facility for evaluation.

LONG-TERM ANGINA PREVENTION Three classes of drugs are used, frequently in combination:

Long-acting nitrates: May be administered by many routes (Table 65-1); start at the lowest dose to limit tolerance and side effects of headache, light-headedness, tachycardia.

Beta blockers (Table 59-1): All have antianginal properties; β_1-selective agents are less likely to exacerbate pulmonary or peripheral vascular disease. Dosage should be titrated to resting heart rate of 50–60 beats/min. *Contraindications* to beta blockers include CHF, AV block, bronchospasm, "brittle" diabetes. Side effects include fatigue, bronchospasm, depressed LV function, impotence, depression, and masking of hypoglycemia in diabetics.

Calcium antagonists (Table 65-2): Useful for stable and unstable angina, as well as coronary vasospasm. Combination with other antianginal agents is beneficial, but verapamil should be administered very cautiously or not at all to pts on beta blockers or disopyramide (additive effects on LV dysfunction).

TABLE 65-2 **Calcium antagonists**

	Dosage	Side effects
Diltiazem	30–90 mg PO tid-qid	(Uncommon) hypotension, AV block
Nifedipine	10–40 mg PO qid	Peripheral edema, hypotension, flushing
Verapamil*	80–120 mg PO tid	AV block, heart failure, constipation

* Avoid combination of verapamil with beta blockers or disopyramide (Norpace).

Percutaneous coronary angioplasty (PTCA) is effective in anatomically suitable stenoses of native vessels and bypass grafts; should be reserved mainly for pts who are refractory to or have inadequate response or troublesome side effects with standard medical therapy.

CORONARY ARTERY BYPASS SURGERY (CABG) For angina refractory to medical therapy or when the latter is not tolerated (and when lesions are not amenable to PTCA) or if severe CAD is present (left main, three-vessel disease with impaired LV function).

UNSTABLE AGINA

Includes (1) new onset of severe angina, (2) angina at rest or with minimal activity, (3) recent increases in frequency and intensity of chronic angina, (4) recurrent angina within several days of acute MI without reelevation of cardiac enzymes.

TREATMENT

- Identify and treat exacerbating factors (hypertension, arrhythmias, CHF, acute infection)
- Rule out MI by ECG and cardiac enzymes
- Maximize therapy with oral nitrates, beta blockers, calcium antagonists
- For refractory pain: IV TNG; titrate dosage to maintain systolic BP $\geq$ 100 mmHg
- Anticoagulation: IV heparin infusing (aim for PTT 1.5–2× control)
- Refractory unstable angina warrants coronary arteriography and consideration of PTCA or CABG.

CORONARY VASOSPASM

Caused by intermittent focal spasm of a coronary artery; often associated with atherosclerotic lesion near site of spasm. Chest discomfort is similar to angina but more severe and occurs typically at rest, with transient ST-segment elevation. Acute infarction or malignant arrhythmias may develop during spasm-induced ischemia. Evaluation includes observation of ECG (or ambulatory Holter monitor tracing) for transient ST elevation; diagnosis confirmed at cardiac catheterization using provocative IV ergonovine testing. *Treatment* consists of long-acting nitrates and calcium antagonists.

For more detailed discussion of this topic, see Selwyn AP, Braunwald E: Ischemic Heart Disease, Chap. 189, in HPIM-11. p. 975

66 COR PULMONALE

Right ventricular enlargement resulting from *primary* lung disease; leads to RV hypertrophy and eventually to RV failure. Etiologies include the following:

Pulmonary parenchymal or airway disease: Chronic obstructive lung disease (COPD), interstitial lung diseases, bronchiectasis, cystic fibrosis (Chaps. 75–77).

Pulmonary vascular disease: Recurrent pulmonary emboli, primary pulmonary hypertension (PHT), sickle cell anemia.

Inadequate mechanical ventilation: Kyphoscoliosis, neuromuscular disorders, marked obesity, sleep apnea.

SYMPTOMS Depend on underlying disorder, but include dyspnea, cough, fatigue, and sputum production (in parenchymal diseases).

PHYSICAL EXAM Tachypnea, cyanosis, clubbing are common. RV impulse along left sternal border, loud P_2, right-sided S_4. If RV failure develops, elevated jugular venous pressure, hepatomegaly with ascites, pedal edema.

LABORATORY **ECG:** RV hypertrophy and RA enlargement, tachyarrhythmias are common.

CXR: RV and pulmonary artery enlargement; if PHT present, tapering of the pulmonary artery branches. PFTs (Chap. 71) and ABGs characterize intrinsic pulmonary disease.

Echocardiogram: RV hypertrophy; LV function typically normal. If pulmonary emboli suspected, obtain radionuclide lung scan.

TREATMENT Aimed at underlying pulmonary disease. If RV failure is present, treat as CHF, instituting low-sodium diet and diuretics (Chap. 58); digoxin must be administered cautiously (toxicity increased due to hypoxemia, hypercapnia, acidosis). Supraventricular tachyarrhythmias are common and treated with digoxin, quinidine, or verapamil (*not* beta blockers). Chronic anticoagulation with warfarin is indicated when pulmonary hypertension is accompanied by RV failure.

For more detailed discussion of this topic, see Fishman AP: Cor Pulmonale, Chap. 191, in HPIM-11, p. 993

67 PERICARDIAL DISEASE

ACUTE PERICARDITIS (Table 67-1)

HISTORY Chest pain, which may be intense, mimicking AMI, but characteristically sharp, pleuritic, and positional; fever and palpitations are common.

PHYSICAL EXAM Rapid or irregular pulse, coarse pericardial friction rub, which may vary in intensity.
ECG: Diffuse ST elevation (concave upwards) usually present in all leads except aVR and V_1; PR-segment depression may be present; *days* later (unlike AMI) ST returns to baseline and T-wave inversion develops.
CXR: Increased size of cardiac silhouette if pericardial effusion present.
Echocardiogram: Most sensitive test for detection of pericardial effusion, which commonly accompanies acute pericarditis.

TREATMENT Aspirin 650–975 mg qid or NSAIDs; for severe pain resistant to preceding, prednisone 40–60 mg is used and tapered over several weeks or months. Intractable, prolonged pain may require pericardiectomy.

CARDIAC TAMPONADE

Life-threatening emergency resulting from accumulation of pericardial fluid under pressure; impaired filling of cardiac chambers and decreased cardiac output.

ETIOLOGY Previous pericarditis (most commonly metastatic tumor, uremia, AMI, viral or idiopathic pericarditis), cardiac trauma, or myocardial perforation during catheter or pacemaker placement.

HISTORY Hypotension may develop suddenly; subacute symptoms include dyspnea, weakness, confusion.

PHYSICAL EXAM Tachycardia, hypotension, pulsus paradoxus (inspiratory fall in systolic blood pressure > 10 mmHg), jugular venous distention with preserved *x* descent, but loss of *y* descent; heart sounds distant. If tamponade develops subacutely, peripheral edema, hepatomegaly, and ascites are frequently present.

TABLE 67-1 **Most common causes of pericarditis**

Idiopathic
Infections (particularly viral)
AMI
Metastatic neoplasm
Radiation therapy for tumor (up to 20 years earlier)
Chronic renal failure
Connective-tissue disease (rheumatoid arthritis, SLE)
Drug reaction (e.g., procainamide, hydralazine)
"Immunologic" following heart surgery or myocardial infarction (several weeks/months later)

ECG: Low limb lead voltage; large effusions may cause electrical alternans (alternating size of QRS complex due to swinging of heart).
CXR: Enlarged cardiac silhouette if effusion present.
Echocardiogram: Swinging motion of heart within large effusion; prominent respiratory alteration of RV dimension with RA and RV collapse during diastole.
Cardiac catheterization: Confirms diagnosis; shows equalization of diastolic pressures in all four chambers; pericardial = RA pressure.

TREATMENT Immediate pericardiocentesis and IV volume expansion.

CONSTRICTIVE PERICARDITIS

Rigid pericardium leads to impaired cardiac filling, elevation of systemic and pulmonary venous pressures, and decreased cardiac output. Results from healing of previous pericarditis. Viral, TBC, uremia, neoplastic are most common etiologies.

HISTORY Gradual onset of dyspnea, fatigue, pedal edema, abdominal swelling; symptoms of LV failure uncommon.

PHYSICAL EXAM Tachycardia, jugular venous distention (prominent *y* descent) which increases further in inspiration (Kussmaul's sign); hepatomegaly, ascites, peripheral edema are common; sharp diastolic sound, "pericardial knock," following S_2 sometimes present.
ECG: Low limb lead voltage; atrial arrhythmias are common.
CXR: Rim of pericardial calcification in 50% of patients.
Echocardiogram: Thickened pericardium, normal ventricular contraction.
Cardiac catheterization: Equalization of diastolic pressures in all chambers; ventricular pressure tracings show "dip and plateau" appearance (to distinguish from restrictive cardiomyopathy; see Table 68-1). Patients with constrictive pericarditis should be investigated for TBC.

TREATMENT Surgical stripping of the pericardium.

APPROACH TO ASYMPTOMATIC PERICARDIAL EFFUSION OF UNKNOWN CAUSE

If careful history and physical exam do not suggest etiology, the following may lead to diagnosis:

- Skin test and cultures for TBC (Chap. 42)
- Serum albumin and urine protein measurement (nephrotic syndrome)
- Serum creatinine and BUN (renal failure)
- Thyroid function tests (myxedema)
- ANA (SLE and other collagen-vascular disease)
- Search for primary tumor

For more detailed discussion of this topic, see Braunwald E: Pericardial Disease, Chap. 194, in HPIM-11, p. 1008

68 CARDIOMYOPATHIES AND MYOCARDITIS

DILATED CARDIOMYOPATHY (CMP)

Symmetrically dilated left ventricle (LV), with poor systolic contractile function; right ventricle (RV) commonly involved.

ETIOLOGY Previous myocarditis or "idiopathic" most common; also toxins (ethanol, doxorubicin), connective tissue disorders, muscular dystrophies, "peripartum." Severe coronary disease/infarctions or chronic aortic/mitral regurgitation may behave similarly.

SYMPTOMS Congestive heart failure (Chap. 58); advanced arrhythmias or peripheral emboli from left ventricular mural thrombus occur.

PHYSICAL EXAM Jugular venous distention, rales, diffuse and dyskinetic LV apex, S_3, hepatomegaly, peripheral edema; murmurs of mitral and tricuspid regurgitation are common.

LABORATORY FINDINGS **ECG:** Left bundle-branch block and ST-T-wave abnormalities common.
CXR: Cardiomegaly, pulmonary vascular redistribution, pulmonary effusions common.
Echocardiogram: LV and RV enlargement with globally impaired contraction. Regional wall motion abnormalities suggest CAD rather than primary cardiomyopathy.

TREATMENT Standard therapy of CHF (Chap. 58); chronic anticoagulation with warfarin, if no contraindications; antiarrhythmic drugs (Chap. 60). Possible trial of immunosuppressive drugs, if active myocarditis present on RV biopsy. In select patients, consider cardiac transplantation.

RESTRICTIVE CARDIOMYOPATHY

Increased myocardial "stiffness" impairs ventricular relaxation; diastolic ventricular pressures are elevated. Causes include infiltrative disease (amyloid, sarcoid, hemochromatosis, eosinophilic disorders), myocardial fibrosis, and fibroelastosis.

SYMPTOMS Are those of CHF, although right-sided heart failure often predominates with peripheral edema and ascites.

PHYSICAL EXAM Signs of right-sided heart failure: JVD, hepatomegaly, peripheral edema, murmur of tricuspid regurgitation. Left-sided signs also may be present.

LABORATORY FINDINGS **ECG:** Low limb lead voltage, sinus tachycardia, ST-T-wave abnormalities.
CXR: Mild LV enlargement.
Echocardiogram: Bilateral atrial enlargement; increased ventricular thickness ("speckled pattern") in cardiac amyloidosis. Systolic function is usually normal, but may be mildly reduced.

Cardiac catheterization: Increased LV and RV diastolic pressures with "dip and plateau" pattern; RV biopsy useful in detecting infiltrative disease (rectal biopsy useful in diagnosis of amyloidosis).

Note: Must distinguish restrictive cardiomyopathy from constrictive pericarditis, which is surgically correctable (see Table 68-1).

TREATMENT

- Salt restriction and diuretics; digitalis is not indicated unless systolic function impaired or atrial arrhythmias present. *Note:* Increased sensitivity to digitalis in amyloidosis.
- Anticoagulation, particularly in patients with eosinophilic endomyocarditis.
- For specific therapy of hemochromatosis see HPIM-11, Chap. 310, and sarcoidosis see HPIM-11, Chap. 270.

HYPERTROPHIC OBSTRUCTIVE CARDIOMYOPATHY (HOCM)

Marked LV hypertrophy; often asymmetric, without underlying cause. Systolic function is normal; increased LV stiffness results in elevated diastolic filling pressures.

SYMPTOMS Secondary to elevated diastolic pressure, dynamic LV outflow obstruction, and arrhythmias; dyspnea on exertion, angina, and presyncope; sudden death may occur.

PHYSICAL EXAM Brisk carotid upstroke with pulsus bisferiens; S_4, harsh systolic murmur along left sternal border, blowing murmur of mitral regurgitation at apex; murmur changes with Valsalva and other maneuvers (see Chap. 56).

LABORATORY FINDINGS ECG: LV hypertrophy with prominent "septal" Q waves in leads I, aVL, V_{5-6}.

TABLE 68-1 **Restrictive cardiomyopathy vs. constrictive pericarditis**

	Constrictive pericarditis	Restrictive cardiomyopathy
Prominent palpable cardiac apex	No	Yes
Cardiac size	Normal	May be enlarged
S_3, S_4	Absent (pericardial knock possible)	Often present
Calcification of pericardium on x-ray	Frequent	Absent
Systolic function	Normal	May be depressed
"Dip and plateau"	Yes	Yes
LV vs. RV diastolic pressure	Equal	LV usually higher
RV biopsy	Normal	Abnormal: may show infiltrative disease

Echocardiogram: LV hypertrophy, asymmetrical septal hypertrophy (ASH) and $\geq 1.3 \times$ thickness of LV posterior wall; LV contractile function excellent with small end-systolic volume. If LV outflow tract obstruction is present, systolic anterior motion (SAM) of mitral valve and midsystolic partial closure of aortic valve are present. Doppler shows early systolic accelerated blood flow through LV outflow tract. Carotid pulse tracing shows "spike and dome" configuration.

TREATMENT Beta blockers, verapamil, or disophyramide used individually to reduce symptoms. Digoxin, other inotropes, diuretics, and vasodilators are *contraindicated.* Endocarditis antibiotic prophylaxis (Chap. 63) is necessary when outflow obstruction or mitral regurgitation is present. Antiarrhythmic agents, especially amiodarone, may suppress atrial and ventricular arrhythmias. Surgical myectomy in patients refractory to medical therapy.

MYOCARDITIS

Inflammation of the myocardium most commonly due to acute viral infection; may progress to chronic dilated cardiomyopathy.

HISTORY Fever, fatigue, palpitations; if LV dysfunction is present, then symptoms of CHF are present. Viral myocarditis may be preceded by URI.

PHYSICAL EXAM Fever, tachycardia, soft S_1; S_3 common.

LABORATORY FINDINGS **ECG:** Transient ST-T-wave abnormalities.
CXR: Cardiomegaly; CK-MB isoenzyme may be elevated in absence of MI. Convalescent antiviral antibody titers may rise.
Echocardiogram: Depressed LV function; pericardial effusion present if accompanying pericarditis present.

TREATMENT Rest; treat as CHF (Chap. 58); immunosuppressive therapy (steroids and azathioprine) may be considered if RV biopsy shows active inflammation. This treatment is experimental, and should not be given early in the course.

For more detailed discussion of this topic, see Wynne J, Braunwald E: The Cardiomyopathies and Myocarditides, Chap. 192, in HPIM-11, p. 998

69 DISEASES OF THE AORTA

AORTIC ANEURYSM

Abnormal widening of the abdominal or thoracic aorta; in ascending aorta most commonly secondary to cystic medial necrosis or atherosclerosis; aneurysms of descending thoracic and abdominal aorta are primarily atherosclerotic.

HISTORY May be clinically silent, but thoracic aortic aneurysms often result in deep, diffuse chest pain, dysphagia, hoarseness, hemoptysis, dry cough; abdominal aneurysms result in abdominal pain or thromboemboli to the lower extremities.

PHYSICAL EXAM Abdominal aneurysms are often palpable, most commonly in periumbilical area. Patients with ascending thoracic aneurysms may show features of Marfan's syndrome (see HPIM-11, Chap. 319).

LABORATORY FINDINGS *CXR:* enlarged aortic silhouette (thoracic aneurysm); confirm abdominal aneurysm by *abdominal plain film* (rim of calcification), *ultrasound,* or *CT scan.* Contrast aortography is performed preoperatively. If clinically suspected, obtain serologic test for syphilis, especially if ascending thoracic aneurysm shows thin shell of calcification.

TREATMENT Control of hypertension (Chap. 59) is essential. Surgical resection of aortic aneurysms > 6 cm in diameter, for persistent pain despite BP control, or evidence of rapid expansion.

DISSECTION OF THE AORTA

Potentially life-threatening condition in which disruption of aortic intima allows dissection of blood into vessel wall; may involve ascending aorta (type II), descending aorta (type III) or both (type I). Involvement of the ascending aorta is most lethal form.

ETIOLOGY Ascending aortic dissection associated with hypertension, cystic medial necrosis, Marfan's syndrome (see HPIM-11, Chap. 319); descending dissections commonly associated with atherosclerosis or hypertension.

SYMPTOMS Sudden onset of severe anterior or posterior chest pain, with "ripping" quality; maximal pain may travel if dissection propagates. Additional symptoms relate to obstruction of aortic branches (stroke, MI), dyspnea (acute aortic regurgitation), or symptoms of low cardiac output due to cardiac tamponade (dissection into pericardial sac).

PHYSICAL EXAM Sinus tachycardia common; if cardiac tamponade develops, hypotension, pulsus paradoxus, and pericardial rub appear. Asymmetry of carotid or brachial pulses, aortic regurgitation, and neurologic abnormalities associated with interruption of carotid artery flow are common findings.

LABORATORY FINDINGS *CXR:* widening of mediastinum; dissection can be confirmed by *CT scan* or *ultrasound.* However, once dissection is strongly suspected clinically, aortography is indicated.

TREATMENT Antihypertensive therapy to maintain systolic BP below 120 mmHg, using IV agents, e.g., sodium nitroprusside (20 to 400 μg/min) or propranolol (0.5 mg IV q 5 min), followed by oral therapy. Ascending aortic dissection requires immediate surgical repair. Descending aortic dissections are stabilized medically with oral antihypertensive agents (especially beta blockers); immediate surgical repair is not necessary unless recurrent pain or extension of dissection is observed (serial CT scans).

OTHER ABNORMALITIES OF THE AORTA

ATHEROSCLEROSIS OF ABDOMINAL AORTA Particularly common in presence of diabetes mellitus or cigarette smoking. Symptoms include intermittent claudication of the buttocks and thighs and impotence (Lerische's syndrome); diagnosis confirmed by aortography. Aortic-femoral bypass surgery is required for symptomatic treatment.

TAKAYASU'S ("PULSELESS") DISEASE Arteritis of aorta and major branches in young women. Anorexia, weight loss, fever, and night sweats occur. Localized symptoms relate to occlusion of aortic branches (cerebral ischemia, claudication, and loss of pulses in arms). ESR is increased; diagnosis confirmed by aortography. Corticosteroid therapy may be beneficial, but mortality is high.

For more detailed discussion of this topic, see Dalen JE: Diseases of the Aorta, Chap. 197, in HPIM-11, p. 1037

[illegible]

OTHER ABNORMALITIES OF THE AORTA

[illegible]

70 PERIPHERAL VASCULAR DISEASE

Occlusive or inflammatory disease that develops within the peripheral arteries, veins, or lymphatics.

ARTERIOSCLEROSIS OF PERIPHERAL ARTERIES

HISTORY *Intermittent claudication* is muscular cramping with exercise; quickly relieved by rest. Pain in buttocks and thighs suggests aortoiliac disease; calf muscle pain implies femoral or popliteal artery disease. More advanced arteriosclerotic obstruction results in pain at rest; painful ulcers of the feet (painless in diabetics) may result.

PHYSICAL EXAM Decreased peripheral pulses, blanching of affected limb with elevation, dependent rubor (redness). Ischemic ulcers or gangrene of toes may be present.

LABORATORY FINDINGS Doppler ultrasound of peripheral pulses before and during exercise localizes stenoses; contrast arteriography performed only if reconstructive surgery is planned.

TREATMENT Most patients can be managed medically with daily exercise program, careful foot care (especially in diabetics), low-cholesterol/low-saturated-fat diet, and local debridement of ulcerations. Abstinence from cigarettes is mandatory. Patients with severe claudication, rest pain, or gangrene are candidates for arterial reconstructive surgery; percutaneous transluminal angioplasty can be performed in selected patients.

Other conditions which impair peripheral arterial flow:

1 *Arterial embolism:* Due to thrombus or vegetation within the heart or aorta or paradoxically formed venous thrombus through a right-to-left intracardiac shunt. *History:* sudden pain or numbness in an extremity in absence of previous history of claudication. *Physical exam:* absent pulse, pallor, and decreased temperature of limb distal to the occlusion. Lesion is identified by angiography and requires immediate anticoagulation and surgical embolectomy.

2 *Vasospastic disorders:* Manifest by Raynaud's phenomenon in which cold exposure results in triphasic color response: blanching of the fingers, followed by cyanosis, then redness. Usually a benign disorder. However, suspect an underlying disease (e.g., scleroderma) if tissue necrosis occurs, if disease is unilateral, or if it develops after age 50. *Treatment:* keep extremities warm; calcium channel blockers (nifedipine 10–40 mg PO tid–qid) may be effective.

3 *Thromboangiitis obliterans (Buerger's disease):* Occurs in young men who are heavy smokers and involves both upper and lower extremities; nonatheromatous inflammatory reaction develops in veins and small arteries leading to superficial thrombophlebitis and arterial obstruction with ulceration or gangrene of digits. Abstinence from tobacco is essential.

VENOUS OCCLUSION

SUPERFICIAL THROMBOPHLEBITIS Benign disorder characterized by erythema, tenderness, and edema along involved vein. Conservative therapy includes local heat, elevation, and anti-inflammatory drugs such as aspirin. More serious conditions such as cellulitis or lymphangitis may mimic this, but these are associated with fever, chills, lymphadenopathy, and red superficial streaks along inflamed lymphatic channels.

DEEP VENOUS THROMBOSIS (DVT) More serious condition which may lead to pulmonary embolism (Chap. 77). Particularly common in patients on prolonged bed rest, those with chronic debilitating disease, and those with malignancies.
History: Pain or tenderness in calf, usually unilateral; may be asymptomatic, with pulmonary embolism as primary presentation.
Physical exam: Often normal; local swelling or tenderness to deep palpation may be present over affected vein.
Laboratory findings: Noninvasive impedance plethysmography useful in detecting DVT; definitive diagnosis is made by peripheral venography.
Treatment: Systemic anticoagulation with heparin (5000 to 10,000 U bolus, followed by continuous IV infusion to maintain PTT at 2 to 2.5 × normal) for 7–10 days, followed by warfarin PO for 3 months.

DVT can be prevented by early ambulation following surgery or with low-dose heparin during prolonged bed rest (5000 U SC bid-tid).

For more detailed discussion of this topic, see Strandness DE Jr.: Vascular Diseases of the Extremities, Chap. 198, in HPIM-11, p. 1040

SECTION IV
RESPIRATORY DISEASE

71 DISTURBANCES OF RESPIRATORY FUNCTION

The prime function of the lung is to exchange gas between inspired air and venous blood. No gas exchange occurs in conducting airways (anatomic dead space). Alveolar gas participates in gas exchange.

VENTILATION

Resting ventilation: Normal tidal volume is about 500 mL, and normal frequency about 15 breaths/minute, making *total ventilation* 7.5 L/minute. Because of dead space, *alveolar* ventilation is only 5 L.

Control of ventilation: Chief regulation of rhythmic breathing is by medullary chemoreceptors, which respond to changes in arterial P_{CO_2} (possibly via induced changes in extracellular fluid pH). Arterial hypoxemia increases ventilation through its action on peripheral chemoreceptors in the carotid body.

Hypoventilation: Alveolar ventilation inadequate to supply sufficient O_2 to keep pace with consumption and remove sufficient CO_2 to match production. Often occurs with normal lungs (see Chap. 81). Arterial P_{CO_2} rises and P_{O_2} falls.

Hyperventilation: Arterial P_{CO_2} falls when alveolar ventilation exceeds CO_2 production. May occur when chemoreceptors are stimulated by acidosis.

DIFFUSION ACROSS BLOOD-GAS BARRIER

O_2 and CO_2 move across the blood-gas barrier by simple physical diffusion. Exercise and alveolar hypoxia stress diffusion capacity of lung.

Measurement of diffusing capacity of lung ($D_{L_{CO}}$): Carried out with low concentration of carbon monoxide (CO) during a single 10-s breath-holding period or during 1 minute of steady breathing. $D_{L_{CO}}$ is decreased by (1) diseases that thicken the alveolar membrane (e.g., interstitial fibrosis, sarcoidosis, asbestosis, alveolar cell carcinoma); (2) reduction of area of alveolar-capillary membrane (e.g., postpneumonectomy, emphysema); and (3) reduction of capillary blood volume or number of RBCs in the capillaries (e.g., pulmonary embolism, anemia).

VENTILATION-PERFUSION RELATIONS

Normal distribution of perfusion (Q): In normal upright lung, Q/unit of lung volume increases from top to bottom. Uneven distribution of blood flow normally is a result of hydrostatic pressure differences in the lung.

Normal distribution of ventilation (V): V also increases down the upright lung, but changes are less marked than for blood flow. However, V to dependent regions is reduced at low lung volumes (important in obesity and following abdominal surgery). Lung volume at which lower-zone airways close (closing volume) increases with age and lung disease and may encroach on normal breathing range, resulting in poorly ventilated regions.

V/Q ratio: Decreases greatly down the upright lung; this ratio critically determines the P_{O_2} in end-capillary blood.

Overall gas exchange: Lung units overperfused in relation to ventilation, which therefore have a low P_{O_2}, contribute a disproportionate amount of blood flow to systemic arterial blood. This may depress arterial P_{O_2} by 50 mmHg, but P_{CO_2} is often maintained at normal level by increased ventilation. *Alveolar-arterial* P_{O_2} difference reflects V/Q inequality (ideal alveolar P_{O_2} = arterial P_{O_2}). *Physiologic shunt* (reflecting lung units with low V/Q) and *physiologic dead space* (reflecting lung units with high V/Q) can also be calculated.

MECHANICS OF BREATHING

Lung and chest wall: Lung is elastic and will collapse if pressure is not applied to keep it expanded. Chest wall, also elastic, tends to recoil outward. Inspiration occurs when active contraction of respiratory muscles lowers intrathoracic (and alveolar) pressure below atmospheric.

Muscles of respiration: Diaphragm is the major inspiratory muscle, descending 1 to 10 cm with a breath. Other inspiratory muscles include intercostals, scalenes, and sternocleidomastoids. Expiration is passive during quiet breathing, but abdominal muscles and intercostals may play an active role.

Compliance: Refers to change in lung volume for a change in pressure, reflecting the elastic properties of lung and chest wall. Elasticity of lung reflects the amount of elastic tissue and the surface tension of alveoli.

Airway resistance: During ventilation, force is required to overcome elasticity and resistance to airflow. Most resistance is in airways $<$ 2 mm in diameter. Resistance is greater during expiration and at low lung volumes. Asthma and emphysema increase resistance.

Measurements of mechanics: Single forced expiration gives information about airways resistance, compliance, and muscle function (Fig. 71-1) and is required for the diagnosis of obstructive lung disease. Measurements of total lung capacity and other lung volumes are required for diagnosis of restrictive lung disease.

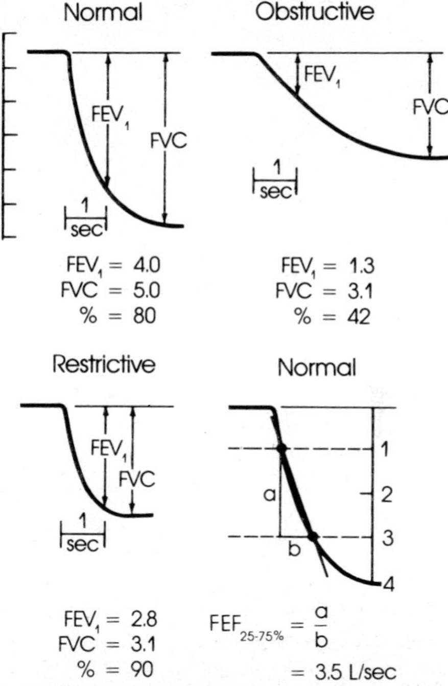

FIG. 71-1 *Measurement of the forced expiratory volume, FEV_1; forced vital capacity, FVC; and maximum midexpiratory flow, $FEF_{25-75\%}$. The patient makes a full inspiration and then exhales as hard and as fast as possible. As the patient exhales the pen moves down. The FEV_1 is the volume exhaled in 1 s; the FVC is the total volume exhaled. $FEF_{25-75\%}$ is the mean flow rate measured over the middle half of the FVC. Note the differences between the normal, obstructive, and restrictive patterns. (Reproduced from West JB: HPIM-11, p. 1055.)*

HYPOXEMIA AND HYPERCAPNIA

Hypoxemia: Four main causes: (1) V/Q inequality, (2) right-to-left shunt, (3) hypoventilation, and (4) impaired diffusion. Of these, V/Q inequality is most common and responsible for hypoxemia in chronic obstructive lung disease. Hypoxemia of shunt is not abolished by inspiring 100% O_2. Hypoventilation always causes hypoxemia and hypercapnia. Impaired diffusion is a rare cause of hypoxemia.

Hypercapnia: Caused either by V/Q inequality or hypoventilation.

For more detailed discussion of this topic, see West JB: Disturbances of Respiratory Function, Chap. 200, in HPIM-11, p. 1049

72 DIAGNOSTIC PROCEDURES IN RESPIRATORY DISEASE

NONINVASIVE PROCEDURES

Radiographic procedures: No CXR pattern is sufficiently specific to *establish* a diagnosis; instead, the CXR serves to *detect* disease, assess magnitude, and guide further diagnostic investigation. Fluoroscopy provides a dynamic image of the chest and is particularly helpful in localizing lesions poorly visible on the CXR. Both fluoroscopy and standard tomography have largely been supplanted by thoracic CT, which is now routine in evaluation of patients with pulmonary nodules and masses. Contrast enhancement also makes thoracic CT useful in differentiating tissue masses from vascular structures.

Skin tests: Specific skin test antigens are available for TBC, histoplasmosis, coccidioidomycosis, blastomycosis, trichinosis, toxoplasmosis, and aspergillosis. A positive delayed reaction (type IV) to a tuberculin test indicates only prior infection, not active disease. Immediate (type I) and late (type III) dermal hypersensitivity to *Aspergillus* antigen supports diagnosis of allergic bronchopulmonary aspergillosis in pts with a compatible clinical illness.

Sputum exam: Sputum is distinguished from saliva by presence of bronchial epithelial cells and alveolar macrophages. Sputum exam should include gross inspection for blood, color, and odor, as well as microscopic inspection of carefully stained smears. Culture of expectorated sputum may be misleading owing to contamination with oropharyngeal flora.

Pulmonary function tests: May indicate abnormalities of airway function, alterations of lung volume, and disturbances of gas exchange. Specific patterns of pulmonary function may assist in differential diagnosis. PFTs also may provide objective measures of therapeutic response, e.g., to bronchodilators.

Pulmonary scintiphotography: Scans of pulmonary ventilation and perfusion aid in the diagnosis of pulmonary embolism. Quantitative ventilation-perfusion scans also are used to assess surgical resectability of lung cancer in pts with diminished respiratory function. *Gallium scanning* may be used to identify inflammatory disease of the lungs or mediastinal lymph nodes. Inflammatory activity of the lungs detected with gallium may be associated with diffuse interstitial infections. Gallium uptake by the lungs also may occur in *Pneumocystis carinii* pneumonia.

INVASIVE PROCEDURES

Bronchoscopy: Permits visualization of airways, identification of endobronchial abnormalities, and collection of diagnostic specimens by lavage, brushing, or biopsy. The fiberoptic bronchoscope permits exam of smaller, more peripheral airways than the rigid bronchoscope, but the latter permits greater control of the airways and provides more effective suctioning. These features make rigid bronchoscopy particularly useful in pts with central obstructing tumors, foreign bodies, or massive hemoptysis. The fiberoptic bronchoscope increases the diagnostic potential of bronchoscopy, permitting biopsy of peripheral nodules and diffuse infiltrative diseases as well as aspiration and lavage of airways and airspaces.

Bronchography: Performed to outline congenital malformations or acquired forms of tracheobronchial distortion and to delineate bronchiectatic airways.

Transtracheal, catheter-brush, and percutaneous needle aspiration of the lung: These procedures provide microbiologic specimens from lung while avoiding contamination with oropharyngeal flora. All procedures involve risks and should be performed only by experienced individuals.

Thoracentesis and pleural biopsy: Thoracentesis should be performed as an early step in the evaluation of any pleural effusion of uncertain etiology. Analysis of pleural fluid helps differentiate transudate from exudate (Chap. 80). Pleural fluid pH (<7.2) suggests that an exudate associated with an infection is an empyema and will almost certainly require drainage. WBC count and differential; glucose, P_{CO_2}, amylase, Gram stain, culture, and cytologic exam should be performed on all specimens. Closed pleural biopsy also can be done when a pleural effusion is present; particularly useful when TBC is suspected.

Pulmonary angiography is the definitive test for pulmonary embolism; also may reveal AV malformations.

Bronchial arteriography is performed to identify and possibly embolize arterial sites in pts with massive hemoptysis.

Mediastinoscopy: Diagnostic procedure of choice in pts with disease involving mediastinal lymph nodes. However, lymph nodes in left superior mediastinum must be approached via *mediastinotomy*.

Lung biopsy: Closed biopsies are performed percutaneously with a cutting needle or with a fiberoptic bronchoscope; open biopsies require thoracotomy. The cutting needle is favored over the bronchoscope for small peripheral lesions, whereas transbronchial biopsy is preferred for diffuse disease. Open biopsy is favored when histologic diagnosis is difficult and when an accurate tissue diagnosis must be made rapidly.

For more detailed discussion of this topic, see Moser KM: Diagnostic Procedures in Respiratory Diseases, Chap. 201, in HPIM-11, p. 1056

---

73 ASTHMA AND HYPERSENSITIVITY PNEUMONITIS

ASTHMA

DEFINITION Disease of lower airways characterized by increased responsiveness of tracheobronchial tree to multiple stimuli; episodic, and by definition, airway obstruction is reversible; may range in severity from mild without limitation of patient's activity to severe and life-threatening. Obstruction persisting for days or weeks is known as *status asthmaticus.*

ETIOLOGY AND PATHOGENESIS Basic abnormality is airway hyperresponsiveness to both specific and nonspecific stimuli. All pts demonstrate enhanced bronchoconstriction in response to inhalation of methacholine or histamine (nonspecific bronchoconstrictor agents). Some pts may be classified as having *allergic asthma;* these experience worsening of symptoms on exposure to pollens or other allergens. They characteristically give personal and/or family history of other allergic diseases, such as rhinitis, urticaria, and eczema. Skin tests to allergens are positive; serum IgE may be ↑. If performed, bronchoprovocation studies may demonstrate positive responses to inhalation of specific allergens.

A significant number of asthmatic pts have negative allergic histories and do not react to skin or bronchoprovocation testing with specific allergens. These pts are said to have *idiosyncratic* or *intrinsic asthma.*

Some pts experience worsening of symptoms on *exercise* or exposure to *cold air* or *occupational* stimuli. Many note increased wheezing following *viral URI* or in response to *emotional stress.* **Miscellaneous triggering factors:** Aspirin, beta-adrenergic blocking agents (e.g., propranolol, timolol), sulfiting agents in food or beverages, air pollution.

APPROACH TO PATIENT

History

• Symptoms: wheezing, dyspnea, cough, fever, sputum production, other allergic disorders. • Duration of current symptoms and possible precipitating factors (allergens, infection, etc.). • Current and previous medicine usage. • Course of previous attacks (e.g., need for hospitalization, steroid treatment).

Physical Exam

• General: tachypnea, tachycardia, use of accessory respiratory muscles, cyanosis, pulsus paradoxus. • Lungs: adequacy of aeration, symmetry of breath sounds, wheezing, prolongation of expiratory phase, hyperinflation. • Heart: evidence for CHF. • ENT/skin: evidence of allergic nasal, sinus, or skin disease.

Laboratory

• PFTs: while PFT findings are not diagnostic, they are very helpful in judging severity of airway obstruction and in following response to therapy in both chronic and acute situations. FVC, FEV_1, MMEFR, PEFR, FEV_1/FVC are decreased; RV and TLC increased during episodes of obstruction; DL_{CO} usually normal or slightly increased. • CBC may show eosinophilia. • IgE may show mild elevations; marked elevations may suggest evidence of allergic bronchopulmonary aspergillosis (ABPA). • Sputum examination: eosinophilia, Curschmann's spirals (casts of small airways), Charcot-Leyden crystals; presence of large numbers of neutrophils suggests bronchial infection. • ABGs: uniformly show hypoxemia during attacks; usually hypocarbia and respiratory alkalosis present; normal or elevated P_{CO_2} worrisome as may suggest respiratory muscle fatigue and severe airways obstruction. • CXR not always necessary: may show hyperinflation, patchy infiltrates due to atelectasis behind plugged airways; important when complicating infection is a consideration.

DIFFERENTIAL DIAGNOSIS "All that wheezes is not asthma": CHF; chronic bronchitis/emphysema; upper airway obstruction due to foreign body, tumor, laryngeal edema; carcinoid tumors; recurrent pulmonary emboli; eosinophilic pneumonia; vocal cord dysfunction; systemic vasculitis with pulmonary involvement.

THERAPY

• Elimination of provoking allergen(s) from environment. • Beta-adrenergic agonists: inhaled route provides most rapid effect and best therapeutic index; isoetharine, albuterol, terbutaline, metaproterenol, or isoproterenol may be given by nebulizer or metered-dose inhaler. • Epinephrine 0.3 mL of 1:1000 solution SC (for use in acute situations in absence of cardiac history). • Methylxanthines: theophylline and various salts; adjust dose to maintain blood level between 10 and 20 μg/mL; may be given PO or IV (as aminophylline). • Glucocorticoids: prednisone 40 to 60 mg PO daily followed by tapering schedule; hydrocortisone 4 mg/kg IV loading dose followed by 3 mg/kg q 6 h; methylprednisolone 50 to 100 mg IV q 6 h. • Inhaled glucocorticoid preparations are important adjuncts to chronic therapy; not useful in acute attacks. • Cromolyn sodium: for chronic therapy, not useful during acute attacks; administered as metered-dose inhaler or nebulized powder. • Anticholinergics: aerosolized atropine and related compounds.

HYPERSENSITIVITY PNEUMONITIS

DEFINITION Hypersensitivity pneumonitis (HP) or extrinsic allergic alveolitis is an immunologically mediated inflammation of lung parenchyma involving alveolar walls and terminal airways secondary to repeated inhalation of a variety of organic dusts by a susceptible host.

ETIOLOGY A variety of inhaled substances have been implicated (see Table 203-1 in HPIM-11). These substances are usually organic antigens but may include inorganic compounds.

CLINICAL MANIFESTATIONS Symptoms may be acute, subacute, or chronic; in acute form, cough, fever, chills, dyspnea appear 6–8 h after exposure to antigen; in subacute and chronic forms, temporal relationship to antigenic exposure may be lost and insidiously increasing dyspnea may be predominant symptom.

DIAGNOSIS History: Symptoms; history of possible exposures and relationship to symptoms are very important; occupational history.

Physical Exam: Nonspecific; may reveal rales in lung fields, cyanosis in advanced cases.

Laboratory

• Serum precipitins to offending antigen may be present. • CXR: nonspecific changes in interstitial structures; pleural changes or hilar adenopathy rare. • PFTs and ABGs: restrictive pattern possibly associated with airway obstruction; diffusing capacity decreased; hypoxemia with rest or exercise. • Bronchoalveolar lavage may show increased lymphocytes of suppressor-cytotoxic phenotype. • Lung biopsy may be necessary in some patients who do not have sufficient other criteria; transbronchial biopsy may suffice, but open lung biopsy is frequently necessary.

DIFFERENTIAL DIAGNOSIS Other interstitial lung diseases, including sarcoidosis, idiopathic pulmonary fibrosis, lung disease associated with collagen-vascular diseases, drug-induced lung disease; eosinophilic pneumonia; allergic bronchopulmonary aspergillosis; silo-fillers' disease; "pulmonary mycotoxicosis" or "atypical" farmer's lung; infection.

TREATMENT Avoidance of offending antigen; corticosteroids: prednisone 1 mg/kg per day followed by tapering schedule to lowest possible dose.

For more detailed discussion of these topics, see McFadden ER Jr: Asthma, Chap. 202, and Hunninghake GW, Richerson HB: Hypersensitivity Pneumonitis, Chap. 203, in HPIM-11, pp. 1060 and 1065

APPROACH TO PATIENT

Ask about workplace and work history in detail: Specific contaminants? Availability and use of protection devices? Ventilation? Do coworkers have similar complaints? Ask about every job; short-term exposures may be significant. CXR may over- or underestimate functional impact of pneumoconioses. PFTs may both quantify impairment and suggest the nature of exposure.

An individual's dose of an environmental agent is influenced by intensity as well as by physiologic factors (ventilation rate and depth).

OCCUPATIONAL EXPOSURES AND PULMONARY DISEASE

INORGANIC DUSTS **Asbestosis:** Exposures may occur in mining, milling, and manufacture of asbestos products, construction trades (pipefitting, boilermaking), and manufacture of safety garments, filler for plastic material, and friction materials (brake and clutch linings). Major health effects of asbestos include pulmonary fibrosis (asbestosis) and cancers of the respiratory tract, pleura, and peritoneum.

Asbestosis is a diffuse interstitial fibrosing disease of the lung that is directly related to intensity and duration of exposure, usually requiring ≥ 10 years of moderate to severe exposure. PFTs show a restrictive pattern. CXR reveals irregular or linear opacities, greatest in lower lung fields. *Pleural plaques* indicate past exposure. Excess frequency of *lung cancer* occurs 15 to 20 years after first asbestos exposure. Smoking substantially increases risk of lung cancer after asbestos exposure but does not alter risk of *mesotheliomas*, which peaks 30 to 35 years after initial exposure.

Silicosis: Exposure to free silica (crystalline quartz) occurs in mining, stone cutting, abrasive industries, blasting, quarrying, farming. Short-term, high-intensity exposures (as brief as 10 months) may produce acute silicosis—rapidly fatal pulmonary fibrosis with radiographic picture of profuse miliary infiltration or consolidation. Longer-term, less-intense exposures are associated with upper lobe fibrosis and hilar adenopathy ≥ 15 years after exposure. Fibrosis is nodular and may lead to pulmonary restriction and airflow obstruction. Pts with silicosis are at higher than normal risk for TBC.

Coal worker's pneumoconiosis (CWP): Symptoms of simple CWP are additive to the effects of cigarette smoking on chronic bronchitis and obstructive lung disease. X-ray signs of simple CWP are small, irregular opacities (reticular pattern) which may progress to small, rounded opacities (nodular pattern). Complicated CWP is indicated by roentgenographic appearance of nodules > 1 cm in diameter in upper lung fields; $D_{L_{CO}}$ is reduced.

Berylliosis: Beryllium exposure may produce acute pneumonitis or chronic interstitial pneumonitis. Histology is indistinguishable from sarcoidosis.

ORGANIC DUSTS **Cotton dust (byssinosis):** Exposures occur in production of yarns for cotton, linen, and rope making. (Flax, hemp, and jute produce a similar syndrome.) Chest tightness occurs typically on first day of work week. After 10 years, recurrent symptoms are associated with airflow obstruction. Therapy includes bronchodilators, antihistamines, and elimination of exposure.

Grain dust: Farmers and grain elevator operators are at risk. Symptoms are those of cigarette smokers—cough, mucus production, wheezing, and airflow obstruction.

Farmer's lung: Persons exposed to moldy hay with spores of thermophilic actinomycetes may develop a hypersensitivity pneumonitis. Acute farmer's lung causes fever, chills, malaise, cough, and dyspnea 4 to 8 h after exposure. Chronic low-intensity exposure causes interstitial fibrosis.

TOXIC CHEMICALS Many toxic chemicals can affect the lung in the form of vapor and gases.

Smoke inhalation: Kills more fire victims than does thermal injury. Severe cases may show pulmonary edema. CO poisoning causing O_2 desaturation may be fatal.

Agents used in the manufacture of synthetic materials may produce sensitization to isocyanates, aromatic amines, and aldehydes. Repeated exposure causes some workers to develop productive cough, asthma, or low-grade fever and malaise.

Fluorocarbons, transmitted from a worker's hands to cigarettes, may be volatilized. The inhaled agent causes fever, chills, malaise, and sometimes wheezing. Occurring in plastics workers, the syndrome is termed *polymer fume fever*.

For more detailed discussion of this topic, see Speizer FE: Environmental Lung Diseases, Chap. 204, in HPIM-11, p. 1068

---

75 CHRONIC BRONCHITIS, EMPHYSEMA, AND AIRWAYS OBSTRUCTION

DEFINITIONS **Chronic bronchitis:** Excessive tracheobronchial mucus secretion sufficient to cause cough with expectoration for at least 3 months of the year for 2 consecutive years.

Simple chronic bronchitis: Characterized by mucoid sputum production.

Chronic mucopurulent bronchitis: Characterized by recurrent purulent sputum in the absence of localized suppurative disease (e.g., bronchiectasis).

Chronic asthmatic bronchitis: Cough and mucus hypersecretion associated with dyspnea and wheezing with acute respiratory infections or exposure to inhaled irritants.

Emphysema: Distention of air spaces distal to the terminal bronchioles with destruction of alveolar septa.

Chronic obstructive lung disease (COLD): Condition with chronic expiratory airflow obstruction due to chronic bronchitis and/or emphysema. Obstruction is assessed by the expiratory FVC maneuver (see Fig. 71-1). Severity of obstruction may fluctuate in COLD, but some degree of obstruction is always present.

PATHOLOGY AND PATHOGENESIS

PATHOLOGY Chronic bronchitis is associated with hyperplasia and hypertrophy of submucosal mucus glands. There is Goblet-cell hyperplasia, mucosal edema and inflammation, and increased smooth muscle in small airways. Emphysema may be panacinar (affecting both central and peripheral portions of the acinus) or centriacinar (primary involvement of respiratory bronchioles and alveolar ducts and little involvement of peripheral acina). Panacinar and centriacinar emphysema may exist in the same lung, and both produce similar physiologic changes, primarily increased wasted ventilation.

PATHOGENESIS

1 *Cigarette smoking:* Responsible for most cases of chronic bronchitis and emphysema; also causes obstruction of small airways in young, asymptomatic persons. Although exacerbations of chronic bronchitis and mortality rates from emphysema and bronchitis are associated with air pollution, the role of pollutants in the pathogenesis of COLD is unclear.

2 *Occupational exposures:* Dust or gases such as cotton dust and toluene diisocyanate accelerate decline of pulmonary function in COLD.

3 *Acute infections:* May contribute to exacerbations of COLD and lead to chronic obstruction.

4 *Familial aggregation of emphysema:* Occurs with deficiency of α_1-antitrypsin, a protease inhibitor.

CLINICAL MANIFESTATIONS

COLD is a progressive disorder even when contributing factors are eliminated and aggressive therapy is instituted. Although most patients demonstrate features of both bronchitis and emphysema, two distinct syndromes exist (see Table 75-1).

PREDOMINANT EMPHYSEMA ("PINK PUFFER") Scant sputum production but prominent exertional dyspnea; asthenic body build, tachypnea, prolonged expiration, hyperresonant chest, diminished breath sounds. Gas exchange is impaired with mildly reduced arterial P_{O_2} and low or normal P_{CO_2}. PFTs show reduced maximal flow rates and diffusing capacity and evidence of gas trapping. Cor pulmonale and hypercapneic respiratory failure occur late in the course.

PREDOMINANT BRONCHITIS ("BLUE BLOATER") Chronic cough and mucus production; dyspnea is less prominent. Pts are often cyanotic and overweight; auscultation reveals coarse rhonchi and wheezes. RV heave, RV S_3, and edema are present. Arterial blood gases are severely deranged, both arterial P_{O_2} and P_{CO_2} (in mmHg) may be in high 40s to low 50s. Maximal expiratory

TABLE 75-1 Chronic obstructive lung disease: Salient features of the two types

	Predominant emphysema	Predominant bronchitis
Age at time of diagnosis, yrs	60±	50±
Dyspnea	Severe	Mild
Cough	After dyspnea starts	Before dyspnea starts
Sputum	Scanty, mucoid	Copious, purulent
Bronchial infections	Less frequent	More frequent
Respiratory insufficiency episodes	Often terminal	Repeated
Chest film	"Hyperinflation" ± bullous changes, small heart	Increased bronchovascular markings at bases, large heart
Chronic Pa_{CO_2}, mmHg	35–40	50–60
Chronic Pa_{O_2}, mmHg	65–75	45–60
Hematocrit, %	35–45	50–55
Pulmonary hypertension:		
Rest	None to mild	Moderate to severe
Exercise	Moderate	Worsens
Cor pulmonale	Rare, except terminally	Common
Elastic recoil	Severely decreased	Normal
Resistance	Normal to slight increase	High
Diffusing capacity	Decreased	Normal to slight decrease

From Ingram RH Jr.: HPIM-11, p. 1090.

flow rates are reduced, residual volume is moderately elevated, and diffusing capacity normal or slightly ↓. Episodes of respiratory failure are frequent, but recovery usually occurs with therapy.

PRINCIPLES OF MANAGEMENT

Because emphysema is untreatable, therapeutic efforts are directed at prevention and management of reversible airways obstruction.

Assessment: In addition to Hx and physical exam, pts should receive a CXR as well as PFTs (spirometry, lung volumes, $D_{L_{CO}}$, arterial blood gases). Effects of inhaled bronchodilator should be assessed after acute administration and PFTs should be repeated regularly with and between exacerbations.

Prevention: COLD is progressive; however, the decline is accelerated by smoking, and all pts should be urged to quit. Eliminate aerosol sprays and occupational factors which may accelerate disease. Administer yearly influenza vaccinations.

Infections: Increases in sputum purulence, volume, and viscosity suggest infection. Nonbacterial infections precipitate most exacerbations, but antibiotics lower intensity and duration of symptoms.

Bronchodilators: Methylxanthines (theophylline), sympathomimetics, and anticholinergics (atropine) may alleviate symptoms by reducing bronchial tone. Selective β_2-stimulating drugs (albuterol and metoproterenol) given by inhalation are most effective and are associated with fewest side effects. Glucocorticoids should be employed when other measures are insufficient and only with objective documentation of improvement.

Other: Bronchopulmonary drainage is important in pts with mucus hypersecretion. Continuous O_2 should be given when severe hypoxia is present ($P_{O_2} < 55$ mmHg) and/or there is evidence of cor pulmonale. Exercise programs do not improve lung function but may increase task-specific exercise tolerance.

ACUTE RESPIRATORY FAILURE

Diagnosis: Made on the basis of arterial blood gas from baseline (P_{O_2} drop ≥ 10–15 mmHg and/or increase in P_{CO_2} associated with pH ≤ 7.30).

Precipitating factors: Infection, exacerbation of bronchospasm, pneumothorax, pulmonary thromboembolism, and sedative administration all may precipitate respiratory failure.

Treatment: (1) Maintain oxygenation with low-flow O_2 therapy. If O_2 results in a large increase in arterial P_{CO_2} with acidosis, mechanical ventilation is required; do not stop O_2 administration abruptly. (2) Treat infection (antibiotics), remove secretions (postural drainage), reverse bronchoconstriction (bronchodilators).

Complications: Arrhythmias, heart failure, pulmonary thromboembolism, GI hemorrhage.

For more detailed discussion of this topic, see Ingram RH Jr.: Chronic Bronchitis, Emphysema and Airways Obstruction, Chap. 208, in HPIM-11, p. 1087

76 PNEUMONIA AND LUNG ABSCESS

PNEUMONIA

Clinical manifestations

• ± Cough, fever, chest pain, dyspnea, sputum. • Physical exam: ↓ respiratory excursion, high-pitched end-inspiratory crackles from fluid-filled alveoli; bronchial breath sounds (↑ inspiratory and expiratory phases) from consolidation with patent bronchus.

X-rays

• Alveolar: nonsegmental consolidation with air bronchograms (pneumococcal pneumonia). • Bronchopneumonia: segmental involvement without bronchograms (staphylococcal). • Interstitial: reticular pattern (*Mycoplasma*).

Diagnosis

• Gram's stain of sputum with > 25 WBC per low-power field. • Specimens expectorated (not for anaerobic cultures), transtracheal aspiration, bronchoscopy, transthoracic needle aspiration, lung biopsy. • Cultures of blood, skin lesions, joint effusions, CSF.

Community-acquired pneumonias

• Pneumococcal (see Chap. 34). • Streptococcal (see Chap. 36). • *S. aureus* (see Chap. 35). • *H. influenzae* (see Chap. 40). • *Klebsiella pneumoniae:* middle-aged or elderly patients with underlying alcoholism or diabetes; abrupt fever, rigors, productive cough (± bloody sputum); CXR—usually upper-lobe air space pneumonia with abscess and pleural effusion ± bulging or interlobar fissure. • Anaerobic (see Chap. 37). • Legionnaire's disease (see Chap. 55). • *Mycoplasma pneumoniae* (see Chap. 52). • Viral pneumonia (see Chap. 43).

Hospital-acquired pneumonia: Most often gram-negative bacilli; diagnosis in intubated patient requires purulent sputum plus fever, leukocytosis, new or progressive infiltrate.

Treatment

• Outpatient without sputum: erythromycin 500 mg qid × 7–14 days; follow-up CXR in 6 weeks. • Hospitalize with: hypoxia, empyema, extrapulmonary focus, severe systemic manifestations. • Pneumococcal most common—2.4 million U penicillin IV or IM. • Aspiration: penicillin 10–12 million U IV qd; clindamycin 300 mg IV q 6 h. • Postviral (pneumococcal or staphylococcal)—oxacillin or nafcillin 8–12 g qd. • Chronic bronchitis with pneumonia (pneumococcus, *H. influenzae*): ampicillin 2–6 g qd or tetracycline 2 g qd. • Hospital-acquired pneumonia: good sputum cultures and blood cultures critical; predominant gram-negative rods on Gram's stain—ticarcillin or carbenicillin + gentamicin; gram-positive cocci—vancomycin, nafcillin. • Compromised hosts (see Chap. 27).

LUNG ABSCESS

Symptoms: Cough productive of moderate to large amounts of purulent, sometimes foul sputum, fever, chest pain, dyspnea, anorexia, weight loss.

Laboratory findings: ↑ WBC ± anemia, hypoalbuminemia; CXR—consolidation with radiolucency and surrounding wall or border.

Treatment: Anaerobic abscess—penicillin 10–12 million U IV, then penicillin V 750 mg–1 g qid or clindamycin 600 mg q 8 h IV, then oral 300 mg qid × 6 weeks.

For more detailed discussion of this topic, see Hirschmann JV, Murray JF: Pneumonia and Lung Abscess, Chap. 205, in HPIM-11, p. 1075

---

77 PULMONARY THROMBOEMBOLISM

PULMONARY EMBOLISM (see Fig. 77-1)

NATURAL HISTORY Immediate result is obstruction of pulmonary blood flow to the distal lung. Respiratory consequences include (1) wasted ventilation (lung ventilated but not perfused), (2) atelectasis that occurs 2–24 h following PE; and (3) widened alveolar-arterial P_{O_2} gradient, usually with arterial hypoxemia. Hemodynamic consequences may include (1) pulmonary hypertension, (2) acute RV failure, and (3) decline in cardiac output. These occur only when significant fraction of pulmonary vasculature is obstructed. Infarction of lung tissue is uncommon, occurring only with underlying cardiac or pulmonary disease.

SYMPTOMS Sudden onset of dyspnea most common; chest pain, hemoptysis accompany infarction; syncope may indicate massive embolism.

PHYSICAL EXAM Tachypnea and tachycardia common; RV gallop; loud P_2 and prominent jugular *a* waves suggest RV failure; temperature >39°C uncommon. Hypotension suggests massive PE.

LABORATORY FINDINGS Routine studies contribute little to diagnosis; normal CXR does not exclude PE, but normal perfusion scintiscan is not seen with a clinically significant embolism; a segmental or larger perfusion defect with normal ventilation ("mismatch") is highly suggestive of PE; pulmonary angiography remains definitive test.

TREATMENT IV heparin by continuous infusion is therapy of choice for most pts; usual goal is to maintain activated PTT 1.5–2.0 × control; heparin is continued 7 to 10 days for deep venous thrombosis (DVT) and 10 days for thromboembolism. Most patients receive minimum of 3 months of oral coumadin therapy after PE. Thrombolytic therapy hastens resolution of venous thrombi and is probably indicated for pts with massive embolism and systemic hypotension. Surgical therapy is rarely employed for DVT or acute PE. IVC interruption (clip or filter) is used in pts with recurrent PE despite anticoagulants and in those who cannot tolerate anticoagulants. Surgical extraction of old emboli may be helpful in pts with chronic pulmonary hypertension due to repeated PE without spontaneous resolution.

PRIMARY PULMONARY HYPERTENSION (PPH)

HISTORY Usual pt is female between ages of 20 and 40. At presentation, symptoms are usually of recent onset and natural history is ordinarily less than 5 years. Early symptoms are nonspecific—hyperventilation, chest discomfort, anxiety, weakness, fatigue. Later, dyspnea develops and precordial pain on exertion occurs in 25–50%. Effort syncope occurs very late and signifies ominous prognosis.

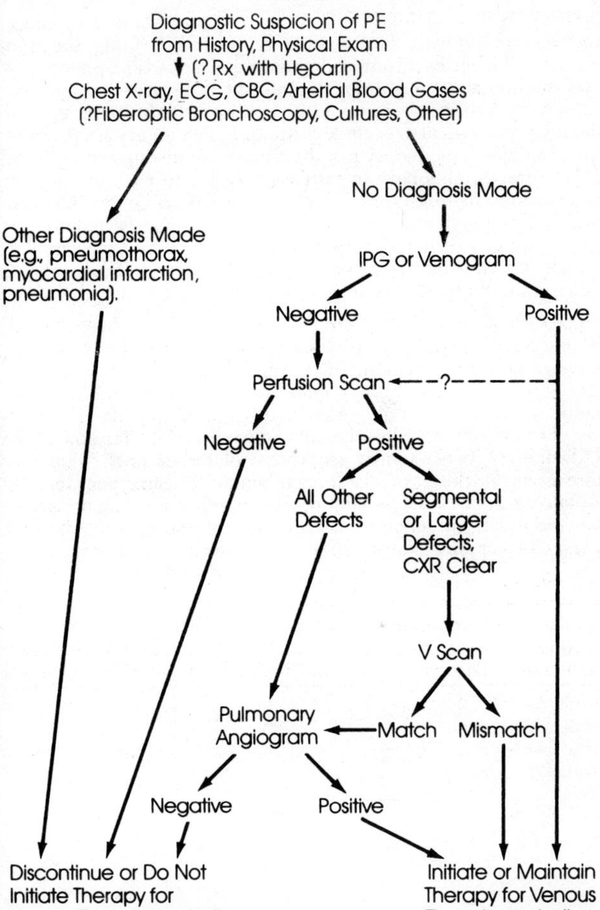

FIG. 77-1 *Flow chart used in diagnosis of pulmonary embolism (PE). IPG, impedance plethysmogram; V scan, ventilation scan. (Reproduced from Moser KM: HPIM-11, p. 1107.)*

PHYSICAL EXAM Prominent *a* wave in jugular venous pulse, right ventricular heave, narrowly split S_2 with accentuated P_2. Terminal course is characterized by signs of right-sided heart failure. *CXR:* RV and central pulmonary arterial prominence. Pulmonary arteries taper sharply. *ECG:* RV enlargement, right axis deviation, and RV hypertrophy. *Echocardiogram:* RA and RV enlargement and tricuspid regurgitation.

DIFFERENTIAL DIAGNOSIS Other disorders of heart, lungs, and pulmonary vasculature must be excluded. Lung function studies will identify chronic pulmonary disease causing pulmonary hypertension and cor pulmonale. Interstitial diseases and hypoxic pulmonary hypertension should be excluded. Perfusion lung scan should be performed to exclude chronic PE. Pulmonary arteriogram and even open lung biopsy may be required to distinguish PE from PPH. Rarely, pulmonary hypertension is due to parasitic disease (schistosomiasis, filariasis). Cardiac disorders to be excluded include pulmonary artery and pulmonic valve stenosis. Pulmonary artery and ventricular and atrial shunts with pulmonary vascular disease (Eisenmenger reaction) should be sought. Silent mitral stenosis should be excluded by echocardiography.

THERAPY Course is usually one of progressive deterioration despite treatment; therapy is palliative. If begun within 12 months of diagnosis, anticoagulants may improve survival. In some pts, other pharmacologic therapy may produce clinical and hemodynamic improvement. Categories of drugs used include (1) direct vascular smooth muscle relaxants (nitroglycerin, diazoxide, hydralazine), (2) beta agonists (isoproterenol, terbutaline), (3) alpha-adrenergic blocking agents (phentolamine, phenoxybenzamine), (4) calcium antagonists (nifedipine, verapamil), and (5) angiotensin-converting enzyme inhibitors. Careful drug testing is required to assess efficacy and detect unfavorable effects. Heart-lung transplantation is a potential therapy in selected patients.

For more detailed discussion of these topics, see Ross J Jr.: Primary Pulmonary Hypertension, Chap. 210, p. 1102, and Moser KM: Pulmonary Thromboembolism, Chap. 211, p. 1105, in HPIM-11

---

78 INTERSTITIAL LUNG DISEASE (ILD)

Chronic, nonmalignant, noninfectious diseases of the lower respiratory tract characterized by inflammation and derangement of the alveolar walls; >180 separate diseases.

CLINICAL FEATURES **History:** First symptoms are usually exertional—fatigue, malaise, dyspnea in everyday activities. Systemic symptoms are infrequent.
Physical exam: Late inspiratory crackles at posterior lung bases. Signs of pulmonary hypertension and clubbing occur late in course.
Laboratory findings: ESR may be elevated. Hypoxemia is common, but polycythemia is rare. Abnormalities of lung parenchyma on CXR in 90%. However, a normal CXR does *not* exclude the possibility of significant infiltrative lung disease.
Scintigraphic findings: Gallium lung scanning is usually positive with diffuse inflammation.
PFTs: Typically restrictive pattern (see Fig. 71-1) with reduced total lung capacity. DL_{CO} often decreased; mild hypoxemia, which worsens with exercise.
Bronchoalveolar lavage: Cells recovered (alveolar macrophages, lymphocytes, neutrophils, eosinophils) may reflect the type of alveolar inflammation in specific disorders.

DIAGNOSTIC EVALUATION Rarely, clinical syndrome can be related to causative agent, but histologic exam is usually necessary. With exception of sarcoidosis, which can often be diagnosed by transbronchial biopsy, most infiltrative diseases require open lung biopsy for diagnosis. Gallium scans and bronchoalveolar lavage do not yield a specific diagnosis but help to document the extent and character of inflammation.

THERAPY Most important is removal of causative agent. With exception of pneumoconioses, which are generally not treated, specific therapy is directed toward suppressing the inflammatory process, usually with prednisone. Other anti-inflammatory and anti-immune agents are used for specific disorders. When $P_{O_2} <$ 55 mmHg, supplemental O_2 is used.

INDIVIDUAL ILDs **Idiopathic pulmonary fibrosis:** Chronic, usually progressive disorder affecting only the lower respiratory tract. Males and females equally affected. Usually fatal within 5 years after onset of symptoms. Corticosteroids usually used.
ILD associated with collagen-vascular disorders: Usually follows development of collagen-vascular disorder; typically mild but occasionally fatal.
Rheumatoid arthritis (RA): 50% of pts with RA have abnormal lung function, 25% have abnormal CXR. Rarely causes symptoms.
Progressive systemic sclerosis: Fibrosis with little inflammation; poor prognosis. Must be distinguished from pulmonary vascular disease.
SLE: Uncommon complication. When it occurs, it is most often an acute, inflammatory patchy process.

Histiocytosis X: Disorder of mononuclear phagocyte system, related to Letterer-Siwe and Hand-Shüller-Christian diseases. In adults, often called eosinophilic granuloma. Develops between 20 and 40 years of age; 90% are present or former smokers. Complicated frequently by pneumothoraces. No therapy available.
Chronic eosinophilic pneumonia: Affects females more than males. Often have history of chronic asthma. Symptoms include weight loss, fever, chills, fatigue, dyspnea. CXR shows "photo-negative pulmonary edema" pattern with central sparing. Very responsive to corticosteroids.
Idiopathic pulmonary hemosiderosis: Characterized by recurrent pulmonary hemorrhage; may be life-threatening. Not associated with renal disease.
Goodpasture's syndrome: Relapsing pulmonary hemorrhage, anemia, and renal failure. Adult males most commonly affected. Circulating anti-basement membrane antibodies.
Inherited disorders: ILD may be associated with tuberous sclerosis, neurofibromatosis, Gaucher's disease, Hermansky-Pudlak syndrome, and Nieman-Pick disease.

For more detailed discussion of this topic, see Crystal RG: Interstitial Lung Disorders, Chap. 209, in HPIM-11, p. 1095

79 CARCINOMA OF THE LUNG

CLASSIFICATION AND CLINICAL CHARACTERISTICS Four major types account for 95% of primary lung cancers: epidermoid (squamous), adenocarcinoma (including bronchioloalveolar), large cell, small cell (including oat cell). Major treatment decisions are made on basis of whether tumor is classified histologically as small cell or non-small cell. Small cell is usually widely disseminated at presentation, while non-small cell may be localized. Epidermoid most common type in males; adenocarcinoma most common type in females. Epidermoid and small cell typically present as central masses, while adenocarcinomas and large cell usually present as peripheral nodules or masses. Epidermoid and large cell cavitate in 20 to 30% of pts.

CLINICAL MANIFESTATIONS Most pts have signs or symptoms of disease at presentation. Central endobronchial tumors cause cough, hemoptysis, wheeze, stridor, dyspnea, pneumonitis. Peripheral lesions cause pain, cough, dyspnea, symptoms of lung abscess resulting from cavitation. Metastatic spread of primary lung cancer may cause tracheal obstruction, dysphagia, hoarseness, Horner's syndrome. Other problems of regional spread include superior vena cava syndrome, pleural effusion, respiratory failure. Extrathoracic metastatic disease affects 50% of pts with epidermoid cancer, 80% with adenocarcinoma and large cell, over 95% with small cell. Clinical problems result from brain metastases, pathologic fractures, liver invasion, and spinal cord compression. Paraneoplastic syndromes may be a presenting finding of lung cancer or first sign of recurrence. Systemic symptoms include weight loss, anorexia, fever. Endocrine syndromes include hypercalcemia (epidermoid), syndrome of inappropriate antidiuretic hormone secretion (small cell), gynecomastia (large cell). Hypertrophic pulmonary osteoarthropathy is most associated with adenocarcinoma.

STAGING Two parts to staging: (1) determination of location (anatomic staging); (2) assessment of pt's ability to withstand antitumor treatment (physiologic staging). Non-small cell tumors are staged by TNM (tumor, node, metastasis) system. Small cell tumors are staged by two-stage system: limited stage disease—confined to one hemithorax and regional lymph nodes; extensive disease—involvement beyond this. General staging procedures include careful ENT exam, CXR, and chest CT scanning. Routine radionuclide scans are not obtained in asymptomatic pts. If mass lesion on CXR and no obvious contraindications to curative surgical approach, mediastinum should be investigated. Major contraindications to curative surgery include extrathoracic metastases, superior vena cava syndrome, vocal cord and phrenic nerve paralysis, malignant pleural effusions, metastases to contralateral lung, and histologic diagnosis of small cell cancer.

TABLE 79-1 Summary of treatment approach to lung cancer patients

Non-small cell lung cancer:
- Resectable:
  - Surgery
  - Radiotherapy for "nonoperable" patients
  - Postoperative radiotherapy for N2 disease (pos. mediastinal disease)
- Nonresectable:
  - Confined to chest: high-dose chest radiotherapy (RT) if possible
  - Extrathoracic: RT to symptomatic local sites; chemotherapy (CT) (for good-performance-status patients, with evaluable lesions)

Small cell lung cancer:
- Limited stage (good performance status):
  - High-dose combination chemotherapy ± chest RT
- Extensive stage (good performance status):
  - High-dose combination chemotherapy
- Complete tumor responders all stages:
  - Prophylactic cranial RT
- Poor-performance-status patients (all stages):
  - Modified dose combination chemotherapy
  - Palliative RT

All patients:
- Radiotherapy for brain metastases, spinal cord compression, weight-bearing lytic bony lesions, symptomatic local lesions (never paralyses, obstructed airway, hemoptysis in non-small cell lung cancer and in small cell cancer not responding to chemotherapy)
- Appropriate diagnosis and treatment of other medical problems and supportive care during chemotherapy
- Encouragement to stop smoking

Reproduced from Minna JD: HPIM-11, p. 1119.

TREATMENT (Table 79-1)

1 Surgery in pts with localized disease and non-small cell cancer; however, majority initially thought to have "curative" resection ultimately succumb to metastatic disease.

2 Solitary pulmonary nodule: risk factors favoring resection include cigarette smoking, age ≥ 35, relatively large (>2 cm) lesion, lack of calcification, chest symptoms, and growth of lesion compared to old CXR.

3 For unresectable non-small cell cancer, metastatic disease, or refusal of surgery: consider for radiation therapy; there is no consensus for "debulking" surgery or adjuvant chemotherapy.

4 Small cell cancer: combination chemotherapy is standard mode of therapy; response after 6 to 12 weeks predicts median- and long-term survival.

5 Laser obliteration of tumor through bronchoscopy in presence of bronchial obstruction.

PROGNOSIS At time of dignosis, only 20% of pts have localized disease. Even in those with apparent localized disease, overall 5-year survival is 30% for males and 50% for females; rates—unchanged over past 20 years.

For more detailed discussion of this topic, see Minna JD: Neoplasms of the Lung, Chap. 213, in HPIM-11, p. 1115

80 DISEASES OF THE PLEURA, MEDIASTINUM, AND DIAPHRAGM

PLEURAL DISEASE

Pleuritis Inflammation of pleura may occur with pneumonia, TBC, pulmonary infarction, and neoplasm. Pleuritic pain without physical and x-ray findings suggests epidemic pleurodynia (viral inflammation of intercostal muscles); hemoptysis and parenchymal involvement on CXR suggest infection or infarction. Pleural effusion without parenchymal disease suggests postprimary TBC, subdiaphragmatic abscess, mesothelioma, or primary bacterial infection of pleural space.

PLEURAL EFFUSION May or may not be associated with pleuritis. In general, effusions due to pleural disease resemble plasma (exudates); effusions with normal pleura are ultrafiltrates of plasma (transudates). Exudates have high protein content (>3 g/100 mL), pleural-to-serum LDH activity ratio > 0.6, and many WBCs (>100,000/mm³). With pleural infection, pH < 7.3 and glucose ↓. If neoplasm or TBC is considered, closed pleural biopsy should be performed (see Fig. 80-1). Despite full evaluation, no cause for effusion will be found in 25% of pts.

FIG. 80-1 *Approach to the diagnosis of pleural effusions. The special tests (Table 214-1) can be found in HPIM-11, p. 1125. (Reproduced from Ingram RH, Jr.: HPIM-11, p. 1125.)*

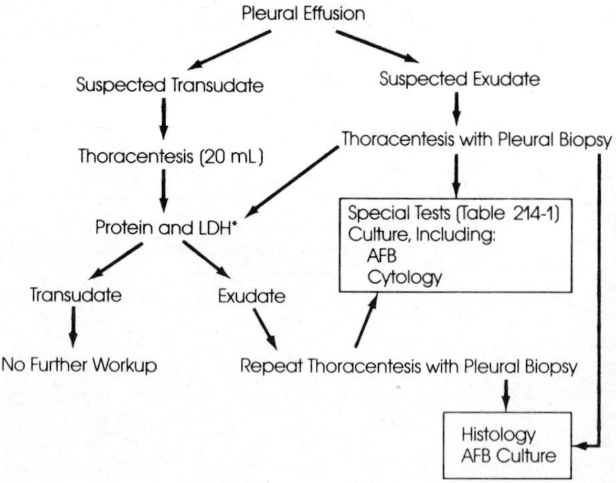

POSTPRIMARY TBC EFFUSIONS Fluid is exudative with predominant lymphocytosis; bacilli are rarely seen on smear and fluid culture is positive in fewer than 20%; closed biopsy required for diagnosis.

NEOPLASTIC EFFUSIONS Fluid is exudative; fluid cytology and pleural biopsy will confirm diagnosis in 60%; pleural sclerosis with tetracycline or cytotoxic agents may be required for management.

RHEUMATOID ARTHRITIS (RA) Exudative effusions may precede articular symptoms; low glucose and pH; usually males.

PANCREATITIS Typically left-sided; up to 15% of pts with pancreatitis; high pleural fluid amylase is suggestive but also may occur with effusions due to neoplasms, infection, and esophageal rupture.

EOSINOPHILIC EFFUSION Defined as more than 10% eosinophils; nonspecific finding may occur with viral, bacterial, traumatic, and pancreatic effusions and may follow prior thoracentesis.

HEMOTHORAX Most commonly follows blunt or penetrating trauma. Pts with bleeding disorders may develop hemothorax following trauma or invasive procedures on pleura. Adequate drainage mandatory to avoid fibrothorax and "trapped" lung.

EMPYEMA An infected pleural effusion or frank pus in pleural space. Usually results from spread of infection from contiguous space. Chest pain, fever, night sweats, cough, and weight loss are common. Thick liquid with loculations, high leukocyte count, and low pH suggest that drainage is required in addition to antibiotics. If closed drainage does not result in marked symptomatic improvement in several days, limited thoracotomy and open drainage are indicated.

PNEUMOTHORAX (PNTX) Spontaneous PNTX most commonly occurs between 20 and 40 years of age; causes sudden, sharp chest pain and dyspnea. Treatment depends on size—if small, observation is sufficient; if large, closed drainage with chest tube is necessary. 50% suffer recurrence, and application of irritants so that surfaces become adherent (pleurodesis) may be required. Complications include hemothorax, cardiovascular compromise secondary to tension PNTX, and bronchopleural fistula. Many interstitial and obstructive lung diseases may predispose to PNTX.

MEDIASTINAL DISEASE

TUMORS AND CYSTS Most common mediastinal masses in adults are metastatic carcinomas and lymphomas. Sarcoidosis, infectious mononucleosis, and AIDS may produce mediastinal lymphadenopathy. Neurogenic tumors, teratodermoids, thymomas, and bronchogenic cysts account for two-thirds of remaining mediastinal masses. Specific locations for specific etiologies (see Table 80-1). Evaluation includes CXR, CT scan, and when diagnosis remains in doubt, mediastinoscopy and biopsy.

TABLE 80-1 **Nature of masses in various locations in mediastinum**

Superior	Anterior and middle	Posterior
Lymphoma	Lymphoma	Neurogenic tumors
Thymoma	Metastatic carcinoma	Lymphoma
Retrosternal thyroid	Teratodermoid	Hernia (Bochdalek)
Metastatic carcinoma	Bronchogenic cyst	Aortic aneurysm
Parathyroid tumors	Aortic aneurysm	
Zenker's diverticulum	Pericardial cyst	
Aortic aneurysm		

NEUROGENIC TUMORS Most common primary mediastinal neoplasms; majority are benign; vague chest pain and cough.

TERATODERMOIDS Anterior mediastinum; 10–20% undergo malignant transformation.

THYMOMAS 10% primary mediastinal neoplasms; one-quarter are malignant; myasthenia gravis occurs in half.

SUPERIOR VENA CAVA SYNDROME Dilation of veins of upper thorax and neck, plethora, facial and conjuctival edema, headache, visual disturbances, and reduced state of consciousness; most often due to malignant disease—75% bronchogenic carcinoma, most others lymphoma.

DISORDERS OF DIAPHRAGM

DIAPHRAGMATIC PARALYSIS **Unilateral paralysis:** Usually caused by phrenic nerve injury due to trauma or mediastinal tumor, but nearly half are unexplained; usually asymptomatic; suggested by CXR, confirmed by fluoroscopy.
Bilateral paralysis: May be due to high cervical cord injury, motor neuron disease, poliomyelitis, polyneuropathies, bilateral phrenic involvement by mediastinal lesions, after cardiac surgery, dyspnea; paradoxical abdominal motion should be sought in supine pts.

For more detailed discussion of this topic, see Ingram RH Jr.: Diseases of the Pleura, Mediastinum, and Diaphragm, Chap. 214, in HPIM-11, p. 1123

81 DISORDERS OF VENTILATION

HYPOVENTILATION

Cardinal feature is CO_2 retention. Major causes are listed in Table 81-1.

CO_2 RETENTION CAUSED BY HYPOVENTILATION WITH NORMAL LUNGS **Conditions affecting the respiratory center:** Drugs are among the most common causes of hypoventilation. Anesthetics, barbiturates, morphine, and their derivatives all depress the respiratory center; assisted ventilation may be lifesaving. **Brainstem abnormalities:** Inflammation, hemorrhage, trauma, and rarely neoplasms of the brainstem may cause hypoventilation; initial irregularities of respiratory rhythm and apnea often may appear during sleep; pts can voluntarily reduce P_{CO_2} to normal. **Thoracic cage abnormalities:**

1 *Crushed chest:* Trauma, particularly to sternum and multiple ribs, often necessitates prompt intubation and ventilatory assistance.

2 *Scoliosis:* Severe spinal curvature may lead to exertional dyspnea followed by CO_2 retention, hypoxemia, and cor pulmonale; therapy is supportive.

3 *Other thoracic cage abnormalities:* Ankylosing spondylitis and pectus excavatum distort thoracic cage but are generally associated with hypoventilation.

Obstruction of upper airways: Tracheal stenosis, upper airway tumors, and foreign bodies may cause airway obstruction, stridor, and hypoventilation with CO_2 retention.

TABLE 81-1 **Causes of carbon dioxide retention**

Pure hypoventilation (normal lungs):
Respiratory center depression—morphine derivatives, barbiturates, some general anesthetics
Diseases of the brainstem—encephalitis, hemorrhage, trauma, neoplasm (rare)
Abnormalities of spinal cord conducting pathways—high cervical dislocation
Anterior horn cell disease—poliomyelitis
Diseases of nerves to respiratory muscles—Guillain-Barré syndrome, diphtheria
Diseases of the myoneural junction—myasthenia gravis, anticholinesterase poisoning
Diseases of the respiratory muscles—progressive muscular dystrophy
Thoracic cage abnormalities—crushed chest, kyphoscoliosis (lungs may be abnormal)
Upper airway obstruction—thymoma, aortic aneurysm
Hypoventilation associated with extreme obesity (Pickwickian syndrome)
Idiopathic hypoventilation
Other causes—metabolic alkalosis
CO_2 retention associated with chronic lung disease

Reproduced from West JB: HPIM-11, p. 1130.

Hypoventilation with extreme obesity: Association with obesity, somnolence, and polycythemia (Pickwickian syndrome); sleep apnea frequent; ventilatory response to inhaled CO_2 is decreased; dramatic improvement occurs with weight loss.
Metabolic alkalosis: A few pts with severe metabolic alkalosis hypoventilate; compensation is incomplete and arterial pH remains elevated.

SLEEP APNEA Central apnea: May occur during sleep due to transient (>10 s) cessation of inspiratory muscle activity with absence of airflow.
Obstructive sleep apnea: Involves upper airway due to enlarged tonsils, backward movement of tongue, or collapse of pharyngeal tissues with persistent activity of inspiratory muscles recorded by transducers around chest wall and abdomen; pts also demonstrate hypersomnolence, fatigue, morning headaches; a small number of pts, usually with coexisting chronic obstructive lung disease (COLD), may develop hypoventilation.

CO_2 RETENTION ASSOCIATED WITH CHRONIC LUNG DISEASE Occurs most often in pts with COLD. Increased CO_2 is not due to pure hypoventilation only but also to ventilation-perfusion inequality. Ventilatory response to CO_2 is reduced either due to increased work of breathing or reduced neural output of respiratory center. Further CO_2 retention may follow O_2 administration, particularly in pts experiencing an exacerbation of airways obstruction.

HYPERVENTILATION

DEFINITION Increased ventilation, causing a decreased P_{CO_2}. Causes include lesions of the CNS, metabolic acidosis, anxiety, drugs (e.g., salicylates), hypoxemia, hypoglycemia, hepatic coma, and sepsis. Hyperventilation also may occur with some types of lung disease, particularly interstitial disease and pulmonary edema.

For more detailed discussion of this topic, see West JB: Disorders of Ventilation, Chap. 215, in HPIM-11, p. 1129

DISEASES OF THE UPPER RESPIRATORY TRACT

ANOSMIA (LOSS OF OLFACTORY SENSE) When *transient,* it is usually due to acute infections of the upper respiratory tract. When *chronic,* it is usually due to congenital defects, tumors, trauma, nasal polyps, or chronic nasal obstruction.

RHINITIS (NASAL DISCHARGE) May be caused by hay fever, vasomotor rhinitis, acute coryza, chronic use of vasoconstrictor drugs, and upper respiratory manifestations of measles, syphilis, TBC.

NASAL OBSTRUCTION When *acute,* it is usually due to viral infection, whereas *chronic* obstruction may be due to allergic reactions or deviated septum. Treatment depends on cause.

EPISTAXIS Most commonly due to trauma, especially "nose picking." Also occurs with viral infections, typhoid fever, malaria. Noninfectious causes include bleeding diatheses, polycythemia vera, acute sinusitis, tumors.

NASAL FURUNCULOSIS Most common organism is *Staphylococcus aureus.* Potentially life-threatening because of threat of spread to cavernous sinus. Treatment consists of antistaphylococcal antibiotics. Lesions *must* not be squeezed; incision and drainage discouraged except for large or painful lesions.

PHARYNX

ACUTE PHARYNGITIS Symptoms range from "scratchy throat" to severe pain with difficulty swallowing. Lingual tonsillitis associated with streptococcal pharyngitis may cause pain on moving tongue. Findings may range from simple erythema to vascular congestion, exudate, and lymphoid hypertrophy. Presence of exudate does not establish a specific etiology. Single throat culture yields *Streptococcus pyogenes* in only 70% of pts with pharyngitis due to this organism. Following culture, initial treatment may be based on clinical diagnosis, with modifications based on results of culture.

PERITONSILLAR CELLULITIS AND ABSCESS A complication of acute pharyngitis. First sign is tonsillar enlargement, which may progress to occlusion of upper airway. May progress from cellulitis to abscess; diagnosis based on PE. Initial treatment consists of antibiotics, with incision and drainage if large abscess persists.

PARAPHARYNGEAL ABSCESS Also a complication of acute pharyngitis. Bacterial invasion of tonsil leads to intratonsillar abscess and inflammation of parapharyngeal space; usually unilateral. May spread to jugular vein causing septic thrombophlebitis. Treatment with antibiotics is followed, if necessary, by incision and drainage if large abscess persists.

RETROPHARYNGEAL ABSCESS Most common under age 4. In adults, may follow acute otitis, dental disease, regional trauma. May complicate cervical or cervicodorsal vertebral osteomyelitis. Diabetes mellitus, immunosuppression are predisposing factors. Treatment as for paraphyngeal abscess.

CHRONIC SORE THROAT May be symptom of upper airway neoplasm. Also caused by mouth breathing (often with sleep apnea), cigarette smoking, subacute thyroiditis.

TABLE 82-1 **Differential diagnosis of hoarseness and other manifestations of laryngeal dysfunction**

Intralaryngeal disease:
- Infectious:
  - Common cold
  - Viral laryngitis
  - *Haemophilus influenzae*
  - Membranous laryngitis *(Streptococcus pyogenes, Pseudomonas, Fusobacterium)*
  - Diphtheria (laryngeal membrane)
  - Herpes simplex
- Noninfectious:
  - Trauma (edema or hematoma)
  - Vocal cord nodules (singer's nodes)
  - Papillomas of vocal cords
  - Pachyderma of vocal cords
  - Inhalation of smoke, fire, irritating gases, tobacco smoke
  - Leukoplakia of vocal cords
  - Tumors (benign or malignant)
  - Foreign bodies

Extralaryngeal disease:
- Lesions in neck:
  - Hemorrhages and/or edema due to trauma, severe traction of neck, thyroidectomy, tracheostomy, and biopsy of scalene node
  - Tumors of hypopharynx
- Local and systemic disorders outside neck (produce hoarseness by pressure on laryngeal nerves anywhere along the course outside the neck, or paresis or paralysis of the vocal cords as a manifestation of generalized neurologic dysfunction):
  - Local lesions:
    - Bacterial meningitis
    - Meningovascular syphilis
    - Infectious mononucleosis (enlarged mediastinal nodes)
    - Angioneurotic edema
    - Aneurysms of arch of aorta, carotid or innominate arteries
    - Tumors of mediastinal structure
    - Tumors of parotid gland
    - Relapsing polychondritis
  - Systemic disorders:
    - Diphtheria (peripheral neuritis)
    - Poliomyelitis (bulbar)
    - Infectious mononucleosis (nervous system involvement)
    - Herpes zoster
    - Mucoviscidosis

Modified from Weinstein L: HPIM-11, p. 1114.

SINUSES

ACUTE SINUSITIS Most common organisms are *S. pneumoniae, S. pyogenes,* and *H. influenzae.* Most common predisposing factor is viral URI. *Diagnosis* is made clinically; localized pain and tenderness, nasal obstruction, recurrent headaches, fever, and chills. *Therapy* includes antibiotics, intranasal vasoconstrictors, and in some cases, surgical drainage. Failure to respond to therapy or relapse should prompt a search for a complicating condition such as fracture, tumor, Wegener's granulomatosis. *Complications* include osteomyelitis, meningitis, as well as infection and thrombosis of cavernous and sagittal veins.

CHRONIC SINUSITIS A difficult diagnosis to establish. Symptoms include headaches, nasal obstruction, and tenderness. X-ray exams of paranasal sinuses reveal thickening of mucus membranes. Allergic background frequent.

LARYNX

Principal symptom of laryngeal disease is hoarseness, which may be due to inflammatory lesions, functional disturbances (hysterical aphonia), and local or generalized neurologic disease (see Table 82-1); cough is common. Stridor and dyspnea are uncommon and suggest obstruction.

EPIGLOTTITIS Uncommon in adults; men are affected more than women. Immunosuppression predisposes to epiglottitis. Organisms include *H. influenzae, S. pneumoniae, S. pyogenes, E. coli,* and anaerobes. Bacteremia occurs in 50%. Sore throat is always present. Fever, dyspnea, dysphagia, and hoarseness also occur. Antibiotics are mandatory; tracheostomy may be necessary.

TBC LARYNGITIS Usually in older men. Hoarseness nearly always present. Pulmonary TBC may be absent. Hyperemia and edema may be only signs on exam.

CANCER OF LARYNX Develops at average age of 60; 10 times more common in men. Therapy includes radiation or surgery.

For more detailed discussion of this topic, see Weinstein L: Diseases of the Upper Respiratory Tract, Chap. 212, in HPIM-11, p. 1111

83 ADULT RESPIRATORY DISTRESS SYNDROME (ARDS)

ARDS is a descriptive term applied to many acute, diffuse infiltrative lung lesions of diverse etiologies (see Table 83-1) with severe arterial hypoxemia.

CLINICAL CHARACTERISTICS AND MANAGEMENT Earliest sign is often tachypnea followed by dyspnea. Arterial blood gas shows reduction of P_{O_2} and P_{CO_2} with widened alveolar-arterial O_2 difference. Physical exam and CXR may be normal initially. Initial therapy is O_2, but as disease worsens, mechanical ventilation and positive end-expiratory pressure may be required. Goal of therapy is to maintain O_2 delivery to tissues with arterial $P_{O_2} \geq$ 60 mmHg. Rationale behind mechanical ventilation is to improve oxygenation by increasing mean lung volume. Pulmonary artery catheter insertion permits more accurate assessment of filling pressures, hemodynamics, and O_2 transport in critically ill pts.

ARDS increases lung water without increasing hydrostatic forces. Toxic gases (chlorine, NO_2, smoke) and gastric acid aspiration damage the alveolar-capillary membrane directly, whereas sepsis increases alveolar-capillary permeability by producing activation and aggregation of formed blood elements.

COMPLICATIONS

1 *LV failure* is a common, easily missed complication, particularly in pts receiving mechanical ventilation.

2 *Secondary bacterial infection* may be obscured by the diffuse roentgenographic changes.

3 *Bronchial obstruction* may be caused by endotracheal or tracheostomy tubes.

4 *Pneumothorax and pneumomediastinum* may cause abrupt deterioration in pts receiving mechanical ventilation.

TABLE 83-1 **Conditions which may lead to the adult respiratory distress syndrome**

Diffuse pulmonary infections (e.g., viral, bacterial, fungal, *Pneumocystis*)
Aspiration (e.g., gastric contents, water with near drowning)
Inhalation of toxins and irritants (e.g., chlorine gas, NO_2, smoke, ozone, high concentrations of O_2)
Narcotic overdose pulmonary edema (e.g., heroin, methadone, morphine, dextropropoxyphene)
Nonnarcotic drug effects (e.g., nitrofurantoin)
Immunologic response to host antigens (e.g., Goodpasture's syndrome, systemic lupus erythematosus)
Effects of nonthoracic trauma with hypotension ("shock lung")
In association with systemic reactions to processes initiated outside the lung (e.g., gram-negative septicemia, hemorrhagic pancreatitis, amniotic fluid embolism, fat embolism)
Postcardiopulmonary bypass ("pump lung," "postperfusion lung")

Reproduced from Ingram RH Jr.: HPIM-11, p. 1135.

PROGNOSIS Overall mortality rate is 50% and varies with the intrinsic mortality of the underlying condition. If ARDS occurs as a result of extrapulmonic sepsis, multiple organ failure often supervenes.

For more detailed discussion of this topic, see Ingram RH Jr.: Adult Respiratory Distress Syndrome, Chap. 216, in HPIM-11, p. 1134

SECTION V
RENAL DISEASE

84 APPROACH TO PATIENT WITH RENAL DISEASE

Despite the complexity of homeostatic and excretory functions of the healthy kidney, diseases of the kidney and urinary tract give rise to a finite number of clinical syndromes (see Table 84-1). The approach to the pt with renal disease begins with recognition of a particular syndrome and its causes based on findings such as presence or absence of azotemia, proteinuria, hypertension, edema, abnormal UA, electrolyte disorders, abnormal urine volumes, or infection.

ACUTE RENAL FAILURE (Chap. 85) Clinical syndrome with diverse causes characterized by a rapid, severe decrease in GFR (a rise in serum creatinine and BUN), frequently with reduced urine output. Volume expansion occurs, leading to edema, hypertension, and CHF. Hyperkalemia, hyponatremia, and acidosis are frequent. Etiologies include ischemia, nephrotoxic injury due to drugs or endogenous pigments, sepsis, severe renovascular disease, or conditions related to pregnancy. Prerenal and postrenal failure are potentially reversible causes of ARF.

Rapidly progressive glomerulonephritis (RPGMN): Loss of renal function occurs over weeks to months. Those who present early are nonoliguric and may complain of recent flulike symptoms; later, oliguric renal failure with uremic symptoms supervenes. Pulmonary manifestations ranging from mild infiltrates to life-threatening hemoptysis are common. UA shows hematuria, proteinuria, and RBC casts.

Acute glomerulonephritis (Chap. 88): An acute illness with sudden onset of hematuria, edema, hypertension, oliguria, and elevated BUN and creatinine. Mild pulmonary congestion may be present. An antecedent or concurrent infection or multisystem disease may be the causative factor; some cases consist of glomerular disease alone. Hematuria with proteinuria and pyuria are present in the majority, and RBC casts confirm the diagnosis. Serum complement may be decreased.

CHRONIC RENAL FAILURE (Chap. 86) Progressive permanent loss of renal function over months to years. Because of adaptive mechanisms, symptoms of uremia do not appear until GFR is reduced to about 25% of normal. Hypertension may be an early finding. Later, the broad array of signs and symptoms includes anorexia, nausea, vomiting, insomnia, weight loss, weakness, paresthesias, bleeding, serositis, anemia, acidosis, and hyperkalemia. Features of a *specific* cause also may be present (diabetes,

TABLE 84-1 Initial clinical and laboratory data base for defining major syndromes in nephrology

Syndromes	Important clues to diagnosis	Findings which are common but not of diagnostic value
Acute or rapidly progressive renal failure	Anuria Oliguria Documented recent decline in GFR	Hypertension, hematuria Proteinuria, pyuria Casts, edema
Acute nephritis	Hematuria, RBC casts Azotemia, oliguria Edema, hypertension	Proteinuria Pyuria Circulatory congestion
Chronic renal failure	Azotemia for > 3 months Prolonged symptoms or signs of uremia Symptoms or signs of renal osteodystrophy Kidneys reduced in size bilaterally Broad casts in urinary sediment	Hematuria, proteinuria Casts, oliguria Polyuria, nocturia Edema, hypertension Electrolyte disorders
Nephrotic syndrome	Proteinuria > 3.5 g per 1.73 m^2 per 24 h Hypoalbuminemia Hyperlipidemia Lipiduria	Casts Edema
Asymptomatic urinary abnormalities	Hematuria Proteinuria (below nephrotic range) Sterile pyuria, casts	
UTI	Bacteriuria > 10^5 colonies per milliliter Other infectious agent documented in urine Pyuria, leukocyte casts Frequency, urgency Bladder tenderness, flank tenderness	Hematuria Mild azotemia Mild proteinuria Fever
Renal tubule defects	Electrolyte disorders Polyuria, nocturia Symptoms or signs of renal osteodystrophy Large kidneys Renal transport defects	Hematuria "Tubular" proteinuria Enuresis
Hypertension	Systolic/diastolic hypertension	Proteinuria, casts, azotemia

(*continued*)

TABLE 84-1 **Initial clinical and laboratory data base for defining major syndromes in nephrology (continued)**

Syndromes	Important clues to diagnosis	Findings which are common but not of diagnostic value
Nephrolithiasis	Previous history of stone passage or removal Previous history of stone seen by x-ray Renal colic	Hematuria Pyuria Frequency, urgency
Urinary tract obstruction	Azotemia, oliguria, anuria Polyuria, nocturia, urinary retention Slowing of urinary stream Large prostate, large kidneys Flank tenderness, full bladder after voiding	Hematuria Pyuria Enuresis, dysuria

Modified from Coe FL, Brenner BM: HPIM-11, p. 1140.

long-standing hypertension, urinary tract obstruction, interstitial nephritis). Indications of chronicity include long-standing azotemia, shrunken kidneys, renal osteodystrophy by x-ray, or findings on renal biopsy.

NEPHROTIC SYNDROME (Chap. 88) Defined as heavy proteinuria (>3.5 g/day in the adult) due to albuminuria; may be accompanied by edema, hypoalbuminemia, and hyperlipidemia. May be idiopathic or due to a variety of drugs, infections, neoplasms, multisystem or hereditary diseases. Varying degrees of renal insufficiency may be present. Complications include severe edema, thromboembolic events, infection, and protein malnutrition.

ASYMPTOMATIC URINARY ABNORMALITIES May consist of hematuria, proteinuria, or pyuria. Hematuria may be due to neoplasms, stones, or infection at any level of the urinary tract, or it may be due to sickle cell disease or analgesic abuse. Renal parenchymal causes are suggested by RBC casts, proteinuria, or dysmorphic RBCs in urine. Pattern of gross hematuria may be helpful in localizing site. Hematuria with low-grade proteinuria may be benign recurrent hematuria or due to IgA nephropathy. Modest proteinuria may be an isolated finding due to conditions such as fever, exertion, CHF, or upright posture. Renal causes include diabetes mellitus, amyloidosis, or other mild forms of glomerular disease. Pyuria as a sole finding may occur with mild renal inflammation (interstitial nephritis, SLE, transplant rejection), UTI, or may be "sterile" and due to treated infection, TBC, prostatitis, urethritis, or unusual urinary pathogens.

UTI (Chap. 90) Generally defined as bacteriuria greater than 10^5 bacteria/mL of urine. Levels above 10^2/mL may indicate infection in some symptomatic pts but are commonly due to poor sample collection, especially if mixed flora are present. Adults at risk are sexually active females or anyone with urinary tract obstruction, reflux, catheterization, or neurogenic bladder. Prostatitis, urethritis, and vaginitis may be distinguished by quantitative urine culture. Flank pain, nausea, vomiting, fever, and chills indicate renal infection. UTI is a common cause of sepsis.

RENAL TUBULAR DEFECTS (Chap. 59) Generally inherited, they include anatomic defects (polycystic kidneys, medullary cystic disease, medullary sponge kidney) detected in the evaluation of hematuria, flank pain, infection, or renal failure of unknown cause; as well as tubular disorders of transport resulting in glucosuria, aminoaciduria, stones, or rickets. Fanconi syndrome is a generalized tubular defect acquired from drugs, heavy metals, multiple myeloma, amyloidosis, or renal transplantation. Nephrogenic diabetes insipidus (polyuria, polydypsia, hypernatremia, hypernatremic dehydration) and renal tubular acidosis are other tubular disorders.

HYPERTENSION (Chap. 59) Blood pressure > 140/90 mmHg may affect 20% of the U.S. adult population and when inadequately controlled is an important contributor to cerebrovascular accident, MI, CHF, and renal failure. By itself, hypertension is usually asymptomatic until cardiac, renal, or neurologic symptoms appear. Most cases are idiopathic, without identifiable cause, and occur between the ages of 25 and 45 years.

NEPHROLITHIASIS (Chap. 92) Patients with colicky pain, UTI, hematuria, dysuria, or unexplained pyuria. Unsuspected stones may be found on routine x-ray. Most are radiopaque Ca stones, commonly with a high level of urinary Ca excretion as underlying cause. Staghorn calculi are large, branching radiopaque stones within kidney due to recurrent infection. Uric acid stones are radiolucent. UA may reveal hematuria, pyuria, or pathologic crystals.

URINARY TRACT OBSTRUCTION (Chap. 93) Presents variable symptoms depending on whether it is acute or chronic, unilateral or bilateral, or complete or partial and on underlying etiology. It is an important reversible cause of unexplained renal failure. Upper tract obstruction may produce flank pain, hematuria, and evidence of renal infection, or it may be silent. Bladder symptoms may be present in lower tract obstruction. Functional consequences include polyuria, anuria, nocturia, acidosis, hyperkalemia, or hypertension. A flank or suprapubic mass may be found on physical exam.

For more detailed discussion of this topic, see Coe FL, Brenner BM: Approach to the Patient with Diseases of the Kidneys and Urinary Tract, Chap. 217, in HPIM-11 p. 1139

$$Cl_{Crea}(est)\ \frac{(140-age)\times Wt(Kg)}{72\times[Crea]_{ser}\ mg/dL}$$

85 ACUTE RENAL FAILURE (ARF)

CAUSES OF ARF (see Table 85-1) These are categorized as prerenal, intrinsic renal, or postrenal. Only about half of pts with ARF have anuria-oliguria; those with preserved urine output usually have a milder disorder and a better prognosis.

Prerenal failure, the most common cause of acute azotemia, results from inadequate perfusion of kidneys. This may be due to severe hemorrhage, volume contraction, extracellular fluid sequestration, low cardiac output, vascular pooling, or renal artery obstruction. NSAIDS may also cause functional prerenal azotemia, especially in patients with chronic renal failure (CRF), nephrotic syndrome, CHF, cirrhosis, those on diuretics, and the elderly. Prolonged renal hypoperfusion is a risk factor for ARF due to acute tubular necrosis (ATN).

Intrinsic renal causes include renovascular disease (Chap. 91), glomerulonephritis (Chap. 88), and interstitial nephritis (Chap. 89). Some are amenable to specific treatment.

Postrenal causes of ARF are those producing urinary obstruction at any level from the kidneys to the urethra (Chap. 93). ARF due to urinary obstruction above the bladder requires simultaneous bilateral involvement or unilateral disease with an absent or impaired contralateral kidney.

ATN: This is due to ischemic or toxic injury acting on renal vessels, glomeruli, and/or tubules causing ↓ GFR and ↑ intratubular pressure.

Ischemic ATN may follow abrupt hypoperfusion or evolve from any condition causing severe prerenal failure, particularly in elderly pts or when nephrotoxins are present.

Nephrotoxic ATN may result from exogenous or endogenous sources. Common exogenous nephrotoxins are (1) aminoglycoside antibiotics (dose-related, in elderly, dehydrated pts or those with prior renal impairment), and (2) contrast dye (in elderly, diabetics,

TABLE 85-1 **Causes of ARF**

Disorder	Causes
Prerenal failure:	
Hypovolemia	Diarrhea, vomiting, hemorrhage, overdiuresis, pancreatitis, peritonitis
Vasodilatation	Sepsis, drugs, anaphylaxis
Cardiovascular	CHF, MI, tamponade
Renal hypoperfusion	Renal artery obstruction, NSAIDs
Intrarenal failure (Intrinsic renal disease)	Hypotension, sustained prerenal failure, postoperative, rhabdomyolysis, aminoglycosides, contrast dye, NSAIDs, glomerulonephritis, vasculitis, interstitial nephritis
Postrenal failure:	
Intrarenal	Crystals, calculi, papillary necrosis
Extrarenal	Prostate, pelvic, bladder neoplasm, retroperitoneal neoplasm or fibrosis, urethral or bladder neck obstruction

pts with prior renal impairment, dehydration, myeloma; can be prevented by volume expansion and use of minimal dose). Endogenous nephrotoxins causing ATN include myoglobin released after muscle trauma or with coma or heat stroke. Intravascular hemolysis may cause ARF in the setting of hypotension or sepsis.

Pathophysiologic theories of ATN include obstruction or backleak through damaged tubules and diminished glomerular perfusion secondary to afferent arteriolar vasoconstriction. Histopathologic lesions are variable. Specific evidence of glomerulonephritis, vasculitis, or interstitial nephritis may be present. Tubular necrosis may be present to varying extent with normal glomeruli and blood vessels.

CLINICAL FEATURES Pts with *prerenal failure* have clinical features of volume contraction, hypotension, or impaired cardiac function. Dx may become obvious only when renal perfusion improves, as occurs with volume repletion or improvement in cardiac function.

Postrenal failure may be evident from a distended bladder, large prostate, pelvic mass, or hydronephrosis. The pattern of urinary flow may suggest total (anuria) or partial (polyuria) obstruction. Crystals or urinary infection may be present in urinary sediment. Early (hours) obstruction results in urinary indices identical to those of prerenal failure; later, obstruction will resemble the indices of ATN (Table 21-1).

ARF due to *intrinsic renal diseases* may require a renal biopsy for diagnosis. RBC casts and heavy proteinuria suggest glomerulonephritis (GN) or vascular inflammatory disease. Pts with interstitial nephritis may have fever, skin eruption, and pyuria with eosinophils on Wright's stain of urinary sediment.

With ATN, brown cellular casts and renal tubular epithelial cells may be present in urine sediment. ATN with a low U_{Na} may be due to contrast dye, acute GN, burns, or myoglobinuria. Toxic ATN due to rhabdomyolysis is suggested by a heme-positive dipstick in the absence of microscopic hematuria and a markedly elevated serum CK.

Clinical course: ATN begins with diminished urine output apparent within a day of the insult; anuria may be present in some cases; oliguria lasts for 10–14 days. If oliguria persists >2–3 weeks, other diagnoses should be increasingly considered. The daily increments in BUN and creatinine average 10–20 and 0.5–1.0 mg/dL, respectively, but will be greater in catabolic pts.

Complications: These include salt and water overload, hypertension, and CHF. Hyperkalemia results from impaired K excretion. Retention of acid causes an anion gap metabolic acidosis. Other complications include hyperphosphatemia, hypocalcemia, anemia, infection, GI bleeding, ileus, pericarditis, and neurologic abnormalities.

During the recovery phase of ARF, urine volume increases progressively; BUN and creatinine plateau, then begin to fall. However, major complications of ARF may first appear during this stage. Fluid and electrolyte depletion may occur during postobstructive diuresis and post ATN.

TABLE 85-2 Approach to patient with ARF

1. Search for and correct prerenal and postrenal causes.
2. Search for evidence of ischemic or nephrotoxic injury or renal parenchymal disease.
3. Attempt to establish a urine output with volume challenge or furosemide.
4. Conservative therapy:
   - Discontinue indwelling catheter
   - Measure intake and output
   - Daily weights
   - Limit fluids to 400 mL + previous day's losses
   - Alter medication doses as indicated
   - Add phosphate binders
   - Treat hyperkalemia and acidosis
5. Dialysis for volume overload, pericarditis, GI bleeding, symptomatic uremia, severe hyperkalemia or acidosis.

Principles of *therapy* of acute renal failure are listed in Table 85-2.

For more detailed discussion of this topic, see **Anderson RJ, Schrier RW: Acute Renal Failure, Chap. 219, in HPIM-11, p. 1149**

86 CHRONIC RENAL FAILURE (CRF) AND UREMIA

CRF refers to the permanent loss of renal function, which, when advanced, results in the signs and symptoms of *uremia.* Unlike ARF, from which recovery is frequent, CRF is not reversible and may lead to a vicious cycle with progressive loss of remaining nephrons. Most common causes of CRF are glomerulonephritis, diabetes mellitus, hypertension, chronic interstitial nephritis, and polycystic kidney disease.

CAUSES The specific causes of the uremic syndrome are unknown. In addition to failure of renal excretion of solutes and products of metabolism, it represents loss of metabolic and endocrine function of the healthy kidney. The most likely retained toxins causing this syndrome are breakdown products of proteins and amino acids. Urea itself is the most abundant and may account, in part, for malaise, anorexia, and vomiting. Another nitrogenous compound, guanidinosuccinic acid, contributes to platelet dysfunction. Larger compounds ("middle molecules") have been implicated in uremic neuropathy. A variety of polypeptide hormones, including PTH, circulate at high levels in CRF and contribute to the uremic syndrome.

CONSEQUENCES The consequences of CRF and uremia include effects on cellular functions and metabolism, as well as on volume and composition of body fluids. Defective membrane transport may result in dysfunction of RBCs and skeletal muscle. Protein malnutrition and inadequate caloric intake are common. Hypertriglyceridemia is typical in uremic pts, although cholesterol levels are usually normal.

With progressive nephron loss, the range of osmolalities which the diseased kidney can achieve narrows, resulting in isosthenuria. Impaired concentrating ability may lead to polyuria and nocturia and makes fluid restriction potentially hazardous; impaired diluting capacity may result in hyponatremia due to water retention.

External Na balance is maintained in CRF by an increase in fractional Na excretion, due to altered peritubular factors, osmotic diuresis due to retained solutes, and perhaps atrial natriuretic hormone. Late in CRF the range of Na excretion by remaining nephrons is restricted, so that dietary salt is retained, resulting in hypertension and volume overload. Severe Na restriction may cause Na depletion, with worsening of renal function due to superimposed prerenal azotemia.

Little or no change in arterial pH, plasma HCO_3, or P_{CO_2} occurs until CRF is far advanced. Metabolic acidosis results in part from diminished real NH_3 production. However, the positive H balance causes only mild nonprogressive metabolic acidosis, probably because of enhanced bone buffering. In moderate renal failure, hyperchloremic acidosis occurs because sulfate and phosphate

TABLE 86-1 Consequences of CRF

Volume and composition of body fluids:	Neuromuscular:
Na retention or depletion	Encephalopathy
Hyponatremia	Peripheral neuropathy
Hyperkalemia	Dialysis dementia
Metabolic acidosis	Dialysis disequilibrium
Hyperphosphatemia	Gastrointestinal:
Hypocalcemia	Anorexia, nausea, vomiting
Hypermagnesemia	Gastroenteritis
Hyperuricemia	Peptic ulcer
Cardiopulmonary:	Ascites
CHF	Diverticulosis
Hypertension	Viral hepatitis
Pericarditis	Endocrine:
Accelerated atherosclerosis	Secondary hyperparathyroidism
Pneumonitis	Vitamin D disorders
Pleuritis	Glucose intolerance
Hematologic:	Amenorrhea
Anemia	Impotence
Poor hemostasis	Skin:
Leukocyte abnormalities	Pruritus
	Ecchymosis
	Hyperpigmentation

anions are not retained. Retention of these and other unmeasured anions in severe CRF results in an anion gap acidosis.

With advancing renal disease, phosphate balance is achieved by reduced fractional phosphate reabsorption, mediated by enhanced PTH secretion; the latter is due to ↓ in serum Ca^{2+}, associated with retention of phosphate, as GFR falls. Elevated PTH levels cause many of the bone changes of renal osteodystrophy. Other abnormalities in CRF include skeletal resistance to PTH and reduced circulating 1,25-dihydroxyvitamin D_3 levels.

Clinical spectrum of abnormalities in uremia are listed in Table 86-1. Signs and symptoms typically appear late in the course of CRF, when GFR $< 25\%$ of normal.

Excessive salt ingestion leads to CHF, hypertension, and edema; when extrarenal fluid losses occur, extracellular volume depletion may result. Excessive water ingestion results in hyponatremia. Hyperkalemia results from excessive K intake, antikaliuretic drugs, acidosis, or when oliguria supervenes. Hyperphosphatemia and hypocalcemia develop when GRF falls to $<25\%$ of normal. Hypermagnesemia is a hazard in pts given Mg-containing antacids or cathartics.

In addition to CHF, pulmonary edema due to ↑ capillary permeability may be observed in the absence of volume overload. Both forms respond to dialysis. Pericarditis may be due to inadequate dialysis or a systemic disease. There is a high incidence of accelerated atherosclerosis in dialysis pts. Normochromic normocytic anemia results from diminished erythropoiesis, shortened RBC survival, and, in some cases, blood loss. Abnormalities in hemostasis, characterized by prolonged bleeding time, lower platelet factor III activity, and platelet function abnormalities, may produce hemorrhagic complications; GI bleeding is common. Mild thrombocytopenia may be present. The hemostatic defect responds to effective dialysis. Cryoprecipitate may be useful. A variety of changes in WBC function also occurs.

Signs and symptoms of mild uremic encephalopathy and peripheral neuropathy are common in advanced CRF and improve with dialysis. GI symptoms of uremia include anorexia, nausea, and vomiting, especially in the morning. Shallow mucosal ulcers, peptic ulcers, and diverticulitis may be sites of GI bleeding. Overproduction of PTH contributes to bone changes of osteitis fibrosa cystica. Skeletal abnormalities due to abnormal vitamin D metabolism may include a form of rickets and osteomalacia. Glucose intolerance results largely from resistance to insulin. Amenorrhea and impotence are common.

Uremic pruritus, ecchymosis, a yellow hyperpigmentation due to retention of urochromes, and discoloration due to hemachromatosis are skin abnormalities seen in CRF.

For more detailed discussion of this topic, see Brenner BM, Lazarus JM: Chronic Renal Failure: Pathophysiologic and Clinical Considerations, Chap. 220, in HPIM-11, p. 1155

---

87 DIALYSIS AND TRANSPLANTATION

CHRONIC HEMODIALYSIS

Most prevalent therapy for end-stage renal disease (ESRD); accomplished by perfusing patient's blood and a dialysate solution on opposite sides of a membrane. Both diffusion of solutes, such as urea, and extraction of salt and water by hyperfiltration occur. Efficiency of dialysis depends on solute size, blood and dialysate flow rates, and characteristics of dialysis membrane.

INDICATIONS These include ARF (Chap. 85), CRF in pts in whom early transplantation is planned, and other pts with CRF in whom the quality of life has deteriorated. Most pts are dialyzed for 4 h three times per week and are maintained on a 40–60 g protein diet with Na and K restriction. Phosphate-binding antacids, folate, and multivitamins are added.

ACCESS Commonly achieved by creation of a subcutaneous AV fistula or shunt. Alternatives include prosthetic fistulas and percutaneous subclavian or femoral catheters. In pts with CRF access, surgery should be performed when the serum creatinine level has reached 7–9 mg/dL, since the native fistula cannot be used for several weeks. Shunts and catheters are temporary devices. Prosthetic fistulas are more likely to cause infection, thrombosis, and aneurysm. Other complications of access sites and of dialysis are shown in Table 87-1. Access infections are usually staphylococcal and may lead to sepsis and/or endocarditis.

Many manifestations of uremia may persist in pts on chronic hemodialysis, although they are less severe. Anemia may be aggravated by blood loss and folate deficiency. Accelerated atherosclerosis is common in pts on chronic hemodialysis. Pericarditis, diverticulosis, hepatitis (most frequently non-A, non-B), sexual dysfunction, and acquired renal cysts are other complications.

TABLE 87-1 **Complications of dialysis**

Access:
Infection
Thrombosis
Vascular compromise
High-output CHF
Carpal tunnel syndrome
Recirculation of blood flow
Dialysis procedure:
Hemorrhage
Hypotension
Cardiac ischemia
Cramps, nausea, vomiting
Seizures
Hypoventilation, hypoxemia
Anticoagulation
Air embolus
Hemolysis

Dialysis dementia, a syndrome of speech dyspraxia, seizures, and myoclonus, linked to aluminum intoxication is usually fatal. *Disequilibrium* refers to CNS symptoms ranging from nausea to seizures related to volume depletion and osmolar shifts, and usually occurs with early treatments. Renal osteodystrophy may progress or appear in the form of osteomalacia with bone pain and fractures.

PERITONEAL DIALYSIS An alternative to chronic hemodialysis this has the advantage of safety, lack of need for blood access, lack of blood loss, less cardiovascular stress, and pt independence. The major complication is peritonitis, most commonly staphylococcal. Malnutrition due to protein loss, hypertriglyceridemia, hypernatremia, hyperglycemia, obesity, and cardiopulmonary compromise are other complications.

RENAL TRANSPLANTATION Now a commonplace therapy for ESRD. Although immunologic rejection is still the major hazard in graft survival, recent advances have improved transplant success and lessened recipient risk.

Graft acceptance is determined by genetic compatibility of donor and recipient, based on matching of antigens (Ag) of *HLA* genes. Class I Ag are detected by a lymphocyte assay; class II Ag ("DR") by the mixed lymphocyte culture (MLC). HLA genes are inherited as a haplotype from each parent. Graft survival in living related transplants improves with matching of class I Ag. Class II Ag matching is more important to success of cadaveric transplants. Presensitization, in the presence of antibody against donor ABO or class I Ag, is detected by a positive cross-match, and is a contraindication to transplantation. Pretransplant blood transfusion enhances graft survival, although it risks sensitization in the minority of pts.

Contraindications to transplantation include presensitization; major extrarenal diseases (such as coronary artery disease, CVA, respiratory failure, or malignancy), active infection, advanced age, active glomerulonephritis, and correctable renal disease (see Table 87-2).

TABLE 87-2 **Contraindications to kidney transplantation**

Absolute contraindications:
- Reversible renal involvement
- Ability of conservative measures to maintain useful life
- Advanced forms of major extrarenal complications (cerebrovascular or coronary disease, neoplasia)
- Active infection
- Active glomerulonephritis
- Previous sensitization to donor tissue

Relative contraindications:
- Age
- Presence of vesical or urethral abnormalities
- Iliofemoral occlusive disease
- Diabetes mellitus
- Psychiatric problems
- Oxalosis

Reproduced from Carpenter CB, Lazarus JM: HPIM-11, p. 1162.

TABLE 87-3 **Complications of immunosuppressive therapy**

Azathioprine:
- Bone marow suppression
- Hepatitis
- Malignancy

Steroids:
- Infection
- Diabetes mellitus
- Adrenal suppression
- Euphoria, psychosis
- Peptic ulcer disease
- Hypertension
- Osteoporosis
- Myopathy

Cyclosporine:
- Nephrotoxicity
- Hepatotoxicity
- Tremor
- Hirsutism
- Lymphoma

REJECTION May be (1) hyperacute (immediate graft failure due to presensitization); (2) acute (within weeks to months with a rise in creatinine, hypertension, fever, graft tenderness, volume overload, and low urine output, treated by intense immunosuppression); or (3) chronic (months to years with ongoing loss of function and hypertension).

IMMUNOSUPPRESSIVE THERAPY Used to prevent or impede allograft rejection (see Table 87-3). Azathioprine, begun at transplantation and continued throughout, is useful in preventing acute rejection. CBC must be monitored. If renal function worsens, smaller doses may be required. Toxicity is indicated by low WBC. Steroids are used for maintenance and are given in higher doses to reverse acute rejection; chronic rejection is often steroid-resistant. Cyclosporine has improved survival rates, decreased severity of acute rejection episodes, and allowed lower doses of prednisone. The most important limiting factor is dose-dependent nephrotoxicity which does not correlate well with blood levels. Manifestations include posttransplant oliguria, an insidious rise in serum creatinine, hypertension, hyperkalemia, and renal tubular acidosis. Other complications are hepatotoxicity, tremor, and hirsutism.

Efficacies of antithrombocyte globulin and monoclonal antibodies are being studied.

In addition to acute rejection, other causes of early posttransplant oliguria include volume depletion, ureteral obstruction or leak, and renal artery stenosis. Workup includes renal ultrasound and radioisotope scan. Acute rejection may begin several days after transplant. Urinary Na may be low. A renal transplant biopsy may be preferable to empirically treating suspected rejection.

Glomerular diseases found in transplants include recurrent glomerulonephritis, chronic rejection, and CMV glomerulopathy with nephrotic syndrome.

For more detailed discussion of this topic, see Carpenter CB, Lazarus JM: Dialysis and Transplantation in the Treatment of Renal Failure, Chap. 221, in HPIM-11, p. 1162

ACUTE GLOMERULONEPHRITIS (AGN)

Characterized by development, over days, of azotemia, hypertension, edema, hematuria, proteinuria, and sometimes oliguria. Salt and water retention are due to reduced GFR and may result in circulatory congestion. RBC casts on UA confirm Dx. Proteinuria usually < 3 g/day. Most forms of AGN are mediated by humoral immune mechanisms. Clinical course depends on underlying lesion (see Table 88-1).

ACUTE POSTSTREPTOCOCCAL GN The prototype; the most common cause in childhood. Nephritis develops 1–3 weeks after pharyngeal or cutaneous infection with nephritogenic strains of group A-hemolytic streptococci. Dx depends on a positive pharyngeal or skin culture, rising antibody titers, and hypocomplementemia. Renal biopsy reveals diffuse proliferative GN. Treatment

TABLE 88-1 **Glomerulonephritis**

Cause	Diagnosis	Treatment
Poststreptococcal	Sore throat, impetigo, +ASO, low complement (C), especially C_3	Supportive, antibiotics in pts with strep. infection
SLE	Rash, arthralgias, pleurisy, pericarditis, +ANA, low C, renal biopsy	Prednisone, cytoxan, plasmapheresis
Infective endocarditis	Murmur, fever, emboli, splenomegaly, +BC, low C_3	Antibiotics
Hepatitis B	Jaundice, history of exposure, abnormal LFT, + serology, renal biopsy	
Wegener's granulomatosis	Infilrates on CXR, sinusitis, arthralgias, + nasal or lung biopsy	Cyclophosphamide plus prednisone
Hypersensitivity vasculitis	Palpable purpura, history of drug exposure, dyspnea, eosinophilia, + skin biopsy	Discontinue offending drug; prednisone
Goodpature's syndrome	Hemoptysis, abnormal CXR, + anti-GBM	Steroids, plasma exchange
Henoch-Schönlein purpura	Purpura, abdominal pain, arthralgias, + skin biopsy, renal biopsy	Symptomatic: sometimes, prednisone, cyclophosphamide
Polyarteritis nodosa	Hypertension, arthralgias, neuropathy, abdominal pain, + angiogram	Prednisone, cyclophosphamide

consists of correction of fluid and electrolyte imbalance. In most cases the disease is self-limited, although the prognosis is less favorable and urinary abnormalities more likely to persist in adults.

POSTINFECTIOUS GN Also may follow other bacterial, viral, and parasitic infections. Examples are bacterial endocarditis, sepsis, hepatitis B, and pneumococcal pneumonia. Clinical features are milder than with poststreptococcal GN. Control of primary infection usually produces resolution of GN.

AGN may be a prominent feature of several *multisystemic diseases*. In SLE, renal involvement is common, due to deposition of circulating immune complexes. Clinical features include arthralgias, skin rash, serositis, hair loss, and CNS disease. Renal manifestations include mesangial, focal, or diffuse GN and membranous nephropathy; nephrotic syndrome with renal insufficiency is typical. Correlation of clinical findings and biopsy is variable. Diffuse GN, the most common finding, is characterized by an active sediment, heavy proteinuria, and progressive renal insufficiency and may have an ominous prognosis. Pts have a positive ANA, anti-dsDNA, and ↓ complement. Treatment includes oral steroids, pulses of IV steroids, and cytotoxic agents.

GOODPASTURE'S SYNDROME Characterized by lung hemorrhage, GN, and circulating antibody to basement membrane, usually in young males. Hemoptysis may precede nephritis. Rapidly progressive renal failure is typical. Circulating anti-GBM antibody and linear immunofluorescence on renal biopsy establish Dx. Linear IgG is also present on lung biopsy. Plasma exchange may produce remission. Severe lung hemorrhage is treated with pulses of IV steroids.

HENOCH-SCHÖNLEIN PURPURA (HSP) A generalized vasculitis causing GN, purpura, arthralgias, and abdominal pain; occurs mainly in children. Renal involvement is manifested by hematuria and proteinuria. Serum IgA is increased in half of pts. Renal biopsy is useful for prognosis. Treatment is symptomatic in most cases.

VASCULITIS Several distinct syndromes cause GN. *Polyarteritis nodosa* causes hypertension, arthralgias, neuropathy, and renal failure. Similar features plus palpable purpura and asthma are common in *hypersensitivity angiitis. Wegener's granulomatosis* involves upper respiratory tract and kidney and responds to cyclophosphamide.

RAPIDLY PROGRESSIVE GLOMERULONEPHRITIS (RPGN)

Characterized by gradual onset of hematuria, proteinuria, and renal failure, which progresses over a period of weeks to months. Crescentic GN is found on renal biopsy. The disorder may occur secondary to infection (bacterial endocarditis, poststreptococcal GN) or multisystem disease (SLE, Goodpasture's vasculitis, HSP). Idiopathic RPGN is a heterogeneous group with three pathologic subgroups: (1) linear deposits of IgG; (2) immune complex (IC) deposition; and (3) without linear or IC deposits. Plasmapheresis may be effective for removal of anti-GBM antibodies. All three groups may respond to pulsed steroids, cytotoxins, and antithrombotic agents.

NEPHROTIC SYNDROME (NS)

Characterized by albuminuria (>3.5 g/day) and hypoalbuminemia (<3 g/dL) and accompanied by edema, hyperlipidemia, and lipiduria. Complications include renal vein thrombosis and other thromboembolic events, infection, vitamin D deficiency, protein malnutrition, and drug toxicities due to decreased protein binding.

In adults, a minority of cases are secondary to diabetes, SLE, amyloidosis, drugs, neoplasia, or other disorders (see Table 88-2). By exclusion, the remainder are idiopathic. Renal biopsy is required to determine accurate diagnosis and therapy in idiopathic NS.

MINIMAL CHANGE DISEASE Causes about 15% of idiopathic NS in adults. Blood pressure is normal; GFR is normal or slightly reduced; urinary sediment is benign or may show few RBCs. Protein selectivity is variable in adults. Recent URI, allergies, or immunizations are present in some cases. ARF may rarely occur. Renal biopsy shows only foot process fusion on electron microscopy. Remission of proteinuria with steroids carries a good prognosis; cytotoxic therapy may be required for relapse. Progression to renal failure is uncommon. Later focal sclerosis has been suspected in some cases.

MEMBRANOUS GN Characterized by subepithelial IgG deposits; accounts for 45% of adult NS. Pts present with edema, nephrotic proteinuria, and normal BP, GFR, and urine sediment, but with hypertension, mild renal insufficiency, and an abnormal urine sediment developing later. Renal vein thrombosis is common. Underlying diseases such as SLE, hepatitis B, and solid tumors and exposure to such drugs as captopril or penicillamine should be sought. Steroids may reduce the decline in renal function if given

TABLE 88-2 **Causes of nephrotic syndrome (NS)**

- Systemic causes (25%):
  - Diabetes mellitus, SLE, amyloidosis
  - Drugs:
    - Gold, penicillamine, probenecid, street heroin, captopril, NSAIDs
  - Infections:
    - Bacterial endocarditis, hepatitis B, shunt infections, syphilis, malaria
  - Malignancy:
    - Hodgkin's and other lymphomas, leukemia, carcinoma of breast, GI tract
  - Allergic reactions
- Glomerular disease (75%):
  - Membranous (40%)
  - Minimal change disease (15%)
  - Focal glomerulosclerosis (15%)
  - Membranoproliferative GN (7%)
  - Mesangioproliferative GN (5%)

Modified from Glassock RJ, Brenner BM: HPIM-11, p. 1178.

TABLE 88-3 **Evaluation of nephrotic syndrome**

24-h urine for protein; creatinine clearance
Serum albumin
Cholesterol
Complement
Urine electrophoresis
Rule out SLE, diabetes mellitus
Review drug exposure
Renal biopsy
Consider malignancy (in elderly pt with membranous GN or minimal change disease)
Consider renal vein thrombosis (if membranous GN or symptoms of pulmonary embolism are present)

prior to renal insufficency, but they do not induce full remission of proteinuria. Some pts progress to end-stage renal disease.

FOCAL GLOMERULOSCLEROSIS Involves fibrosis of portions of some (primarily juxtamedullary) glomeruli and is found in 15% of pts. Hypertension, reduced GFR, and hematuria are typical. Some cases may be a late stage of minimal change disease or be due to heroin abuse, vesicoureteral reflux, or AIDS. Fewer than half undergo remission with steroids. Half progress to renal failure in 10 years; may recur in a renal transplant. Pressure of azotemia or hypertension reflects poor prognosis. Role of dietary protein restriction is unclear.

MEMBRANOPROLIFERATIVE GLOMERULONEPHRITIS (MPGN) Mesangial expansion and proliferation extends into the capillary loop. Two ultrastructural variants exist. Decreased serum complement levels are characteristic. MPGN affects young adults; blood pressure and GFR are abnormal and the urine sediment is active. Some present with acute nephritis or hematuria. Similar lesions occur in SLE and hemolytic-uremic syndrome. Renal function declines over several years. Steroids may delay progression. ASA plus dipyridamole appears beneficial in some pts. May recur in allografts.

DIABETIC NEPHROPATHY Common among secondary forms of NS. Pathologic changes include diffuse and/or nodular glomerulosclerosis, nephrosclerosis, chronic pyelonephritis, and papillary necrosis. *Clinical features* include proteinuria, hypertension, azotemia, and bacteriuria. Duration of diabetes is variable, but proteinuria may develop 10–15 years after onset of diabetes, progress to NS, and then progress to renal failure over 3–5 years. Retinopathy is nearly universal. Tight glucose control may delay onset of nephropathy. Aggressive management of hypertension and restriction of dietary protein may retard decline of renal failure. Mortality rates on dialysis are high, and successful transplantation is somewhat less frequent than in nondiabetics.

Evaluation of NS is shown in Table 88-3.

For more detailed discussion of these topics, see Glassock RJ, Brenner BM: Immunopathogenic Mechanisms of Renal Injury, Chap. 222, p. 1170; Glassock RJ, Brenner BM: The Major Glomerulopathies, Chap. 223, p. 1173; and Glassock RJ, Brenner MB: Glomerulopathies Associated with Multisystem Diseases, Chap. 224, p. 1183, HPIM-11

89 RENAL TUBULAR DISEASES

Tubulointerstitial diseases form a diverse group of acute and chronic hereditary and acquired disorders involving renal tubules and supporting structures. Functionally, they may result in nephrogenic DI with polyuria, nocturia, non-anion gap acidosis, salt-wasting, and hypo- or hyperkalemia. Azotemia is frequently present, owing to associated glomerulofibrosis or ischemia. Compared to glomerulopathies, proteinuria is modest, hypertension less common, but anemia more severe.

ACUTE INTERSTITIAL NEPHRITIS (IN) Drugs are a leading cause of this increasingly recognized cause of renal failure (RF), identifiable by acute oliguria and sometimes an allergic reaction with fever, rash, and arthralgias. In addition to azotemia, tubular dysfunction may be present. Common causes are methicillin, other penicillins, sulfonamides, diuretics, rifampin, cimetidine, cephalosporin, and allopurinol; NSAIDs cause IN with nephrotic syndrome asociated with minimal change disease and may lack allergic manifestations.

Eosinophilia is common; UA shows RBCs, pyuria, and eosinophiliuria on Wright's stain. On renal biopsy, interstitial edema with WBC infiltration is present. RF commonly responds to withdrawal of offending drug, and most pts have good recovery. Uncontrolled studies support more rapid and complete renal recovery with steroids, which may outweigh their risk.

Acute bacterial pyelonephritis may cause acute IN but does not generally cause RF unless complicated by dehydration, sepsis, or urinary obstruction.

CHRONIC INTERSTITIAL NEPHRITIS Analgesic nephropathy is now recognized as an important cause of RF that results from prolonged consumption of combination analgesics (5–10 tablets/day for 3 years), usually of phenacitin and aspirin. Nephropathy may be manifested as chronic IN, uremia, acute papillary necrosis in nondiabetics, sterile pyuria, or renal calculi. Pts are often females with headaches, anemia, and GI symptoms. Renal function stabilizes with total cessation of drugs.

Other drugs causing chronic IN include lithium (polyuria is common but risk of RF due to chronic IN is small in the absence of toxic levels), cisplatin (nephrotoxicity reduced by saline diuresis), and methyl-CCNU. Metabolic causes of chronic IN include (1) chronic hypercalcemia (fibrosis with tubular Ca deposits; causes early nephrogenic DI and late chronic RF); (2) hypokalemia (may cause fibrosis after many years); and (3) uric acid nephropathy (acute RF due to acute hyperuricemia or chronic RF due to chronic hyperuricemia, hypertension, and uric acid stones).

Chronic IN also may be due to multiple myeloma, in which progressive RF follows light-chain precipitation in tubules and fibrosis ("myeloma kidney") and correlates with Bence-Jones proteinuria. Other renal manifestations of myeloma include ARF, proteinuria, amyloidosis, tubular defects, and hypercalcemic nephropathy. Chronic IN is also caused by Sjögren's syndrome, sarcoidosis, TBC, and radiation nephritis. *Medullary sponge kidney* is a disorder, usually sporadic, of ectatic collecting ducts which presents as hematuria, urinary infection, distal RTA, and/or nephrolithiasis in the fourth and fifth decades. Dx is made by IVP. RF is rare.

Several *inherited* disorders affect the renal tubules and interstitium. *Polycystic kidney disease* is a frequent cause of CRF; inheritance is autosomal dominant, and males and females are equally affected. Symptoms of flank pain, nocturia, hematuria, and urinary infection appear in the third or fourth decade. Kidneys are palpable. Hepatic cysts and intracranial aneurysms also may be present. Progressive azotemia occurs in most pts. Dx is by IVP or ultrasound. Dialysis and transplantation are routinely used in treatment. In medullary cystic disease, polyuria, acidosis, and salt wasting precede slowly progressive RF. Genetics are variable, the Dx may be made by IVP or may require arteriography or renal biopsy.

Congenital disorders of tubular transport include

1 *Bartter's syndrome:* Hypokalemia due to renal K wasting, weakness, polyuria, beginning in childhood; autosomal recessive; high renin and aldosterone, often responsive to indomethacin.

2 *Renal tubular acidosis (RTA):*

Distal (type I) RTA: Patients are unable to lower urine pH normally despite acidosis; autosomal dominant but frequently sporadic due to autoimmune disease, obstruction, or amphotericin; associated with hypokalemia, hypercalciuria, and osteomalacia.

Proximal (type II) RTA: A defect in HCO_3 reabsorption, usually associated with glucosuria, aminoaciduria, phosphaturia; may also be due to myeloma, drugs, or renal transplant; requires large amounts of HCO_3, which aggravates hypokalemia.

Type IV RTA: Occurs with hyperkalemia and usually low renin and aldosterone levels and is generally associated with diabetes, advanced age, chronic IN, or nephrosclerosis.

For more detailed discussion of this topic, see Brenner BM, Hostetter TH: Tubulointerstitial Diseases of the Kidney, Chap. 226, in HPIM-11, p. 1195

URINARY TRACT INFECTIONS (UTI)

ETIOLOGY

• 80% *E. coli;* increased with calculi—*Proteus* (positive urease) and *Klebsiella.* • *Staphylococcus saprophyticus* 10–15% in young women. • A third of women with $<10^5$ organisms/mL of urine → three-quarters have usual pathogens; others have *Chlamydia, Neisseria gonorrhoeae,* herpes simplex.

Increased risk: sexually active women, prostatitis, prostatic hypertrophy, pregnancy (20–30% with asymptomatic bacteriuria develop pyelonephritis), obstruction, neurogenic bladder dysfunction, vesicoureteral reflux.

CLINICAL PRESENTATION

- Cystitis: dysuria, frequency, urgency, suprapubic pain, 30% bloody urine.
- Acute pyelonephritis: fever, chills, nausea, vomiting, costovertebral angle tenderness.
- Urethritis: dysuria, frequency but no or nonsignificant bacterial growth; frequently sexually transmitted infection.
- Catheter-associated infections: risk of infection 5% per day of catheterization; usually *E. coli, Proteus, Pseudomonas, Klebsiella, Serratia.*

TREATMENT

1 *Cystitis (E. coli):* Amoxacillin 3.0 g, trimethoprim-sulfamethoxazole 2–3 double-strength, sulfa 2.0 g in reliable patients; treat for 7 days in children, pregnant women.

2 *Acute pyelonephritis:* Most *E. coli;* IV aminoglycoside, cephalosporin, trimethoprim-sulfamethoxazole for several days then PO × 10–14 days; 20–30% *E. coli* ampicillin-resistant; if relapse (within 2 weeks), investigate for calculi or urologic disease.

3 *Asymptomatic bacteriuria:* Document twice before treatment orally × 7 days; if it persists, follow without further treatment unless neutropenic, renal transplant, or previous pyelonephritis—6 weeks oral therapy.

4 *Catheter-associated UTI:* Cure unlikely unless catheter removed; if asymptomatic, do not treat unless at risk for sepsis (1–2%) with old age, underlying disease, diabetes, pregnancy.

Urologic evaluation: IVP and cystoscopy only for women with relapsing infection, history of childhood infections, stones, recurrent pyelonephritis; investigate all men or any patient with symptoms suggestive of obstruction or stones.

Prophylaxis: >2 infections q 6 months; single-dose trimethoprim-sulfamethoxazole or nitrofurantoin 50 mg qd after urine sterilized.

CHRONIC PYELONEPHRITIS Diagnosis: recurrent UTIs, impaired renal function, pyuria with WBC casts, bacteriuria, IVP with irregularly outlined renal pelvis with cortical scars; symptoms often minimal; hypertension; progression to uremia.

PAPILLARY NECROSIS

• Increased risk: gout, diabetes, phenacetin-containing analgesic mixtures, sickle cell, alcoholism, vascular disease. • Symptoms: hematuria, flank pain, chills, fever. • Treatment: with overwhelming infection, if unilateral, may require nephrectomy.

PROSTATITIS

1 *Acute bacterial prostatitis:* usually young males or indwelling catheter; PE: fever, chills, dysuria, boggy or tender prostate; diagnose by urine gram stain and culture (prostatic massage may cause bacteremia); usually gram-negative rods or *S. aureus;* treat with IV cephalosporin, trimethoprim-sulfamethoxazole, or aminoglycoside.

2 *Chronic bacterial prostatitis:* Usually no symptoms, normal prostate, pyuria; prostatic massage may cause bacteremia; treat with prolonged courses of trimethoprim-sulfamethoxazole or nitrofurantoin.

For more detailed discussion of this topic, see Stamm WE, Turck M: Urinary Tract Infection, Pyelonephritis, and Related Conditions, Chap. 225, in HPIM-11, p. 1189

91 RENOVASCULAR DISEASE

Vascular occlusion of the large and small renal arteries produces ischemic injury whose expression depends on the rate, site, severity, and duration of vascular compromise. Signs and symptoms range from painful infarction to ARF, impaired GFR, hematuria, or tubular dysfunction. Renal ischemia of any etiology may cause renin-mediated hypertension.

ACUTE OCCLUSION OF A RENAL ARTERY May be due to thrombosis or embolism (from valvular disease, endocarditis, mural thrombi, or atrial arrhythmias). Large renal infarcts cause pain, vomiting, nausea, hypertension, fever, proteinuria, hematuria, and elevated LDH and SGOT. Renal functional loss depends on contralateral function. IVP or radionuclide scan shows unilateral hypofunction; ultrasound is normal. Renal arteriography establishes diagnosis. With occlusions of large arteries, surgery may be the initial therapy; with occlusions of small arteries, anticoagulation should be used.

RENAL ATHEROEMBOLISM Usually arises when aortic angiography or surgery causes cholesterol embolization of small renal vessels. Renal insufficiency may develop suddenly or gradually. Other findings are GI or retinal ischemia with cholesterol emboli visible on fundoscopic examination, neurologic deficits, livido reticularis, toe gangrene, and hypertension. UA is negative, and U_{Na} may be low. Skin or renal biopsy may be necessary for diagnosis. Heparin is contraindicated.

RENAL ARTERY STENOSIS Main cause of renovascular hypertension; due to (1) atherosclerosis (two-thirds of cases, usually males >60 years, advanced retinopathy) or (2) fibromuscular dysplasia (a third of cases, Caucasian females <45 years, brief history of hypertension). Renal hypoperfusion activates renin-angiotensin-aldosterone axis. Suggestive clinical features include onset of hypertension <30 or >50 years, bruits, hypokalemic alkalosis, acute onset of hypertension or malignant hypertension, and hypertension resistant to medical therapy.

To identify treatable patients, IVP is a useful screening test (small kidney, delayed appearance, and late concentration of contrast) but lacks sensitivity. Radioisotope studies are no more accurate. Digital subtraction angiography may be a superior screening test. Renal arteriography is definitive diagnostic method, and renal vein renins are necessary to show functional significance (ipsilateral elevation with contralateral suppression); captopril will reduce false-negative results.

Surgical revascularization: Achieves best results in fibromuscular disease. Those with localized atherosclerosis do well, but mortality is higher; surgery in patients with diffuse or bilateral lesions is best reserved for urgent cases which have failed medical management.

Angioplasty: Also most successful with fibromuscular disease and nonoccluded, nonostial atherosclerotic lesions; has a low complication rate and cost. In many pts (the elderly, those with impaired renal function, or those with high surgical risk), pharmacotherapy is employed. Converting-enzyme inhibitors are ideal drugs except in pts with bilateral stenosis or disease in solitary kidney.

Malignant hypertension (Chap. 59) also may be caused by renal vascular occlusion with severe hypertension, papilledema, headache, malaise, encephalopathy, and renal impairment. Nitroprusside or calcium antagonists are generally effective in lowering BP.

In some pts with previously stable scleroderma (Chap. 110), sudden oliguric renal failure and severe hypertension occur due to small vessel occlusion. Aggressive control of BP with converting-enzyme inhibitors and dialysis improves survival and may restore renal function.

Sludging of blood in the renal medulla causes hematuria in pts with sickle cell anemia or trait. It may cause nephrogenic diabetes insipidus, papillary necrosis, proteinuria, and mild renal insufficiency.

HEMOLYTIC-UREMIC SYNDROME Characterized by ARF, microangiopathic hemolytic anemia, and thrombocytopenia; increasingly recognized in adults; may be preceded by a prodrome of bloody diarrhea and abdominal pain. Fibrin deposition leads to small vessel occlusion. Lack of fever or CNS involvement helps to distinguish it from thrombotic thrombocytopenic purpura. Treatment is symptomatic; prognosis for recovery of renal function is poor.

PREECLAMPSIA Characterized by hypertension, proteinuria, and edema after 24 weeks of gestation; *eclampsia* is the further development of seizures. Glomerular swelling causes renal insufficiency. Coagulation abnormalities and ARF may occur. Treatment consists of bed rest, sedation, and control of hypertension. In severe cases, $MgSO_4$ and termination of pregnancy are indicated.

Renal complications of *vasculitis* are frequent and severe in polyarteritis nodosa, Wegener's granulomatosis, hypersensitivity, and other forms of vasculitis (Chap. 111). Therapy consists of steroids and cyclosphosphamide in Wegener's.

For more detailed discussion of this topic, see Hollenberg NK: Vascular Injury to the Kidney, Chap. 227, in HPIM-11, p. 1200

Renal stones form a common (1% of population) and recurrent (50–85%) group of disorders that are increasingly preventable. Stone formation begins when urine becomes supersaturated with insoluble component(s) due to excessive excretion or factors that diminish solubility. Stone composition [Ca, 75%; struvite (magnesium-ammonium-phosphate), 15%; uric acid, 5%; cystine, 1%] reflects the variety of metabolic disorders from which they arise.

SYMPTOMS Similar for most types of stones. Those attached in the renal pelvis may be asymptomatic or cause hematuria, and obstruction may occur at any site. On passage, severe colicky migrating pain and hematuria are typical. Symptoms of UTI or obstruction can occur. Staghorn calculi present with recurrent infection.

STONE COMPOSITION Most stones are composed of *Ca oxalate;* 30% of these are associated with hypercalciuria, whereas hyperoxaluria is rare. Hypercalciuria without hypercalcemia is usually idiopathic, i.e., without specific etiology (sarcoidosis, immobilization, furosemide, RTA, Cushing's syndrome). The abnormality in idiopathic hypercalciuria ranges from excessive GI Ca absorption to increased renal Ca excretion and appears to be familial. Standard treatment of both GI and renal forms is high fluid intake and thiazide diuretics.

Other causes of Ca oxalate stones include (1) hyperuricosuria due to dietary purine excess (uric acid initiates Ca oxalate crystal formation); treatment is low purine diet and allopurinol; (2) primary hyperparathyroidism (hypercalcemic hypercalciuria with high PTH); parathyroidectomy prevents stones; (3) distal RTA (renal acidosis causes hypercalciuria; with alkaline urine and low urine citrate, Ca phosphate stones form, along with nephrocalcinosis); treat with alkali; (4) hyperoxaluria (usually due to excess GI absorption associated with steatorrhea); therapy is correction of fat malabsorption, oral Ca lactate and/or cholestyramine; and (5) idiopathic (normocalciuric); treat with hydration and dietary Ca restriction.

Struvite stones form in the collecting system when infection with urea-splitting organisms (usually *Proteus*) is present. High urine pH (8–9), magnesium, ammonium, and carbonate levels result, producing struvite ($MgNH_4PO_4$) stones. It is the most common cause of staghorn calculi and causes obstruction. Risk factors include urinary catheters, neurogenic bladder, and repeated instrumentation. Mandelamine and antibiotics are useful for lowering urine pH, suppressing infection, and preventing stone growth and/or recurrence. Cure usually requires surgical removal. Partial dissolution may occur with chronic antibacterial therapy. Irrigation of renal pelvis with renacidin is newer therapy.

Uric acid stones occur when urine is saturated with uric acid in the presence of an acid urine pH and dehydration. Occur in pts with (1) gout, where they may precede arthritis; (2) myeloproliferative disorders, particularly when chemotherapy increases uricosuria; (3) diarrhea, inflammatory bowel disease, or ileostomy; or (4) idiopathic. Treatment is with fluids, alkalinization of urine, and allopurinol. When hyperuricosuria (>1 g/day) is present, reduced purine intake is indicated.

CYSTINURIA A rare inherited disorder of defective renal (and intestinal) transport resulting in overexcretion of cystine. Stones begin to form in childhood and are a rare cause of staghorn calculi. Hexagonal cystine crystals identified in urine should be further assessed by measurement of urine cystine excretion. Treatment is with high urine volume, alkali therapy (urine pH > 7.5). Penicillamine, which binds cystine, is reserved for refractory cases.

EVALUATION OF PATIENT Yields an identifiable cause in many and should be offered to all stone formers. History may reveal prior episodes or positive family history of dietary excess or low fluid intake, UTI, gout, bowel disease, or a specific cause of hypercalciuria. Serum Ca, HCO_3, and creatinine should be measured. Cystine, struvite, or other crystals may be found in urine; a culture should be done if infection is suggested. Abdominal film (KUB) and IVP will reveal stone location, quantity, size, and opacity, as well as presence of obstruction. Obtained stones should always be analyzed. No matter what the composition, urine volume should be increased by high fluid intake.

All patients with infection, uric acid, or cystine stones should be evaluated and specific therapy instituted. For Ca stone formers, hypercalcemia and hyperparathyroidism should be ruled out. 24-hour urines should be obtained to detect hypercalciuria (>300 mg in males, >250 mg in females); urine pH and excretion of uric acid and oxalate may guide specific therapy.

Management of stones already present in kidney and urinary tract depends on their location and whether they are obstructing or causing infection or impairing renal function. Stone migration and risk of removal should be assessed. Lithotripsy, if available, is a useful alternative to surgical lithotomy.

For more detailed discussion of this topic, see Coe FL, Favus MJ: Nephrolithiasis, Chap. 229, in HPIM-11, p. 1211

---

93 URINARY TRACT OBSTRUCTION (UTO)

UTO is a potentially reversible cause of renal failure; should be considered in all cases of acute renal failure (ARF) or when chronic renal failure (CRF) worsens abruptly. Consequences depend on duration and severity and whether obstruction is unilateral or bilateral.

UTO may occur at any level from collecting tubule to urethra. In adults, UTO is preponderant in females (pelvic tumors), elderly males (prostatic disease), diabetics (papillary necrosis, neurogenic bladder), and those with retroperitoneal disease, vesicoureteral reflux, stones, or functional urinary retention.

The initial effect of renal function is a prompt increase in renal blood flow (RBF) in an attempt to preserve GFR. Later RBF and GFR ↓ and tubular pressures ↑. As a result, oliguria with low U_{Na} and high osmolality (similar to prerenal azotemia) develop followed by indices similar to ARF (Chap. 85). Complete and bilateral obstruction causes anuria. The effects of chronic UTO on renal function resemble other forms of CRF; Na wasting and impaired K secretion are prominent.

CLINICAL MANIFESTATIONS Pain due to distention of upper urinary tract or bladder, renal colic, prostatic symptoms, nocturia, and diminished urine output. UTO should be considered in pts with UTI (Chap. 90) and stones (Chap. 92) and in all pts with unexplained azotemia.

PHYSICAL EXAM May reveal large bladder, palpable kidneys, prostatic or pelvic disease, rectal mass, or abnormal sphincter tone. Suspected lower tract obstruction may be confirmed by large residual urine on bladder catheterization.

On UA, pyuria, hematuria, bacteriuria, or crystalluria may be found without heavy proteinuria. Opaque stones should be sought on x-ray. Abdominal ultrasound should be performed to assess bladder and kidney size, the presence of hydronephrosis, and degree of preservation of renal parenchyma. Dilatation may be absent in UTO due to tubular obstruction, upper tract encasement by tumors or retroperitoneal fibrosis, staghorn calculus, very early ARF, or antecedent CRF with small kidneys. Unilateral hydronephrosis may be responsible for azotemia when contralateral kidney is diseased or absent.

IVP may be employed to determine level of obstruction and its cause. IVP should not be attempted in severe renal failure. To examine the renal pelvis and ureter in patient with RF, either retrograde or antegrade pyelography should be performed. CT scan is helpful in elucidating etiology, particularly in pts with retroperitoneal disease causing UTO without hydronephrosis.

ARF due to UTO requires rapid intervention, since return of renal function depends in part on duration of obstruction. Bladder catheterization and nephrostomy relieve obstruction in lower and upper tracts, respectively. Infection should be treated aggressively. Dialysis is indicated in severe RF due to reversible UTO.

Relief of severe bilateral obstruction is typically followed by physiologic *diuresis* lasting several days, with excretion of large quantities of water and electrolytes. Volume depletion, hypokalemia, hyponatremia, and hypomagnesemia may result. IV fluids (one-half normal saline with added K and Mg prn) should be used to replace urinary losses. Close monitoring of fluid balance is mandatory.

For more detailed discussion of this topic, see Brenner BM, Milford EL, Seifter JL: Urinary Tract Obstruction, Chap. 230, in HPIM-11, p. 1215

---

94 TUMORS OF THE URINARY TRACT

Of renal tumors, 85% are *renal cell carcinomas;* the remainder arise in the renal pelvis. Occur typically in males in sixth decade; cigarette smoking is a risk factor. Rare forms are inherited (in von Hippel–Lindau disease) and some are due to chromosomal translocations. Renal cysts in hemodialysis patients may become malignant.

CLINICAL MANIFESTATIONS Include hematuria (gross or microscopic), flank pain, abdominal mass (and systemic symptoms), fever, fatigue, weight loss, cachexia, anemia. Paraneoplastic syndromes include FUO, hypercalcemia, galactorrhea, Cushing's syndrome, erythrocytosis, or hypertension. LFTs may be abnormal.

DIAGNOSIS Usually begins with discovery of a flank mass by IVP (space-occupying lesion, distorted collecting system), often in patient with systemic symptoms or manifestations of metastases. When renal mass is detected, CT and ultrasound are performed to differentiate benign cysts from tumor. Percutaneous needle aspiration for cytology is frequently helpful. CT may reveal solid mass, occasionally with extension into renal vein. Renal arteriography may show hypervascular tumor. *Staging* begins with search for metastatic disease (CXR, bone and liver scans). If negative, radical nephrectomy is indicated. Five-year survival rates range from about 70% (tumor confined to kidney) to under 5% (distant spread). Metastatic disease is resistant to hormonal and/or chemotherapy. Cure is occasionally achieved by excision of solitary metastasis.

Tumors of *renal pelvis* are usually *transitional cell carcinomas.* Risk factors include smoking, chemical exposure, and analgesic abuse; present with painless gross hematuria; IVP and urine cytology are positive. Treatment of advanced disease is radical nephroureterectomy. Survival is 10–50% after 5 years. Close follow-up is required.

Tumors metastatic to kidney (principally liver cancer and lymphoma) are rarely evident clinically.

Bladder (transitional cell) carcinoma is most common in males over age 40. Risk factors are smoking and chemical exposure. Bladder cancer also may follow cyclophosphamide therapy or chronic *Schistosoma haematobium* infection. Hematuria or other bladder symptoms are present in majority. Dx is by urine cytology and cystoscopy with biopsy. Prognosis depends on depth of invasion of bladder and systemic involvement. Superficial disease is treated by endoscopic resection with frequent follow-up; recurrences are common and may require intravesical chemotherapy. Metastatic disease may remit with surgery and combination chemotherapy.

For more detailed discussion of this topic, see Garnick MB, Brenner BM: Tumors of the Urinary Tract, Chap. 231, in HPIM-11, p. 1218

SECTION VI
GASTROINTESTINAL DISEASES

95 ESOPHAGEAL DISEASES

DYSPHAGIA

OROPHARYNGEAL: Difficulty initiating swallowing; food sticks at level of suprasternal notch; nasopharyngeal regurgitation; aspiration. Not to be confused with globus hystericus, the sensation of a lump in the throat.
Solids only: Carcinoma, aberrant vessel, congenital web (Plummer-Vinson syndrome), lye stricture.
Solids and liquids: Cricopharyngeal achalasia, Zenker's diverticulum, myasthenia gravis, steroid myopathy, thyrotoxic myopathy, myotonic dystrophy, amyotrophic lateral sclerosis, multiple sclerosis, parkinsonism, bulbar and pseudobulbar palsy.

ESOPHAGEAL Food sticks in mid or lower sternal area; odynophagia (pain on swallowing); regurgitation; aspiration.
Solids only: *Intermittent:* lower esophageal (Schatski) ring; *progressive:* peptic stricture (with heartburn), carcinoma (no heartburn).
Solids and liquids: *Intermittent:* diffuse esophageal spasm (with chest pain); *progressive:*scleroderma (with heartburn), achalasia (no heartburn).

ESOPHAGEAL MOTOR DISORDERS

Patients with esophageal motility disturbances may have a spectrum of manometric findings ranging from nonspecific abnormalities to defined clinical entities.

ACHALASIA (1) Inadequate relaxation of lower esophageal sphincter (LES); (2) loss of peristalsis in smooth-muscle portion of esophageal body.
Causes: Primary or secondary: Chagas' disease, lymphoma, carcinoma, chronic idiopathic intestinal pseudo-obstruction, ischemia, neurotropic viruses, drugs, toxins, radiation, postvagotomy.
Diagnosis: CXR: absence of gastric air bubble; barium swallow: dilated esophagus with distal narrowing and air-fluid level; endoscopy: exclude tumor; manometry: decreased LES relaxation ± absent peristalsis.
Treatment: Trial of calcium antagonists; pneumatic (forceful) balloon dilatation; Heller's extramucosal myotomy of LES.

DIFFUSE ESOPHAGEAL SPASM Multiple spontaneous and swallow-induced contractions of the esophageal body that are of simultaneous onset, high amplitude, long duration, and repetitive occurrence.

Causes: Primary or secondary: reflux esophagitis, emotional stress, diabetes, alcoholism, neuropathy, radiation, ischemia, collagen-vascular disease, aging (presbyesophagus).

Diagnosis: Barium swallow: corkscrew esophagus, pseudodiverticula; manometry: contractions in esophageal body that are of simultaneous onset, high amplitude, long duration, and repetitive occurrence; possible provocation with edrophonium, ergonovine, bethanecol, etc. (first exclude CAD).

Treatment: Trials of anticholinergics, nitrates, Ca antagonists; longitudinal myotomy.

NUTCRACKER ESOPHAGUS High-amplitude peristaltic contractions; may be associated with pain or dysphagia.

SCLERODERMA (1) Aperistalsis due to atrophy of esophageal smooth muscle ± fibrosis; (2) incompetent LES leading to reflux esophagitis, stricture.

GASTROESOPHAGEAL REFLUX

PATHOPHYSIOLOGY **Reflux episode:** (1) Increased gastric volume (after meal, gastric stasis, acid hypersecretion); (2) contents near gastroesophageal junction (bending, recumbency); (3) increased gastric pressure (obesity, tight clothes, pregnancy, ascites); (4) loss of LES-gastric pressure gradient: LES pressure decreased by smoking, anticholinergics, Ca antagonists, pregnancy, scleroderma; role of hiatal hernia unclear.

Heartburn: Occurrence may depend on amount refluxed and frequency; esophageal clearance by gravity and peristalsis; neutralization by salivary secretion.

Esophagitis: Results when refluxed acid (or bile) overwhelms mucosal defenses.

CLINICAL FEATURES Heartburn, dysphagia due to stricture, aspiration; complications: esophageal ulcer, bleeding, Barrett's esophagus (replacement of squamous with columnar epithelium, premalignant), adenocarcinoma.

DIAGNOSIS History often suffices; further testing in atypical or refractory cases.

- Barium swallow: frequent false-negatives for reflux or esophagitis; detects strictures.
- Endoscopy: detects esophagitis, Barrett's esophagus.
- Bernstein test: reproduction of symptoms with 0.1 *N* HCl but not normal saline infused by tube into esophagus.
- ^{99m}Tc sulfur colloid scintiscan: to document and quantitate reflux.
- Esophageal luminal pH recording (24-h or nocturnal): possibly most sensitive test for reflux.

TREATMENT General: weight reduction; sleeping with elevated head of bed; avoidance of smoking, large meals, caffeine, alcohol, chocolate, fatty foods, citrus juices.
Medical therapy: Antacids, H-2-receptor blockers, or sucralfate (doses as for peptic ulcer; Chap. 96); in unresponsive cases add agent to increase LES pressure and enhance gastric emptying—metoclopramide 10–20 mg PO ac + hs (side effects: tremor, spasms, parkinsonism, elevated prolactin) or bethanecol 25 mg PO ac + hs (side effects: dry mouth, urinary retention; avoid in glaucoma, prostatism). Dilate strictures. *Surgical therapy* in severe and refractory cases.

OTHER FORMS OF ESOPHAGITIS

HERPES ESOPHAGITIS In immunocompromised hosts (e.g., AIDS); may present with odynophagia, dysphagia, fever, bleeding; diagnosis by endoscopy with biopsy, brush cytology, culture; treatment—often self-limited; viscous Xylocaine for pain; acyclovir in prolonged cases.

***CANDIDA* ESOPHAGITIS** In immunocompromised hosts (e.g., AIDS), malignancy, diabetes, hypoparathyroidism, hemoglobinopathy, SLE, corrosive esophageal injury; may present with odynophagia, dysphagia, oral thrush (in 50%); diagnosis by barium swallow (large filling defects), endoscopy with brushings (KOH stain), biopsy, culture; treatment—oral nystatin (100,000 U/mL) 5 mL q 4 h; if necessary, miconazole, ketoconazole, or amphotericin B (500 mg total).

PILL-RELATED ESOPHAGITIS Doxycycline, tetracycline, aspirin, NSAIDs, KCl, quinidine, ferrous sulfate.

ESOPHAGEAL CANCER (see Chap. 99)

For more detailed discussion of this topic, see Goyal RK: Dysphagia, Chap. 32, and Diseases of the Esophagus, Chap. 234, in HPIM-11, pp. 169 and 1231

96 PEPTIC ULCER DISEASE, GASTRITIS, AND ZOLLINGER-ELLISON SYNDROME

PEPTIC ULCER DISEASE

Most commonly in duodenal bulb (DU) and stomach (GU). May also occur in esophagus, pyloric channel, duodenal loop, jejunum, Meckel's diverticulum. Results from imbalance between "aggressive" factors (gastric acid, pepsin) and "defensive" factors involved in mucosal resistance (gastric mucus, bicarbonate, microcirculation, prostaglandins, mucosal "barrier").

RISK FACTORS AND ASSOCIATIONS **General:** Heredity, smoking, gastrinoma (Zollinger-Ellison syndrome), hypercalcemia, mastocytosis, gastric campylobacter (*C. pylori*). (*Unproven:* Stress, coffee, alcohol.)
DU: Corticosteroids, chronic renal failure, renal transplantation, cirrhosis, chronic lung disease.
GU: Gastritis, salicylates, NSAIDs, achlorhydria.

CLINICAL FEATURES **DU:** Burning epigastric pain 90 min to 3 h after meals, often nocturnal, relieved by food.
GU: Burning epigastric pain made worse or unrelated to food; anorexia, food aversion, weight loss (in 40%). Great individual variation. Similar symptoms may occur in persons without demonstrated peptic ulcers (nonulcer or ulcer-like dyspepsia); less responsive to standard therapy.

COMPLICATIONS Bleeding, obstruction, penetration causing acute pancreatitis, perforation, intractability.

DIAGNOSIS **DU:** Upper endoscopy or upper GI barium radiography.
GU: Upper endoscopy often preferable to exclude possibility that ulcer is malignant (brush cytology, ≥6 pinch biopsies of ulcer margin). Radiographic features suggesting malignancy: ulcer within a mass, folds that do not radiate from ulcer margin, a large ulcer (>2.5–3 cm); however, 1% of radiographically benign-appearing ulcers prove to be malignant.

TREATMENT **Medical:** Dietary restriction unnecessary with contemporary drugs; smoking prevents healing and should be stopped. Available drugs (in U.S.A.) equally effective (80–90% healing of DUs and 60% healing of GUs in 6 weeks; larger ulcers heal more slowly) (see Table 96-1).

Maintenance therapy: After healing (cimetidine 300 mg hs, ranitidine 150 mg hs, famotidine 20 mg hs, sucralfate 1 g bid) lowers 1-year relapse rate from 60–70% to 20%; reserved for patients with frequent recurrences.
Surgery: For complications (persistent or recurrent bleeding, obstruction, perforation) or intractability (check serum gastrin to exclude gastrinoma). For *DU* see Table 96-2. For *GU* perform

TABLE 96-1

Drug	Mechanism	Dose	Side effects
Antacids	Acid neutralization	140 meq 1 h + 3 h pc + hs (e.g., 30 mL Maalox); lower doses appear to be as effective	Diarrhea (Mg), constipation (Al), osteomalacia, milk-alkali syndrome
Cimetidine	H-2-receptor blockade	300 mg qid or 400 mg bid or 800 mg hs	Antiandrogen, confusion, ↑ creatinine, ↓ hepatic drug metabolism, ↑ serum aminotransferase levels, rare hematologic
Ranitidine	H-2-receptor blockade	150 mg bid or 300 mg hs	As for cimetidine but antiandrogen, mental status and drug metabolism effects are less frequent
Famotidine	H-2-receptor blockade	40 mg hs	Probably as for ranitidine
Sucralfate	Ulcer coating, pepsin binding	1 g 1 h ac + hs or 2 g bid	Constipation, binding to coadministered drugs

subtotal gastrectomy.

Complications of surgery: (1) Obstructed afferent loop (Billroth II), (2) bile reflux gastritis, (3) dumping syndrome (rapid gastric emptying + postprandial vasomotor symptoms), (4) postvagotomy diarrhea, (5) bezoar, (6) anemia (iron, B_{12}, folate malabsorption), (7) malabsorption (poor mixing of gastric contents, pancreatic juices, bile; bacterial overgrowth), (8) osteomalacia and osteoporosis (vitamin D and Ca malabsorption), (9) gastric remnant carcinoma.

GASTRITIS

EROSIVE GASTRITIS (Hemorrhagic gastritis, multiple gastric erosions) Caused by aspirin, NSAIDs, alcohol, severe stress (burns, sepsis, trauma, surgery, shock, or respiratory, renal, or liver failure). May be asymptomatic or associated with epigastric discomfort,

TABLE 96-2

Operation	Recurrence rate	Complication rate
Vagotomy + antrectomy (Billroth I or II)*	1%	Highest
Vagotomy and pyloroplasty	10%	Intermediate
Parietal cell (proximal gastric, superselective) vagotomy	10%	Lowest

Billroth I = gastroduodenostomy; Billroth II = gastrojejunostomy.

nausea, hematemesis, or melena. Diagnosis by upper endoscopy. Treatment/prevention by removing offending agent and liquid antacids ± H-2-receptor antagonist to maintain gastric pH ≥ 4.

NONEROSIVE GASTRITIS **Fundal gland gastritis:** Three patterns: superficial gastritis, atrophic gastritis, gastric atrophy. Generally asymptomatic, common in elderly; atrophic types may be associated with achlorhydria, pernicious anemia, and increased risk of gastric cancer (value of screening endoscopy uncertain).
Pyloric gland gastritis: May result from regurgitation of duodenal contents. Generally asymptomatic, but may be associated with gastric ulcers.

SPECIFIC TYPES OF GASTRITIS Ménétrier's disease (hypertrophic gastropathy), eosinophilic gastritis, granulomatous gastritis, Crohn's disease, sarcoidosis, infections (TBC, syphilis, fungi, viruses, parasites), pseudolymphoma, radiation, corrosive gastritis.

ZOLLINGER-ELLISON (Z-E) SYNDROME (GASTRINOMA)

Consider when ulcer disease is severe, refractory to therapy, associated with ulcers in atypical locations, or associated with diarrhea. Tumors usually pancreatic, often multiple, slowly growing; > 60% malignant; 20–25% associated with multiple endocrine neoplasia type I.

DIAGNOSIS **Suggestive:** Basal acid output > 15 meq/h; basal/maximal acid output > 60%; upper GI radiograph: large mucosal folds.
Confirmatory: serum gastrin > 1000 pg/mL or rise in gastrin of 200 pg/mL following IV secretin (see Table 96-3).

DIFFERENTIAL DIAGNOSIS **Increased gastric acid secretion:** Z-E syndrome, antral G-cell hyperplasia, postgastrectomy retained antrum, renal failure, massive small bowel resection, chronic gastric outlet obstruction.
Normal or decreased gastric acid secretion: Pernicious anemia, chronic gastritis, gastric cancer, vagotomy, pheochromocytoma.

TREATMENT High-dose H-2-receptor antagonist ± anticholinergic agent; exploratory laparotomy with resection of primary

TABLE 96-3

Condition	Fasting gastrin	Gastrin response to	
		IV Secretin	Food
DU	N* (≤150 pg/mL)	NC†	Slight ↑
ZE	↑ ↑ ↑	↑ ↑ ↑	NC
Antral G (gastrin) cell hyperplasia	↑	↑, NC	↑ ↑ ↑

* N = normal.
† NC = no change.

tumor and solitary metastases when possible; chemotherapy for metastatic tumor.

For more detailed discussion of this topic, see McGuigan JE: Peptic Ulcer, Chap. 235, p. 1239; and MacDonald WC, and Rubin CE: Gastric Tumors, Gastritis, and Other Gastric Disorders, Chap. 236, p. 1253 in HPIM-11

---

97 PANCREATITIS

ACUTE PANCREATITIS

Differentiation between acute and chronic is based on clinical criteria. In acute pancreatitis there is restoration of normal pancreatic function; in the chronic form there is permanent loss of function and pain may predominate. There are three pathologic types of acute pancreatitis: edematous, hemorrhagic, and necrotizing.

ETIOLOGY Most common causes are alcohol and cholelithiasis. Others include abdominal trauma, peptic ulcer perforation, medications (e.g., azathioprine, estrogens, furosemide, thiazides, and sulfonamides), hyperlipidemia, hypercalcemia, hyperparathyroidism, pancreas divisum, viruses (mumps, Coxsackie), and idiopathic.

SYMPTOMS AND SIGNS Can vary from mild abdominal pain to shock.
Common symptoms: (1) Midepigastric pain radiating to the back; (2) nausea, vomiting; (3) low-grade fever.
Physical exam: (1) Low-grade fever, tachycardia, hypotension; (2) erythematous skin nodules due to subcutaneous fat necrosis; (3) basilar rales, pleural effusion (often on the left); (4) abdominal tenderness, diminished bowel sounds; (5) Cullen's sign—blue discoloration in the periumbilical area due to hemoperitoneum; (6) Turner's sign—blue-red-purple or green-brown discoloration of the flanks due to tissue catabolism of hemoglobin.

LABORATORY

1 *Serum amylase:* Large elevations (2–3 times normal) virtually ensure the diagnosis if salivary gland disease and intestinal perforation/infarction are excluded. However, normal serum amylase does *not* exclude the diagnosis of acute pancreatitis.

2 *Urinary amylase-creatinine clearance ratio* may be helpful in distinguishing between pancreatitis and other causes of hyperamylasemia (e.g., macroamylasemia), but it is invalid in the presence of renal failure. Simultaneous serum and urine amylase values are used: $C_{am}/C_{Cr} = (am_{urine} \times Cr_{serum})/(am_{serum} \times Cr_{urine})$. Normal value is less than 4%.

3 *Serum lipase* tends to parallel serum amylase and is more specific for pancreatic disease.

4 *Other tests: Hypocalcemia* occurs in approximately 25% of patients. *Leukocytosis* (15,000–20,000/mm^3) occurs frequently. *Hypertriglyceridemia* occurs in 15% of cases and can cause a spuriously normal serum amylase level.

IMAGING

1 *Abdominal radiographs* are abnormal in 50% of patients but are not specific for pancreatitis. Common findings include total or partial ileus ("sentinel loop") and spasm of transverse colon. Useful for excluding other diagnoses such as intestinal perforation.

2 *Ultrasound* often fails to visualize the pancreas because of overlying intestinal gas but may detect gallstones or edema or enlargement of the pancreas.

3 *CT* can confirm diagnosis of pancreatitis (edematous pancreas) and is useful for predicting and identifying late complications.

DIFFERENTIAL DIAGNOSIS Intestinal perforation, cholecystitis, acute intestinal obstruction, mesenteric ischemia, appendicitis, renal colic, myocardial ischemia, and aortic dissection.

TREATMENT Most cases subside over a period of 3–7 days. Conventional measures: (1) analgesics, such as meperidine; (2) intravenous fluids; (3) nasogastric suction; (4) treatment of hypocalcemia, if symptomatic; (5) antibiotics only if there is established infection; (6) cimetidine and/or antacids to prevent stress ulceration.

COMPLICATIONS **Early:** Shock, GI bleeding, common duct obstruction, ileus, splenic infarction or rupture, DIC, subcutaneous fat necrosis, ARDS, pleural effusion, hematuria, acute renal failure. **Late:** (1) *Pancreatic pseudocyst* in patients who develop recurrent pain within 7–10 days or fail to improve; can be detected by abdominal ultrasound or CT scan. Treatment is supportive; if there is no resolution within 6 weeks, consider surgical drainage or resection. (2) *Pancreatic abscess* (signaled by fever, pain after 2–3 weeks) is most often due to *E. coli.* Treatment consists of antibiotic therapy and surgical drainage.

CHRONIC PANCREATITIS

Chronic pancreatitis may occur as recurrent episodes of acute inflammation superimposed on a damaged pancreas or as chronic damage with pain and malabsorption.

ETIOLOGY Chronic alcoholism most frequent; also hypertriglyceridemia, hypercalcemia, hereditary pancreatitis, hemochromatosis, and cystic fibrosis.

SYMPTOMS AND SIGNS *Pain* is cardinal symptom. Weight loss, steatorrhea, and other signs and symptoms of malabsorption common. Physical examination often unremarkable.

LABORATORY No specific laboratory test available. Serum amylase and lipase levels are often normal. Steatorrhea late in the course. The bentiromide test, a simple, effective test of pancreatic exocrine function, may be helpful. Impaired glucose tolerance is present in over 50% of patients.

IMAGING (1) *Plain films of the abdomen* reveal pancreatic calcifications in 30–60%. (2) *Ultrasound* and *CT scans* may show pseudocysts or dilation of the pancreatic duct. (3) *Endoscopic retrograde cholangiopancreatography* often reveals irregular dilation of the main pancreatic duct and pruning of the branches.

DIFFERENTIAL DIAGNOSIS Important to distinguish from pancreatic carcinoma; may require radiographically guided biopsy.

TREATMENT Aimed at controlling pain and malabsorption. Narcotic use with subsequent addiction is common. Malabsorption is managed with a low-fat diet and pancreatic enzyme replacement (e.g., Viokase or its equivalent). Because pancreatic enzymes are inactivated by acid, bicarbonate or H-2-receptor antagonists (e.g., cimetidine) may improve their efficacy. Insulin may be necessary to control serum glucose. Alcohol must be avoided. Surgery may control pain if there is a ductal stricture. Subtotal pancreatectomy also may control pain but at the cost of exocrine insufficiency and diabetes.

For more detailed discussion of this topic, see Greenberger NJ, Toskes PP: Approach to the Patient with Pancreatic Disease, Chap. 254, p. 1368, and Greenberger NJ, Toskes PP, Isselbacher KJ: Diseases of the Pancreas, Chap. 255, p. 1372, in HPIM-11

Chronic inflammatory disorders of unknown etiology involving the GI tract.

ULCERATIVE COLITIS (UC)

Pathology: Colonic *mucosal* inflammation, crypt abscesses, ulcers; continuous involvement (no skip areas); rectum almost always involved.
Clinical manifestations: Bloody diarrhea, mucus, fever, abdominal pain, tenesmus, weight loss; spectrum of severity (majority of cases are mild, limited to rectosigmoid).
Complications: Toxic megacolon, colonic perforation, cancer–risk related to extent and duration of colitis; preceded by dysplasia (precancer), which may be detected on surveillance colonoscopic biopsies.
Diagnosis: Sigmoidoscopy/colonoscopy: mucosal erythema, granularity, friability, exudate, hemorrhage, ulcers, pseudopolyps (regenerating mucosa). Barium enema: loss of haustrations, mucosal irregularity, ulcerations.

CROHN'S DISEASE (CD)

Pathology: Any part of GI tract, usually terminal ileum and/or colon; *transmural* inflammation, bowel wall thickening, linear ulcerations leading to cobblestone pattern; discontinuous involvement (skip areas); granulomas, fissures, fistulas.
Clinical manifestations: Fever, abdominal pain, diarrhea (often without blood), fatigue, weight loss, growth retardation in children; acute ileitis mimicking appendicitis; anorectal fissures, fistulas, abscesses.
Complications: Intestinal obstruction (edema vs. fibrosis); rarely toxic megacolon or perforation; intestinal fistulas to bowel, bladder, vagina, skin, soft tissue; bile salt malabsorption leading to cholesterol gallstones and/or oxalate kidney stones; intestinal malignancy.
Diagnosis: Sigmoidoscopy/colonoscopy, barium enema, upper GI and small bowel series: nodularity, rigidity, ulcers that may be deep or longitudinal, cobblestoning, skip areas, strictures, fistulas.

DIFFERENTIAL DIAGNOSIS

Infectious enterocolitis: *Shigella, Salmonella, Campylobacter, Yersinia, Gonorrhea, Lymphogranuloma venereum, Clostridium difficile.*
Others: Ischemic bowel disease, diverticulitis, radiation enterocolitis, bleeding colonic lesion (e.g., neoplasm), irritable bowel syndrome (no bleeding).

EXTRAINTESTINAL MANIFESTATIONS (UC AND CD)

1 *Joint:* Peripheral arthritis—parallels activity of bowel disease; ankylosing spondylitis and sacroiliitis (associated with HLA-B27)—activity independent of bowel disease.

2 *Skin:* Erythema nodosum, aphthous ulcers, pyoderma gangrenosum.

3 *Eye:* Episcleritis, iritis, uveitis.

4 *Liver:* Pericholangitis, sclerosing cholangitis, cholangiocarcinoma, chronic hepatitis.

5 *Others:* Autoimmune hemolytic anemia, phlebitis, pulmonary embolus.

TREATMENT

Supportive: Antidiarrheal agents in mild disease; hydration and blood transfusions in severe disease; parenteral nutrition (effective as primary therapy in CD, although high relapse rate when oral feeding is resumed; should not replace drug therapy; important role in preoperative preparation).

Sulfasalazine: Active component 5-aminosalicylic acid (5-ASA) linked to sulfapyridine carrier; useful in colonic disease of mild to moderate severity (1–1.5 g PO qid); maintenance of remission in UC (500 mg PO qid). Toxicity (generally due to sulfapyridine component): dose-related—nausea, headache, rarely hemolytic anemia; idiosyncratic—fever, rash, neutropenia, pancreatitis, hepatitis, etc.; miscellaneous—oligospermia. New alternative drugs: 5-ASA linked to other carriers, in slow release form, or as enema.

Corticosteroids: Useful in severe disease and ileal or ileocolonic CD. Prednisone 40–60 mg PO qd, then taper; IV hydrocortisone 100 mg tid or equivalent in hospitalized patients; IV ACTH drip (120 U per day) may be preferable in first attacks of UC. Nightly retention enemas in proctosigmoiditis.

Immunosuppressive agents: (Azathioprine, 6-mercaptopurine 50 mg PO qd.) Useful as steroid-sparing agents and in intractable CD (may require 4- to 8-month trial period). Toxicity—immunosuppression, pancreatitis, ? carcinogenicity.

Metronidazole: Appears effective in colonic CD (500 mg PO bid) and refractory perineal CD (up to 20 mg/kg PO qd). Toxicity—peripheral neuropathy, metallic taste, ? carcinogenicity.

Surgery: *UC:* Colectomy (curative) for intractability, toxic megacolon, cancer, severe dysplasia. *CD:* Resection for fixed obstruction (or stricturoplasty), abscesses, persistent symptomatic fistulas, intractability.

For more detailed discussion of this topic, see Glickman RM: Inflammatory Bowel Disease, Chap. 238, in HPIM-11, p. 1277

99 TUMORS OF THE INTESTINAL TRACT

ESOPHAGEAL CARCINOMA

Fifth most common cancer in men; less frequent in women. Highest incidence in focal regions of China, Iran, Soviet Union. In U.S. blacks more frequently affected than whites; 5-year survival <5%.

Pathology: 90% squamous cell carcinoma, most commonly in upper two-thirds; <10% adenocarcinoma, usually in distal third, arising in region of columnar metaplasia (Barrett's esophagus), glandular tissue, or as direct extension of proximal gastric adenocarcinoma; lymphoma and melanoma rare.

Etiology and risk factors: Cause unknown; major risk factors for squamous cell carcinoma: ethanol abuse, smoking (combination is synergistic); other risks: lye ingestion and esophageal stricture, radiation exposure, head and neck cancer, achalasia, Plummer-Vinson syndrome, tylosis.

Clinical features: Progressive dysphagia (first with solids, then liquids), rapid weight loss common, chest pain (from mediastinal spread), pulmonary aspiration (obstruction, tracheoesophageal fistula), hoarseness (laryngeal nerve palsy), hypercalcemia; bleeding infrequent, occasionally severe; examination often unremarkable.

Diagnosis: Double-contrast barium swallow useful for screening; flexible esophagogastroscopy most sensitive and specific test; pathologic confirmation by endoscopic biopsy and cytologic examination of mucosal brushings.

Therapy: *Squamous cell carcinoma:* Surgical resection after chemotherapy (5-fluorouracil, cisplatin) prolongs survival and provides greatest chance of cure. *Adenocarcinoma:* Curative resection rarely possible; palliative measures include laser ablation, mechanical dilatation, radiotherapy, and bypass surgery.

GASTRIC CARCINOMA

Common worldwide, although incidence decreasing in U.S. Male:female = 2:1; peak incidence sixth and seventh decades; overall 5-year survival less than 15%.

Etiology and risk factors: Cause unknown; several dietary factors correlated with increased incidence: nitrates, smoked foods, heavily salted foods; genetic component suggested by increased incidence in first-degree relatives of affected patients; other risk factors: atrophic gastritis, Billroth II gastrectomy, adenomatous gastric polyps, pernicious anemia, hyperplastic gastric polyps (latter two associated with atrophic gastritis).

Pathology: Adenocarcinoma is greater than 90%; usually focal (polypoid, ulcerative), less commonly diffusely infiltrative (linitis plastica) or superficial spreading; spreads primarily to local nodes, liver, peritoneum; systemic spread uncommon; lymphoma accounts for 5% and leiomyosarcoma less than 3% of gastric malignancies.

Clinical features: Most commonly presents with progressive upper abdominal discomfort, frequently with weight loss, anorexia, nausea; acute or chronic GI bleeding (mucosal ulceration) common; dysphagia (location in cardia); vomiting (pyloric and widespread disease); examination often unrevealing early in course; later, abdominal tenderness, pallor, and cachexia most common signs; palpable mass uncommon; metastatic spread may be manifest by hepatomegaly, ascites, left supraclavicular or scalene adenopathy, periumbilical, ovarian, or prerectal mass (Blummer's shelf), low-grade fever, skin abnormalities (nodules, dermatomyositis, acanthosis nigricans, or multiple seborrheic keratoses); laboratory findings: iron deficiency anemia in two-thirds of patients; fecal occult blood in 80%; rarely associated with pancytopenia (from marrow replacement) or leukemoid reaction.
Diagnosis: Double-contrast barium swallow useful for screening; gastroscopy most sensitive and specific test; pathologic confirmation by biopsy and cytologic examination of mucosal brushings; important to differentiate benign from malignant gastric ulcers with multiple biopsies and follow-up examinations to demonstrate ulcer healing.
Treatment: Gastrectomy offers only chance of cure; in absence of obvious metastatic spread, CT may aid in determining tumor resectability. Palliative therapy for pain, obstruction, and bleeding includes surgery, endoscopic dilatation, radiation, chemotherapy; unresectable gastric lymphoma treated with radiation and chemotherapy, with occasional long-term survival.

BENIGN GASTRIC TUMORS

Much less common than malignant gastric tumors; hyperplastic polyps most common, with adenomas, hamartomas, and leiomyomas rare; 30% of adenomas and occasional hyperplastic polyps are associated with gastric malignancy; polyposis syndromes include Peutz-Jeghers and familial polyposis (hamartomas and adenomas), Gardner's (adenomas), and Cronkhite-Canada (cystic) (see Colonic Polyps below).
Clinical features: Usually asymptomatic; occasionally present with bleeding or vague epigastric discomfort.
Treatment: Endoscopic or surgical excision.

SMALL BOWEL TUMORS

Clinical features: Uncommon tumors; usually present with bleeding, abdominal pain, weight loss, or intestinal obstruction; increased incidence in patients with gluten-sensitive enteropathy, small bowel Crohn's disease.
Pathology: Usually benign; adenomas, leiomyomas, and lipomas most common; most prevalent malignant tumors are adenocarcinoma, usually in duodenum (at or near ampulla of Vater) or jejunum; leiomyosarcomas frequently large at diagnosis; lymphomas occur as focal mass or diffuse infiltration (Mediterranean type), can present as intestinal malabsorption; carcinoid tumors

rare, usually asymptomatic; carcinoid syndrome limited to patients with metastatic spread to liver.

Diagnosis: Barium x-ray examination best diagnostic test; direct small bowel instillation of contrast (enteroclysis) occasionally reveals tumors not seen with routine small bowel radiography; laparotomy often required for diagnosis.

Treatment: Surgical excision.

COLONIC POLYPS

TUBULAR ADENOMAS Present in 2 to 15% of adults; pedunculated or sessile; usually asymptomatic; may cause bleeding or, rarely, obstruction; risk of malignant degeneration correlates with size; 65% found in rectosigmoid colon; diagnosis by barium enema or colonoscopy. *Treatment:* Endoscopic resection (surgery if polyp large or inaccessible by colonoscopy); follow-up surveillance by colonoscopy every 2–3 years.

VILLOUS ADENOMAS Generally larger than tubular adenomas at diagnosis; often sessile; high risk of malignancy (up to 50% when greater than 2 cm); more prevalent in left colon; may be associated with potassium-rich secretory diarrhea. *Treatment:* As for tubular adenomas.

HYPERPLASTIC POLYPS Asymptomatic; usually incidental finding at colonoscopy; rarely greater than 5 mm; no malignant potential. *No treatment* required.

HEREDITARY POLYPOSIS SYNDROMES

1 *Familial polyposis coli (FPC):* Diffuse pancolonic adenomatous polyposis (up to several thousand polyps); autosomal dominant inheritance; colon carcinoma from malignant degeneration of polyp in 100% by age 40. *Treatment:* Prophylactic colectomy before age 30.

2 *Gardner's syndrome:* Variant of FPC with associated soft tissue tumors (sebaceous cysts, osteomas, lipomas, desmoids), gastroduodenal polyps, ampullary adenocarcinoma. Potential for malignant degeneration mandates prophylactic colectomy.

3 *Juvenile polyposis:* Multiple colonic and small bowel hamartomas; frequently bleed; other symptoms: abdominal pain, diarrhea; occasional intussusception; rarely recur after excision; diffuse polyposis associated with increased incidence of colon cancer from malignant degeneration of interspersed *adenomatous* polyps. Prophylactic colectomy controversial.

4 *Peutz-Jehgers syndrome:* Numerous hamartomatous polyps of entire GI tract; polyps more prevalent in small bowel than colon; GI bleeding common; increased risk for the development of cancer at gastrointestinal and non-gastrointestinal sites. Prophylactic surgery not recommended.

COLON CANCER

Second most common internal cancer in humans; accounts for 20% of cancer-related deaths in U.S., incidence increases above age 40, equal in men and women.

Etiology and risk factors: Cause unknown; dietary factors (low fiber, high animal fat) suggested by increased prevalence in developed countries; risk increased in first-degree relatives of patients, families with increased prevalence of cancer, and pts with history of breast or gynecologic cancer, familial polyposis syndromes, ulcerative colitis, Crohn's colitis, asbestosis.

Pathology: Nearly always adenocarcinoma; 75% located distal to the splenic flexure; may be polypoid, sessile, fungating, or constricting; subtype and degree of differentiation do not correlate with course; degree of invasiveness at surgery (Dukes' classification) single best predictor of prognosis: >90% 5-year survival for cancer confined to mucosa and submucosa (class A); 60–75% with extension to serosa; 30–40% with regional lymph node involvement; 5% for metastatic cancer (liver, bone, lung); rectosigmoid tumors may spread to lungs early because of systemic venous drainage of this area.

Clinical features: Left-sided colon cancers present most commonly with rectal bleeding, altered bowel habits (narrowing, constipation, intermittent diarrhea, tenesmus), and abdominal or back pain; cecal and ascending colon cancers more frequently present with symptoms of anemia, occult blood in stool, or weight loss; other complications: perforation, fistula, volvulus, inguinal hernia; laboratory findings: anemia in 50% of right-sided lesions; determination of serum carcinoembryonic antigen (CEA) useful to follow therapy and assess recurrence.

Diagnosis: Early diagnosis aided by screening asymptomatic persons with fecal occult blood testing (see below); more than half of all colon cancers are within reach of a 60-cm flexible sigmoidoscope; air-contrast barium enema will diagnose approximately 80% of colon cancers not within reach of sigmoidoscope; colonoscopy most sensitive and specific, but incurs somewhat greater expense.

Treatment: Surgical resection of colonic segment containing tumor; resection of isolated hepatic metastases possible in selected cases; intrahepatic arterial fluorodeoxyuridine (FUDR) for diffuse hepatic spread (marginally prolongs survival); radiotherapy and systemic chemotherapy for palliation of metastatic disease.

Prevention: Early detection of colon carcinoma may be facilitated by routine screening of stool for occult blood (Hemoccult II, ColoTest, etc.); false positives: ingestion of red meat, iron, aspirin; upper GI bleeding; false negatives: vitamin C ingestion, intermittent bleeding; annual testing recommended for patients over age 40–50; *screening* flexible sigmoidoscopy recommended every 3 years; careful evaluation of patients with positive fecal occult blood tests (flexible sigmoidoscopy *and* air-contrast barium enema or colonoscopy) reveals polyps in 20–40% and carcinoma in approximately 5%; screening of asymptomatic persons allows earlier detection of colon cancer (i.e., earlier Dukes' stage), greater resectability rate; however, routine fecal occult blood testing not yet shown to affect overall mortality.

For more detailed discussion of these topics, see Goyal RK: Diseases of the Esophagus, Chap. 234, p. 1231; MacDonald WC, Rubin CE: Gastric Tumors, Gastritis, and Other Gastric Diseases, Chap. 236, p. 1253; and LaMont JT, Isselbacher KJ: Diseases of the Small and Large Intestine, Chap. 239, p. 1290, in HPIM-11

IRRITABLE BOWEL SYNDROME

Three variants: (1) spastic colon (chronic abdominal pain and constipation), (2) alternating constipation and diarrhea, and (3) chronic, painless diarrhea.

Pathophysiology: Alteration in colonic motility (increased resting colonic motility in spastic colon; decreased motility in diarrhea); motility increases in response to stress, cholinergic drugs, cholecystokinin; psychologic disturbances in some patients—depression, hysteria, obsessive-compulsive traits; specific food intolerances in a few cases.

Clinical manifestations: Onset often before age 30; females:males = 2:1; pasty stools, ribbony or pencil-thin stools, mucus in stools (no blood), heartburn, bloating, back pain, weakness, faintness, palpitations, urinary frequency.

Diagnosis: Often by history; consider sigmoidoscopy and barium radiographs to exclude inflammatory bowel disease or malignancy; consider excluding giardiasis, intestinal lactase deficiency, hyperthyroidism.

Treatment: Reassurance, avoidance of stress or precipitating factors, dietary bulk (fiber, psyllium extract, e.g., Metamucil 1 tbsp bid-tid); occasional trials of loperamide, diphenoxylate (Lomotil), cholestyramine, anticholinergics.

DIVERTICULAR DISEASE

Herniations or saclike protrusions of the mucosa through the muscularis at points of nutrient artery penetration; possibly due to increased intraluminal pressure, low-fiber diet; most common in sigmoid colon.

Clinical presentations and treatment:

1 *Asymptomatic*

2 *Pain:* Recurrent left lower quadrant pain relieved by defecation; alternating constipation and diarrhea. Diagnosis by barium enema. *Treatment:* high-fiber diet, psyllium extract, anticholinergics.

3 *Diverticulitis:* Pain, fever, altered bowel habits, tender colon, leukocytosis. *Treatment:* nothing by mouth, IV fluids, antibiotics (e.g., IV cefoxitin), surgical resection in refractory or frequently recurrent cases. *Complications:* pericolic abscess, perforation, fistula (to bladder, vagina, skin, soft tissue), liver abscess, stricture.

4 *Hemorrhage:* Usually in absence of diverticulitis, often from ascending colon and self-limited. If persistent, manage with mesenteric arteriography and intraarterial infusion of vasopressin or surgery.

INTESTINAL PSEUDO-OBSTRUCTION

Recurrent attacks of nausea, vomiting, and abdominal pain and distention mimicking mechanical obstruction; may be complicated by steatorrhea due to bacterial overgrowth.

Causes: *Primary:* Familial visceral neuropathy, familial visceral myopathy, idiopathic. *Secondary:* Scleroderma, amyloidosis, diabetes, celiac disease, parkinsonism, muscular dystrophy, drugs, electrolyte imbalance, postsurgical.
Treatment: Acute attacks—intestinal decompression with long tube. Oral antibiotics for bacterial overgrowth. Avoid surgery. In refractory cases, consider long-term parenteral hyperalimentation.

VASCULAR DISORDERS (SMALL AND LARGE INTESTINES)

MECHANISMS OF MESENTERIC ISCHEMIA (1) *Occlusive:* arterial thrombus (atherosclerosis); embolus (atrial fibrillation, valvular heart disease); venous thrombosis (trauma, neoplasm, infection, cirrhosis, oral contraceptives, antithrombin-III deficiency); vasculitis (SLE, polyarteritis, rheumatoid arthritis); (2) *nonocclusive:* hypotension, heart failure, arrhythmia.

ACUTE MESENTERIC ISCHEMIA Periumbilical pain out of proportion to tenderness, nausea, vomiting, distention, GI bleeding, altered bowel habits. Abdominal x-ray shows bowel distention, air-fluid levels, thumbprinting (submucosal edema). Peritoneal signs indicate infarcted bowel requiring surgical resection. In suspected arterial embolus, consider early celiac and mesenteric arteriography and embolectomy.

CHRONIC MESENTERIC INSUFFICIENCY "Abdominal angina"—dull, crampy periumbilical pain 15–30 min after a meal for several hours; weight loss. Evaluate with arteriography for possible bypass graft surgery.

ISCHEMIC COLITIS Usually due to nonocclusive disease in patient with atherosclerosis. Severe lower abdominal pain, rectal bleeding, hypotension. Abdominal x-ray shows colonic dilatation, thumbprinting. Sigmoidoscopy shows submucosal hemorrhage, friability, ulcerations. Conservative management (NPO, IV fluids); surgical resection for infarction or postischemic stricture.

COLONIC POLYPS AND COLON CANCER

(See Chap. 99)

ANORECTAL DISEASES

HEMORRHOIDS Due to increased hydrostatic pressure in hemorrhoidal venous plexus (straining at stool, pregnancy, portal hypertension). May be external, internal, thrombosed, acute (prolapsed or strangulated), or bleeding. Treat pain with bulk laxative and stool softeners (psyllium extract, dioctyl sodium sulfosuccinate 100–900 mg/day), sitz baths 1–4/day, witch hazel compresses, analgesics as needed. Bleeding may require rubber band ligation or injection sclerotherapy. Operative hemorrhoidectomy in severe or refractory cases.

ANAL FISSURES Medical therapy as for hemorrhoids. Internal anal sphincterotomy in refractory cases.

PRURITUS ANI Often of unclear cause; may be due to poor hygiene, fungal or parasitic infection. Treat with thorough cleansing after bowel movement, topical corticosteroid, antifungal agent if indicated.

For more detailed discussion of this topic, see LaMont JT; Isselbacher KJ: Diseases of the Small and Large Intestine, Chap. 239, in HPIM-11, p. 1290

---

101 CHOLELITHIASIS, CHOLECYSTITIS, AND CHOLANGITIS

CHOLELITHIASIS

There are three major types of gallstones: cholesterol, pigment, and mixed stones. In the U.S. 80% of stones are cholesterol or mixed, 20% pigment.

Epidemiology: One million new cases of cholelithiasis per year in the U.S. Increased incidence in American Indians, and with obesity, diabetes, ileal disease, pregnancy, estrogen or oral contraceptive use, type IV hyperlipidemia, and cirrhosis. Females:males = 4:1.

Symptoms and signs: Many gallstones are "silent," i.e., formed in asymptomatic pts. Symptoms occur when stones produce inflammation or obstruction of the cystic or common bile ducts. Major symptoms: (1) biliary colic which is usually constant, RUQ or epigastric pain that occurs 30–90 min after meals, lasts for several hours, and occasionally radiates to the right scapula or back; and (2) nausea and vomiting. Physical examination may be normal or show epigastric or RUQ tenderness.

Laboratory: Occasionally, mild and transient elevations in bilirubin (<5 mg/dL) accompany biliary colic.

Imaging: Only 10% of gallstones are radiopaque. Ultrasonography is best diagnostic test. The oral cholecystogram (OCG) requires a functioning gallbladder and serum bilirubin <3 mg/dL.

Differential diagnosis: Includes peptic ulcer disease, gastroesophageal reflux, irritable bowel syndrome, and hepatitis.

Treatment: Since risk of developing complications requiring surgery is small in asymptomatic patients, elective cholecystectomy should be reserved for (1) symptomatic patients [i.e., biliary colic despite dietary restriction (low-fat diet)], (2) persons with previous complications of cholelithiasis (see below), and (3) asymptomatic patients with an increased risk of complications (diabetes, calcified or nonfunctioning gallbladder). Oral dissolution agents (chenodeoxycholic acid, ursodeoxycholic acid) partially or completely dissolve radiolucent stones in 50% of patients. However, they are ineffective in dissolving large, radiopaque or pigment stones, and recurrence is likely if the medication is stopped.

Complications: See Acute Cholecystitis below.

ACUTE CHOLECYSTITIS

Acute inflammation of the gallbladder usually caused by cystic duct obstruction by an impacted stone.

Etiology: 90% calculous; 10% acalculous; latter caused by prolonged acute illness, fasting, hyperalimentation leading to gallbladder stasis, vasculitis, carcinoma of gallbladder or common bile duct.

Symptoms and signs: (1) RUQ or epigastric pain, (2) nausea, vomiting, anorexia, and (3) fever. Examination typically reveals RUQ tenderness; palpable RUQ mass found in 20% of pts.

Laboratory: Mild leukocytosis; serum bilirubin, alkaline phosphatase, and SGOT may be mildly elevated.
Imaging: Ultrasonography is useful for demonstrating gallstones and occasionally a phlegmonous mass surrounding the gallbladder. Radioisotope scans (HIDA, DISIDA, etc.) may identify cystic duct obstruction.
Differential diagnosis: Includes acute pancreatitis, appendicitis, pyelonephritis, peptic ulcer disease, hepatitis, and hepatic abscess.
Treatment: Bowel rest, nasogastric suction, IV fluids, analgesics (meperidine), and antibiotics (ampicillin and gentamicin) are the mainstays of treatment. Surgery is definitive and should be performed within 24–48 h of admission.
Complications: Empyema, hydrops, perforation, fistulization.

CHRONIC CHOLECYSTITIS

Etiology: Chronic cholecystitis usually caused by gallstones.
Symptoms and signs: Often nonspecific; include dyspepsia, fatty food intolerance, and abdominal pain.
Laboratory: All tests are usually normal.
Imaging: Ultrasonography preferred; usually shows gallstones within a contracted gallbladder.
Differential diagnosis: Peptic ulcer disease, esophagitis, irritable bowel syndrome.
Treatment: Surgery is the treatment of choice if symptomatic.

CHOLEDOCHOLITHIASIS/CHOLANGITIS

Symptoms and signs: Choledocholithiasis may present as an incidental finding, biliary colic, obstructive jaundice, cholangitis, or pancreatitis. Cholangitis usually presents as fever, RUQ pain, and jaundice (Charcot's triad).
Laboratory: Elevations in serum bilirubin, alkaline phosphatase, and SGOT.
Imaging: Ultrasonography may reveal dilated bile ducts but is not sensitive for detecting common duct stones. Endoscopic retrograde cholangiopancreatography or transhepatic cholangiography will confirm diagnosis.
Differential diagnosis: Acute cholecystitis, renal colic, perforated viscus, pancreatitis.
Treatment: Surgery or endoscopic papillotomy with stone extraction are procedures of choice. Cholangitis treated like acute cholecystitis; bowel rest, hydration, and analgesia are the mainstays; stones should be removed surgically or endoscopically.
Complications: Cholangitis, obstructive jaundice, and gallstone-induced pancreatitis.

PRIMARY SCLEROSING CHOLANGITIS (PSC)

PSC is a sclerosing inflammatory process involving the biliary tree.
Etiology: Males outnumber females, and most patients are 25–45 years old. Associations: ulcerative colitis (60% of cases of PSC), rarely Crohn's disease and retroperitoneal fibrosis.

Symptoms and signs: Pruritus, RUQ pain, jaundice, fever, weight loss, and malaise. May progress to cirrhosis with portal hypertension.
Laboratory: Evidence of cholestasis (elevated bilirubin and alkaline phosphatase) common.
Radiology/endoscopy: Transhepatic or endoscopic cholangiograms reveal stenosis and dilation of the intrahepatic and extrahepatic bile ducts.
Differential diagnosis: Cholangiocarcinoma, Caroli's disease (cystic dilation of bile ducts). Fasciola hepatica (see HIPM-11, Chap. 167), echinococcosis, and ascariasis.
Treatment: No satisfactory therapy. Cholangitis should be treated as outlined above. Liver transplantation should be considered in patients with endstage cirrhosis (see Chap. 105).

For more detailed discussion of this topic, see McPhee MS, Greenberger NJ: Diseases of the Gallbladder and Bile Ducts, Chap. 253, in HPIM-11, p. 1358

---

102 TUMORS OF THE PANCREAS AND HEPATOBILIARY TREE

PANCREATIC CARCINOMA

Fourth most common cause of cancer death in the U.S., accounts for 10% of GI tumors; peak incidence in seventh decade; male:female = 1.5:1.

Etiology and risk factors: Cause unknown; incidence increased in smokers, diabetics, and pts with chronic calcific pancreatitis; relationship to coffee or caffeine ingestion not substantiated; may be associated with diet high in grilled meats.

Pathology: 65% in head, 35% in body and tail; almost always ductal adenocarcinoma; 85% already locally invasive or metastatic at time of initial diagnosis.

Clinical features: Weight loss, anorexia, abdominal pain, back pain, depression common; painless jaundice (with dark urine, clay-colored stools, occasional pruritus) frequent presenting feature of tumors in pancreatic head. Examination commonly reveals jaundice, hepatomegaly, abdominal mass, or abdominal tenderness, but may be unremarkable; enlarged, palpable gallbladder (Courvoisier's) in about 25%. Complications include portal vein thrombosis (leading to splenomegaly, gastric varices, GI bleeding) and duodenal invasion (causing GI bleeding, obstruction); occasionally, hyperglycemia due to new-onset diabetes and elevated amylase and lipase levels from associated pancreatitis.

Diagnosis: Ultrasound useful screening test; shows abnormalities in about 75% of pts; most sensitive for lesions over 2 cm in head and body; CT most accurate noninvasive test (80% sensitivity; frequently able to detect lesions in tail); cholangiography (endoscopic or transhepatic) most sensitive test for pts with carcinoma in pancreatic head. Pathologic confirmation by aspiration of biliary secretions during cholangiography or percutaneous needle biopsy of mass under sonographic or CT guidance; serum tumor markers (e.g., carcinoembryonic antigen) insensitive, still too nonspecific for population screening.

Treatment: Surgical resection by partial pancreatectomy or pancreaticoduodenectomy (Whipple procedure) potentially curative; however, tumor resectable in only 15% of pts and curable in less than 3%. Intraoperative irradiation may improve survival from unresectable local disease. Palliative relief of biliary obstruction provided by surgical bypass or endoscopic or transhepatic stent placement; stenting preferable in elderly pts with multiple medical problems and those with advanced disease and short life expectancy; benefit of combination chemotherapy in pts with inoperable disease unproven.

OTHER PANCREATIC TUMORS

ISLET CELL TUMORS Second most common class of pancreatic neoplasms; often suspected because of clinical effects of the hormones secreted (see HPIM-11, Chap. 329); "nonsecreting" islet cell tumors produce no discernible endocrine abnormalities. Most often in body and tail of pancreas, can grow to 10 cm or more before causing pain, palpable mass, weight loss, or splenomegaly (from splenic vein compression). Therapy includes surgical resection, pharmacologic inhibition of hormonal effects, and chemotherapy (streptozotocin, 5-fluorouracil) for unresectable tumor.

CYSTADENOCARCINOMA Rare, slow-growing, cystic neoplasms; symptoms caused by mass effect. Two pathologic forms: mucinous (malignant) and serous (benign); differentiation by CT and chemical analysis of cyst fluid. *Treatment*: surgical resection.

BENIGN PANCREATIC MASSES Pseudocysts complicating pancreatitis, true cysts (isolated or in association with polycystic kidney and liver disease; usually asymptomatic), and abscesses (which usually present with fever or signs of sepsis; see Chap. 97).

BILIARY TRACT CANCERS

Less common than pancreatic carcinoma; usually present with obstructive jaundice, pruritus, RUQ pain, weight loss.

CHOLANGIOCARCINOMA Adenocarcinoma of bile duct epithelium; highest incidence in fifth to seventh decades; male:female = 1.5:1. Predisposing factors: choledochal (biliary) cysts, primary sclerosing cholangitis, ulcerative colitis, chronic biliary parasitic infestation, but *not* gallstones. Usually presents with obstructive jaundice, occasionally with GI bleeding from hematobilia; usually unresectable at time of diagnosis. *Treatment:* similar to carcinoma of head of pancreas.

AMPULLARY CARCINOMA Tumor of papilla of Vater or ampullary involvement of duodenal adenocarcinoma. Usual presentation is obstructive jaundice and GI bleeding; stools occasionally silver (combination of acholic and melenic). Papillary tumors rare but slow-growing and commonly resectable (Whipple procedure); duodenal carcinoma less often resectable.

GALLBLADDER CARCINOMA Rare complication of chronic cholelithiasis; male:female = 1:4. May be found incidentally at laparotomy (usually cholecystectomy) or autopsy (1% prevalence). Advanced tumor usually presents in seventh to eighth decades with RUQ pain, mass, jaundice, and weight loss; preoperative diagnosis occasionally made by ultrasound or CT. *Treatment:* surgical resection or palliation; cure rate of advanced or symptomatic tumors less than 5%.

HEPATOCELLULAR CARCINOMA

Most common form of internal cancer worldwide; highest incidence in areas where hepatitis B virus infection endemic (esp. Southeast Asia, sub-Saharan Africa); far less common in U.S. (1–2% of malignant tumors). Peak incidence fifth and sixth decades in U.S., fourth and fifth in endemic areas; male:female = 2:1–4:1.

Etiology and risk factors: Strong correlation with chronic hepatitis B infection suggests causative role of this virus in majority of cases. Neonatal infection carries highest risk of subsequent carcinoma; other risk factors: cirrhosis, hemochromatosis, α_1-antitrypsin deficiency, tyrosinosis, ingested fungal metabolites (e.g., aflatoxin), use of anabolic steroids, administration of Thorotrast (radiologic contrast agent used in 1940s and 1950s).

Clinical features: In cirrhotic pts, often presents as decompensation of underlying liver disease; weight loss, RUQ pain (occasionally acute due to tumor hemorrhage or rupture); jaundice rare except in terminal stages. Examination commonly reveals tender hepatomegaly; palpable liver mass, ascites (often blood-tinged) present in about 25% at time of diagnosis. Laboratory studies: elevated alkaline phosphatase, often out of proportion to other liver tests; elevated serum α-fetoprotein (AFP; often > 400 ng/mL) in 80% of pts (fewer in U.S.). Other causes of elevated AFP include cirrhosis, acute or chronic hepatitis, liver metastases (all with mild elevations), normal pregnancy, malignant teratomas.

Diagnosis: CT, MRI most sensitive for detection of liver mass; radionuclide scanning (e.g., gallium, ethiotol) may suggest primary hepatocellular carcinoma; angiography often reveals typical vascularity of lesions and may detect small tumors. Pathologic confirmation by radiologically guided percutaneous liver biopsy, laparoscopy, or laparotomy.

Treatment: Curative resection possible in fewer than 5% of patients; liver transplantation may benefit selected patients with small tumors confined to the liver; radiation therapy for palliation of pain; systemic and intraarterial chemotherapy of no proven benefit. Prevention may ultimately be achieved by effective global immunization against hepatitis B infection.

OTHER LIVER TUMORS

Most common liver tumors in U.S. population are metastases from other primary cancers; liver second most common site of metastases after lymph nodes; most common primaries are tumors of GI tract, lung, breast, and melanoma.

Clinical features: Metastatic liver tumors usually asymptomatic or associated with nonspecific symptoms (weight loss, fever, weakness, etc.); hepatomegaly less common; ascites, jaundice, liver dysfunction rare. Laboratory findings: elevated alkaline phosphatase, anemia, hypoalbuminemia.

Diagnosis: As for hepatocellular carcinoma; CT-guided biopsy most sensitive means of tissue diagnosis short of laparotomy; role of MRI undefined.

Treatment: On rare occasions, resection of isolated hepatic metastases and primary tumor can be curative; usual therapy is palliative, either by surgery, radiation, or chemotherapy. Direct hepatic artery FUDR administration for hepatic metastases of primary colon carcinoma and for carcinoma of unknown primary may improve survival slightly.

BENIGN LIVER TUMORS

1 *Hemangiomas:* Most common benign hepatic tumors; usually single and small, but may present as large mass. Diagnosis by MRI, CT with intravenous contrast, angiography. Surgical resection for symptomatic tumors only.

2 *Adenomas:* Increased incidence in women taking oral contraceptives; lesions often regress after stopping these agents; biopsy required to exclude malignancy. Major complications include bleeding, rupture. Curative therapy by surgical excision.

3 *Focal nodular hyperplasia:* Usually asymptomatic, incidental finding at laparotomy; not caused by oral contraceptives, but may enlarge and become hypervascular under influence of estrogen; rarely bleed or rupture. Surgical resection required only to exclude adenoma or carcinoma.

For more detailed discussion of these topics, see Alpert E, Isselbacher KJ: Tumors of the Liver, Chap. 250, p. 1351; McPhee MS, Greenberger NJ: Diseases of the Gallbladder and Bile Ducts, Chap. 253, p. 1358; and Greenberger NJ, Toskes PP, Isselbacher KJ: Diseases of the Pancreas, Chap. 255, p. 1372, in HPIM-11

---

103 ACUTE HEPATITIS

VIRAL HEPATITIS

Clinically characterized by malaise, nausea, vomiting, diarrhea, and low-grade fever followed by dark urine, jaundice, and tender hepatomegaly; may be subclinical and detected on basis of elevated aspartate and alanine aminotransferase (AST and ALT) levels. Hepatitis B may be associated with immune complex phenomena, including arthritis, glomerulonephritis, and polyarteritis nodosa. Hepatitis-like illnesses may be caused not only by hepatotropic viruses (A, B, D, non-A, non-B), but also by other viruses (Epstein-Barr, cytomegalovirus, coxsackievirus, etc.), alcohol, drugs, hypotension and ischemia, and biliary tract disease.

HEPATITIS A (HAV) 27-nm enterovirus (picornavirus) with single-stranded RNA genome. Course: See Fig. 103-1.
Outcome: Recovery within 6–12 months, rare fatalities (fulminant hepatitis), no chronic carrier state.
Diagnosis: IgM anti-HAV in acute or early convalescent serum sample.
Epidemiology: Fecal-oral transmission; endemic in underdeveloped countries; food-borne and waterborne epidemics; outbreaks in day-care centers, residential institutions.
Prevention: After exposure—immune globulin 0.02 mL/kg IM within 2 weeks to household and institutional contacts (not casual contacts at work). No vaccine yet.

HEPATITIS B (HBV) 42-nm hepadnavirus with outer surface coat (HBsAg), inner nucleocapsid core (HBcAg), DNA polymerase, and partially double-stranded DNA genome. Circulating form of

FIG. 103-1 *Scheme of typical clinical and laboratory features of HAV. (Reproduced from Dienstag JL, Wands JR, Koff RS, HPIM-11, p. 1326.)*

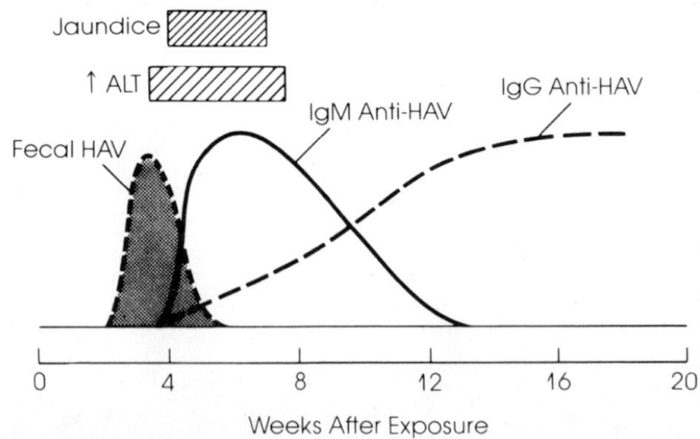

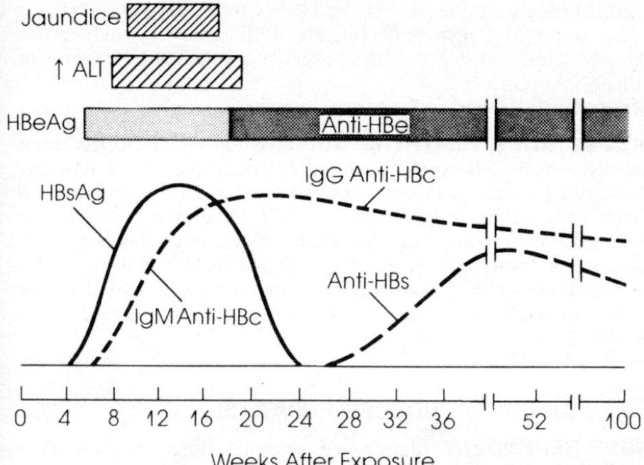

FIG. 103-2 *Scheme of typical clinical and laboratory features of HBV. (Reproduced from Dienstag JL, Wands JR, Koff RS, HPIM-11, p. 1327.)*

HBcAg is HBeAg, a marker of viral replication and infectivity. Course: see Fig. 103-2.

Outcome: Recovery 90%, fulminant hepatitis (<1%), chronic hepatitis or carrier state (10%), cirrhosis and hepatocellular carcinoma (especially following chronic neonatal infection) (Chap. 105).

Diagnosis: HBsAg in serum (acute or chronic infection); IgM anti-HBc (early anti-HBc indicative of acute or recent infection).

Epidemiology: Percutaneous (needlestick), sexual, or perinatal transmission. Endemic in sub-Saharan Africa and Southeast Asia, where up to 20% of population acquire infection, usually early in life.

Prevention: After exposure—hepatitis B immune globulin (HBIG) 0.06 mL/kg IM immediately after needlestick, within 14 days of sexual exposure, or at birth (HBsAg+ mother) plus vaccine series. Before exposure—hepatitis B vaccine 20 μg (plasma-derived vaccine) or 10 μg (recombinant vaccine) IM (half dose to young children) at 0, 1, and 6 months to high-risk groups (e.g., health workers, gay men, IV drug users, hemodialysis patients, hemophiliacs, all neonates in endemic areas, or high-risk neonates in lower-risk areas).

HEPATITIS D (HDV, DELTA AGENT) Defective 37-nm RNA virus that requires HBV for its replication; either *coinfects* with HBV or *superinfects* a chronic HBV carrier. Enhances severity of HBV infection (acceleration of chronic hepatitis to cirrhosis, occasionally fulminant acute hepatitis).

Diagnosis: Anti-HD in serum (acute hepatitis D—often in low titer, transient; chronic hepatitis D—in higher titer, sustained).

Epidemiology: Endemic among HBV carriers in Mediterranean basin, areas of South America, etc. Otherwise spread percutaneously among HBsAg + IV drug users or gay men or by transfusion in hemophiliacs.
Prevention: Hepatitis B vaccine (noncarriers only).

NON-A, NON-B HEPATITIS Virus(es) not yet identified. Incubation period 7–8 weeks. Course often marked by fluctuating elevations of serum aminotransferase levels; >50% likelihood of chronicity leading to cirrhosis in 15%. Diagnosis by exclusion. Percutaneous transmission (similar to HBV). Accounts for >90% of cases of tranfusion-associated hepatitis in U.S. (10–12% incidence). Prevention by excluding commercial (paid) blood donors and those with raised serum ALT levels or anti-HBc (surrogate markers).

TOXIC AND DRUG-INDUCED HEPATITIS

DOSE-DEPENDENT (direct hepatotoxins) Onset within 48 h, predictable, necrosis around terminal hepatic venule—carbon tetrachloride, benzene derivatives, mushroom poisoning, acetaminophen.

IDIOSYNCRATIC Variable dose and time of onset, small number of exposed persons affected, may be associated with fever, rash, arthralgias, eosinophilia—methyldopa, isoniazid. In some cases mechanism may involve toxic metabolite determined on genetic basis—halothane, phenytoin.

ACUTE HEPATIC FAILURE

Massive hepatic necrosis with impaired consciousness occurring within 8 weeks of the onset of illness.
Causes: Infections (viral, including HAV, HBV, HDV, non-A, non-B, bacterial, rickettsial, parasitic), drugs and toxins, ischemia (shock), Budd-Chiari syndrome, idiopathic chronic active hepatitis, acute Wilson's disease, microvesicular fat syndromes (Reye's syndrome, acute fatty liver of pregnancy).
Clinical manifestations: Neuropsychiatric changes—delirium, personality change, stupor, coma, decerebrate rigidity (due to cerebral edema), deep jaundice, coagulopathy, bleeding, renal failure, hypoglycemia, acute pancreatitis, cardiorespiratory failure.
Adverse prognostic indicators: Older age, absence of removable cause (e.g., virus), coma (survival < 20%), rapid reduction in liver size, respiratory failure, marked prolongation of PT.
Treatment: Endotracheal intubation often required. Monitor serum glucose—IV D10 or D20 as necessary. Prevent gastrointestinal bleeding with H-2 receptor antagonists and antacids (gastric pH $\geq$ 4). Value of intracranial pressure monitoring and dexamethasone for cerebral edema unclear; IV mannitol may be beneficial (value of monitoring intracranial pressure unclear). Liver transplantation if timing permits.

For more detailed discussion of this topic, see Dienstag JL, Wands, JR, Koff RS: Acute Hepatitis, Chap. 247, in HPIM-11, p 1325

104 CHRONIC HEPATITIS

A group of disorders characterized by a chronic inflammatory reaction in the liver for at least 6 months.

CLASSIFICATION (Table 104-1)

Etiology: Hepatitis B virus (HBV), hepatitis D virus (HDV, delta agent), non-A, non-B hepatitis (NANB), drugs (methyldopa, nitrofurantoin, isoniazid), Wilson's disease, alpha$_1$ antitrypsin deficiency, idiopathic (autoimmune, "lupoid").

CHRONIC HEPATITIS B

Follows 10% of cases of acute hepatitis B. Spectrum of severity: asymptomatic antigenemia, CPH, and CAH; *early phase* often associated with continued symptoms of hepatitis, elevated aminotransferase levels, presence in serum of HBeAg, and presence in liver of replicative form of HBV; *later phase* in some patients may be associated with clinical and biochemical improvement, disappearance of HBeAg and appearance of anti-HBe in serum, and integration of HBV DNA into host hepatocyte genome. May lead to cirrhosis (particularly in patients with HDV superinfection) and hepatocellular carcinoma (particularly when chronic infection is acquired early in life).

Extrahepatic manifestations (immune-complex–mediated): Rash, urticaria, arthritis, polyarteritis, polyneuropathy, glomerulonephritis, cryoglobulinemia.

TABLE 104-1

Histology	Chronic persistent (CPH)	Chronic active (CAH)
Portal zone infiltrate of lymphocytes and plasma cells	+ +	+ + +
Piecemeal necrosis (extension of portal infiltrate into hepatic lobule with erosion of limiting plate of hepatocytes surrounding portal zones)	–	+ + +
Bridging necrosis (from portal zone to portal zone or portal zone to central vein)	–	±
Multilobular necrosis (extensive inflammation and hepatocyte necrosis)	–	±
Cirrhosis	–	±
Symptoms	Mild or absent	Common
Prognosis	Good	Depends on severity, cause, treatment

Treatment: Experimental—interferons, adenine arabinoside, acyclovir; antiviral agent following prednisone withdrawal.

CHRONIC NON-A, NON-B HEPATITIS

Follows at least 50% of cases of transfusion-associated NANB hepatitis; less frequent after sporadic (non-transfusion-related) cases. Clinically mild, often waxing and waning aminotransferase elevations; mild CAH on liver biopsy. May lead to cirrhosis in 15% of cases. No available treatment.

IDIOPATHIC CAH

Clinical manifestations: 80% women, third to fifth decades. Abrupt onset (acute hepatitis) in a third. Insidious onset in two-thirds: progressive jaundice, anorexia, hepatomegaly, abdominal pain, epistaxis, fever, fatigue, amenorrhea. Leads to cirrhosis; >50% 5-year mortality if untreated.
Extrahepatic manifestations: Rash, arthralgias, keratoconjunctivitis sicca, thyroiditis, hemolytic anemia, nephritis.
Serologic abnormalities: Hypergammaglobulinemia, smooth-muscle antibody (40–80%), ANA (20–50%), LE prep (10–20%), antimitochondrial antibody (10–20%).
Treatment: Indicated for symptomatic disease with biopsy evidence of severe CAH (bridging necrosis) and marked aminotransferase elevations (5–10-fold). Prednisone or prednisolone 30 mg PO qd tapered to 10–15 mg qd over several weeks. Monitor LFTs monthly and liver biopsy every 6 months. If no response, consider adding azathioprine 50 mg PO qd. Withdrawal of corticosteroids can be attempted following remission for 1–2 years; relapse in 50–90% of cases (re-treat).

For more detailed discussion of this topic, see Wands JR, Koff RS, and Isselbacher KJ: Chronic Hepatitis, Chap. 248, in HPIM-11, p. 1338

---

105 CIRRHOSIS AND ALCOHOLIC LIVER DISEASE

Chronic disease of the liver characterized by fibrosis, disorganization of the lobular and vascular architecture, and regenerating nodules of hepatocytes.

CAUSES Alcohol, viral hepatitis [B, D (delta), non-A, non-B; see Chap. 103], primary or secondary biliary cirrhosis, hemochromatosis (Chap. 146), Wilson's disease (Chap. 146), $alpha_1$ antitrypsin deficiency, chronic active hepatitis (Chap. 103), Budd-Chiari syndrome, chronic CHF (cardiac cirrhosis), drugs and toxins, schistosomiasis, cryptogenic.

CLINICAL MANIFESTATIONS May be absent.
Symptoms: Anorexia, nausea, vomiting, diarrhea, fatigue, weakness, fever, jaundice, amenorrhea, impotence, infertility.
Signs: Spider telangiectases, palmar erythema, parotid and lacrimal gland enlargement, nail changes (Muehrcke lines, Terry's nails), clubbing, Dupuytren's contracture, gynecomastia, testicular atrophy, hepatosplenomegaly, ascites, gastrointestinal bleeding (e.g., varices), hepatic encephalopathy.
Laboratory findings: Anemia (microcytic due to blood loss, macrocytic due to folate deficiency), pancytopenia (hypersplenism), prolonged PT, rarely DIC; hyponatremia, hypokalemic alkalosis, glucose disturbances, hypoalbuminemia.
Other associations: Gastritis; duodenal ulcer; gallstones; altered drug metabolism because of decreased drug clearance, metabolism (e.g, by cytochrome P_{450}), and elimination; hypopalbuminemia; and portosystemic shunting.

DIAGNOSTIC STUDIES (choices depend on clinical setting) Serum: HBsAg, anti-HBc, anti-HBs, anti-HD, Fe, total iron binding capacity, ferritin, antimitochondrial antibody (AMA), smooth-muscle antibodies (SMA), ANA, ceruloplasmin, $alpha_1$ antitrypsin (and pi typing); abdominal ultrasound, liver scan, portal venography, and wedged hepatic vein pressure measurement. Definitive diagnosis often depends on liver biopsy (percutaneous or open); may be precluded by coagulopathy.

ALCOHOLIC LIVER DISEASE

Three forms: fatty liver, alcoholic hepatitis, cirrhosis; may coexist. History of excessive alcohol use often denied. Severe forms (hepatitis, cirrhosis) associated with ingestion of 80–160 g/day for >5–10 years.

FATTY LIVER May follow even brief periods of ethanol use. Often presents as asymptomatic hepatomegaly and mild elevations in biochemical liver tests. Reverses on withdrawal of ethanol; does not lead to cirrhosis.

ALCOHOLIC HEPATITIS Clinical presentation ranges from asymptomatic to severe liver failure with jaundice, ascites, GI bleeding, and encephalopathy. Typically anorexia, nausea, vomiting, fever, jaundice, tender hepatomegaly. Occasional cholestatic picture mimicking biliary obstruction. Aspartate aminotransferase (AST) usually less than 300 U and > twofold higher than alanine aminotransferase (ALT). Bilirubin may be >10 mg/dL. WBC may be as high as 20,000/mm³. Diagnosis defined by liver biopsy findings: hepatocyte swelling, alcoholic hyaline (Mallory bodies), infiltration of PMNs, necrosis of hepatocytes, pericentral venular fibrosis.

Other metabolic consequences of alcoholism (increased NADH/NAD ratio): Lacticacidemia, ketoacidosis, hyperuricemia, hypoglycemia.

Adverse prognostic factors: *Short-term:* PT > 5 s above control despite vitamin K, bilirubin > 10 mg/dL, encephalopathy, hypoalbuminemia, azotemia. *Long-term:* severe hepatic necrosis and fibrosis, portal hypertension, continued alcohol consumption.

Treatment: Abstinence is essential; 2000–3000 kcal diet with 1 g/kg protein (less if encephalopathy). Daily multivitamin, thiamine 100 mg, folic acid 1 mg. Correct potassium and magnesium deficiencies. Transfusions of packed red cells, plasma as necessary. Monitor glucose (hypoglycemia in severe liver disease). Prednisone or prednisolone 40 mg PO qd × 1 month may be beneficial in severe alcoholic hepatitis with encephalopathy.

PRIMARY BILIARY CIRRHOSIS

Progressive nonsuppurative destructive intrahepatic cholangitis. Affects middle-aged women. Presents as asymptomatic elevation in alkaline phosphatase (often nonprogressive, good prognosis) or with pruritus, progressive jaundice, and ultimately cirrhosis and liver failure.

CLINICAL MANIFESTATIONS Pruritus, jaundice, xanthelasma, xanthomata, osteoporosis, steatorrhea, skin pigmentation, hepatosplenomegaly, portal hypertension, elevations in serum alkaline phosphatase, bilirubin, cholesterol, and IgM levels.

ASSOCIATED DISEASES Sjögren's syndrome, collagen-vascular diseases, thyroiditis, glomerulonephritis.

DIAGNOSIS AMA in >90–95%. Liver biopsy: stage 1—destruction of interlobular bile ducts, granulomas; stage 2—ductural proliferation; stage 3—fibrosis; stage 4—cirrhosis.

TREATMENT Cholestyramine 4 g PO with meals for pruritus. Vitamin K 10 mg IM qd × 3 (then once a month) for elevated PT due to intestinal bile salt deficiency. Vitamin D 100,000 U IM q 4 weeks plus oral calcium 1 g qd for osteoporosis (often unresponsive). Vitamin A 25–50,000 U PO qd or 100,000 U IM q 4 weeks and zinc 220 mg PO qd may help night blindness. Vitamin E 10 mg IM or PO qd. Substituting dietary fat with medium-chain triglycerides (MCTs) may reduce steatorrhea. Experimental: D-penicillamine, azathioprine, colchicine, chlorambucil.

LIVER TRANSPLANTATION

Consider for chronic, irreversible, progressive liver disease or fulminant hepatic necrosis when no alternative therapy is available.

CONTRAINDICATIONS **Absolute:** Portal vein thrombosis, hypoxemia ($P_{O_2} < 60$ mmHg), extrahepatobiliary sepsis or malignancy, cardiopulmonary or renal disease (except hepatorenal syndrome), active alcoholism, lack of patient understanding. **Relative:** Age > 55, HBsAg and $HBeAg^+$, hepatobiliary sepsis, extensive previous abdominal surgery.

INDICATIONS (guidelines) Expected death in 3–6 months; preferably in anticipation of major complication (variceal bleeding, irreversible encephalopathy, severe malnutrition and incapacitating weakness, hepatorenal syndrome); bilirubin > 10–20 m/dL, albumin < 2 g/dL, worsening coagulopathy; poor quality of life.

For more detailed discussion of this topic, see Podolsky DK, Isselbacher, KJ: Cirrhosis, Chap. 249, p. 1341; Schmid, R: Liver Transplantation, Chap. 252, p. 1356, in HPIM-11

---

106 PORTAL HYPERTENSION

Any increase in portal vein pressure due to anatomic or functional obstruction to blood flow in the portal venous system.

Normal portal vein pressure is 5–10 mmHg. Indicators of portal hypertension are:

- Intraoperative portal vein pressure — >30 cm saline
- Intrasplenic pressure — >17 mmHg
- Wedged hepatic vein pressure — >4 mmHg above IVC pressure

CLASSIFICATION (Table 106-1)

CONSEQUENCES (1) Increased collateral circulation between high-pressure portal venous system and low-pressure systemic venous system: lower esophagus/upper stomach (varices), rectum (hemorrhoids), anterior abdominal wall (caput Medusae; flow away from umbilicus), parietal peritoneum, splenorenal; (2) increased lymphatic flow; (3) increased plasma volume; (4) ascites (Chap. 20); (5) splenomegaly, possible hypersplenism; (6) portosystemic shunting (incl. hepatic encephalopathy).

ESOPHAGOGASTRIC VARICES

Bleeding is major life-threatening complication; risk correlates with variceal size above minimal portal venous pressure > 12 mmHg. Mortality correlates with severity of underlying liver disease (hepatic reserve).

DIAGNOSIS *Upper GI series:* tortuous, beaded filling defects in lower esophagus. *Esophagogastroscopy:* procedure of choice for

TABLE 106-1

	Pressure		
Site of obstruction	Portal	Corrected wedged hepatic vein (wedged hepatic vein minus inferior vena cava pressure)	Examples
Presinusoidal	↑	Normal	Splenic AV fistula, portal or splenic vein thrombosis, schistosomiasis
Sinusoidal	↑	↑	Cirrhosis, hepatitis
Postsinusoidal	↑	↑ (May be unmeasurable due to hepatic vein occlusion)	Budd-Chiari syndrome, veno-occlusive disease

acute bleeding. *Celiac and mesenteric arteriography:* when massive bleeding precludes endoscopy and to evaluate portal vein patency (portal vein also may be studied by ultrasound).

TREATMENT See Chapter 18 for general measures to treat GI bleeding.

Control of acute bleeding: (1) Intravenous vasopressin up to 0.4–0.9 U/min, then taper slowly (0.1 U/min q 6–12 h); add nitroglycerin up to 0.6 mg SL q 30 min to prevent coronary and renal vasoconstriction. (2) Blakemore-Sengstaken balloon tamponade: can be inflated for up to 24–48 h; complications—obstruction of pharynx, asphyxiation, esophageal ulceration. (3) Endoscopic sclerotherapy—may be procedure of choice (not suitable for gastric varices); variety of techniques, sclerosants; >90% success rate; complications—esophageal ulceration and stricture, mediastinitis, pleural effusions, aspiration.

Prevention of recurrent bleeding: (1) Repeated endoscopic sclerotherapy (e.g., q 2–4 weeks until obliteration). Long-term efficacy unclear; does not prevent all recurrent bleeding but may improve overall survival rate and compares favorably to shunt surgery. (2) Propranolol—portal venous antihypertensive; most effective in well-compensated cirrhotics; generally given bid in dose that reduces heart rate by 25%. (3) Splenectomy (for splenic vein thrombosis). (4) Portosystemic shunt surgery: portacaval (total decompression) or distal splenorenal (Warren) (selective; contraindicated in ascites; ? lower incidence of hepatic encephalopathy). Alternative procedure—devascularization of lower esophagus and upper stomach (Sugiura).

PROGNOSIS (AND SURGICAL RISK) Correlated with classification of Child and Turcotte; see Table 106-2.

HEPATIC ENCEPHALOPATHY

A state of disordered CNS function associated with severe acute or chronic liver disease; may be acute and reversible or chronic and progressive.

CLINICAL FEATURES Mild—day-night reversal of sleep cycle, somnolence, confusion, personality change, asterixis. More severe—stupor, coma, dementia, occasionally extrapyramidal signs. Characteristic EEG abnormalities.

TABLE 106-2

	Class		
	A	B	C
Serum bilirubin (mg/dL)	<2	2–3	>3
Serum albumin (g/dL)	>3.5	3.0–3.5	<3.0
Ascites	None	Easily controlled	Poorly controlled
Encephalopathy	None	Mild	Advanced
Nutrition	Excellent	Good	Poor
Prognosis	Good	Fair	Poor

PATHOPHYSIOLOGY Failure of liver to detoxify agents noxious to CNS (ammonia, mercaptans, fatty acids, α-aminobutyric acid) due to decreased hepatic function and portosystemic shunting. False neurotransmitters also may enter CNS due to increased aromatic and decreased branched-chain amino acid levels in blood. Blood ammonia most readily measured marker, although may not always correlate with clinical status.

PRECIPITANTS GI bleeding (100 mL = 14–20 g protein), azotemia, constipation, high-protein meal, hypokalemic alkalosis, CNS depressant drugs (e.g., benzodiazepines), hypoxia, hypercarbia, sepsis.

TREATMENT Remove precipitants; reduce protein intake (20–30 g/day, vegetable sources); enemas/cathartics to clear gut. Lactulose (converts NH_3 to unabsorbed NH_4^+, produces diarrhea, alters bowel flora) 30–45 mL PO q 2 h until diarrhea, then tid-qid prn 2–3 loose stools/day. In coma, give as enema (300 mL in 700 mL H_2O). In refractory cases, add neomycin 1 g PO bid.

For more detailed discussion of this topic see Podolsky DK, Isselbacher KJ: Cirrhosis, Chap. 249, in HPIM-11, p. 1341

SECTION VII
ALLERGY, CLINICAL IMMUNOLOGY, AND RHEUMATOLOGY

107 ANAPHYLAXIS AND DISEASES OF IMMEDIATE TYPE HYPERSENSITIVITY

DEFINITION

Diseases of immediate type hypersensitivity result from IgE-dependent release of mediators from sensitized basophils and mast cells on contact with appropriate antigen (allergen). Associated disorders include anaphylaxis, allergic rhinitis, urticaria, asthma, and eczematous (atopic) dermatitis. *Atopic allergy* implies a familial tendency to the development of these disorders singly or in combination.

PATHOPHYSIOLOGY IgE binds to surface of mast cells and basophils through a high-affinity receptor. Cross-linking of this IgE by antigen causes cellular activation with the subsequent release of preformed and newly synthesized mediators. These include histamine, prostaglandins, leukotrienes (including leukotrienes C_4, D_4, and E_4, collectively known as slow-reacting substance of anaphylaxis, SRS-A), acid hydrolases, neutral proteases, and proteoglycans. These mediators have been implicated in many pathophysiologic events associated with immediate-type hypersensitivity, such as vasodilatation, increased vasopermeability, smooth-muscle contraction, and chemotactic attraction of neutrophils and other inflammatory cells. The clinical manifestations of each allergic reaction depend largely on the anatomic site(s) and time course of this mediator release.

ANAPHYLAXIS

DEFINITION A life-threatening systemic reaction to contact with an allergen; may appear within minutes of exposure to offending substance. Manifestations include respiratory distress, pruritus, urticaria, mucous membrane swelling, gastrointestinal disturbances (including nausea, vomiting, pain, and diarrhea), and vascular collapse. The more common inciting allergens are proteins such as antisera, hormones, pollen extracts, *Hymenoptera* venom, foods, drugs (especially antibiotics), and diagnostic agents.

CLINICAL MANIFESTATIONS Time to onset is variable, but symptoms may occur within seconds to minutes.

- *Respiratory*: Mucous membrane swelling, hoarseness, stridor, wheezing

- *Cardiovascular*: Tachycardia, hypotension
- *Cutaneous*: Pruritis, urticaria, angioedema

DIAGNOSIS History of exposure to offending substance with subsequent development of characteristic complex of signs and symptoms.

PREVENTION AND THERAPY

• Epinephrine 0.2 to 0.5 mL of 1:1000 solution SC with repeat doses at 3-min intervals as necessary. • Epinephrine IV infusion of 1:50,000 solution to treat hypotension. • IV fluids and volume expanders. • Antihistamines such as diphenhydramine 50 to 80 mg IM or IV. • Aminophylline 0.25 to 0.5 g IV for bronchospasm. • Oxygen. • Corticosteroids IV; not useful for acute manifestations but may help control persistent hypotension or bronchospasm. • *Prevention*: avoidance of offending antigen, where possible; skin testing and desensitization to materials such as penicillin and *Hymenoptera* venom, if necessary.

URTICARIA AND ANGIOEDEMA

DEFINITION May occur together or separately. *Urticaria* involves superficial dermis and presents as circumscribed wheals with raised serpiginous borders and blanched centers; wheals may coalesce. *Angioedema* involves deeper layers of skin and may include subcutaneous tissue. These disorders may be classified as (1) IgE-dependent, including atopic, secondary to specific allergens, and physical stimuli, especially cold, (2) complement-mediated (including hereditary angioedema and hives related to serum sickness or vasculitis), (3) nonimmunologic due to direct mast cell-releasing agents or drugs that influence mediator release, and (4) idiopathic.

PATHOPHYSIOLOGY Characterized by massive edema formation in the dermis (and subcutaneous tissue in angioedema). Presumably the edema is due to increased vasopermeability caused by mediator release from mast cells or other cell populations.

DIAGNOSIS

• *History*: special attention to possible offending exposures and/or ingestion. • Skin testing to food and/or inhalant antigens. • Physical provocation, e.g., challenge with vibratory or cold stimuli. • *Laboratory examination*: complement levels, ESR; C1-esterase inhibitor levels if history suggests hereditary angioedema; cryoglobulins, hepatitis B antigen and antibody studies; autoantibody screen. • Skin biopsy may be necessary.

DIFFERENTIAL DIAGNOSIS Atopic dermatitis, cutaneous mastocytosis (urticaria pigmentosa), systemic mastocytosis.

PREVENTION AND TREATMENT

• Identification and avoidance of offending agent(s). • Antihistamines: both H1 and H2 blockers may be useful.

ALLERGIC RHINITIS

DEFINITION An inflammatory condition of the nose characterized by sneezing, rhinorrhea, and obstruction of nasal passages; may be associated with conjunctival and pharyngeal itching, lacrimation, and sinusitis. *Seasonal* allergic rhinitis is commonly caused by exposure to pollens, especially from grasses, trees, weeds, and molds. *Perennial* allergic rhinitis is frequently due to contact with house dust (containing dust mite antigens) and animal danders.

PATHOPHYSIOLOGY Impingement of pollens and other allergens on nasal mucosa of sensitized individual results in IgE-dependent triggering of mast cells with subsequent release of mediators which cause development of mucosal hyperemia, swelling, and fluid transudation. Inflammation of nasal mucosal surface probably allows penetration of allergens deeper into tissue, where they contact perivenular mast cells. Obstruction of sinus ostia may result in development of secondary sinusitis, with or without bacterial infection.

DIAGNOSIS

- Accurate *history* of symptoms correlated with time of pollination of plants in a given locale; special attention must be paid to other potentially sensitizing antigens such as pet danders.
- *Physical examination*: nasal mucosa may be boggy or erythematous; nasal polyps may be present; sinuses may demonstrate decreased transillumination; conjunctivae may be inflamed or edematous; manifestations of other allergic conditions (e.g., asthma, eczema) may be present.
- Skin tests to inhalant and/or food antigens.
- Nasal smear may reveal large numbers of eosinophils; presence of neutrophils may suggest infection.
- Total and specific serum IgE may be elevated.

DIFFERENTIAL DIAGNOSIS Vasomotor rhinitis, URI irritant exposure, pregnancy with nasal mucosal edema, rhinitis medicamentosa, nonallergic rhinitis with eosinophilia.

PREVENTION AND THERAPY

• Identification and avoidance of offending antigen(s). • Antihistamines. • Oral decongestants. • Nasal corticosteroids. • Nasal cromolyn sodium • Hyposensitization therapy if more conservative therapy is unsuccessful.

For more detailed discussion of this topic, see Austen KF: Diseases of Immediate Type Hypersensitivity, Chap. 260 in HPIM-11, p. 1407

DEFINITION Disorders involving the cell-mediated (T-cell) or antibody-mediated (B-cell) arm of immune system; some disorders may manifest abnormalities of both pathways. Patients are prone to development of recurrent infections and, in certain disorders, lymphoproliferative neoplasms. *Primary disorders* may be congenital or acquired; some are familial in nature. *Secondary disorders* are not caused by intrinsic abnormalities of immune cells but may be due to infection (such as in AIDS; see HPIM-11, Chap. 257), treatment with cytotoxic drugs, radiation therapy, or lymphoreticular malignancies. Patients with disorders of antibody formation are chiefly prone to infection with encapsulated bacterial pathogens (e.g., streptococci, *Haemophilus,* meningococcus) and *Giardia.* Individuals with T-cell defects are generally susceptible to infections with viruses, fungi, and protozoa.

CLASSIFICATION **Severe combined immunodeficiency (SCID):** Congenital (autosomal recessive or X-linked); affected infants rarely survive beyond 1 year. Dysfunction of both cellular and humoral immunity:

- Swiss-type: autosomal recessive; severe lymphopenia involving B and T cells.
- Adenosine deaminase deficiency: autosomal recessive.
- X-linked patterns: some patients have normal numbers of B-cells but few or no circulating T cells.

Bone marrow transplantation is useful in some patients.

T-cell immunodeficiencies:

1 *DiGeorge syndrome:* Maldevelopment of organs derived embryologically from third and fourth pharyngeal pouches (including thymus); associated with congenital cardiac defects, parathyroid hypoplasia with hypocalcemic tetany, abnormal facies, thymic aplasia; serum Ig levels may be normal, but specific antibody responses are impaired.

2 *Ataxia-telangiectasia:* Autosomal recessive; cerebellar ataxia, oculocutaneous telangiectasia, immunodeficiency; not all patients have immunodeficiency; lymphomas common; IgG subclasses may be abnormal.

Immunoglobulin deficiency syndromes:

1 *X-linked agammaglobulinemia:* Marked deficiency of circulating lymphocytes; all Ig classes low; arthritis associated with *Mycoplasma* and chronic echovirus encephalitis are common complications.

2 *Transient hypogammaglobulinemia of infancy:* This occurs between 3 and 6 months of age as maternally derived IgG levels decline.

3 *Isolated IgA deficiency:* Most common immunodeficiency; many affected patients do not have increased infections; antibodies against IgA may lead to anaphylaxis during transfusion of blood or plasma; may be associated with deficiencies of IgG subclasses.

4 *X-linked immunodeficiency with increased IgM.*

5 *Isolated deficiency of IgM.*

6 *Common varied immunodeficiency:* Heterogeneous group of syndromes characterized by panhypogammaglobulinemia, deficiency of IgG and IgA, or selective IgG deficiency; associated conditions include lymphoreticular neoplasms, arthritis, ulcerative colitis.

7 *Immunodeficiency with thymoma.*

8 *Wiskott-Aldrich syndrome:* X-linked genetic disorder characterized by eczema, thrombocytopenia, and infections.

Miscellaneous immunodeficiency syndromes:
• Mucocutaneous candidiasis. • Immunodeficiency associated with serum lymphocytotoxins. • Selective IgG subclass deficiency. • X-linked lymphoproliferative syndrome.

PRELIMINARY EVALUATION

• CBC with differential. • Quantitative immunoglobulin levels. • Isoagglutinins, diphtheria and tetanus antibody titers. • Complement levels (C3, C4, and CH_{50}). • Skin tests for T-cell function (PPD, *Candida, Trichophyton, tetanus toxoid).*

TREATMENT Treatment of T-cell disorders is complex and largely investigational. Therapy of humoral immunodeficiencies with intravenous IgG preparations should aim to keep IgG levels near low-normal range.

For more detailed discussion of this topic, see Cooper MD, Lawton AR III: Immune Deficiency Diseases, Chap. 256, in HPIM-11, p. 1385

---

109 ACQUIRED IMMUNODEFICIENCY SYNDROME (AIDS)

DEFINITION Originally defined empirically by the Centers for Disease Control (CDC) as "presence of a reliably diagnosed disease that is at least moderately indicative of an underlying defect in cell-mediated immunity." Examples are Kaposi's sarcoma in individual <60 years old or a life-threatening opportunistic infection such as *Pneumocystis carinii* pneumonia. Following recognition of the causative virus, human immunodeficiency virus (HIV) (formerly called HTLV-III/LAV), diagnosis is now excluded if tests for presence of the virus or its antibodies are negative and number of T-helper lymphocytes is normal.

In the *absence* of classic opportunistic infection (required by original case definition) and in *presence* of positive serologic or virologic tests for HIV, any of the following diseases is considered indicative of AIDS: disseminated histoplasmosis; isosporosis causing chronic diarrhea; bronchial or pulmonary candidiasis; non-Hodgkin's (lymphocytic) lymphoma of high-grade pathologic type and of B-cell or unknown immunologic phenotype; Kaposi's sarcoma diagnosed by biopsy in pts ≥ 60 years old when diagnosed; histologically confirmed chronic lymphoid interstitial pneumonitis in a child < 13 years of age; and diagnosis of a lymphoreticular malignancy > 3 months after appearance of an opportunistic disease used as a marker for AIDS. (These pts were excluded under original case definition on the presumption that malignancy could have caused the immunosuppression which led to the opportunistic infection.)

ETIOLOGY AIDS is caused by infection with HIV. This virus is lymphotropic and selectively infects human T-lymphocytes of the helper/inducer subset (designated by the T4 or Leu 3 phenotypic marker). The infection causes a cytopathic effect on these cells with a decline in their number or function. Virus is passed through sexual contact; through contact with blood, blood products, or other bodily fluids (as in drug abusers who share contaminated IV needles); or perinatally from mother to infant. There is no evidence that virus can be passed through casual or family contact.

EPIDEMIOLOGY AIDS first appeared in the U.S. in the late 1970s and was first recognized in 1981, when CDC announced the unexplained occurrence of *P. carinii* pneumonia and Kaposi's sarcoma in previously healthy homosexual men from New York City and Los Angeles. There has since been a geometric increase in number of cases; it is anticipated that there will have been > 270,000 cases in the U.S. by 1991. The disease is occurring elsewhere with increased frequency, particularly in Europe and Africa.

Among adult cases in the U.S., 66% have occurred in homosexual or bisexual men; 17% in IV drug abusers; 8% in men who are both homosexual and IV drug abusers; 1% in hemophiliacs who have received large volumes of factor VIII concentrates; 4% in heterosexual partners of individuals with AIDS or at risk for AIDS; and 2% in nonhemophiliacs who have received blood products. There are at least 400 cases of pediatric AIDS reported; the vast majority were born of parents with AIDS or at increased risk for AIDS.

Exact prevalence of infection with HIV in general population is not known. In contrast to high rates of seropositivity among certain groups of homosexual men, drug abusers, and individuals with hemophilia, <0.05% of general blood donor pool is antibody-positive. It is estimated that 20–30% of asymptomatic seropositive individuals will develop AIDS within 5 years.

PATHOPHYSIOLOGY AND IMMUNOPATHOGENESIS Characteristic immunologic feature of AIDS is a profound defect in cell-mediated immunity caused by infection of helper/inducer subset of T lymphocytes by HIV. There is particular depletion of this cellular subset; cytotoxic/suppressor T cells may be normal or slightly increased or decreased in number.

Because of central role of helper/inducer T-cell subset in inducing and coordinating many components of immune response, global defects of immune function are present in AIDS pts, including defects in natural killer cells, monocytes, virus-specific cytotoxic T cells and B cells. B cells are polyclonally activated, resulting in hypergammaglobulinemia with elevated levels of IgG, IgM, and IgA. Monocytes also can be infected.

In addition to effects on immune system, HIV may directly infect other organ systems and cause pathology. This is particularly true of CNS; neuropsychiatric manifestations directly related to HIV infection may be seen in as many as 30% of AIDS pts. Virus has been isolated from semen, saliva, plasma, tears, vaginal secretions, and CSF.

CLINICAL MANIFESTATIONS

- *Primary infection:* may be acute illness in some pts 3–6 weeks after primary infection; characterized by fever, rigors, arthralgias, myalgias, rash, abdominal cramps, diarrhea; symptoms last 2–3 weeks and resolve spontaneously.
- *AIDS-related complex:* group of infected individuals who do not fulfill criteria for full-blown syndrome; symptoms may include fever, weight loss, diarrhea, fatigue, night sweats, lymphadenopathy, immunologic abnormalities.
- *Neuropsychiatric manifestations:* wide range of neurologic findings; acute or chronic meningitis; progressive dementia with or without localizing signs.
- *Kaposi's sarcoma:* a multifocal neoplasm; presents as vascular nodules on skin and other organs; course may be indolent or fulminant; may involve any organ system, but skin, mucous membranes, GI, lymph node, and pleuropulmonary involvement are most common; Dx by biopsy.
- *P. carinii* pneumonia (PCP): may present with fever, dyspnea, and hypoxemia; however, compared to nonAIDS patients with

PCP, presentation in AIDS may be indolent; Dx by bronchoscopy with biopsy and/or lavage.

- *Cytomegalovirus* (CMV): may present as fever and disseminated organ involvement; colitis, chorioretinitis, pneumonitis most prominent.
- *Candida albicans:* thrush and esophagitis common.
- Smoldering infection with *Mycobacterium avium-intracellulare;* rarely a cause of death.
- *Herpes simplex virus:* severe mucocutaneous involvement (esp. perianal).
- CNS infection with *Toxoplasma gondii* or *Cryptococcus neoformans;* needs to be distinguished from CNS Kaposi's or lymphoma.
- Pediatric patients have higher incidence of bacterial infections.
- Diarrheal syndromes, particularly due to the protozoan *Cryptosporidium.*
- Hypercatabolic wasting syndrome even in absence of demonstrable infection.
- Other malignancies such as lymphomas and certain carcinomas.
- Lymphoid interstitial pneumonitis.
- Immune-mediated thrombocytopenia.

DIAGNOSIS AND TREATMENT

- Diagnosis requires demonstration of infection with AIDS retrovirus by serologic (ELISA test confirmed by Western blot analysis if necessary) or virologic means *plus* diagnosis of the empirically defined secondary complications of immune dysfunction (see above).
- Treatment of infection with HIV is still investigational and includes use of agents such as 3′-azido-3′-deoxythymidine (AZT).
- Enhancement and reconstitution of immune system are under investigation.

APPROACH TO PATIENT

- Careful history and PE with special reference to possible risk factors for AIDS and clues to opportunistic infections or malignancies.
- CBC, platelet count.
- Chemistry profile.
- Chest radiograph.
- Immune testing: T-cell subsets and numbers, quantitative immunoglobulins, anergy screening.
- Special further testing if necessary: biopsies of skin lesions, bronchoscopy, GI endoscopy, stool for ova and parasites, cultures of urine for CMV, CT scanning of head with and without contrast, lumbar puncture, cultures of blood and other fluids for *Mycobacterium avium-intracellulare.*
- Treatment of specific infections with antimicrobial agents.
- Treatment of Kaposi's sarcoma and other malignancies with appropriate chemo- and/or radiotherapy.

PROGNOSIS Typical clinical course is repeated bouts of opportunistic infections and/or progression of malignancies until death occurs from specific complications or general wasting. Some individuals may remain quite well for many months. There has been no report of spontaneous reversal of underlying immune deficiency.

For more detailed discussion of this topic, see Fauci AS, Lane HC: The Acquired Immunodeficiency Syndrome (AIDS), Chap. 257, in HPIM-11, p. 1392

110 CONNECTIVE TISSUE DISEASES

Heterogeneous disorders which share certain common features, including inflammation of skin, joints, and other structures rich in connective tissue, as well as altered patterns of immunoregulation, including production of autoantibodies and abnormalities of cell-mediated immunity. While certain distinct clinical entities may be defined, manifestations may vary considerably from one patient to the next and overlap of clinical features between and among specific diseases is common.

SYSTEMIC LUPUS ERYTHEMATOSUS (SLE)

Definition and pathogenesis: Disease of unknown etiology in which tissues and cells are damaged by deposition of pathogenic antibodies and immune complexes. Genetic, environmental, and sex hormonal factors are likely of pathogenetic importance. B-cell hyperactivity, production of autoantibodies with specificity for nuclear antigenic determinants, and abnormalities of T-cell function occur.

Clinical manifestations: May involve virtually any organ system. Course of disease is one of periods of exacerbation and remission. *Common features* include fatigue, fever, malaise, weight loss, skin rashes (especially malar "butterfly" rash), photosensitivity, arthritis, myositis, oral ulcers, vasculitis, alopecia, anemia (may be hemolytic), neutropenia, thrombocytopenia, lymphadenopathy, splenomegaly, organic brain syndromes, seizures, psychosis, pleuritis, pericarditis, myocarditis, pneumonitis, nephritis, venous or arterial thrombosis, mesenteric vasculitis, sicca syndrome. Antinuclear antibodies are usually present. Syndrome may be *drug-induced* (especially by procainamide, hydralazine, isoniazid).

Evaluation: Hx and PE, appropriate radiographic studies, ECG, UA, CBC, ESR, serum immunoglobulins, antinuclear antibodies and subtypes (dsDNA, ssDNA, anti-Sm, anti-Ro, anti-La, antihistone), complement levels (C3, C4, CH_{50}), VDRL, PT, PTT.

Treatment: No cure; treatment is directed at controlling inflammation. Useful drugs include salicylates and NSAIDs, hydroxychloroquine; glucocorticoids may be necessary for life-threatening or severely disabling manifestations; cytotoxic agents (cyclophosphamide, azathioprine) may be required for manifestations not successfully controlled by acceptable doses of steroids.

RHEUMATOID ARTHRITIS (RA)

Definition and pathogenesis: A chronic multisystem disease of unknown etiology characterized chiefly by persistent inflammatory synovitis, usually involving peripheral joints in a symmetrical fashion. Cartilaginous destruction, bony erosions, and joint deformation are hallmarks of persistent synovial inflammation. Pathogenesis is not well understood; synovial hyperplasia and hypertrophy, lymphocytic infiltration of synovial tissue, joint infiltration by neutrophils, protease release, and chondrocyte activation occur.

Clinical manifestations: Hallmark is symmetrical polyarthritis of peripheral joints with pain, tenderness, and swelling of affected joints; morning stiffness is common; PIP and MCP joints frequently involved; joint deformities may develop after persistent inflammation. *Extraarticular manifestations* include rheumatoid nodules, rheumatoid vasculitis, pleuropulmonary inflammation, scleritis, sicca syndrome, Felty's syndrome (splenomegaly and neutropenia), osteoporosis.

Evaluation: Hx and PE with careful examination of all joints; CBC, ESR, rheumatoid factor, complement levels, synovial fluid analysis, chest and joint radiographs.

Treatment: (1) Aspirin and NSAIDs are mainstays of therapy; (2) disease-modifying drugs (gold, D-penicillamine, antimalarials); (3) glucocorticoids should be avoided unless absolutely necessary; (4) cytotoxic agents when other modalities fail.

PROGRESSIVE SYSTEMIC SCLEROSIS (PSS)

Definition and pathogenesis: Multisystem disorder characterized by inflammatory, vascular, and fibrotic changes of skin and various internal organ systems (chiefly GI tract, lungs, heart, and kidney). Pathogenesis not clear; primary event may be endothelial cell injury with eventual intimal proliferation, fibrosis, and vessel obliteration.

Clinical manifestations: Raynaud's phenomenon, fibrosis of the skin (scleroderma), telangiectasis, calcinosis, esophageal hypomotility, arthralgias and/or arthritis, intestinal hypofunction, pulmonary fibrosis, hypertension, renal failure (leading cause of death).

Evaluation: Hx and PE, ESR, CXR, barium swallow, ANA (specific antibodies may include antibodies to nucleolar antigens, ribonucleoprotein, centromere, and Scl-70), ECG, UA, skin biopsy.

Treatment: No definitive therapy. Calcium channel blockers may be useful for Raynaud's phenomenon; antacids and H-2 antihistamines may relieve esophageal discomfort; glucocorticoids may be useful for acute myositis; aggressive treatment of hypertension is important in delaying renal dysfunction—captopril (an angiotensin converting enzyme inhibitor) is an effective drug.

MIXED CONNECTIVE TISSUE DISEASE (MCTD)

Definition and pathogenesis: Syndrome characterized by a combination of clinical features similar to those of SLE, PSS, polymyositis, and RA; unusually high titers of circulating antibodies to a nuclear ribonucleoprotein (RNP) are found. Pathogenic mechanisms are unknown, but evidence exists for abnormal immunoregulation and proliferative intimal and/or medial vascular lesions resulting in narrowing of vessel lumens.

Clinical manifestations: Raynaud's phenomenon, polyarthritis, swollen hands or sclerodactyly, esophageal dysfunction, pulmonary fibrosis, inflammatory myopathy. Renal involvement is less common than in PSS. Laboratory abnormalities include high-titer

ANAs, positive rheumatoid factor in >50% of patients, very high titers of antibody to RNP component of extractable nuclear antigen.
Evaluation: Similar to that for SLE and PSS.
Treatment: Similar to that for SLE; directed at controlling inflammatory manifestations of disease.

SJÖGREN'S SYNDROME

Definition and pathogenesis: An immunologic disorder characterized by progressive destruction of exocrine glands leading to mucosal and conjunctival dryness (sicca syndrome); may be primary or in association with other autoimmune diseases; affected tissues demonstrate lymphocytic infiltration and immune-complex deposition.
Clinical manifestations: Xerostomia and keratoconjunctivitis sicca, nephritis, vasculitis (usually cutaneous), polyneuropathy, interstitial pneumonitis, pseudolymphoma, autoimmune thyroid disease, congenital cardiac conduction defects in children born to women with anti-Ro (SSA) antibodies.
Evaluation: Hx and PE, with special attention to determining extent of disease and presence of other autoimmune disorders; CBC, UA, CXR, ECG, thyroid function tests, Schirmer's test, ESR, cryoglobulins.
Treatment: Symptomatic relief of dryness with artificial tears, ophthalmic lubricating ointments, nasal saline sprays, frequent sips of water, moisturizing skin lotions; treatment of associated autoimmune phenomena.

For more detailed discussion of these topics, see Hahn, BH: Systemic Lupus Erythematosus, Chap. 262, p. 1418; Lipsky PE: Rheumatoid Arthritis, Chap. 263, p. 1423; Gilliland BC: Progressive Systemic Sclerosis (Diffuse Scleroderma), Chap. 264, p. 1428; Sharp GC: Mixed Connective Tissue Disease, Chap. 265, p. 1432; and Lane HC, Fauci AS: Sjögren's Syndrome, Chap. 266, p. 1433, in HPIM-11.

---

111 VASCULITIS

DEFINITION AND PATHOGENESIS

A clinicopathologic process characterized by inflammation of and damage to blood vessels, compromise of vessel lumen, and resulting ischemia. Clinical manifestations of ischemic damage depend on size and location of vessel. May be primary or sole manifestation of a disease or secondary to another disease process.

Most vasculitic syndromes appear to be mediated in whole or in part by immune mechanisms, particularly deposition of immune complexes in vessel walls.

CLASSIFICATION **Systemic necrotizing vasculitis:**

1 *Classic polyarteritis nodosa* (PAN): Small and medium-sized muscular arteries involved, esp. branch points; commonly involves kidney, heart, liver, GI tract, peripheral nerves, skin; lungs usually spared.

2 *Allergic angiitis and granulomatosis* (Churg-Strauss disease): Granulomatous vasculitis of multiple organ systems, particularly the lung; similar to PAN but with higher frequency of involvement of lungs and vessels of multiple sizes and types; eosinophilic tissue infiltration, peripheral eosinophilia, and association with severe asthma.

3 *Polyangiitis overlap syndrome:* Overlap of PAN, allergic angiitis and granulomatosis, and manifestations of small-vessel hypersensitivity vasculitis.

Hypersensitivy vasculitis: Heterogeneous group of disorders; common feature is small-vessel involvement; skin disease usually predominates.

Exogenous stimuli proved or suspected:

• Henoch-Schönlein purpura. • Serum sickness and serum sickness-like reactions. • Drug-induced vasculitis. • Vasculitis associated with infectious diseases.

Endogenous antigens likely involved:

• Vasculitis associated with neoplasms. • Vasculitis associated with connective tissue disorders. • Vasculitis associated with other underlying diseases. • Vasculitis associated with congenital deficiencies of complement system.

Wegener's granulomatosis: Granulomatous vasculitis of upper and lower respiratory tracts together with glomerulonephritis; paranasal sinus congestion and pain, drainage, purulent or bloody nasal discharge. Mucosal ulceration, septal perforation, and cartilaginous destruction (saddle nose deformity) may result. Lung involvement may be asymptomatic or cause cough, hemoptysis, or dyspnea; eye involvement may occur; renal involvement accounts for most deaths.

Giant cell arteritis:

1 *Temporal arteritis:* Inflammation of medium- and large-sized arteries; temporal artery usually involved, but systemic involvement

may occur; fever, high ESR, anemia, musculoskeletal symptoms (polymyalgia rheumatica), sudden blindness are major manifestations; steroid therapy necessary to prevent ocular complications. 2 *Takayasu's arteritis:* Vasculitis of medium- and large-sized arteries with strong predilection for aortic arch and its branches; most common in young women; presents with inflammatory or ischemic symptoms in arms and neck, systemic inflammatory symptoms, AR.

Miscellaneous vasculitic syndromes:
• Mucocutaneous lymph node syndrome (Kawasaki's disease). • Isolated vasculitis of the central nervous system. • Thromboangiitis obliterans (Buerger's disease).

EVALUATION

- Thorough Hx and PE, with special reference to ischemic manifestations and systemic inflammatory signs/symptoms.
- CBC, ESR, serum chemistries, UA, ECG.
- Quantitative serum immunoglobulins.
- ANA, rheumatoid factor, VDRL, hepatitis B antigen and antibody, immune complexes, complement levels.
- Radiographic studies, including angiography of affected organs when necessary.
- Biopsy of affected organ system(s) necessary to establish diagnosis.

THERAPY Once diagnosis is established, therapy may be necessary with corticosteroids and/or cytotoxic agents. Cytotoxic agents are particularly important in syndromes with life-threatening organ system involvement, including Wegener's granulomatosis, PAN, allergic angiitis and granulomatosis, and isolated CNS vasculitis. Steroids alone may control temporal arteritis and Takayasu's arteritis. Some of the small-vessel syndromes may be particularly resistant to therapy. *Useful medications:*

- Prednisone 1 mg/kg per day initially, then tapered.
- Cyclophosphamide 2 mg/kg per day, adjusted to avoid severe leukopenia.
- Azathioprine 2 mg/kg per day, adjusted to avoid severe leukopenia; used when side effects of cyclophosphamide are prohibitive.

For more detailed discussion of this topic, see Fauci AS: The Vasculitis Syndromes, Chap. 269, in HPIM-11, p. 1438

112 SARCOIDOSIS

DEFINITION A systemic granulomatous disease of unknown etiology. Affected organs are characterized by an accumulation of lymphocytes and mononuclear phagocytes, noncaseating epithelioid granulomas, and derangements of normal tissue architecture.

PATHOPHYSIOLOGY Mononuclear cells, mostly T-helper lymphocytes and mononuclear phagocytes, accumulate in affected organs followed by formation of granulomas. No evidence that this process by itself permanently injures parenchyma of organ system; however, distortion of organ architecture from accumulation of these inflammatory components occurs. Granulomatous inflammation is maintained by secretion of mediators (including interleukin 2 and γ-interferon) by the activated T-helper lymphocytes. Severe damage of parenchyma can lead to irreversible fibrosis, which can alter further the structural integrity of organ and in advanced cases lead to serious organ dysfunction.

CLINICAL MANIFESTATIONS

- May be asymptomatic and discovered on routine CXR as hilar adenopathy and slight infiltrative disease of lung parenchyma.
- Constitutional symptoms: fever, weight loss, anorexia, fatigue.
- Lung: hilar adenopathy, alveolitis, interstitial pneumonitis, cough, dyspnea; pleural disease and hemoptysis rare; airways may be involved and cause obstruction to airflow; lung most commonly involved organ—90% with sarcoidosis will have abnormal CXR some time during course.
- Lymph nodes: intrathoracic and peripheral lymph nodes may be enlarged.
- Skin: 25% will have skin involvement; lesions include erythema nodosum, plaques, maculopapular eruptions, subcutaneous nodules, and lupus pernio (indurated blue-purple shiny lesions on face, fingers, and knees).
- Eye: uveitis in approximately 25%; may progress to blindness.
- Bone marrow and spleen: mild anemia and thrombocytopenia may occur.
- Liver: involved on biopsy in 60 to 90%; rarely important clinically.
- Kidney: may have parenchymal disease or more commonly nephrolithiasis secondary to abnormalities of calcium metabolism.
- Nervous system: may involve CNS, cranial nerves, peripheral nerves.
- Heart: may involve left ventricular wall or conduction system, causing disturbances of rhythm and/or contractility.

COMPLICATIONS Major morbidity and mortality related to progressive respiratory dysfunction in association with severe interstitial lung disease; eye involvement (including blindness) is most common extrapulmonary complication, but is manageable with corticosteroid treatment.

EVALUATION

- Hx and PE to rule out exposures and other evidence of interstitial lung disease.
- CBC, Ca^{++}, angiotensin converting enzyme, PPD and control skin tests, LFTs.
- CXR, ECG, PFTs.
- Bronchoalveolar lavage and gallium scan of lungs to help decide when treatment is indicated and to follow therapy.

TREATMENT Many cases remit spontaneously; therefore, deciding when treatment is necessary is difficult and controversial. Progressive lung involvement, eye disease, and cardiac disease are unequivocal indications for treatment. Bronchoalveolar lavage and gallium scanning may help to identify individuals with high risk of progression to end-stage lung stage; however, these are not uniformly accepted. Corticosteroids are mainstay of therapy. In patients with progressive disease failing steroid therapy, cytotoxic drugs may be helpful.

For more detailed discussion of this topic, see Crystal RG: Sarcoidosis, Chap. 270, in HPIM-11, p. 1445

---

113 APPROACH TO PATIENT WITH MUSCULOSKELETAL DISEASE

Musculoskeletal complaints are extremely common among patients seen in outpatient medical practice and are among the leading causes of disability and absenteeism from work. Musculoskeletal complaints must be evaluated in a uniform, thorough, and logical fashion to ensure the best chance of accurate diagnosis and to plan appropriate follow-up testing and therapy.

HISTORIC FEATURES

- Age, sex, race, family history.
- Mode of onset: characteristically acute in infection or gout, more chronic in osteoarthritis, rheumatoid arthritis.
- Duration of symptoms.
- Precipitating events: e.g., trauma, drug administration, associated illnesses.
- Number and pattern of involved structures: symmetrical? one joint or more than one? migratory? intermittent or continuous?
- Associated features: fever, rash, morning stiffness, involvement of other organ systems.

PHYSICAL EXAMINATION

- Complete examination with special attention to eyes, skin, mucuous membranes, heart, lungs, nails (may reveal characteristic pitting in psoriasis), nervous system.
- Careful and thorough examination of involved and uninvolved joints and periarticular structures; this should proceed in an organized fashion from head to foot or from extremities inward toward axial skeleton; special attention should be paid to identifying the presence or absence of (1) warmth, erythema, swelling; (2) joint or bursal effusions; (3) subluxation, dislocation, joint deformity; (4) synovial thickening; (5) joint instability; (6) limitations to active and passive range of motion; (7) crepitus.

ADDITIONAL INVESTIGATIONS

- CBC, ESR, serum uric acid.
- Joint radiographs.
- ANA, rheumatoid factor, ASO titer, complement levels.
- Synovial fluid aspiration and analysis; especially important in acute monarthritis or when crystal-induced or septic arthritis is suspected. Should be examined for (1) appearance, viscosity; (2) cell count; (3) glucose, protein; (4) crystals using polarizing microscope; (5) Gram's stain, cultures.

For more detailed discussion of this topic, see Cush JJ, Lipsky PE: Approach to Disorders of the Joints and Musculoskeletal Disorders, Chap. 273, in HPIM-11, p. 1454

114 ANKYLOSING SPONDYLITIS

DEFINITION Also known as rheumatoid spondylitis and Marie-Strümpell disease, this is a chronic and progressive inflammatory disease of spinal joints, sacroiliac joints, hips, shoulders, and occasionally peripheral joints. Most frequently presents in young men in third decade; strong association with histocompatibility antigen HLA-B27.

PATHOLOGY Earliest changes found in sacroiliac joints. Synovitis resembles that seen in RA with synovial hyperplasia, lymphoid cell accumulation, bony erosions, cartilage destruction followed by fibrosis and bony ankylosis (fusion). Ossification of the annulus fibrosis of intervertebral disks and anterior longitudinal ligament causes "bamboo spine" appearance on spine radiographs. Inflammation at insertion of tendons, ligaments, and capsules into bone is called "enthesitis." Focal medial necrosis at root of aorta may be seen.

CLINICAL MANIFESTATIONS

- Morning back pain and stiffness; peripheral joint pain (esp. hip).
- Chest pain from involvement of thoracic skeleton and muscular insertions.
- Aortic valve incompetence and regurgitation in 3%.
- Cardiac conduction defects.
- Acute anterior uveitis in 20–30%; may be recurrent.
- Constitutional symptoms may be severe: fever, anemia, fatigue, weight loss.
- Rare: amyloidosis, bilateral upper lobe lung fibrosis.
- Cauda equina syndrome: buttock or leg pain; leg weakness; loss of bladder or rectal sphincter control.
- Physical findings: tenderness over involved joints, diminished chest expansion, diminished anterior flexion of lumbar spine (Schober test).

LABORATORY FINDINGS

- ESR elevated in majority; normal in 20% of pts with mild disease; rheumatoid factor negative; mild anemia.
- Radiographs: early may be normal but will soon show progressive sclerosis of sacroiliac joints; spinal x-rays show straightening of lumbar spine, squaring of vertebrae, syndesmophytes ("bamboo spine").

DIFFERENTIAL DIAGNOSIS RA; juvenile RA; spondylitis associated with Reiter's syndrome, psoriatic arthritis, inflammatory bowel disease; diffuse idiopathic skeletal hyperostosis.

TREATMENT Maintenance of good posture; exercise; NSAIDs are mainstays of therapy; gold and chloroquine not useful; intraocular steroids for iritis; surgery to correct deformities.

For more detailed discussion of this topic, see Gilliland BC: Ankylosing Spondylitis, Chap. 267, in HPIM-11, p. 1434

115 DEGENERATIVE JOINT DISEASE

DEFINITION Osteoarthritis (OA) is a disorder characterized by progressive deterioration and loss of articular cartilage accompanied by proliferation of new bone and soft tissue in and around involved joint. Most common form of arthritis, OA affects almost all joints, especially weight-bearing and frequently used joints. In *primary* (idiopathic) OA no underlying cause is apparent. In *secondary* OA, a predisposing factor such as trauma, congenital abnormality, or metabolic disorder is present.

PATHOGENESIS Unknown events (? microfractures in subchondral bone from repeated impact of weight-bearing; ? primary changes in cartilage with secondary bony changes) stimulate chondrocytes and changes in structure of cartilage. Degradation of existing cartilage exceeds capacity of reparative processes and progressive cartilage loss occurs. Breakdown products of cartilage stimulate release of collagenase and other hydrolytic enzymes. Immune complexes and crystals of hydroxyapatite and/or calcium pyrophosphate may play a role in inducing inflammation.

CLINICAL MANIFESTATIONS

- Pain usually limited to one or a few joints, but may be generalized.
- Stiffness in morning or after rest may occur but usually brief.
- Pain at night or with weather changes may occur; patients may note crepitus.
- With progressive disease, joint motion becomes limited; subluxation and deformity may occur.
- Heberden's or Bouchard's nodes may occur at interphalangeal joints.
- Hip involvement more common in men than women; may be unilateral at first; internal rotation most limited in early stages.
- OA of knee may involve medial, lateral, or patellofemoral compartments; pain may be diffuse or localized to one compartment.
- Spine involvement may affect intervertebral disks, apophyseal joints, and paraspinal ligaments.
- Lumbar stenosis may cause cord compression due to posterior vertebral osteophytes; symptoms provoked by hyperextension of lumbar spine, relieved by flexion; laminectomy may be required if symptoms progress.
- Secondary OA due to traumatic, systemic, or congenital disorders may be unilateral, appear at early age, or involve joints not usually seen in OA.

LABORATORY FINDINGS

- Routine lab work usually normal.
- ESR usually normal but may be elevated in patients with primary generalized or erosive OA.

- Joint fluid is straw-colored with good viscosity; fluid WBCs < 2000; calcium pyrophosphate or hydroxyapatite crystals may be found in some fluids.
- Radiographs may be normal at first but as disease progresses may show joint space narrowing, subchondral bone sclerosis, osteophytes, joint surface erosions.
- Rheumatoid factor, ANA studies normal.

DIAGNOSIS Usually established on basis of pattern of joint involvement, normal laboratory tests, synovial fluid findings, and radiographic features. Differential diagnosis includes rheumatoid arthritis and crystal-induced arthritides.

TREATMENT Patient education, weight reduction, appropriate use of cane and other supports, isometric exercises to strengthen muscles around affected joints. Medical treatment includes salicylates or NSAIDs, intraarticular steroid injections; surgery and/or splinting may be necessary.

For more detailed discussion of this topic, see Gilliland BC: Degenerative Joint Disease, Chap. 274, in HPIM-11, p. 1456

---

116 GOUT, PSEUDOGOUT, AND RELATED DISEASES

GOUT

The term *gout* is applied to a spectrum of disorders which may encompass (in their fully developed states) five cardinal features which may occur singly or in combination:

1 Increased serum urate concentration
2 Recurrent arthritic attacks with urate crystals demonstrable in synovial fluid leukocytes
3 Appearance of tophi, aggregated deposits of monosodium urate monohydrate
4 Renal disease involving interstitial tissues and blood vessels
5 Uric acid nephrolithiasis

Pathogenesis: Hyperuricemia may arise from the overproduction or reduced excretion of uric acid or a combination of the two. Uric acid represents the end product of degradation of purine nucleotides; thus uric acid production is closely linked to pathways of purine metabolism, with the intracellular concentration of 5-phosphoribosyl-1-pyrophosphate (PRPP) being the major determinant of the rate of uric acid biosynthesis.

Primary hyperuricemia may occur from undefined metabolic defects or as the result of two inborn metabolic errors, partial hypoxanthine-guanine phosphoribosyltransferase (HGPRT) deficiency or PRPP synthetase superactivity.

Secondary hyperuricemia may be due to an increased rate of purine biosynthesis, type I glycogen storage disease, certain myeloproliferative and lymphoproliferative disorders, hemolytic anemias, thalassemia, certain hemoglobinopathies, pernicious anemia, infectious mononucleosis, and some carcinomas. Reduced excretion of uric acid may arise from renal causes, diuretic therapy, treatment with certain drugs, volume depletion, and competition by certain organic acids (e.g., in starvation ketosis, diabetic ketoacidosis, and lactic acidosis).

Acute gouty arthritis results from release of monosodium urate crystals into joint space, phagocytosis of these crystals by leukocytes, recruitment of additional phaygocytes into joint space, and inflammation of joint induced by activation of kallikrein and complement systems and release of lysosomal products and other toxins into synovial fluid.

Clinical manifestations:

1 *Asymptomatic hyperuricemia*: Nearly all pts with gout are hyperuricemic; however, only about 5% of hyperuricemic pts develop gout.

2 *Acute gouty arthritis*: Usually an exquisitely painful monarthritis but may be polyarticular and accompanied by fever; podagra (attack in the great toe) may occur eventually in 90% and may

be site of first attack in half; attack will generally subside spontaneously after days to weeks; during the subsequent intercritical period, pt is asymptomatic; diagnosis of acute gouty arthritis made by demonstration of characteristic monosodium urate crystals in joint fluid by polarizing microscopy.

3 *Tophi and chronic gouty arthritis*: Nodular (tophaceous) deposits of monosodium urate may develop after long periods of untreated hyperuricemia; commonly involve helix and antihelix of ears, ulnar surface of forearm, Achilles tendon; incidence has fallen due to effective antihyperuricemic therapy.

4 *Nephropathy*: May be due to deposition of monosodium urate crystals in renal interstitium or to obstruction of collecting system and ureter by urate crystals.

5 *Nephrolithiasis.*

Evaluation:

• Quantitation of urine uric acid. • Abdominal flat plate, possibly IVP. • Chemical analysis of renal stones. • Joint x-rays and synovial fluid analysis. • If overproduction is suspected, measurement of erythrocyte HGPRT and PRPP levels may be indicated.

Treatment:

- Necessity for treatment of asymptomatic hyperuricemia is controversial; probably not indicated unless pt becomes symptomatic; has strong family history of gout, renal disease, or stones; or excretes $>$ 1100 mg uric acid per day.
- Treatment of acute gouty attack: colchicine or NSAIDs (especially indomethacin).
- Prophylaxis with chronic colchicine or indomethacin; avoidance of precipitating factors (e.g., alcohol, purine-rich foods); antihyperuricemic therapy.
- Uricosuric agents: probenecid, sulfinpyrazone.
- Allopurinol: decreases uric acid synthesis by inhibiting xanthine oxidase.

PSEUDOGOUT

Definition and pathogenesis: Calcium pyrophosphate deposition disease (CPDD) characterized by acute and chronic inflammatory joint disease, usually affecting older individuals. The knee and other large joints most commonly affected. Calcium deposits in articular cartilage (chondrocalcinosis) may be seen radiographically.

CPDD may be classified into three categories: (1) a hereditary type; (2) a form associated with metabolic disorders, including hyperparathyroidism, hemochromatosis, hypophosphatasia, hypomagnesemia, hypothyroidism, gout, ochronosis, and Wilson's disease; and (3) an idiopathic form.

Crystals are not thought to form in synovial fluid but probably are shed from articular cartilage into joint space, where similar to gout they are phagocytosed by neutrophils and incite the characteristic inflammatory response.

Clinical manifestations: Acute *pseudogout* occurs in approximately 25% of pts with CPDD; knee is most frequently involved, but other joints may be affected; involved joint is erythematous, swollen, warm, and painful; most pts have evidence of chondrocalcinosis.

A minority will have involvement of multiple joints (*pseudorheumatoid disease*). Approximately half of pts with CPDD will have *chronic disease* with progressive degenerative changes in multiple joints. These pts may also have intermittent acute attacks.
Diagnosis: Made by demonstration of calcium pyrophosphate dihydrate crystals (appearing as short blunt rods, rhomboids, and cuboids with weak positive birefringence) in synovial fluid and finding of chondrocalcinosis in joint radiographs.
Treatment: Indomethacin or other NSAIDs; intraarticular injection of glucocorticosteroids; colchicine is variably effective.

HYDROXYAPATITE ARTHROPATHY

Crystal-induced arthritis may be observed due to calcium hydroxyapatite crystals; described mainly in knee and shoulder. Hydroxyapatite crystals may coexist with pyrophosphate crystals and must be identified using EM or x-ray diffraction studies. Radiographic appearance resembles CPDD. Treatment involves NSAIDs, repeated joint aspiration, and rest of affected joint.

For more detailed discussion of these topics, see Kelley WN, Palella TD: Gout and Other Disorders of Purine Metabolism, Chap. 309, p. 1623; and Gilliland BC: Calcium Pyrophosphate (Pseudogout) and Calcium Hydroxyapatite Deposition Diseases, Chap. 275, p. 1458, in HPIM-11

---

117 PSORIATIC ARTHRITIS

Approximately 5% of pts with psoriasis develop arthritis related to their skin disease. Some 50% of pts with psoriasis and spondylitis have the HLA-B27 histocompatibility antigen; however, there is no apparent relation between HLA-B27 and psoriatic peripheral arthritis. Onset of psoriasis usually precedes development of joint disease; approximately 15% of pts develop arthritis prior to onset of skin disease.

PATTERNS OF JOINT INVOLVEMENT

- Approximately 70% of pts have asymmetric oligoarticular arthritis affecting two or three joints simultaneously; proximal joints of hands and feet are frequently affected; "sausage digits" may be present reflecting involvement of interphalangeal joints.
- Some 15% of pts have symmetrical polyarthritis resembling RA; rheumatoid factor is negative.
- Approximately 10% have predominantly DIP involvement with psoriatic changes of adjacent nail.
- Rare pts have aggressive, destructive form of arthritis known as "arthritis mutilans" with severe joint deformities and bony dissolution.
- Approximately 20% of pts with psoriatic arthritis have spondylitis and/or sacroiliitis; spondylitis may occur in absence of peripheral arthritis.

LABORATORY FINDINGS

• Hypoproliferative anemia, elevated ESR. • Negative tests for rheumatoid factor. • Hyperuricemia. • Inflammatory synovial fluid and biopsy without specific findings. • Radiographic features include severe joint destruction with bony ankylosis, osteolysis, whittling of tufts of terminal phalanges, "pencil-in-cup" deformity.

DIAGNOSIS Suggested by presence of inflammatory arthritis in patient with skin and nail changes of psoriasis and in absence of findings characterisitic of other chronic inflammatory arthritides.

TREATMENT

• Aspirin and other NSAIDs. • Intraarticular glucocorticosteroid injections. • Gold salts in some patients. • Methotrexate in some selected patients with severe disease.

For more detailed discussion of this topic, see Gilliland BC: Psoriatric Arthritis and Arthritis Associated with Gastrointestinal Diseases, Chap. 276, in HPIM-11, p. 1460

118 INFECTIOUS ARTHRITIS AND OSTEOMYELITIS

INFECTIOUS ARTHRITIS

Acute bacterial or septic arthritis is a medical emergency requiring prompt diagnosis and therapy.

Etiology and pathogenesis: Bacteria may infect joint space during bacteremia from a penetrating wound, by extension from an adjacent osteomyelitis, or during surgical manipulations or diagnostic procedures. Certain individuals are more prone to development of septic arthritis due to host-defense defects, immunosuppressive therapy, or previous joint trauma.

Common bacterial pathogens include *N. gonorrhoeae, S. aureus, Strep. pneumoniae, Strep. pyogenes, H. influenzae,* and gram-negative bacilli (*E. coli, Salmonella, Pseudomonas* spp.). Less common pathogens include *Brucella,* mycobacteria, fungi, and viruses.

Clinical manifestations: Fever; warmth, erythema, swelling, and pain in affected joint(s); spasm and guarding of adjacent muscle groups; any joint can be involved, but knee, hip, shoulder, wrist, ankle, and elbow are most common. IV drug abusers have predilection for involvement of sternoclavicular or sacroiliac joint. Infection in spine may involve vertebral body, disk space, and apophyseal joint.

Laboratory findings:

- Synovial fluid aspiration should be performed immediately when joint infection is suspected; fluid is cloudy or purulent, WBCs 10,000 to >100,000/mm^3 with more than 90% neutrophils; glucose is low; Gram's stain may be positive for organisms; appropriate cultures must be performed.
- CBC may reveal leukocytosis.
- Radiographs show soft tissue swelling, distention of joint capsule, juxtaarticular osteoporosis, periosteal elevation, joint space narrowing, bony erosions; osteomyelitis may be seen.
- Bone scan may be useful in localizing infection; will be negative in soft tissue infection, while gallium scan will be positive in arthritis or soft tissue infection.

Diagnosis: Made by Gram's stain and/or culture demonstration of organisms in joint fluid. Differential diagnosis includes other causes of acute mono- or oligoarticular arthritis, e.g., gout, pseudogout, rheumatic fever, Reiter's syndrome, psoriatic arthritis, peripheral arthritis associated with inflammatory bowel disease, bursitis, cellulitis of skin adjacent to joint.

Treatment:

- Appropriate antibiotic therapy administered parenterally; instillation of antibiotics into joint is not necessary.

- Drainage is an essential modality of therapy; repeated aspiration will usually suffice; surgical drainage may be necessary in hip infections or if pus becomes loculated.

SPECIAL CASES

1 *Gonococcal arthritis:* Most common cause of arthritis in young adults; polyarthritis associated with bacteremia may evolve into monoarthritis; joint fluid cultures frequently negative; usually good response to antibiotic therapy.

2 *Tuberculous arthritis:* Spine, hips, knees, sacroiliac, wrists, and ankles most frequently involved. Often combined with tuberculous osteomyelitis. Course is insidious, usually monarticular; fever and night sweats may be present; diagnosis made by demonstrating bacilli in fluid or tissue by smear, histology, or culture.

3 *Mycotic arthritis:* In systemic mycoses or actinomycosis.

4 *Syphilitic arthritis:* In congenital, secondary, or tertiary syphilis.

5 *Viral arthritis:* Rubella, hepatitis B, arboviruses, adenoviruses, infectious mononucleosis, varicella.

6 *Lyme disease:* Multisystem disease caused by tick-borne spirochete; arthritis, neurologic and cardiac abnormalities, skin lesions.

OSTEOMYELITIS

May be due to virtually any kind of organism; however, bacterial pathogens are most common. Bacteria can reach bone by (1) hematogenous spread, (2) direct extensions from contiguous site of infection, or (3) directly via trauma (including surgery).

Clinical manifestations: *Hematogenous osteomyelitis:* In adults most commonly involves spine. Symptoms include back pain, fever (may be minimal or absent), muscle spasm, and local tenderness. In other sites, findings are pain and evidence of soft tissue infection overlying affected bone.

Posttraumatic osteomyelitis or osteomyelitis from continguous infection: Features are local pain, draining sinuses, swelling, tenderness, and erythema over infected site. Infected joint prostheses may present with pain and loosening months after surgery.

Diagnosis: Requires isolation of organisms from bone aspiration, biopsy, or blood culture; radiographic studies may be helpful; bone scanning with technetium pyrophosphate usually positive.

Treatment: Rest of affected part; parenteral antibiotics for 4–6 weeks; surgical debridement when necessary; external stabilization may be necessary for spine infections; removal of infected prosthesis generally required.

For more detailed discussion of these topics, see Gilliland BC, Petersdorf RG: Infectious Arthritis, Chap. 277, p. 1462; and Hirschmann JV: Osteomyelitis, Chap. 340, p. 1910, in HPIM-11

119 REITER'S SYNDROME

DEFINITION A disorder characterized by seronegative, oligoarticular, asymmetric arthritis with urethritis and/or cervicitis.

PATHOGENESIS Two clinical forms of syndrome are recognized: postvenereal and postdysenteric (see also Chap. 120). Reiter's syndrome is most common cause of arthritis in young men. Up to 90% of pts carry the HLA-B27 alloantigen.

Syndrome is thought to be triggered in individuals with appropriate genetic background by an infection of urogenital or GI tracts with organisms such as *Chlamydia trachomatis*, *Ureoplasma urealyticum*, *Shigella dysenteriae*, *S. flexneri*, *Salmonella enteritidis*, *Yersinia enterocolitica*, or *Campylobacter jejuni*.

CLINICAL MANIFESTATIONS

- Usually begins with urethritis followed by conjunctivitis and arthritis; urethral discharge intermittent and may be asymptomatic; conjunctivitis, usually minimal; uveitis, keratitis, and optic neuritis rarely present.
- Arthritis usually acute, asymmetric, oligoarticular, involving predominantly lower extremities; plantar fasciitis and Achilles tendonitis common; sacroiliitis may ocur.
- Mucocutaneous lesions: painless lesions on glans penis and oral mucosa in approximately a third of pts; keratoderma blenorrhagica (crusted scaling papules) may occur in postvenereal form but not in postdysenteric variety.
- Uncommon manifestations: pleuropericarditis, aortic regurgitation, neurologic manifestations, secondary amyloidosis.
- Prognosis is variable; a third will have recurrent or sustained disease, with 15 to 25% developing permanent disability.

LABORATORY FINDINGS Nonspecific; rheumatoid factor and ANA negative; mild anemia, leukocytosis, elevated ESR may be seen; synovial fluid analysis nondiagnostic.

DIAGNOSIS Presence of asymmetric seronegative oligoarthritis for >1 month with nonspecific urethritis or cervicitis allows diagnosis with approximately 80% specificity; differential diagnosis includes gonococcal arthritis and psoriatic arthritis.

TREATMENT Analgesics and NSAIDs; local corticosteroid injections may be useful; in severe destructive arthritis, cytotoxic drugs may be necessary.

For more detailed discussion of this topic, see Moutsopoulos HM: Reiter's Syndrome and Behçet's Syndrome, Chap. 268 in HPIM-11, p. 1436

ARTHRITIS ASSOCIATED WITH BOWEL DISEASE

Both peripheral arthritis and spondylitis may be associated with *ulcerative colitis* or *regional enteritis*. Spondylitis associated with inflammatory bowel disease (IBD) is indistinguishable from ankylosing spondylitis. Peripheral arthritis is episodic, asymmetric, and most frequently affects knee and ankle. Attacks usually subside within several weeks and characteristically resolve completely without residual joint damage.

Laboratory findings are nonspecific; rheumatoid factors absent; radiographs of peripheral joints usually normal; spine films resemble ankylosing spondylitis.

Treatment is directed at underlying IBD; aspirin and NSAIDs may alleviate joint symptoms.

Some pts will develop arthritis and/or vasculitis following *intestinal bypass* surgery. Treatment involves reconnection of bowel, if possible, or suppression of bacterial overgrowth with tetracycline or other antibiotics. Aspirin and NSAIDs may be of benefit.

Whipple's disease is characterized by arthritis in approximately two-thirds of pts and usually precedes appearance of intestinal symptoms. GI and joint manifestations respond to antibiotic therapy.

NEUROPATHIC JOINT DISEASE

Also known as Charcot's joint, this is a severe form of osteoarthritis that occurs in joints deprived of pain and position sense; may occur in tabes dorsalis, diabetic neuropathy, meningomyelocele, amyloidosis, or leprosy. Usually begins in a single joint but may spread to involve other joints. *Treatment* involves stabilization of joint; surgical fusion may improve function.

RELAPSING POLYCHONDRITIS

An idiopathic disorder characterized by recurrent inflammation of cartilaginous structures, eyes, ears, and cardiovascular system. Cardinal manifestations include ear and nose involvement with floppy ear and saddle nose deformities, scleritis, conjunctivitis, iritis, oral and/or genital ulcerations, episodic nondeforming polyarthritis, collapse of tracheal and bronchial cartilage rings, aortic regurgitation, and vasculitis of medium or large vessels.

Diagnosis is made clinically and may be confirmed by biopsy of affected cartilage. *Treatment* is glucocorticoids, with addition of cytotoxic agents if disease progresses.

HYPERTROPHIC OSTEOARTHROPATHY

Syndrome consisting of periosteal new bone formation, digital clubbing, and arthritis. Most commonly seen in association with lung carcinoma, but also occurs with chronic lung or liver disease;

congenital heart, lung, or liver disease in children; and idiopathic and familial forms. *Symptoms* include burning and aching pain most pronounced in distal extremities. Radiographs show periosteal thickening with new bone formation of distal ends of long bones. *Treatment* is that of associated disorder.

FIBROSITIS

A common disorder characterized by pain, aching, and stiffness of trunk and extremities, and presence of a number of specific tender sites (trigger points). More common in women than men. Frequently associated with sleep disorders. *Diagnosis* is made clinically; there are no laboratory or radiographic abnormalities. *Treatment* is supportive care, salicylates, NSAIDs, benzodiazepines or tricyclics for sleep disorder, and local measures (heat, massage, injection of trigger points).

REFLEX SYMPATHETIC DYSTROPHY SYNDROME (RSDS)

A syndrome of pain and tenderness, usually of a hand or foot, associated with vasomotor instability, trophic skin changes, and rapid development of bony demineralization. Frequently, development will follow a precipitating event (local trauma, myocardial infarction, stroke, or peripheral nerve injury). Early recognition and treatment can be effective in preventing disability. *Therapeutic options* include pain control, application of heat or cold, exercise, sympathetic nerve block, and short courses of high-dose prednisone in conjunction with physical therapy.

PERIARTICULAR DISORDERS

Bursitis is inflammation of the thin-walled bursal sac surrounding tendons and muscles over bony prominences. The subacromial and greater trochanteric bursae are most commonly involved. *Treatment* involves prevention of aggravating conditions, rest, NSAIDs, and local steroid injections.

Tendonitis may involve virtually any tendon but frequently affects tendons of the rotator cuff around shoulder, especially the supraspinatus. Pain is dull and aching but becomes acute and sharp when tendon is squeezed below acromion. NSAIDs, steroid injection, and physical therapy may be beneficial. The rotator cuff tendons or biceps tendon may rupture acutely, frequently requiring surgical repair.

Calcific tendonitis results from deposition of calcium salts in tendon, usually supraspinatus. The resulting pain may be sudden and severe.

Adhesive capsulitis ("frozen shoulder") results from conditions which enforce prolonged immobility of shoulder joint. Shoulder is painful and tender to palpation, and both active and passive range of motion is restricted. Spontaneous improvement may occur; local injections of steroids, NSAIDs, and physical therapy may be helpful.

For more detailed discussion of these topics, see Gilliland BC: Psoriatric Arthritis and Arthritis Associated with Gastrointestinal Diseases, Chap. 276, p. 1460; and Gilliland BC: Miscellaneous Arthritides and Extraarticular Rheumatism, Chap. 278 p. 1465, in HPIM-11

---

121 AMYLOIDOSIS

DEFINITION A disease characterized by deposition of the fibrous protein amyloid in one or more sites of the body. Clinical manifestations depend on anatomic distribution and intensity of amyloid protein deposition and range from local deposition with little significance to involvement of virtually any organ system with consequent severe pathophysiologic changes.

BIOCHEMISTRY OF AMYLOID FIBRILS Chemical characterization of amyloid fibrils reveals several varieties associated with different clinical situations:

1 *AL:* Associated with primary amyloid and amyloid associated with multiple myeloma; has significant homology to *N*-terminal sequence of immunoglobulin light chains.
2 *AA:* Found in secondary amyloid deposits and patients with familial Mediterranean fever (FMF); formed from serum precursor (SAA); SAA release from hepatocytes induced by interleukin 1.
3 *AF:* Found in familial form; identical to prealbumin except for single amino acid substitution.
4 AE_{mct}: Associated with medullary thyroid carcinoma; fibril is probably a calcitonin precursor.
5 *AS:* May be related to realbumin; found in senile cardiac amyloid.
6 *AP:* P component; found in most systemic forms; distinct from amyloid fibrils.

CLASSIFICATION

1 *Primary amyloidosis:* No evidence for preexisting or coexisting disease; AL type deposits.
2 *Amyloidosis associated with myeloma:* AL type.
3 *Secondary (reactive) amyloidosis:* AA type; associated with chronic infectious or inflammatory diseases.
4 *Heredofamilial amyloidosis:* AF type; amyloidosis associated with FMF (AA type), and a variety of other syndromes (AF type).
5 *Local amyloidosis.*
6 *Senile amyloidosis:* Associated with aging; heart and brain especially involved.

CLINICAL MANIFESTATIONS Major clinical findings may include proteinuria, nephrosis, azotemia, CHF, cardiomegaly, arrhythmias, cutaneous involvement with raised waxy papules, GI obstruction or ulceration, hemorrhage, protein loss, diarrhea, macroglossia, disordered esophageal motility, neuropathy, postural hypotension, arthritis, respiratory obstruction, and selective clotting factor deficiency.

DIAGNOSIS Requires demonstration of amyloid in a biopsy of affected tissue using appropriate stains (e.g., Congo red). Electrophoresis and immunoelectrophoresis of serum and urine may assist in detecting paraproteins.

PROGNOSIS AND TREATMENT Prognosis of generalized amyloidosis is poor, with renal failure most common cause of death. Treatment involves therapy of underlying disease; colchicine may be effective, especially in FMF.

For more detailed discussion of this topic, see Cohen AS: Amyloidosis, Chap. 259, in HPIM-11, p. 1403

SECTION VIII
HEMATOLOGY AND ONCOLOGY

122 THE BLOOD FILM

ERYTHROCYTE (RBC) MORPHOLOGY Normal: 7.5-μm diameter.

- *Reticulocytes* (Wright's stain)—large, grayish-blue, admixed with pink (polychromasia); variation in RBC size (anisocytosis) or abnormal shapes (poikilocytosis) may provide clues to causes of anemia.
- *Acanthocytes* (spur cells)—irregularly spiculated; abetalipoproteinemia, severe liver disease, rarely anorexia nervosa.
- *Echinocytes* (burr cells)—regularly shaped, uniformly distributed spiny projections; uremia, RBC volume loss.
- *Elliptocytes*—elliptical; hereditary elliptocytosis.
- *Schizocytes* (schistocytes)—fragmented cells of varing sizes and shapes; microangiopathic or macroangiopathic hemolytic anemia.
- *Sickled cells*—elongated, crescentic; sickle cell anemias.
- *Spherocytes*—small hyperchromic cells lacking normal central pallor; hereditary spherocytosis, extravascular hemolysis as in autoimmune hemolytic anemia, glucose-6-phosphate dehydrogenase (G6PD) deficiency.
- *Target cells*—central and outer rim staining with intervening ring of pallor; liver disease, thalassemia, hemoglobin C and sickle C diseases.
- *Teardrop cells*—myelofibrosis, other infiltrative processes of marrow (e.g., carcinoma).
- *Rouleaux formation*—alignment of RBCs in stacks; may be artifactual or due to paraproteinemia (e.g., multiple myeloma, macroglobulinemia).

RBC INCLUSIONS

- *Howell-Jolly bodies*—1-μm diameter basophilic cytoplasmic inclusion, usually single; asplenic pts.
- *Basophilic stippling*—multiple, punctate basophilic cytoplasmic inclusions; lead poisoning, thalassemia, myelofibrosis.
- *Pappenheimer (iron) bodies*—resemble basophilic stippling, but also stain with Prussian blue; lead poisoning, other sideroblastic anemias.
- *Heinz bodies*—seen only with supravital stains, such as crystal violet; G6PD deficiency (after oxidant stress such as infection, certain drugs), unstable hemoglobin variants.
- *Parasites*—characteristic intracytoplasmic inclusions; malaria, babesiosis.

LEUKOCYTE INCLUSIONS

- *Toxic granulations*—dark cytoplasmic granules; bacterial infection.
- *Döhle bodies*—1–2 μm blue, oval cytoplasmic inclusions; bacterial infection, Chediak-Higashi anomaly.
- *Auer rods*—eosinophilic, rodlike cytoplasmic inclusions; acute myelogenous leukemia (some cases).

PLATELET ABNORMALITIES

- *Platelet clumping*—an in vitro artifact, often readily detectable on smear; can lead to falsely low platelet count by automated cell counters.

For more detailed discussion of this topic, see Bunn FH: Anemia, Chap. 53, p. 262; Gallin JJ: Disorders of Phagocytic Cells, Chap. 56, p. 278, in HPIM-11

---

123 BONE MARROW EXAMINATION

Aspiration assesses cell morphology. *Biopsy* assesses overall marrow architecture, including degree of cellularity.

INDICATIONS **Aspiration:** Hypoproliferative anemia, unexplained leukopenia or thrombocytopenia, suspected leukemia or myeloma, evaluation of iron stores.

Special tests: Histochemical staining (leukemias), cytogenetic studies (leukemias, lymphomas), microbiology (bacterial, mycobacterial, fungal cultures), Prussian blue (iron) stain (assess iron stores; diagnosis of sideroblastic anemias).

Biopsy: Performed in addition to aspiration for possible pancytopenia (rule out aplastic anemia), metastatic tumor, granulomatous infection (e.g., mycobacteria, brucellosis, histoplasmosis), myelofibrosis, lipid storage disease (e.g., Gaucher's, Niemann-Pick), any case with "dry tap" on aspiration.

Special tests: Histochemical staining (e.g., acid phosphatase for metastatic prostate carcinoma), immunoperoxidase staining (e.g., immunoglobulin detection in multiple myeloma, lysozyme detection in monocytic leukemia), reticulin staining (increased in myelofibrosis), microbiological staining (e.g., acid-fast staining for mycobacteria).

INTERPRETATION **Cellularity:** Varies inversely with age; a simple formula is: Normal marrow cellularity (%) = 100 − age of patient. Therefore, 70% cellularity normal for a 30 year-old patient but abnormally hypercellular for a 70 year-old patient.

Myeloid:erythroid (M:E) ratio: Normally 3:1 to 4:1. The M:E ratio is *increased* in acute and chronic infection, leukemoid reactions (e.g., chronic inflammation, metastatic tumor), acute and chronic myelogenous leukemia, myelodysplastic disorders ("preleukemia") and pure red cell aplasia; *decreased* in agranulocytosis, anemias with erythroid hyperplasia (megaloblastic, iron-deficiency, thalassemia, hemorrhage, hemolysis, sideroblastic), and erythrocytosis (excessive RBC production); *normal* in aplastic anemia (though marrow hypocellular), myelofibrosis (marrow hypocellular), multiple myeloma, lymphoma, anemia of chronic disease.

CYTOGENETIC, HISTOCHEMICAL, AND IMMUNOLOGIC TESTS See HPIM-11, Chaps. 289, 290, 291.

For more detailed discussion of this topic, see Gallin JJ: Disorders of Phagocytic Cells, Chap. 56, in HPIM-11, p. 278

ANEMIA

Blood hemoglobin (Hb) concentration < 14 g/dL or hematocrit (Hct) < 42% in adult males; Hb < 12 g/dL or Hct < 37% in adult females.

Basic evaluations: (1) *reticulocyte index,* (2) review of *blood smear* and *RBC indices* [mean corpuscular volume (MCV), mean corpuscular hemoglobin (MCH), mean corpuscular hemoglobin concentration (MCHC)], and (3) determination of *acuteness* or *chronicity* of anemia.

The *reticulocyte index* (RI) = [reticulocyte count (%) × observed Hct]/(2 × normal Hct). RI < 2% implies inadequate RBC production; RI > 2% implies excessive RBC destruction or loss.

ANEMIA DUE TO EXCESSIVE RBC DESTRUCTION OR LOSS

Blood Loss: Trauma, GI hemorrhage (may be occult); less commonly genitourinary sources (menorrhagia, gross hematuria), retroperitoneal, iliopsoas hemorrhage (e.g., in hip fractures).

Hemolysis:

1 *Hypersplenism* (pancytopenia may be present).

2 *Immunohemolytic anemia* (positive Coombs' test, spherocytes). Two types: (a) *warm* antibody (usually IgG)—idiopathic, lymphomas, chronic lymphocytic leukemia, systemic lupus erythematosus, drugs (e.g., methyldopa, penicillins, quinine, quinidine, isoniazid, sulfonamides); and (b) *cold* antibody—cold agglutinin disease (IgM) due to *Mycoplasma* infection, infectious mononucleosis, lymphoma, idiopathic; paroxysmal cold hemoglobinuria (IgG) due to syphilis, viral infections.

3 *Mechanical trauma* (macro- and microangiopathic hemolytic anemias; schistocytes)—prosthetic heart valves, vasculitis, malignant hypertension, eclampsia, renal graft rejection, giant hemangioma, scleroderma, thrombotic thrombocytopenic purpura, hemolytic-uremic syndrome, DIC, march hemoglobinuria (e.g., marathon runners).

4 *Direct toxic effect*—infections (e.g., malaria, *Clostridia,* toxoplasmosis).

5 *Membrane abnormalities*—spur cell anemia (cirrhosis, anorexia nervosa), paroxysmal nocturnal hemoglobinuria, hereditary spherocytosis (increased RBC osmotic fragility, spherocytes).

6 *Intracellular RBC abnormalities*—enzyme defects [glucose-6 phosphate dehydrogenase deficiency (G6PD), pyruvate kinase deficiency (PK)], hemoglobinopathies, sickle cell anemia and variants, thalassemia, unstable hemoglobin variants.

Laboratory abnormalities: Elevated reticulocyte index, polychromasia and nucleated RBCs on smear; also spherocytes, schistocytes, target, spur, or sickle cells may be present depending on disorder; elevated unconjugated serum bilirubin and lactate de hydrogenase (LDH), elevated plasma hemoglobin, low or absent haptoglobin; look for urine hemosiderin or hemoglobin (latter seen in brisk, *intravascular* hemolysis); Coombs' test (immunohemolytic anemias), osmotic fragility test (hereditary spherocytosis), hemoglobin electrophoresis (sickle cell anemia, thalassemia), G6PD assay (best performed *after resolution* of hemolytic episode to prevent false-negative result).

ANEMIA DUE TO INADEQUATE RBC PRODUCTION Hypochromic anemias (MCHC < 32%): (1) *Iron deficiency* (e.g., blood loss, pregnancy, impaired gut absorption); (2) *thalassemia;* (3) *sideroblastic anemias* (e.g., hereditary, 2° drugs such as alcohol, lead). Anemia of chronic disorders (inflammatory, infectious, neoplastic) is also occasionally hypochromic.

Iron studies may help in the differential diagnosis (see Table 124-1).

Normochromic anemias (MCHC 32–36%): May be *normocytic* (MCV 82–94 fL) or *macrocytic* (MCV > 94 fL).

Normocytic anemias—(1) Anemia of chronic disorders; (2) endocrinopathies (e.g., hypothyroidism, adrenal insufficiency, hyperparathyroidism); (3) chronic renal insufficiency; (4) marrow failure (e.g., irradiation, drugs—chloramphenicol, antineoplastic agents; chemicals—benzene; viral—parvovirus, hepatitis B, human immunodeficiency virus); (5) marrow replacement (e.g., metastatic carcinoma, leukemia, myelofibrosis).

Macrocytic anemias—(1) Chronic hepatic disorders (e.g., cirrhosis, chronic hepatitis); (2) alcoholism; (3) hypothyroidism (anemia may also be normocytic); (4) megaloblastic anemias (e.g., B_{12}, folate deficiencies); (5) myelodysplasia (Chap. 129).

BONE MARROW EXAMINATION FOR ANEMIA See Chap. 123.

TREATMENT OF ANEMIA General approaches: The acuteness and severity determine whether *transfusion therapy* with packed RBCs is indicated. Rapid occurrence of severe anemia (e.g., after acute GI hemorrhage resulting in Hct < 27, following volume repletion) is a general indication for transfusion. For each unit of packed RBCs, Hct should increase 3–4% (Hb by 1 g/dL), assuming no ongoing losses. *Chronic* anemia (e.g., B_{12} deficiency secondary to pernicious anemia), even when severe, may not require trans-

TABLE 124-1

Disorder	Serum iron (Fe)*	Iron-binding capacity*	Fe/IBC (%)*	Ferritin*
Iron-deficiency	D	I	D (<15%)	D
Anemia of chronic disorders	D	D	N (~30%)	N/I
Thalassemia	N	N	N	N
Sideroblastic anemia	I	N	I (>60%)	I

* D = decreased; I = increased; N = normal.

fusion therapy if the patient is compensated and specific therapy (e.g. parenteral B_{12}) is instituted.

Specific disorders: (1) *Autoimmune hemolysis:* corticosteroids, sometimes immunosuppressive agents, danazol, plasmapheresis; (2) *G6PD deficiency:* avoid agents known to precipitate hemolysis (e.g., primaquine, sulfonamides, nitrofurantoin); (3) *aplastic anemia:* antithymocyte globulin, bone marrow transplantation; (4) *iron deficiency:* treat cause of blood loss; oral iron (e.g., $FeSO_4$ 300 mg tid); (5) *B_{12} deficiency:* parenteral B_{12} required in most cases (e.g., pernicious anemia—lack of *intrinsic factor* prevents dietary absorption); vitamin B_{12} 100 μg IM qd for 7 days, then 100–1000 μg IM per month; (6) *folate deficiency:* common in malnourished, alcoholics; folic acid 1 mg PO qd (5 mg qd for patients with malabsorption).

ERYTHROCYTOSIS

Also known as polycythemia, this is an increase above the normal range of RBCs in the circulation. *Relative erythrocytosis*—due to plasma volume loss (e.g., severe dehydration, burns); does not represent a true increase in total RBC mass. *Absolute erythrocytosis*—increase in total RBC mass.

Causes: Polycythemia vera (Chap. 129), erythropoietin-producing neoplasms (e.g., hypernephroma, cerebellar hemangioma), chronic hypoxemia (e.g., high altitude, pulmonary disease), carboxyhemoglobin excess (e.g. smokers), high-affinity hemoglobin variants, Cushing's syndrome, androgen excess.

Complications: Hyperviscosity (with diminished O_2 delivery) with risk of ischemic organ injury.

Treatment: Phlebotomy recommended for Hct $> 55\%$, regardless of cause.

For more detailed discussion of this topic, see Schafer AI, Bunn HF: Anemias of Iron Deficiency and Iron Overload, Chap. 284, p. 1493; Babior BM, Bunn HF: Megaloblastic Anemias, Chap. 285, p. 1498; Bunn HF: Anemia Associated with Chronic Disorders, Chap. 286, p. 1504; Cooper RA, Bunn HF: Hemolytic Anemias, Chap. 287, p. 1506, in HPIM-11

125 LEUKOCYTOSIS

APPROACH Review *smear* (? abnormal cells present) and obtain *differential* count. The normal values for concentration of blood leukocytes are shown in Table 125-1.

NEUTROPHILIA Absolute neutrophil count (polys and bands) > 10,000/mm³.
Causes: (1) *Exercise, stress;* (2) *infections*—esp. bacterial; smear shows increased numbers of immature neutrophils ("left shift"), toxic granulations, Döhle bodies; (3) *burns;* (4) *tissue necrosis* (e.g., myocardial, pulmonary, renal infarction); (5) *chronic inflammatory disorders* (e.g., gout, vasculitis); (6) *drugs* (e.g., glucocorticoids, epinephrine, lithium); (7) *myeloproliferative disorders* (Chap. 129); (8) *metabolic* (e.g., ketoacidosis, uremia); (9) *other*—malignant neoplasms, acute hemorrhage or hemolysis, after splenectomy.

LEUKEMOID REACTION Extreme elevation of leukocyte count (>50,000/mm³) secondary to mature and/or immature neutrophils.
Causes: (1) *Infection* (severe, chronic), esp. in children; (2) *hemolysis* (severe); (3) *malignant neoplasms* (esp. carcinoma of the breast, lung, kidney). May be distinguished from chronic myelogenous leukemia (CML) by measurement of the *leukocyte alkaline phosphatase (LAP) level:* elevated in leukemoid reactions, depressed in CML.

LEUKOERYTHROBLASTIC REACTION Similar to leukemoid reaction with addition of nucleated RBCs on blood smear.
Causes: (1) *Myelophthisis*—invasion of the bone marrow by tumor, fibrosis, granulomatous processes; smear shows "teardrop" RBCs; (2) *hemorrhage or hemolysis* (rarely, in severe cases).

LYMPHOCYTOSIS Absolute lymphocyte count > 5000/mm³.
Causes: (1) *Infection*—infectious mononucleosis, hepatitis, CMV, rubella, pertussis, TBC, brucellosis, syphilis; (2) *endocrine*—thyrotoxicosis, adrenal insufficiency; (3) *neoplastic*—chronic lymphocytic leukemia (CLL), most common cause of lymphocyte count > 10,000/mm³.

MONOCYTOSIS Absolute monocyte count > 800/mm³.
Causes: (1) *Infection*—subacute bacterial endocarditis, TBC, brucellosis, rickettsial diseases (e.g., Rocky Mountain spotted fever),

TABLE 125-1

Cell type	Mean (cells/mm³)	95% confidence limits (cells/mm³)	Percent total WBC
Neutrophil	3650	1830–7250	30–60
Lymphocyte	2500	1500–4000	20–50
Monocyte	430	200–950	2–10
Eosinophil	150	0–700	0.3–5
Basophil	30	0–150	0.6–1.8

Modified from Table A-13, HPIM-11, p. A-10.

malaria, leishmaniasis; (2) *granulomatous diseases*—sarcoidosis, Crohn's disease; (3) *collagen-vascular diseases*—rheumatoid arthritis, SLE, polyarteritis nodosa, polymyositis, temporal arteritis; (4) *hematologic*—leukemias, lymphoma, myeloproliferative and myelodysplastic syndromes, hemolytic anemia, chronic idiopathic neutropenia; (5) *malignant neoplasms.*

EOSINOPHILIA Absolute eosinophil count > 500/mm^3.
Causes: (1) *Drugs;* (2) *parasitic infections;* (3) *allergic diseases;* (4) *collagen-vascular diseases;* (5) *malignant neoplasms;* (6) *hypereosinophilic syndromes.*

BASOPHILIA Absolute basophil count > 100/mm^3.
Causes: (1) *Allergic diseases;* (2) *myeloproliferative disorders* (esp. CML); (3) *chronic inflammatory disorders* (rarely).

For more detailed discussion of this topic, see Adamson JW: The Myeloproliferative Diseases, Chap. 289, p. 1527; Chauplin R, Golde DW: The Leukemias, Chap. 292, p. 1541, HPIM-11

---

126 LEUKOPENIA

DEFINITION Total leukocyte count < 4300/mm^3.

NEUTROPENIA Absolute neutrophil count < 2500/mm^3 (increased risk of bacterial infection with count < 1000/mm^3). **Causes:** (1) *Drugs*—phenytoin, carbamazepine, indomethacin, chloramphenicol, penicillins, sulfonamides, cephalosporins, propylthiouracil, phenothiazines, captopril, methyldopa, procainamide, chlorpropamide, thiazides, cimetidine, allopurinol, colchicine, ethanol, penicillamine, chemotherapeutic and immunosuppressive agents; (2) *infections*—viral (e.g., influenza, hepatitis, infectious mononucleosis, human immunodeficiency virus), bacterial (e.g., typhoid fever, miliary TBC, fulminant sepsis), malaria; (3) *nutritional*—B_{12}, folate deficiencies; (4) *benign*—mild neutropenia common in blacks, no associated risk of infection; (5) *hematologic*—cyclic neutropenia (q 21 days, with recurrent infections common), leukemia, myelodysplasia (preleukemia), aplastic anemia, bone marrow infiltration (uncommon cause), Chediak-Higashi syndrome; (6) *hypersplenism*–e.g., Felty's syndrome, congestive splenomegaly, Gaucher's disease; (7) *autoimmune*—idiopathic, SLE, lymphoma (may see positive anti-neutrophil antibodies).
Management of the febrile, neutropenic patient: In addition to usual sources of infection, consider *"occult" sites* (e.g., paranasal sinuses, oral cavity, anorectal region); empiric therapy with broad-spectrum antibiotics is usually indicated after blood and other appropriate cultures are obtained. Prolonged neutropenia (>14 days) leads to increased risk of disseminated *fungal* infections; may require addition of antifungal chemotherapy (e.g., amphotericin B). Granulocyte transfusions may be helpful (controversial).

LYMPHOPENIA Absolute lymphocyte count < 1000/mm^3. **Causes:** (1) *Acute stressful illness*—e.g., MI, pneumonia, sepsis; (2) *glucocorticoid therapy*; (3) *lymphoma* (esp. Hodgkin's disease); (4) *immune deficiency syndromes*—ataxia telangiectasia, Wiskott-Aldrich, DiGeorge's syndromes; (5) *immunosuppressive therapy*—e.g., antilymphocyte globulin, cyclophosphamide; (6) *after radiotherapy* (esp. for lymphoma); (7) *intestinal lymphangiectasia* (increased lymph loss); (8) *chronic illness*—e.g., CHF, uremia, SLE, disseminated malignancies; (9) *bone marrow failure/replacement*—e.g., aplastic anemia, miliary TBC.

MONOCYTOPENIA Absolute monocyte count < 100/mm^3. **Causes:** (1) *Acute stressful illness*; (2) *glucocorticoid therapy*; (3) *aplastic anemia;* (4) *leukemia* (certain types, e.g., hairy cell leukemia); (5) *chemotherapeutic* and *immunosuppressive* agents.

EOSINOPENIA Absolute eosinophil count < 50/mm^3. **Causes:** (1) *Acute stressful illness;* (2) *Glucocorticoid therapy.*

For more detailed discussion of these topics, see Gallin JJ: Disorders of Phagocytic Cells, Chap. 56, p 278; Masur H, Fauci AS:

Infections in the Compromised Host, Chap. 84, p 466; Rappeport JJ, Bunn HF: Bone Marrow Failure: Aplastic Anemia and Other Primary Bone Marrow Disorders, Chap. 290, p 1533, in HPIM-11

127 BLEEDING AND THROMBOTIC DISORDERS

BLEEDING DISORDERS

Bleeding may result from abnormalities of (1) platelets, (2) blood vessel walls, or (3) coagulation. *Platelet disorders* characteristically produce *petechial* and *purpuric skin lesions* and bleeding from *mucosal* surfaces. *Defective coagulation* results in *ecchymoses, hematomas,* and *mucosal* and, in some disorders, recurrent *joint bleeding* (hemarthroses).

PLATELET DISORDERS Thrombocytopenia: Normal platelet count is 150,000—350,000/mm³. Bleeding is rare if platelet count > 100,000/mm³. *Bleeding time,* a measurement of platelet function, is abnormally increased if platelet count < 100,000/mm³; injury or surgery may provoke excess bleeding. Spontaneous bleeding unusual unless count is < 20,000/mm³; platelet count < 10,000/mm³ often is associated with serious hemorrhage. *Bone marrow examination* shows increased number of megakaryocytes in disorders associated with accelerated platelet destruction; decreased number in disorders of platelet production.

Causes: (1) *Production defects* such as marrow injury (e.g., drugs, irradiation), marrow failure (e.g., aplastic anemia), marrow invasion (e.g., carcinoma, leukemia, fibrosis); (2) *sequestration* due to *splenomegaly;* (3) *accelerated destruction*—causes include:

- *Drugs* such as chemotherapeutic agents, thiazides, ethanol, estrogens, sulfonamides, quinidine, quinine, methyldopa. *Treatment* includes discontinuation of possible offending agents; expect recovery in 7–10 days. *Heparin-induced* thrombocytopenia is seen in 5% of pts receiving > 5 days of therapy; is due to in vivo platelet aggregation. Arterial and occasionally venous *thromboses* may result.
- *Autoimmune* destruction by an *antibody* mechanism; may be idiopathic or associated with SLE, lymphoma, human immunodeficiency virus. *Idiopathic thrombocytopenic purpura* (ITP) has two forms: an *acute,* self-limited disorder of childhood requiring no specific therapy, and a *chronic* disorder of adults (esp. women 20–40 years of age). *Treatment* of chronic ITP—prednisone (initially 1–2 mg/kg per day, then slow taper) to keep the platelet count >60,000/mm³. Splenectomy, danazol (androgen), or other agents (e.g., vincristine, cyclophosphamide) indicated for pts requiring >5–10 mg prednisone daily.
- *Disseminated intravascular coagulation* (DIC)—platelet consumption with coagulation factor depletion (prolonged PT, PTT) and stimulation of fibrinolysis (generation of fibrin split products, FSP). Blood smear shows microangiopathic hemolysis (schistocytes). *Causes*—infection (esp. meningococcal, pneumococcal, gram-negative bacteremias), extensive burns, trauma, or thrombosis; giant hemangioma, retained dead fetus, heat stroke, mismatched blood transfusion, metastatic carcinoma, acute pro-

myelocytic leukemia. *Treatment*—control of underlying disease most important; platelets, fresh frozen plasma (FFP) to correct clotting parameters. Heparin may be beneficial in patients with acute promyelocytic leukemia.

- *Thrombotic thrombocytopenic purpura*—rare disorder characterized by microangiopathic hemolytic anemia, fever, thrombocytopenia, renal dysfunction (and/or hematuria), and neurologic dysfunction. *Treatment*—plasmapheresis and plasma infusions; recovery in two-thirds of cases.
- *Hemorrhage* with extensive *transfusion*.

Pseudothrombocytopenia: Platelet clumping secondary to collection of blood in EDTA (0.3% of patients).

Thrombocytosis: Platelet count > 350,000/mm^3. Either *primary* (thrombocythemia; Chap. 129) or *secondary* (reactive); latter secondary to severe hemorrhage, iron deficiency, surgery, after splenectomy (transient), malignant neoplasms, chronic inflammatory diseases (e.g., inflammatory bowel disease), recovery from acute infection, drugs (e.g., vincristine, epinephrine). *Rebound thrombocytosis* may occur after marrow recovery from cytotoxic agents, alcohol. *Primary* thrombocytosis may be complicated by bleeding and/or thrombosis; secondary rarely causes hemostatic problems.

Disorders of platelet function: Suggested by the finding of prolonged bleeding time with normal platelet count. *Causes:* (1) *Drugs*—aspirin, other NSAIDs, dipyridamole, heparin, penicillins, esp. carbenicillin, ticarcillin; (2) *uremia;* (3) *cirrhosis;* (4) *dysproteinemias;* (5) *myeloproliferative* and *myelodysplastic* disorders; (6) *von Willebrands's disease. Treatment:* Remove or reverse underlying cause.

Platelet Transfusion Therapy: See Chap. 128.

HEMOSTATIC DISORDERS DUE TO BLOOD VESSEL WALL DEFECTS *Causes:* (1) *Aging;* (2) *drugs*—e.g., corticosteroids (chronic therapy), penicillins, sulfonamides; (3) *vitamin C deficiency;* (4) *Henoch-Schönlein purpura;* (5) *paraproteinemias;* (6) *hereditary hemorrhagic telangiectasia* (Osler-Rendu-Weber disease).

DISORDERS OF BLOOD COAGULATION Congenital disorders:

1 *Hemophilia A*—most common hereditary disorder of coagulation (1:10,000); sex-linked recessive deficiency of factor VIII (low plasma factor VIII *coagulant* activity, but normal amount of factor VIII-related antigen–von Willebrand's factor). *Laboratory features*—elevated PTT, normal PT. *Treatment*—factor VIII replacement for bleeding or before surgical procedure; degree of replacement depends on severity of bleeding.

2 *Hemophilia B*—also sex-linked recessive, due to factor IX deficiency. Clinical and laboratory features similar to hemophilia A. *Treatment*—factor IX concentrates (Proplex, Konyne).

3 *von Willebrands's disease*—relatively common, usually auto-

somal dominant; primary defect is reduced synthesis or chemically abnormal factor VIII-related antigen, resulting in *abnormal platelet function*. *Treatment*—cryoprecipitate (plasma product rich in factor VIII); DDAVP (vasopressin analogue) may benefit some pts.

Acquired disorders:

1 *Vitamin K deficiency*—impairs production of factors II (prothrombin), VII, IX, and X; major source of vitamin K is dietary (green vegetables) with minor production by gut bacteria. *Laboratory features*—elevated PT and PTT.

2 *Liver disease*—results in deficiencies of all clotting factors except VIII. *Laboratory features*—elevated PT, normal or elevated PTT. *Treatment*—fresh frozen plasma (FFP).

3 *Other disorders*—DIC, fibrinogen deficiency (liver disease, DIC, L-asparaginase therapy, rattlesnake bites), other factor deficiencies, circulating anticoagulants (lymphoma, SLE, idiopathic), massive transfusion (dilutional coagulopathy).

THROMBOTIC DISORDERS

HYPERCOAGULABLE STATE Consider in patients with recurrent episodes of venous thrombosis (i.e., deep venous thrombosis, DVT; pulmonary embolism). *Causes:* (1) *Venous stasis* (e.g., pregnancy, immobilization); (2) *vasculitis;* (3) *myeloproliferative disorders;* (4) *oral contraceptives;* (5) *lupus anticoagulant*—antibody to platelet phospholipid, *stimulates* coagulation; (6) *heparin-induced thrombocytopenia;* (7) *deficiencies of endogenous anticoagulant factors*—antithrombin III, protein C, protein S; (8) *other*—paroxysmal nocturnal hemoglobinuria, dysfibrinogenemias (abnormal fibrinogen).

ANTITHROMBOTIC THERAPY Anticoagulant agents:

1 *Heparin*—enhances activity of antithrombin III; parenteral agent of choice. In adults, 25,000–40,000 U continuous IV infusion over 24 h following initial IV bolus of 5000 U; monitor by following PTT, should be maintained between 1.5 and 2 times upper normal limit. *Prophylactic* anticoagulation to lower risk of venous thrombosis recommended in some patients (e.g., postoperative, immobilized); dosage is 5000 U SC q 8–12 h. Major *complication* of heparin therapy is *hemorrhage*—manage by discontinuing heparin; for severe bleeding, administer *protamine* (1 mg/100 U heparin); results in rapid neutralization.

2 *Warfarin* (Coumadin)—vitamin K antagonist, decreases levels of factors II, VII, IX, X and anticoagulant proteins C and S. Administered over 2–3 days; initial load of 5–10 mg PO qd followed by titration of daily dose to keep PT 1.5–2 times control PT. *Complications*—hemorrhage, warfarin-induced skin necrosis (rare), teratogenic effects. Warfarin effect reversed by administration of vitamin K; FFP infused if urgent reversal necessary. Numerous drugs potentiate or antagonize warfarin effect. *Potentiating agents*—chlorpromazine, chloral hydrate, sulfonamides,

chloramphenicol, other broad-spectrum antibiotics, allopurinol, cimetidine, tricyclic antidepressants, disulfiram, laxatives, high-dose salicylates, thyroxine, clofibrate. *Antagonizing agents*—vitamin K, barbiturates, rifampin, cholestyramine, oral contraceptives, thiazides.

In-hospital anticoagulation usually initiated with heparin with subsequent maintenance on warfarin after an *overlap* of 3 days.

Fibrinolytic agents: Two agents currently available; *streptokinase* and *urokinase;* mediate *clot lysis* by activating plasmin, which degrades fibrin. *Indications*—treatment of DVT, with lower incidence of postphlebitic syndrome (chronic venous stasis, skin ulceration) than with heparin therapy; massive pulmonary embolism, arterial embolic occlusion of extremity. Under investigation for treatment of acute MI, unstable angina pectoris.

Antiplatelet agents: Aspirin, dipyridamole; may be beneficial in lowering incidence of arterial thrombotic events (stroke, MI) in high-risk patients.

For more detailed discussion of these topics, see Handin RI: Bleeding and Thrombosis, Chap. 54, p. 266; Handin RI: Inherited Thrombotic Disorders and Antithrombotic Therapy, Chap. 281, p. 1480, in HPIM-11

---

128 BLOOD TRANSFUSION AND PHERESIS THERAPY

In general, individual components, not whole blood, should be used. With hemorrhage, packed RBCs, fresh frozen plasma (FFP), and platelets in an approximate ratio of 3:1:10 units are an adequate replacement for whole blood.

TRANSFUSIONS

RED BLOOD CELL TRANSFUSION Indicated for symptomatic anemia unresponsive to specific therapy or requiring urgent correction. In general, transfusions should be withheld when Hb > 9 g/dL (Hct > 27%); may be indicated when Hb is between 7 and 9 g/dL, esp. in pts with ischemic cardiovascular disease. Transfusion almost always necessary when Hb <7 g/dL. One unit of packed RBCs raises the Hb by approximately 1 g/dL.
Other indications: (1) *Hypertransfusion therapy*—e.g., thalassemia, sickle cell anemia; (2) *exchange transfusion*—hemolytic disease of newborn; (3) *transplant recipients*—decreases rejection of cadaveric kidney transplants.
Complications: (1) *Transfusion reaction*—immediate or delayed; IgA-deficient pts at particular risk for severe reaction; (2) *infection*—bacterial (rare), hepatitis, most commonly non-A, non-B (also hepatitis B, CMV), human immunodeficiency virus (HIV), cause of AIDS (antibody screening of donated blood now routinely performed); (3) *pulmonary leukoagglutinin reaction*—rare; (4) *circulatory overload*; (5) *iron overload*—usually after 100 U of RBCs (less in children), in absence of blood loss; can result in *hemochromatosis*—iron chelation therapy with *deferoxamine* indicated.

AUTOLOGOUS TRANSFUSION Use of pt's own stored blood; avoids hazards of donor blood; also useful in pts with multiple RBC antibodies.

GRANULOCYTE TRANSFUSION May be of benefit in severe neutropenia (< 500 granulocytes/mm^3) with bacterial infection unresponsive to appropriate antibiotics; short (<24 h) life span and potential for severe leukoagglutinin reactions limit utility.

PLATELET TRANSFUSION Prophylactic transfusions usually reserved for platelet count < 10,000/mm^3. One unit elevates the count by about 10,000/mm^3 if no platelet antibodies are present as a result of prior transfusions. Efficacy assessed by 1-h and 24-h posttransfusion platelet counts. HLA-matched single-donor platelets may be required in patients with platelet alloantibodies.

THERAPEUTIC HEMAPHERESIS

DEFINITION Removal of a cellular or plasma constituent of blood; specific procedure referred to by the blood fraction removed.

LEUKAPHERESIS Removal of WBCs; most often used in acute leukemia, esp. acute myelogenous leukemia (AML) in cases complicated by marked elevation (>50,000/mm^3) of the peripheral blast count, to lower risk of *leukostasis* (blast-mediated vasoocclusive events resulting in CNS, pulmonary infarction, hemorrhage).

PLATELETPHERESIS Used in some patients with *thrombocytosis* associated with myeloproliferative disorders with bleeding and/or thrombotic complications; not practical for long-term control (Chap. 127). Also used to enhance platelet yield from blood donors.

PLASMAPHERESIS **Indications:** (1) *Hyperviscosity* states (e.g., Waldenström's macroglobulinemia); (2) *thrombotic thrombocytopenic purpura* (Chap. 127); (3) *immune complex and autoantibody disorders*—e.g., Goodpasture's syndrome, rapidly progressive glomerulonephritis, myasthenia gravis; possibly Guillain-Barré, SLE.

For more detailed discussion of these topics, see Giblett ER: Blood Groups and Blood Transfusion, Chap. 282, in HPIM-11, p. 1483

---

129 MYELOPROLIFERATIVE AND MYELODYSPLASTIC DISORDERS

MYELOPROLIFERATIVE DISEASES

Stem cell disorders characterized by autonomous proliferation of one or more hematopoietic cell lines (erythroid, myeloid, megakaryocytic) in the bone marrow; results in excess number of cells in peripheral blood and, in some cases, liver and spleen (extramedullary hematopoiesis). Four basic disorders.

CHRONIC MYELOGENOUS (GRANULOCYTIC) LEUKEMIA Characterized by splenomegaly and leukocytosis (WBC typically 50,000–200,000) with a spectrum of granulocyte precursors and mature granulocytes in blood. Associated with characteristic chromosomal abnormality (Philadelphia chromosome, a 9;22 translocation). Two phases of disease—*chronic phase*, relatively indolent, lasting 2–3 years, followed by *blastic phase*, resembling acute leukemia, usually rapidly fatal.
Treatment: During chronic phase, *cytotoxic agents* (busulfan, hydroxyurea) and/or *interferon* can control granulocyte count, but are not curative; *bone marrow transplantation* may be curative in some patients.

POLYCYTHEMIA VERA Characterized by excessive production of erythroid cells, resulting in elevation of the blood hemoglobin and hematocrit. WBC and platelet overproduction also occurs in >50% of pts. Increased RBC mass results in increased blood volume and blood *viscosity*.
Clinical features: Pruritus, plethoric facies, retinal vein engorgement, impairment of cerebral circulation (headache, tinnitus, dizziness, visual disturbances, transient ischemic events). Accelerated *atherosclerotic and thrombotic disease* are typical (stroke, MI, peripheral vascular disease; uncommonly mesenteric, hepatic vein thrombosis); *hemorrhage* (esp. epistaxis, GI); *splenomegaly* in 75%.
Diagnosis: Exclusion of secondary causes of an elevated RBC mass (e.g., chronic hypoxemia, excess carboxyhemoglobin, erythropoietin-producing neoplasm).
Treatment: Aimed at reducing the RBC mass toward normal, usually with repeated *phlebotomy*, ^{32}P radiotherapy. About 20% of pts progress to *myelofibrosis*, <5% to leukemia (higher if treated with alkylating agents; no longer recommended).

MYELOFIBROSIS (MYELOID METAPLASIA) Fibrosis of bone marrow and extramedullary hematopoiesis (myeloid metaplasia) involving spleen and liver (splenomegaly in all cases; hepatomegaly in one-half).
Clinical features: Thromboses increased, hemorrhage uncommon.
Diagnosis: Anemia, with abnormal blood smear: RBC atypia (teardrops, other poikilocytes, nucleated RBCs, basophilic stip-

pling, giant platelet forms); bone marrow *biopsy* the definitive test—marrow fibrosis can be documented by *reticulin staining.* May also see *osteosclerosis* (increased bone density). *Secondary* causes of myelofibrosis in the differential diagnosis: metastatic tumor, TBC, Paget's disease, Gaucher's disease.
Treatment: Supportive, with median survival about 4 years.

ESSENTIAL THROMBOCYTOSIS (THROMBOCYTHEMIA)

Excessive megakaryocytic proliferation leading to platelet excess; platelet count > 800,000/mm^3. Anemia usually present, often secondary to iron deficiency from blood loss.
Clinical features: Resembles polycythemia vera; recurrent hemorrhage and thrombosis.
Diagnosis: Elevated platelet count and abnormal platelet forms (e.g., giant platelets) on blood smear; exclude secondary causes of an elevated platelet count (Chap. 127).
Treatment: Aimed at lowering the platelet count (alkylating agents, hydroxyurea, ^{32}P). Acute reduction in platelet count by plateletpheresis indicated in occasional patient presenting with severe hemorrhage. Possible benefit of antiplatelet agents (aspirin, dipyridamole) for recurrent thromboses.

MYELODYSPLASTIC SYNDROMES

A *heterogeneous* group of disorders of persons over age 50 characterized by *peripheral cytopenias* (one or more lines) in the presence of a normocellular or hypercellular marrow and *dysplastic maturation* of one or more of the marrow cell lineages; 25–50% of pts progress to *acute myelogenous leukemia* (AML) (Chap. 130); syndromes often referred to as *preleukemia.*
Treatment: Rarely successful after progression to acute leukemia, in contrast to patients with de novo AML.

For more detailed discussion of these topics, see Adamson JW: The Myeloproliferative Diseases, Chap. 289, in HPIM-11, p. 1527

THE LEUKEMIAS

DEFINITION A heterogeneous group of malignant neoplasms developing from hematopoietic (blood-forming) cells. The cells of these neoplasms proliferate in bone marrow and lymphoid tissues and eventually involve peripheral blood and infiltrate other organ systems. These disorders are classified on the basis of the cell line involved as either *myeloid* or *lymphoid* and as acute or chronic depending on the course of progression of the illness.

ETIOLOGY In most cases, the etiology is not known. Congenital syndromes, radiation, and chemical exposure are important factors in some cases. The human T-cell leukemia virus (HTLV I) is associated with adult T-cell leukemia (see HPIM-11, Chap. 293 for additional details).

PATHOPHYSIOLOGY The proliferating cell in acute leukemias is an immature clonal myeloid or lymphoid cell that may demonstrate varying degrees of differentiation. These proliferating cells accumulate in bone marrow primarily because they fail to mature past the myeloblast or promyelocyte level in acute myelogenous leukemia (AML) or the lymphoblast level in acute lymphocytic leukemia (ALL). The neoplastic cells in many forms of acute and chronic leukemia demonstrate characteristic cytogenetic abnormalities. Many pts with leukemia demonstrate pancytopenia, which may result from bone marrow crowding by malignant cells or may be the result of direct effects of the leukemic cells or their interaction with the bone marrow microenvironment. Infiltration of leukemic cells into other organ systems may produce the varied clinical manifestations of advanced leukemia.

ACUTE LEUKEMIA

PATHOLOGY AND CLASSIFICATION Bone marrow in acute leukemia is typically hypercellular and heavily infiltrated with a monomorphic population of leukemic blasts; numbers of normal bone marrow elements are markedly reduced. Prognostic and therapeutic considerations make it crucial to distinguish between AML and ALL. These disorders are classified on the basis of cellular morphology, cytochemical features, immunologic phenotype, and degree of differentiation. A collaborative French-American-British (FAB) group has divided ALL into 3 subtypes (L1, L2, and L3) and AML into 7 subtypes (M1 through M7) based on morphologic features.

Leukemic lymphoblasts in ALL are typically smaller than in AML and have round or convoluted nuclei and small amounts of cytoplasm. In >90% of pts with ALL, these cells contain terminal deoxynucleotidal transferase (TdT), rarely present in AML cells. In approximately 60% of cases, cells express the common ALL antigen (CALLA) but are negative for surface immunoglobulin or T-cell markers. About 20% of ALL cases are of T-cell type, and the cells express T-cell surface markers; some 5% of ALL are of

B-cell type and represent the leukemic form of the B-cell neoplasm, Burkitt's lymphoma (L3 in the FAB classification). Approximately 15% of cases are of null cell type.

AML blasts are usually larger than those seen in ALL and have a lower nuclear-cytoplasmic ratio. Cytoplasm of the cells may stain positive for such enzymatic markers as peroxidase or esterase and may contain Auer rods (abnormal primary granules). Clinical differences among the 7 subtypes of AML in the FAB classification are subtle. Pts with acute promyelocytic leukemia (M3) frequently present with DIC.

CLINICAL AND LABORATORY FEATURES

- Initial symptoms of acute leukemia usually present for less than 3 months; a preleukemic syndrome may be present in some 25% of pts with AML.
- WBC may be low, normal, or markedly elevated; circulating blast cells may or may not be present; with WBC > 100,000 blasts/μL leukostasis in lungs and brain may occur.
- Thrombocytopenia and spontaneous bleeding, especially when platelet count <20,000/μL.
- Bacterial and fungal infection common; risk is heightened when total neutrophil count <500/μL; breakdown of mucosal and cutaneous barriers aggravates susceptibility; infections may be clinically occult in presence of severe leukopenia, and prompt recognition requires a high degree of clinical suspicion.
- Hepatosplenomegaly and lymphadenopathy are common in ALL, less so in AML; leukemic meningitis may present with headache, nausea, seizures, papilledema, cranial nerve palsies; testicular involvement in males with ALL.
- Metabolic abnormalities may include hyponatremia, hypokalemia, elevated serum LDH, hyperuricemia, and (rarely) lactic acidosis.

TREATMENT OF ACUTE LEUKEMIA General considerations: Leukemic cell mass at time of presentation may be 10^{11}–10^{12} cells; when total leukemic cell numbers fall below approximately 10^9, they are no longer detectable in blood or bone marrow and patient appears to be in complete remission. Thus aggressive therapy must continue past the point when initial cell bulk is reduced if leukemia is to be eradicated. Typical phases of chemotherapy include *remission induction, consolidation, maintenance,* and *late intensification.*

Supportive care with transfusions of red cells, granulocytes, and platelets is very important, as are aggressive prevention, diagnosis, and treatment of infections.

Treatment of ALL:

- With current ALL therapy, >50% of children will achieve probable cure; prognosis for adults not as good.
- Remission-induction chemotherapy usually includes vincristine and prednisone plus either L-asparaginase or daunorubicin.
- CNS prophylaxis with radiation or intrathecal chemotherapy is effective in reducing rates of CNS relapse.

- Maintenance chemotherapy for 2 to 3 years or longer should follow the above measures.

Treatment of AML: 60 to 80% of pts with AML will achieve initial remission when treated with regimens including cytarabine and daunorubicin with or without 6-thioguanine; following intensive consolidation and maintenance therapy, 10 to 30% of pts may achieve 5-year disease-free survival and probable cure; duration of remissions induced after relapse is short, and prognosis for pts who have relapsed is poor.
Bone marrow transplantation: Role of bone marrow transplantation in treatment of acute leukemia is controversial; transplantation from identical twin or HLA-identical sibling may be effective in ALL or AML; best results achieved in children and young adults.

CHRONIC LEUKEMIA

CHRONIC LYMPHOCYTIC LEUKEMIA (CLL)

- CLL is a neoplasm characterized by accumulation of mature-appearing lymphocytes in blood and bone marrow; 95% of cases involve B lymphocytes; spleen and lymph nodes may be infiltrated; pts are usually over 50 years old.
- Complications include cytopenia, Coombs-positive hemolytic anemia, hypogammaglobulinemia, infection, evolution into lymphoma (Richter's syndrome).
- Many pts require no therapy; some may need therapy with alkylating agents, steroids, immunoglobulin infusion.

CHRONIC MYELOGENOUS LEUKEMIA (CML)

- CML is usually characterized by splenomegaly and production of increased numbers of granulocytes; course is initially indolent but eventuates in leukemic phase (blast crisis); rate of progression to blast crisis is variable; overall survival averages 3½ years from diagnosis.
- More than 95% of pts have characteristic chromosomal abnormality, Philadelphia chromosome.
- Blastic phase may involve cells of either lymphoid or myeloid origin.
- Treatment of chronic phase involves control of cell counts with alkylating agents or hydroxyurea; blast crisis is usually refractory to most regimens, but ALL or AML programs may be useful; bone marrow transplantation during chronic phase may improve prognosis in some pts.

HAIRY-CELL LEUKEMIA

Hairy-cell leukemia (HCL) is a lymphoid neoplasm marked by cytopenia, splenomegaly, and proliferation of typical cells (with characteristic cytoplasmic projections) in blood and bone marrow. Malignant cells are almost always B cells; T-cell variants are rare. Cells stain positively for tartrate-resistant acid phosphatase (TRAP). *Complications* include vasculitis and frequent infection. Alpha-interferon is of therapeutic benefit for some pts. Prognosis is variable; ≥50% of pts will survive more than 8 years from diagnosis.

For more detailed discussion of these topics, see Champlin R, Golde DW: The Leukemias, Chap. 292, p. 1541; Adamson JW: The Myeloproliferative Diseases, Chap. 289, p. 1527, in HPIM-11

---

131 HODGKIN'S DISEASE AND OTHER LYMPHOMAS

DEFINITION These neoplasms are tumors of the immune system. Previous classification schemes divided lymphomas into Hodgkin's disease and non-Hodgkin's lymphomas; newer and more sophisticated diagnostic techniques have allowed more precise categorization of these disorders. Current thinking divides the general groups of lymphomas into Hodgkin's disease and lymphocytic lymphomas. Diagnosis of both forms requires biopsy of affected tissue.

CELLULAR ORIGINS Approximately 65% of lymphocytic lymphomas are of B-cell origin; 30 to 40% arise from T cells. Follicular lymphomas are derived from the lymphoid follicle, the proliferative compartment of the B-cell system. Diffuse small lymphocytic lymphomas arise from the secretory compartment of medullary cords. T-cell lymphomas may be classified as being of peripheral or thymic origin. Malignant cells in Hodgkin's disease (HD) may arise from the antigen-presenting interdigitating reticulum cell found in the paracortical regions of lymph nodes.

HODGKIN'S DISEASE

CLINICAL MANIFESTATIONS

- Usually presents with asymptomatic lymph node enlargement or with adenopathy associated with fever, night sweats, weight loss, and sometimes pruritus. Mediastinal adenopathy (common in nodular sclerosing HD) may produce cough.
- SVC obstruction or spinal cord compression may be presenting manifestation.
- Visceral involvement of bone marrow, liver, etc., may be seen, especially in advanced disease.

DIFFERENTIAL DIAGNOSIS

- Infection—mononucleosis, viral syndromes, toxoplasma, histoplasma, primary TBC.
- Other malignancies—especially head and neck cancers.
- Sarcoidosis—mediastinal and hilar adenopathy.

IMMUNOLOGIC AND HEMATOLOGIC ABNORMALITIES

- Defects in cell-mediated immunity (remains even after successful treatment of lymphoma); cutaneous anergy; diminished antibody production to capsular antigens of *Haemophilus* and pneumococcus.
- Anemia; elevated ESR; leukemoid reaction; eosinophilia; lymphocytopenia; fibrosis and granulomas in marrow.

STAGING Important to determine extent of disease and guide choice of treatment protocol; should include thorough PE, CXR, lymphangiogram, abdominal CT and ultrasound examinations.

Bone marrow biopsy, laparoscopy, or staging laparotomy should be used in certain selected cases.

TREATMENT More than 70% of patients with HD are curable with radiotherapy, combination chemotherapy, or both. Therapy should be performed by experienced clinicians in centers with appropriate facilities. Treatment and prognosis depend on stage and cell type. Generally, stages I and II are treated with radiotherapy, whereas stages III and IV receive chemotherapy. However, treatment protocols vary, and combinations of radio- and chemotherapy may be employed.

LYMPHOCYTIC LYMPHOMAS

CLINICAL FEATURES Generally present as painless adenopathy with or without hepatosplenomegaly; abdominal masses may be seen. Waldeyer's ring involvement more common than in HD. Systemic symptoms less common than in HD. Average age is older than for HD; otherwise, differential diagnosis is similar and includes infection and other malignancies. Immune function less often depressed than in HD; some patients with diffuse small lymphocytic lymphomas may have monoclonal gammopathy or hypogammaglobulinemia.

STAGING Similar to that described for HD; however, extranodal disease is more common in lymphocytic lymphomas and should be carefully sought and evaluated.

TYPES OF LYMPHOCYTIC LYMPHOMAS

1 *Follicular, predominantly small cleaved cell*: Most common follicular lymphoma; clinical course quite variable; histologic pattern may change as clinical picture progresses.

2 *Low-grade follicular, mixed small cleaved and large cell*: Combination chemotherapy yields good results in significant percentage of patients.

3 *Intermediate-grade follicular, predominantly large cell lymphomas*: Large and poorly differentiated cells, more aggressive growth pattern.

4 *Diffuse lymphomas*: Group of disorders with variable presentation and course; therapy and prognosis vary with cell type and localization.

5 *High-grade diffuse lymphocytic lymphomas*: Cells exhibit T-cell characteristics; some will evolve into acute leukemia; CNS involvement frequent; all stages require chemotherapy; combination chemotherapy with CNS prophylaxis may give long-term disease-free survival.

6 *Burkitt's lymphoma*: B-cell neoplasm; African form associated with Epstein-Barr virus infection; tumor is very responsive to chemotherapy.

TREATMENT Protocols involve radiotherapy, combination chemotherapy, or both modalities; should be guided by experienced oncologists and radiation therapists.

COMPLICATIONS OF LYMPHOMAS AND THEIR THERAPIES

- Infection—opportunistic organisms common.
- Obstruction of SVC, airways, esophagus, urinary or GI tracts.
- Infiltration of CNS, lung, skin, and other organ systems.
- Anemia, leukopenia, leukocytosis, thrombocytopenia, or thrombocytosis.
- Metabolic abnormalities—hypercalcemia, hyperuricemia.
- Radiation toxicity to susceptible organs.
- Secondary malignancies, especially AML, may follow therapy.

For more detailed discussion of this topic, see DeVita VT Jr., Ultmann JE: Hodgkin's Disease and the Lymphocytic Lymphomas, Chap. 294, in HPIM-11, p. 1553

PLASMA CELL MALIGNANCIES

GENERAL PRINCIPLES

Plasma cell disorders are monoclonal malignancies of the B-lymphocyte system characterized by excessive proliferation of plasma cells (antibody-secreting descendants of B lymphocytes) and secretion of cell products (immunoglobulin molecules or subunits or lymphokines).

Serum from pts with plasma-cell tumors frequently contains a monoclonal protein which represents the immunoglobulin molecule (or heavy or light chain) produced by the malignant cells. This protein is called the M component (M for monoclonal), and in any given pt the amount of M component in the serum represents a measure of the pt's tumor burden. Some pts may excrete light chains in their urine (Bence Jones protein); this may be the only evidence of the abnormal protein in certain individuals. M components also may be seen in other neoplasms as well as in some infectious or immune-mediated diseases.

MULTIPLE MYELOMA

DEFINITION Multiple myeloma (also called simply myeloma) is a malignant proliferation of plasma cells chiefly in the bone marrow but also other organ systems. Cells may form solitary tumor masses known as plasmacytomas.

PATHOGENESIS AND CLINICAL MANIFESTATIONS

- Bone pain most common symptom; bone lesions are osteolytic without osteoblastic new bone formation, so are not well-visualized on radioisotopic bone scanning. Pathologic fractures may develop; vertebral body collapse may lead to spinal cord compression.
- Infection—recurrent infection may be presenting complaint in 25% of pts; may be significant *hypogammaglobulinemia* (when M component is excluded).
- Hypercalcemia.
- Renal failure—related to hypercalcemia and toxic effects of light chains on renal tubules.
- Neuropathies may be due to amyloid infiltration of nerves.
- Hyperviscosity syndrome—causes fatigue, headache, visual disturbances, and retinopathy.
- Hematologic disturbances—anemia in approximately 80%; granulocytopenia and thrombocytopenia are rare; clotting abnormalities may be present; cryoglobulins may be present.

DIAGNOSIS Classic triad of myeloma is (1) marrow plasmacytosis (>10%), (2) lytic bone lesions, and (3) a serum and/or urine M component. Studies to determine diagnosis and staging should include:

- CBC, platelet count.
- Bone marrow aspiration and biopsy.
- Serum and urine electrophoresis and immunoelectrophoresis to

detect and quantitate M component. • Skeletal radiographic survey—"punched out" lesions are characteristic of myeloma. • Serum calcium. • Serum viscosity.

Staging systems (see Table 258-2, in HPIM-11) correlate with survival.

Differential diagnosis: Includes benign monoclonal gammopathy (or monoclonal gammopathy of uncertain significance). 11% of pts with monoclonal gammopathy of uncertain significance will go on to develop myeloma.

TREATMENT It is generally felt that cure is not possible in myeloma, so therapy must be tailored to individual case. Some pts will have a very indolent course and not require therapy, but majority will require therapy for an indefinite period of time. Standard therapy usually involves pulses of an alkylating agent (such as L-phenylalanine mustard, cyclophosphamide, or chlorambucil) and prednisone for 4–7 days every 4–6 weeks. Response to treatment may be judged by symptomatic improvement and decrease in serum M component (may lag behind symptomatic relief). Optimal duration of initial course of treatment is uncertain but usually is 1 to 2 years. Supportive care of complications also must be given. Prognosis relates to stage of disease and response to treatment. Approximately 25% of pts may die of diseases unrelated to their myeloma.

WALDENSTRÖM'S MACROGLOBULINEMIA

Also a malignancy of lymphoplasmacytoid cells, but in contrast to myeloma is associated with lymphadenopathy and hepatosplenomegaly; cells secrete IgM; hyperviscosity is main clinical manifestation; bony lesions and hypercalcemia not seen; renal disease not common because size of IgM M component prevents glomerular filtration; cryoglobulinemia occurs in about 10% of pts.

TREATMENT Identical to that of myeloma; plasmapheresis may be necessary for serious hyperviscosity symptoms; absence of serious organ system involvement in Waldenström's improves prognosis compared to that for myeloma.

HEAVY CHAIN DISEASES

Rare lymphoplasmacytic malignancies; clinical manifestations vary with heavy chain isotype secreted.

GAMMA HEAVY CHAIN DISEASE (FRANKLIN'S DISEASE) Characterized by lymphadenopathy, fever, anemia, malaise, hepatosplenomegaly, weakness; palatal edema may result from node involvement of Waldeyer's ring; usually demonstrates rapid downhill course with death from infection; chemotherapy may prolong survival.

ALPHA HEAVY DISEASE (SELIGMANN'S DISEASE) Most common of heavy chain diseases; lymphoplasmacytoid infiltration of intestinal lamina propria causes diarrhea, malabsorption, weight loss, mesenteric and paraaortic adenopathy; clinical course very variable.

MU HEAVY CHAIN DISEASE Appears to be a rare subset of chronic lymphocytic leukemia; tumor cells may have a defect in assembly of heavy and light chains.

For more detailed discussion of this topic, see Longo DL, Broder S: Plasma Cell Disorders. Chap. 258, in HPIM-11, p. 1396

---

133 CANCER CHEMOTHERAPY

BIOLOGY OF TUMOR GROWTH An understanding of the biologic principles of tumor growth is essential to rational therapy of malignancies. The malignant phenotype of a cell is the end result of a series of changes in various aspects of mechanisms controlling growth and cellular development. Among these changes is increased or abnormal expression of certain highly conserved genes known as proto-oncogenes. These genes are found in the normal human genome, their products show partial homology with some growth factors and growth factor receptors, and alterations in their structure or rearrangement in their location in the genome may have profound effects on control of cellular growth.

In addition to uncontrolled growth, malignant cells have the ability to metastasize (spread widely from their primary site). This capacity appears to be related to deregulation of genetic mechanisms once responsible for normal cell adhesion and migration, the ability of malignant cells to express receptors for basement membrane components, and the power of enzymes to disrupt the basement membrane and allow escape of cell from primary site.

Once cells are malignant, their growth kinetics are similar to those of normal cells. Tumor growth kinetics are expressed by a Gompertzian function: as the tumor mass increases, the growth is matched by an exponential retardation of growth. Cancer cells proceed through the same cell-cycle stages as normal cycling cells: G_1 (period of normal cell metabolism without DNA synthesis), S (DNA synthesis), G_2 (tetraploid phase preceding mitosis), and M (mitosis). Some noncycling cells may remain in a G_0 phase for long lengths of time. Certain chemotherapeutic agents are specific for cells in certain phases of the cell cycle, a fact that is important in designing effective chemotherapeutic regimens.

DEVELOPMENT OF DRUG RESISTANCE Drug resistance of cancer cells may be viewed as either temporary or permanent. *Temporary resistance* refers to inability of drugs to kill cells because cells are in wrong phase of cell cycle, are in pharmacologic sanctuaries such as the CNS or testis, or are in the center of a poorly vascularized tumor. *Permanent resistance* arises because of fundamental changes in the way in which the cell transports, activates, deactivates, or repairs damage caused by the drug in question.

The Goldie-Coldman hypothesis postulates that, as in bacteria, permanent drug resistance occurs in tumor cells as the result of random genetic mutations at a rate of perhaps 1 in 10^6 cells. Thus in a tumor of minimally detectable size of approximately 10^9 cells there is a good chance of occurrence of singly or even doubly resistant cell lines. As tumor size and cell number increase, the number of multiply drug-resistant cell lines will increase as well. This is consistent with the observations that reduction of tumor bulk often improves responsiveness to chemotherapy and that initially responsive tumors will regrow during continued exposure to drug therapy. Implications of the Goldie-Coldman hypothesis explain the usefulness of multidrug regimens in overcoming problems of resistance and the importance of early treatment in improving success of chemotherapy.

DISEASES IN WHICH CHEMOTHERAPY HAS MAJOR ACTIVITY

Acute lymphocytic leukemia (ALL)
Acute myelocytic leukemia (AML)
Anal cancer
Medulloblastoma
Adult gliomas
Breast cancer
Choriocarcinoma
Embryonal rhabdomyosarcoma
Ewing's sarcoma
Hairy-cell leukemia
Hodgkin's disease
Small cell lung cancer
Lymphocytic lymphomas
Mycosis fungoides
Ovarian carcinoma
Osteogenic sarcoma
Soft tissue sarcomas
Testicular carcinomas
Wilms' tumor

DISEASES IN WHICH CHEMOTHERAPY HAS MODERATE ACTIVITY

Adrenocortical carcinoma
Bladder carcinoma
Cervical carcinoma
Chronic lymphocytic leukemia
Chronic myelocytic leukemia
Endometrial carcinoma
Gastric carcinoma
Head and neck carcinoma, squamous cell
Islet cell carcinoma
Kaposi's sarcoma (epidemic)
Non-small-cell lung cancer
Multiple myeloma
Neuroblastoma
Prostate carcinoma
Retinoblastoma

DISEASES IN WHICH CHEMOTHERAPY HAS MINOR ACTIVITY

Colorectal carcinoma
Esophageal carcinoma
Hepatic carcinoma
Melanoma
Pancreatic carcinoma
Renal cell carcinoma

CATEGORIES OF CHEMOTHERAPEUTIC AGENTS AND MAJOR TOXICITIES (*Note:* List of toxicities is partial; some toxicities may apply only to certain members of a group of drugs.)

Alkylating agents

Agents	Toxicities
Mechlorethamine (nitrogen mustard) Cyclophosphamide L-Phenylalanine mustard Chlorambucil Dacarbazine (DTIC) Nitrosoureas Thiotepa Busulfan	Nausea and vomiting, bone marrow depression, pulmonary fibrosis, sterility, hemorrhagic cystitis, secondary malignancies, alopecia

Antimetabolites	
Methotrexate Fluorouracil Cytarabine 6-Mercaptopurine Azathioprine 6-Thioguanine	Nausea and vomiting, bone marrow depression, oral and GI ulceration, hepatic toxicity, alopecia, neurologic defects
Vinca alkaloids	
Vincristine Vinblastine	Nausea and vomiting, local pain upon extravasation, bone marrow depression, peripheral neuropathy, alopecia, inappropriate ADH secretion, paralytic ileus
Antibiotics	
Dactinomycin (actinomycin D) Daunorubicin Doxorubicin Bleomycin Mithramycin Mitomycin	Nausea and vomiting, bone marrow depression, cardiotoxicity, pulmonary fibrosis, hypocalcemia, alopecia, hypersensitivity reactions
Enzymes	
L-Asparaginase	Nausea and vomiting, fever, anaphylaxis, CNS changes, pancreatitis, thrombosis, renal and hepatic damage
Miscellaneous agents	
Hydroxyurea Cisplatin Alpha interferon Etoposide Tamoxifen	Nausea and vomiting, bone marrow depression, fever, chills, renal damage, antiestrogen effects

COMPLICATIONS OF THERAPY While the effects of cancer chemotherapeutic agents may be exerted primarily on the malignant cell population, virtually all currently employed regimens have profound effects on normal tissues as well. Every side effect of treatment must be balanced against potential benefits expected, and pts must always be fully apprised of the risks they may undertake. While the duration of certain adverse effects may be short-lived, others, such as sterility and the risk of secondary malignancy, obviously have long-term implications; consideration of these effects is of importance in the use of regimens as adjuvant therapy. The combined toxicity of regimens involving radiotherapy and chemotherapy must be weighed in designing these programs. Teratogenesis is a special concern in treating women of childbearing years with radiation or chemotherapy.

For more detailed discussion of this topic, see DeVita VT Jr.: Principles of Cancer Therapy, Chap. 79, in HPIM-11, p. 431

SECTION IX
ENDOCRINOLOGY AND METABOLISM

134 DISORDERS OF THE ANTERIOR PITUITARY AND HYPOTHALAMUS

The anterior pituitary produces six major hormones: growth hormone (GH), prolactin (PRL), luteinizing hormone (LH), follicle-stimulating hormone (FSH), thyroid-stimulating (TSH), and adrenocorticotropin (ACTH). Production of these hormones is under feedback control by target glands, and hence, hormone levels in blood increase when target glands fail (e.g., elevated TSH in primary hypothyroidism). The pituitary is also under control of the hypothalamus via chemical mediators synthesized in the hypothalamus and transported to the pituitary via hypothalamic portal vessels of the pituitary stalk. With hypothalamic ablation, the levels of GH, LH, FSH, TSH, and ACTH fall, whereas PRL levels increase, indicating that the major hypothalamic influence on the latter is inhibitory.

Anterior pituitary disorders can cause three distinct syndromes.

ENLARGEMENT OF THE SELLA May be an incidental finding on routine skull series or cause symptoms of a space-occupying lesion, such as headache and bitemporal hemianopsia. Differential diagnosis includes tumors (pituitary adenomas, craniopharyngiomas, meningiomas, granulomas, and metastatic tumors) and empty sella syndrome, a nontumorous enlargement resulting from protrusion of arachnoid cavity and CSF into sella. Endocrine function of anterior pituitary is usually not impaired in the latter.

CT scanning, usually with contrast enhancement, is useful in defining lesions at or above the diaphragma sellae, and metrizamide CT cisternography may be required to define lesions within the diaphragma sellae. Evaluation for hyper- and hypofunction should be performed in all pts with a pituitary mass (see below). Bromocriptine, radiation therapy, or surgery can be appropriate therapy, depending on nature of tumor.

PITUITARY HORMONE HYPERSECRETION May involve one or more pituitary hormones and can be caused by microadenomas (<1 cm) and/or macroadenomas that cause enlargement of sella (Table 134-1). PRL is secreted by ≥ 50% of all pituitary tumors and can cause milk production in women (galactorrhea) and hypogonadism due to inhibition of LH and FSH secretion in men and women. Serum PRL level > 300 ng/mL is diagnostic, and 100–300 ng/mL in a man or nonpregnant woman is suggestive of pituitary adenoma. Hyperprolactinemia of lesser degrees can be caused by drugs (phenothiazines, metoclopramide, aldomet, estro-

TABLE 134-1 **Pituitary hormone evaluation**

Hormone	Excess	Deficiency
Growth hormone	Plasma GH 1 h following glucose PO Insulin-like growth factor 1; somatomedin C (IGF1/SMC)	Plasma GH 30, 60, and 120 min after one of the following: *a* Regular insulin 0.1 to 0.15 U/kg IV *b* Levodopa 10 mg/kg PO *c* L-Arginine 0.5 mg/kg IV over 30 min
Prolactin	Basal serum PRL	
TSH	T_4, free T_4 index, T_3, TSH	Measurement of T_4, free T_4, free T_4 index, TSH
Gonadotropins	FSH, LH, testosterone	FSH in postmenopausal women; no measurements in menstruating, ovulating women; testosterone, FSH, and LH in men
ACTH	Urine free cortisol or 8 A.M. plasma cortisol after administration of 1 mg dexamethasone at midnight or 8 A.M. plasma cortisol or 24-h urine 17-hydroxysteroids after 0.5 mg dexamethasone PO q 6 h for 8 doses	Metyrapone response by one of the following: *a* Plasma 11-deoxycortisol at 8 A.M. after 30 mg metyrapone at midnight (maximal dose 2 g) *b* 24-h urinary 17-hydroxycorticoids day of and day after 750 mg metyrapone q 4 h for 6 doses *c* Measurement of 24-h urinary 17-hydroxycorticoids day of and day after 500 mg metyrapone q 2 h for 12 doses

Modified from Daniels GH, Martin JB: HPIM-11, p. 1710.

gens, and opiates), renal failure, primary hypothyroidism, cirrhosis of liver, and disease of the hypothalamus and pituitary stalk. All pts with unexplained hyperprolactinemia require contrast-enhanced CT of hypothalamus and pituitary or MRI of this area. Dopamine agonists (bromocriptine) lower serum PRL levels in most hyperprolactinemic pts. To minimize side effects, dosage should initially be 1.25 mg hs and gradually increased to 2.5 mg bid.

Growth hormone (GH) excess causes *acromegaly,* associated with bony and soft tissue overgrowth shown by increased hand, foot, jaw, and cranial size, enlargement of the tongue, wide spacing of teeth, and coarsening of facial features. Symptoms may be present for many years prior to diagnosis. Thickening of palms, increased skin tags, acanthosis nigricans, and oily skin are common. Obstructive sleep apnea may cause hypersomnolence. Neurologic symptoms include headaches, paresthesias (including carpal tunnel syndrome), muscle weakness, and arthralgias. Insulin resistance is common, and frank diabetes mellitus occurs in a sixth of pts. Basal or random GH levels may be elevated in normal persons, and failure of suppressibility of plasma GH levels by glucose must be documented to diagnose acromegaly. The standard screening test is measurement of serum GH 60–120 minutes after giving 100 g glucose PO; serum GH levels normally fall to <5 ng/mL, but in acromegalics levels remain >10 ng/dL after glucose administration. IGF1/SMC levels are also elevated. Conventional x-rays of the sella turcica are abnormal in 90% of pts with acromegaly, but CT scanning or MRI provides better definition of tumor size. Surgical resection is generally the treatment of choice, although radiation may be used on occasion.

For discussion of Cushing's disease see Chap. 137.

HYPOPITUITARISM Causes variable manifestations, depending on which hormone is lacking. GH deficiency in adults causes minimal changes (fine wrinkling of facial skin and increased sensitivity to insulin in subjects with diabetes mellitus). LH and FSH deficiency cause amenorrhea in women, decreased libido in men, and infertility in both. TSH deficiency causes hypothyroidism in absence of goiter. ACTH deficiency results in cortisol deficiency unassociated with hyperpigmentation or mineralocorticoid deficiency (see Chap. 137).

Hypopituitarism may be due to disease of pituitary itself or of hypothalamus (Table 134-2). The former includes infarction during postpartum period (Sheehan's syndrome), pituitary tumors (with or without infarction), pituitary surgery, and radiation. Hypothalamic or pituitary stalk damage can result from sarcoidosis, metastatic carcinoma, germinoma, histiocytosis, or craniopharyngioma, all of which can also cause diabetes insipidus without hypofunction of anterior pituitary (see Chap. 135). Pituitary insufficiency from conventional radiation to brain or pituitary also may be hypothalamic in origin.

To diagnose GH deficiency, the most reliable GH stimulus is insulin-induced hypoglycemia in which blood glucose falls to

TABLE 134-2 **Causes of hypopituitarism**

Isolated hormone deficiencies (congenital or acquired)
Tumors of pituitary or hypothalamus
Inflammatory and infiltrative diseases (granulomatous, histiocytosis X, hemachromatosis)
Vascular diseases (postpartum necrosis)
Destruction (surgical resection, trauma, radiation)
Developmental anomalies

Modified from Daniels GH, Martin JB: HPIM-11, p. 1712.

<40 mg/dL. A GH concentration >10 ng/mL after hypoglycemia, levodopa, or arginine excludes GH deficiency. The adequacy of ACTH reserve can be assessed with use of metyrapone test (see Chap. 137). Adequacy of TSH secretion can be assessed by simultaneous measurement of serum TSH and thyroxine levels. Estrogen deficiency in women and testosterone deficiency in men in absence of elevated levels of plasma LH and FSH imply gonadotropin deficiency. Most pts with hypopituitarism have deficiencies of more than one hormone.

Cortisol replacement is most important feature of treatment, usually cortisone acetate (20–37.5 mg/day) given as a single or divided dose. Levothyroxine (0.1–0.2 mg/day) is indicated for central hypothyroidism. Glucocorticoid replacement should precede levothyroxine therapy to avoid precipitation of adrenal crisis. Hypogonadism in women is treated with estrogen/progestogen combinations (see Chap. 141), and in men is treated with testosterone esters by injection (see Chap. 140). GH deficiency is not treated in adults.

For more detailed discussion of this topic, see Daniels GH, Martin JB: Neuroendocrine Regulation and Diseases of the Anterior Pituitary and Hypothalamus, Chap. 321, in HPIM-11, p. 1694

135 DISORDERS OF THE POSTERIOR PITUITARY

DIABETES INSIPIDUS Arginine vasopressin (AVP, ADH, antidiuretic hormone) functions to concentrate urine and hence to conserve water. In *central diabetes insipidus,* insufficient AVP is released in response to physiologic stimuli. Causes include (1) neoplastic or infiltrative lesions of hypothalamus such as pituitary tumors that extend upward, metastatic tumors, leukemia, germinomas, pinealomas, histiocytosis X, and sarcoidosis; (2) pituitary or hypothalamic surgery; (3) severe head injury, usually associated with skull fracture; and (4) idiopathic. The onset of polyuria, excessive thirst, and polydipsea may be sudden, and urine volume may be as high as 16–24 L/day. Urine osmolality (<290 mosmol/kg; specific gravity < 1.010) is < that of serum. Increase in serum osmolality stimulates thirst, and dehydration is unusual as long as pts have free access to water. When water intake is inadequate (postoperatively, head trauma, or other CNS dysfunction), rising serum sodium level and osmolality can cause weakness, fever, mental disturbances, prostration, and death.

Comparison of urinary osmolality after dehydration with that after AVP administration (Table 135-1) is a reliable way of defining the cause of polyuria (Table 135-2). Urinary osmolality normally rises by ≤ 9% after injection of vasopressin. In central diabetes insipidus, the increase in urinary osmolality after vasopressin is >9%. Pts with nephrogenic diabetes insipidus or potassium depletion have little change in urine osmolality with dehydration and no further rise with vasopressin.

In absence of brain tumor or systemic disease, treatment is usually successful. For acute therapy of unconscious pts after head trauma or neurosurgery, aqueous vasopressin should be given subcutaneously in doses of 5–10 U q 3–6 h. For long-term therapy, 10–20 μg/day of desmopressin is given intranasally. Chlorpropamide may be useful in patients with partial deficiency of vasopressin.

SYNDROME OF INAPPROPRIATE ANTIDIURETIC HORMONE (SIADH) Causes hyponatremia because of inability to dilute urine; ingested fluids are retained, and extracellular fluid volume is expanded without edema. May occur by three mechanisms: (1) AVP is synthesized and autonomously released from tumors (usually small cell carcinoma of lung); (2) nontumorous tissue

TABLE 135-1 **Dehydration test**

1. Withold fluids until urinary osmolality becomes stable (an increase of <30 mosmol/kg/per hour for at least 3 h); body weight usually decreases by 1 kg.
2. Administration of 5 U aqueous vasopressin or 1 μg desmopressin by SC injection or 10 μg desmopressin intranasally.
3. Measure urine and plasma osmolality before and 1 h after the injection.

TABLE 135-2 **Major polyuric syndromes**

Excessive water intake (primary polydipsia)
Inadequate tubular reabsorption of filtered water:
Vasopressin deficiency (central diabetes insipidus)
Renal tubular unresponsiveness to AVP (nephrogenic diabetes insipidus)
Osmotic diuresis

Modified from Streeten DHP, Moses AM, Miller M: HPIM-11, p. 1727.

acquires capacity to synthesize and release AVP autonomously or to stimulate AVP release by pituitary (as in pulmonary TBC, pneumonias, and other pulmonary diseases); (3) pituitary AVP is released inappropriately due to inflammation, neoplasm, vascular lesions, or drugs such as morphine.

Symptoms: Weight gain, weakness, lethargy, and mental confusion, ultimately progressing to convulsion and coma.

Laboratory features: Low BUN, creatinine, uric acid, and albumin; serum Na < 130 meq/L and plasma osmolality < 270 mosmol/kg; urine almost always hypertonic to plasma, and urinary Na usually > 20 meq/L.

SIADH should be suspected in hyponatremic pts with urine that is hypertonic to plasma.

Differential diagnosis: (1) Depletional hyponatremias, especially due to adrenal insufficiency, salt-losing nephritis, diarrhea, or diuretic therapy; (2) hyponatremic edematous states (CHF, cirrhosis, nephrosis); (3) pseudohyponatremia from hyperlipidemia or severe hyperglycemia; (4) hypothyroidism; and (5) primary polydipsia in which the urine is invariably dilute. Assessment of response to water loading may be useful in establishing diagnosis.

In pts with mild SIADH, fluid intake should be restricted to 0.8–1 L/day. If severe SIADH is life-threatening, 200–300 mL 5% saline solution should be given IV over several hours to raise the serum Na to a level at which symptoms will improve. Demeclocycline interferes with renal action of AVP and may be useful when fluid restriction is impractical.

For more detailed discussion of this topic, see Streeten DHP, Moses AM, Miller M: Disorders of the Neurohypophysis, Chap. 323, in HPIM-11, p. 1722

The thyroid secretes thyroxine (T_4) and triiodothyronine (T_3), which influence basal metabolic rate and cardiac and neurologic function. Diseases of the thyroid may be manifest by quantitative or qualitative alterations in hormone secretion, enlargement of the gland, or both.

The hypothalamus releases thyrotropin-releasing hormone (TRH), which traverses the pituitary stalk and stimulates release of thyroid-stimulating hormone (TSH) from the anterior pituitary. TSH is released into the circulation and controls production and release of T_4 and T_3, which in turn inhibit further TSH release from the pituitary.

Some T_3 is secreted by the thyroid, but most is produced by deiodination of T_4 in peripheral tissues. Both T_4 and T_3 are bound to carrier proteins (principally thyroid-binding globulin, TBG) in the circulation.

Under- or overproduction of thyroid hormones is usually reflected in ↓ or ↑ of serum T_4 and T_3 levels. When TBG is excessive (pregnancy, estrogens) or inadequate (malnutrition, chronic liver disease, steroids), the free thyroxine index (FTI) corrects serum T_4 for alterations in binding protein and thus provides an index of thyroid status.

HYPOTHYROIDISM Insufficient thyroid hormone secretion can result from thyroid failure (primary hypothyroidism) or from pituitary or hypothalamic disease (secondary hypothyroidism). *Symptoms* of lethargy, constipation, cold intolerance, stiffness and cramping of muscles, carpal tunnel syndrome, and menorrhagia may be insidious in onset. Intellectual and motor activity slows, appetite declines, weight increases, hair and skin become dry, and the voice deepens. Obstructive sleep apnea may occur. Cardiomegaly can be due to dilatation or pericardial effusion. Relaxation phase of deep tendon reflexes is prolonged. The ultimate picture is a dull, expressionless face, sparse hair, periorbital puffiness, large tongue, and pale, doughy, cool skin. Pts may progress into a hypothermic, stuporous state (myxedema coma). Factors predisposing to myxedema coma include cold exposure, trauma, infection, and administration of narcotics. Respiratory depression may cause rise in arterial P_{CO_2}.

Decreased serum T_4 is common to all varieties of hypothyroidism. Serum TSH is ↑ in primary and normal or ↓ in secondary hypothyroidism. Increases in serum cholesterol, creatinine phosphokinase and lactic dehydrogenase are common, as are bradycardia, low-amplitude QRS complexes, and flattened or inverted T waves on ECG.

Levothyroxine is preferred *treatment*. In adults the initial daily dose of 25 μg/day is increased by 25–50 μg/day at 2–3 week intervals until serum TSH is within normal range (an average dose of 150 μg/day). When secondary hypothyroidism is suspected, thyroxine should not be administered until adrenal insufficiency has been treated. Treatment should be initiated rapidly in pts with myxedema coma and in hypothyroid pts being prepared for emergency surgery.

THYROTOXICOSIS *Symptoms* include nervousness, palpitations, emotional lability, inability to sleep, tremors, frequent bowel movements, excessive sweating, heat intolerance, oligomenorrhea, amenorrhea, and weight loss despite a well-maintained or increased appetite. Pt appears anxious, restless, and fidgety. Skin is warm, moist, and velvety; palms are erythematous; and fingernails may separate from the nail bed (Plummer's nail). Hair is fine and silky, and a fine tremor may involve fingers and tongue. Eye signs include a stare with widened palpebral fissures, infrequent blinking, and lid lag. Cardiovascular findings include a wide pulse pressure, especially atrial fibrillation, systolic murmurs, and cardiac enlargement.

Several disorders can produce thyrotoxicosis: *Graves' disease* is manifested by a diffuse goiter and infiltrative ophthalmopathy with variable ophthalmoplegia, proptosis, and periorbital swelling. *Treatment* is directed at limiting the amount of hormone the gland can produce. Antithyroid drugs interpose a chemical blockage to hormone synthesis (propylthiouracil 150 mg every 6 or 8 h). Leukopenia is the principal side effect. Ablation of thyroid tissue can be effected by surgery or radioiodine; indications for ablation include relapse or recurrence following drug therapy, large goiter, failure to follow a medical regimen, and unavailability for followup. Radioiodine affords a simple, effective, and economic means of treating thyrotoxicosis; as many as 40–70% of patients eventually become hypothyroid after radioiodine.

Toxic multinodular goiter can cause excess thyroid hormone production, usually in the elderly. The thyrotoxicosis is less severe than in Graves' disease, but impact on the cardiovascular system may be great. Radioactive iodine is the treatment of choice.

Thyrotoxicosis associated with *acute* and *subacute thyroidits* is due to leakage of preformed thyroid hormone from the inflamed gland. Thyroid function eventually returns to normal. Mild cases may be treated with aspirin; prednisone (20–40 mg/day) is reserved for severe cases. Propranolol may control symptoms of thyrotoxicosis.

Rarely, source of excess thyroid hormone is from outside the thyroid, e.g., *thyroid hormone ingestion* or *metastatic thyroid carcinoma*.

SICK EUTHYROID SYNDROME Severe illness, physical trauma, or physiological stress can alter peripheral binding and metabolism of thyroid hormones and regulation of TSH secretion. The most consistent feature is low serum T_3, and serum T_4 may be $\downarrow$, normal, or rarely $\uparrow$. Condition is due to a combination of inhibition of conversion of T_4 to T_3 and inhibition of serum binding of hormones. The importance of this syndrome is that is has to be distinguished from mild hypothyroidism or from mild hyperthyroidism. Measurements of serum T_4 or T_3 in conjunction with assessment of hormone binding are generally the most reliable means of making this distinction. Primary alterations in TBG produce changes in T_3 uptake that are inverse to those in serum T_4 and T_3, and as a result, free levels of the hormone and the FTI remain normal. By contrast, hyper- and hypothyroidism cause changes in free hormone levels in the same directions as those in total serum thyroxine. When the FTI is low (e.g., in severely ill patients), euthyroid state can be confirmed by measuring TSH.

THYROIDITIS **Subacute thyroiditis:** Can be due to any of several viruses, including mumps. *Symptoms* usually follow URI, are due to stretching of the thyroid capsule, and are principally pain over the thyroid or pain referred to lower jaw, ear, or occiput. Onset may be acute, with severe pain over thyroid, accompanied by fever and nodularity over thyroid. ESR may be ↑, and radioactive iodine uptake may be ↓. Early, many patients are mildly thyrotoxic owing to leakage of T_4 from gland. After glandular hormone is depleted, a hypothyroid phase may ensue. Normal thyroid function eventually returns. In mild cases, aspirin controls symptoms. In more severe cases, prednisone is generally effective. Propranolol can be used to control associated thyrotoxicosis. When RAIU returns to normal, therapy can be withdrawn without recurrence of symptoms.
Hashimoto's thyroiditis (lymphadenoid goiter): A chronic inflammation of thyroid, probably autoimmune in nature. Also coexists with other autoimmune diseases, including pernicious anemia, Sjögren's syndrome, chronic hepatitis, SLE, RA, adrenal insufficiency, and diabetes mellitus. Goiter may be asymmetric. Pt may be metabolically normal, but thyroid failure usually supervenes. The latter is evident first in a rise in serum TSH concentration, serum T_4 then declines, and when serum T_3 concentration falls, frank hypothyroidism ensues. High titers of thyroid antimicrosomal antibody are used. Treatment with replacement doses of levothyroxine is indicated. In some pts, such therapy is associated with regression of goiter.

NONTOXIC GOITER Enlargement of thyroid gland (normally 15–25 g) may be generalized or focal and may be associated with ↑, normal, or ↓ hormone secretion. Most commonly, a cause cannot be found. In the case of a nontoxic (euthyroid) goiter, clinical manifestations arise solely from the large gland itself when the metabolic state is normal. Mechanical sequelae include compression and displacement of trachea or esophagus and obstructive symptoms. *Treatment* is generally aimed at reduction in goiter size or prevention of further growth by suppression of TSH and is achieved by graduated dosages of levothyroxine to a maximum of 150–200 μg/day. Surgical resection is rarely indicated.

THYROID CARCINOMA Can involve follicular epithelium or parafollicular cells and usually presents as a single thyroid nodule. Features suggesting carcinoma include recent rapid growth of a nodule, fixation to surrounding structures, lymphadenopathy, and history of radiation to head or neck in infancy or childhood.

Diagnosis should be established by needle or surgical biopsy in suspicious cases.

For more detailed discussion of this topic, see Ingbar SH: Diseases of the Thyroid, Chap. 324, in HPIM, p. 1732

137 DISEASES OF THE ADRENAL CORTEX

CUSHING'S DISEASE Most common cause of glucocorticoid excess is iatrogenic use of corticosteroids. Excess production of cortisol by the adrenal (Cushing's disease) is usually due to bilateral adrenal hyperplasia secondary to hypersecretion of pituitary ACTH (micro- or macroadenomas) or production of ACTH by nonendocrine tumors (small cell carcinoma of lung, medullary carcinoma of thyroid, or tumors of thymus, pancreas, or ovary). Approximately 25% is due to adrenal neoplasm, half of which is malignant.

Glucocorticoid excess causes muscle weakness, cutaneous striae, and easy bruisability and promotes fat deposition in face (moon facies), interscapular areas (buffalo hump), and mesenteric bed (truncal obesity). Hypertension and emotional changes are common, and diabetes mellitus occurs in ≥ 10%.

Plasma and urine cortisol and urinary 17-hydroxycorticoid levels are elevated. Hypokalemia, hypochloremia, and metabolic alkalosis are prominent, particularly with ectopic production of ACTH.

Diagnosis: Requires demonstration of increased cortisol production and of failure to suppress cortisol secretion normally by dexamethasone (See Table 134-1). Overnight dexamethasone test or measurement of urinary free cortisol is an appropriate screening test. Definitive diagnosis requires demonstration of failure of suppression of urinary cortisol to <30 μg/day or plasma cortisol to <5 mg/dL after 0.5 mg dexamethasone q 6 h for 48 h. Once diagnosis is established, further testing is required to determine cause (Table 134-1). Demonstration of low levels of plasma ACTH suggests an adrenal adenoma or carcinoma, but a high plasma ACTH and/or failure of adrenal suppression by high-dose dexamethasone suggests an ACTH-producing tumor (pituitary or ectopic). A head CT scan can be used to differentiate pituitary from ectopic sources of ACTH.

Treatment: For adenoma or carcinoma, surgery; treatment of bilateral adrenal hyperplasia directed at pituitary (transsphenoidal hypophysectomy or radiation) or toward reducing adrenal steroid secretion (bilateral adrenalectomy, metyrapone, aminoglutethimide). On occasion, debulking of a lung carcinoma can cause remission of ectopic Cushing's disease.

PRIMARY HYPERALDOSTERONISM Causes increased tubular exchange of Na for K and H^+ in kidney and results in hypokalemia. Most pts have headaches and mild to moderate hypertension, but edema is not a feature. ECG signs of K depletion include prominent U waves, cardiac arrhythmias, and premature contractions.

Laboratory findings: Depend on duration and severity of K depletion: severe hypokalemia (<3 meq/L) implies body depletion in excess of 300 meq and causes impairment of concentration of urine. Hypernatremia is due to both Na retention and water loss from polyuria. Metabolic alkalosis and elevated serum HCO_3 are due to H^+ movement intracellularly and loss into urine.

Diagnosis: Suggested by persistent hypokalemia in a nonedematous hypertensive pt not receiving K-wasting diuretics (furosemide, ethacrynic acid, thiazides). Diagnostic features are (1) low plasma renin that fails to increase appropriately during volume depletion (upright posture or diuresis), and (2) hypersecretion of aldosterone that fails to suppress appropriately during volume expansion.

After diagnosis is made, a distinction must be made between bilateral adrenal hyperplasia and adrenal adenomas. Adenomas can be identified by abdominal CT scan or by percutaneous transfemoral adrenal vein catheterization with adrenal venography. A 2- to 3-fold increase in plasma aldosterone concentration may be present on involved side.

Treatment: Adenoma is usually treated by surgical excision, but dietary Na restriction and the aldosterone antagonist spironolactone (25–100 mg/day) are effective in many pts. Surgery is indicated for bilateral hyperplasia only if hypokalemia cannot be controlled with medical therapy.

ADRENAL INSUFFICIENCY (ADDISON'S DISEASE) Occurs when ≥90% of adrenal tissue is destroyed, either by TBC, histoplasmosis, coccidioidomycosis and cryptococcosis, or autoimmune mechanisms. Bilateral tumor metastases, amyloidosis, and sarcoidosis are rare causes.

Clinical manifestations: Include fatigability, weakness, anorexia, nausea and vomiting, cutaneous and mucosal pigmentation, hypotension, and occasionally, hypoglycemia. Routine laboratory parameters may be normal, or serum Na, Cl, and HCO_3 can be reduced while serum K is ↑. Extracellular fluid depletion accentuates hypotension.

Diagnosis: Requires assessment of adrenal capacity for steroid production. A rapid screening test is to administer 25 U ACTH (cosyntropin) intravenously and measure plasma cortisol levels before and 30 and 60 minutes later. An increment of <7 μg/dL above baseline suggests adrenal insufficiency. To differentiate primary from secondary adrenal insufficiency, cosyntropin is infused at a rate of 2 U/h for 24 h. In normal subjects, 17-hydroxysteroid excretion is increased by 25 mg/day, and plasma cortisol levels > 40 μg/dL. In secondary disease, the maximal urinary 17-hydroxysteroid is 3–20 mg/per day, and the plasma cortisol ranges from 10–40 mg/dL. Patients with primary disease have smaller responses.

Treatment: Hydrocortisone: in periods of stress, the dosage should be 100–200 mg/day, tapered for long-term replacement to 25–37.5 mg/day. Fludrocortisone (0.1 mg/day) also may be necessary. In emergencies, a bolus of 100 mg IV cortisol is followed by a continuous infusion of 10 mg/h.

PHEOCHROMOCYTOMA (see Chap. 59).

For more detailed discussion of this topic, see Williams GH, Dluhy RG: Diseases of the Adrenal Cortex, Chap. 325, in HPIM-11, p. 1753

DIAGNOSIS Requires a fasting plasma glucose of ≥140 mg/dL on two occasions. Pts with insulin-dependent diabetes (IDDM) develop ketoacidosis in absence of insulin. Those with non-insulin-dependent diabetes (NIDDM) do not develop ketoacidosis and may be treated with diet, oral hypoglycemics, or insulin. Secondary forms of diabetes occur in chronic pancreatitis, pheochromocytoma, acromegaly, and Cushing's syndrome. Hyperglycemia usually causes polyuria, polydipsia, polyphagia, and weight loss, but the first symptom may be ketoacidosis or hyperosmolar nonketotic coma.

Once diagnosis is established, a diet should be instituted that includes an appropriate number of calories based on ideal body weight, adequate protein, and a carbohydrate intake of about 40–60% of total calories. When hyperglycemia in NIDDM cannot be controlled by diet, sulfonylureas may be administered. Insulin is required for pts with IDDM and many with NIDDM. Conventional therapy involves the administration of an intermediate-acting insulin (NPH) once or twice a day with or without small amounts of regular insulin.

DIABETIC KETOACIDOSIS Results from insulin deficiency with a relative or absolute increase in glucagon and may be caused by cessation of insulin therapy or by infection, surgery, or emotional stress. Anorexia, nausea and vomiting, and increased urine output herald the onset, and abdominal pain, altered consciousness, Kussmaul breathing, or frank coma may ensue. Volume depletion can lead to vascular collapse and renal shutdown. Leukocytosis is common. Body temperature is normal or ↓. Fever suggests infection.

Laboratory findings: Include prerenal azotemia, hyperglycemia, and metabolic acidosis due to elevated plasma acetoacetate and β-hydroxybutyrate. Initial serum K and P levels may be normal or ↑ despite depletion of body stores. Mg deficiency may be present. Serum amylase may be ↑, and frank pancreatitis can occur.

Other forms of metabolic acidosis must be excluded: lactic acidosis, uremia, alcoholic ketoacidosis, and certain poisonings. If urine ketones are negative, another cause for acidosis is likely. If urine ketones are positive, plasma ketones should be measured; a strong test in undiluted plasma may be due to starvation whereas a strongly positive reaction beyond a 1:1 dilution is presumptive evidence for ketoacidosis.

Diabetic ketoacidosis cannot be reversed without insulin. Because pts with insulin resistance cannot be identified prospectively, it is preferable to administer 25–50 U/h of regular insulin IV until acidosis is reversed and lesser amounts for several hours thereafter (usually 0.1 U/kg per h). Therapy also requires intravenous fluids; 1–2 L isotonic saline is given initially, and additional amounts are determined by clinical assessment. When plasma glucose falls to about 300 mg/dL, 5% glucose solutions should be started, both as source of free water and to prevent late cerebral edema and hypoglycemia. Potassium must be replaced, but time of administration varies. Initial high serum K falls when glucose oxidation and plasma volume return toward normal. Poor prognostic signs include hypotension, azotemia, deep coma, and associated illness. Bicarbonate should be given when acidosis is severe ($pH \leq 7.0$), especially if hypotension is present. Most pts with diabetic ketoacidosis recover when properly treated. Causes of death include MI and infection, particularly pneumonia.

HYPEROSMOLAR NONKETOTIC COMA Profound dehydration results from sustained osmotic diuresis when pt is unable to drink sufficient water to keep up with urinary fluid losses. Commonly, an elderly diabetic develops a stroke or infection, which worsens hyperglycemia and prevents adequate water intake so that volume depletion causes prerenal azotemia. Seizures may occur. Other causes include tube feedings of high-protein formulas, peritoneal dialysis, high carbohydrate intake, and osmotic agents such as mannitol or urea.

Plasma glucose is generally around 1000 mg/dL. Mild metabolic acidosis may be present. Serum bicarbonate < 10 meq/L and normal plasma ketones suggest lactic acidosis. The serum osmolality is high, but because of hyperglycemia, serum Na may be normal. Serum osmolality can be estimated:

$$\text{Osmolality (mosm/L)} = 2([\text{Na}] + [\text{K}]) + \frac{\text{glucose (mg/dL)}}{18} + \frac{(\text{BUN mg/dL})}{2.8}$$

Average fluid deficit is 10 L. Sufficient IV fluids must be given to support circulation and urine flow. While free water is ultimately needed, 2–3 L isotonic saline should be given over first 1–2 h. Subsequently, half-strength saline can be used. As plasma glucose approaches normal, 5% dextrose can be given as a vehicle for free water. Insulin should be given to control hyperglycemia. Mortality rate is $> 50\%$.

LONG-TERM COMPLICATIONS Cause serious morbidity and mortality. *Peripheral atherosclerosis* may cause intermittent claudication, gangrene, CAD, and stroke. *Cardiomyopathy* can cause heart failure, despite angiographically normal coronary arteries. *Diabetic retinopathy* can be divided into simple (background) and proliferative forms. New vessel formation and scarring can cause vitreal hemorrhage and retinal detachment, so that it is leading cause of blindness. *Renal disease* is a major cause of death and disability. The kidneys are initially enlarged with "superfunction." Microalbuminuria then appears with excretion of albumin in the range of 20–200 mg/day. Once macroalbuminuria begins (>200 mg/day), GFR declines at a rate of about 1 mL/min per month. Ordinarily azotemia begins about 10–12 years after onset of diabetes and may be preceded by nephrotic syndrome. No specific treatment is available, but hypertension must be aggressively controlled. Low-protein diets may be useful.

Peripheral sensory neuropathy causes numbness, paresthesias, severe hypesthesias, and pain that may be deep-seated and severe and is often worse at night. Absent stretch reflexes and diminished vibratory sensation are early signs. A special problem is foot ulcers. Diabetics should be instructed about proper foot care to prevent ulcers. *Autonomic neuropathy* may cause GI complaints (esophageal dysfunction, delayed gastric emptying, constipation, or diarrhea), orthostatic hypotension, bladder dysfunction, incontinence, and (in men) erectile impotence.

For more detailed discussion of this topic, see Foster DW: Diabetes Mellitus, Chap. 327, in HPIM-11, p. 1778

---

139 HYPOGLYCEMIA

The diagnosis requires a plasma glucose <45–50 mg/dL in men and < 35–40 mg/dL in women, symptoms consistent with the diagnosis, and improvement of symptoms with an increase of plasma glucose (Whipple's triad). When diagnosis is strongly suspected, glucose should be administered after drawing blood for diagnostic studies.

Catecholamine secretion causes sweating, tremor, tachycardia, anxiety, and hunger. CNS symptoms include dizziness, visual abnormalities, diminished mental acuity, convulsions, and syncope.

POSTPRANDIAL (REACTIVE) HYPOGLYCEMIA Results when gastrectomy, gastrojejunostomy, pyloroplasty, or vagotomy causes rapid gastric emptying and when brisk absorption of glucose in turn causes excessive insulin release. Plasma glucose falls more rapidly than insulin levels, and hypoglycemia results. Additional causes include fructose intolerance, galactosemia, and leucine sensitivity.

FASTING HYPOGLYCEMIA Results from an imbalance between hepatic production and peripheral glucose utilization. Increased utilization (glucose demand of >200 g/day) usually results from hyperinsulinism (insulinoma, exogenous insulin, sulfonylurea ingestion, or insulin autoimmunity). Glucose overutilization with low plasma insulin can be due to extrapancreatic tumors (fibromas, sarcomas, hepatomas, carcinomas of GI tract, and adrenal tumors). Such tumors either produce insulin-like factors or utilize glucose directly. Hypoglycemia with low plasma insulin also may occur when free fatty acids are not available for oxidation, as in carnitine deficiency and carnitine palmitoyltransferase deficiency. Diminished hepatic glucose production can be due to alcoholism, adrenal insufficiency, or liver disease (i.e., CHF).

Diagnosis of fasting hypoglycemia is established by the simultaneous measurement of serum glucose, insulin, and C-peptide and urine sulfonylurea metabolites during an episode of symptoms consistent with hypoglycemia. If history is suggestive but fasting plasma glucose is normal, hospitalization for a 72-h fast is required; serial measurements are made until symptoms develop or fast is completed. Diagnosis of insulinoma requires a low plasma glucose and inappropriately high insulin. Exogenous insulin is excluded by the simultaneous measurement of C-peptide, and a screen for sulfonylureas eliminates the possibility of oral hypoglycemic agents. The presence of an extrapancreatic tumor is suggested by low glucose and insulin levels.

THERAPY Initial rapid IV administration of 50 mL 50% glucose in water followed by infusion of 10% glucose to keep plasma glucose > 100 mg/dL. Pts with glucose overutilization may require >10 g/h (or a diet containing more than 300 g carbohydrate/day if the patient can eat). Glucagon (1 mg) is less desirable because its transient effects are blunted when hepatic glycogen is depleted.

For more detailed discussion of this topic, see Foster DW, Rubenstein AH: Hypoglycemia, Insulinoma, and Other Hormone-Secreting Tumors of the Pancreas, Chap. 329, in HPIM-11, p. 1800

140 DISORDERS OF THE TESTES AND PROSTATE

Inadequate production of sperm can occur as an isolated defect, whereas inadequate formation of testosterone by the interstitial (Leydig) cells usually impairs spermatogenesis secondarily.

DISORDERS OF ANDROGENS Assessment of androgen status should include documenting timing and extent of sexual maturation at puberty, rate of beard growth, testicular size, current libido, sexual function, and general strength and energy. If Leydig cell dysfunction occurs prior to onset of puberty, sexual maturation will not occur (eunuchoidism), evidenced by an infantile amount and distribution of body hair, poor development of skeletal muscles, and failure of closure of the epiphyses so that the arm span is >5 cm greater than height and lower body segment is >5 cm longer than upper body segment (pubis to crown).

At the completion of puberty, plasma testosterone levels reach the adult level of 3–10 ng/mL throughout the day, and plasma LH and FSH levels are 5–20 IU/dL each. Testicular failure after puberty can be due either to hypothalamic-pituitary defects (secondary hypogonadism) or testicular failure (primary hypogonadism). Detection of Leydig cell failure that occurs after puberty requires a high index of suspicion, commonly presenting as gynecomastia or diminished virilization and libido.

Kallman's syndrome (hypogonadotropic hypogonadism): The most frequent cause of secondary hypogonadism; characterized by familial occurrence, low FSH and LH levels, and (in some) anosmia, midline skeletal defects, and mental retardation. Destruction of pituitary gland by tumors, infections, trauma, or metastatic disease ordinarily causes hypogonadism as a component of panhypopituitarism. Pts with Cushing's syndrome, congenital adrenal hyperplasia, hemochromatosis, and hyperprolactinemia (due to either pituitary adenomas or drugs such as phenothiazines) may have suppressed levels of LH and resultant low testosterone levels.

In men with primary hypogonadism, testosterone levels are ↓ and gonadotropin levels are ↑.

Klinefelter's syndrome: Most frequent cause of primary testicular failure; due to presence of one or more extra X chromosomes, usually 47,XXY karyotype. The testes are small and contain sclerosed tubules; azoospermia is usual. Gynecomastia is common. Variable features include a eunuchoid habitus, mental retardation, and diabetes mellitus.

Acquired primary testicular failure: Usually results from *viral orchitis*, most frequently mumps, but also may be due to trauma, radiation damage, or systemic diseases such as amyloidosis, Hodgkin's disease, and sickle cell anemia. Testicular failure also may result from malnutrition, renal failure, liver disease, and toxins such as lead, alcohol, marijuana, heroin, and methadone. Spironolactone and ketoconazole block the synthesis of testosterone, and spironolactone and cimetidine act as antiandrogens by competing for binding to the androgen receptor.

The aim of androgen therapy in hypogonadal men is to restore normal male secondary sexual characteristics (beard, body hair, external genitalia), male sexual behavior, and somatic development (hemoglobin, muscle mass). Parenteral administration of a long-acting testosterone ester (100–200 mg testosterone enanthate at 1- to 3-week intervals) causes a return of testosterone levels to normal.

MALE INFERTILITY Normal sperm production is dependent on both FSH and testosterone. When damage occurs to seminiferous tubule prior to puberty, testes are small and firm, whereas testes are usually soft following postpubertal damage (the capsule once enlarged does not contract to its previous size). Normal ejaculate volume should be >2 mL, with 20–100 million sperm/mL, >60% of which should be mobile. Plasma FSH usually correlates inversely with spermatogenesis.

In addition to secondary impairment of spermatogenesis by androgen deficiency, isolated spermatogenic tubule dysfunction and impaired spermatogenesis can arise from alterations of temperature of testes (varicocele), cryptorchism, cystic fibrosis, or immotile cilia syndrome. Kartagener's syndrome is a subgroup of the latter with situs inversus.

CARCINOMA OF TESTES Once universally fatal, now usually curable by excision and/or chemotherapy with cisplatin. Manifestations range from an asymptomatic nodule or swelling detected while performing testicular self-examination to symptoms caused by metastases. Any testicular mass in a man requires prompt evaluation to exclude testicular carcinoma.

PROSTATIC HYPERPLASIA Common in men > age 50, and 40% or more of men eventually develop urinary tract obstruction. Symptoms can be minimal if compensatory hypertrophy of detrusor musculature of bladder compensates for resistance to urine flow. With increasing obstruction, diminution in caliber and force of urinary stream, hesitancy in initiating voiding, postvoiding dribbling, sensation of incomplete emptying, and on occasion, urinary retention supervene. These obstructive symptoms must be distinguished from irritative symptoms such as dysuria, frequency, and urgency that can result from inflammatory, infectious, or neoplastic causes. As residual urine increases, nocturia and overflow incontinence may develop.

The prostate is palpated during digital rectal examination. Hyperplasia produces a smooth, firm, elastic enlargement. Bladder neck obstruction is evaluated by cystourethroscopy. Obstruction to outflow is assessed by measurement of urine flow rate and/or residual urine. Treatment is surgical, usually transurethral prostatectomy.

PROSTATIC CARCINOMA Cancer of the prostate is second most common malignancy in men. It can be asymptomatic at diagnosis, but most pts have extensive disease at diagnosis. Common presenting complaints include dysuria, difficulty in voiding, increased urinary frequency, complete urinary retention, back or hip pain, and hematuria.

Importance of the rectal exam in the physical exam of men cannot be stressed too strongly. The posterior surfaces of the lateral lobes, where carcinoma usually begins, are palpable on rectal examination. Carcinoma is characteristically hard, nodular, and irregular.

Biopsy is indicated when a palpable abnormality is detected or when lower urinary tract symptoms occur in men who have no known cause of obstruction. Core-needle biopsy may be performed transperineally or transrectally. Elevated serum acid phosphatase level is present in some localized disease but more commonly with extensive disease.

Surgical staging is the usual modality for identifying lymph node involvement and determining therapy. Radiation therapy and androgen deprivation (orchiectomy or diethylstilbestrol) are indicated for palliation of metastatic disease.

For more detailed discussion of these topics, see Griffin JE III, Wilson JD: Disorders of the Testes, Chap. 330, p. 1807; and Sagalowsky AI, Wilson JD: Hyperplasia and Carcinoma of the Prostate, Chap. 298, p. 1582, in HPIM-11

---

141 DISORDERS OF THE OVARY AND FEMALE GENITAL TRACT

MENSTRUAL DISORDERS **Abnormal uterine bleeding:** When uterine bleeding is suspected, other sources such as rectum, bladder, cervix, and vagina must be excluded. In premenarche period, abnormal uterine bleeding may result from trauma, infection, or precocious puberty. When vaginal bleeding develops following menopause, malignancy must be excluded.

In absence of pregnancy, abnormal uterine bleeding during reproductive years is associated with either ovulatory or anovulatory cycles. Menstrual bleeding with ovulatory cycles is spontaneous, regular in onset, predictable in duration and amount of flow, and usually painful. Abnormal but nevertheless regular cycles are usually due to organic obstruction of uterus, usually leiomyomas, adenomyosis, endometrial polyps, or on occasion, uterine synechiae or scarring. Bleeding between cyclic ovulatory menses can be due to cervical or endometrial lesions.

Menstrual bleeding unassociated with ovulation (dysfunctional uterine bleeding) is painless, irregular in occurrence, and unpredictable as to amount and duration. Transient disruption of hypothalamic-pituitary-ovarian cycle is a common cause of failure of ovulation in menarchial years. Persistent dysfunctional uterine bleeding in reproductive years is usually due to continuous estrogenization of uterus uninterrupted by cyclic progesterone withdrawal, most commonly due to polycystic ovarian disease.

Amenorrhea: All women of childbearing age with amenorrhea should be assumed to be pregnant until proven otherwise. Even when history and PE are not suggestive, it is prudent to exclude pregnancy by a suitable screening test.

Primary amenorrhea is defined as failure of menarche by age 16 regardless of the presence or absence of secondary sexual characteristics, and *secondary amenorrhea* is failure of menstruation for 6 months in a woman with previous periodic menses. However, the causes of primary and secondary amenorrhea overlap, and it is generally more useful classifying the disorder according to etiology (Fig. 141-1). Initial workup involves careful PE, serum prolactin assay, and evaluation of estrogen status.

Anatomic defects of reproductive tract: Defects that prevent vaginal bleeding include absence of vagina, imperforate hymen, transverse vaginal septae, and cervical stenosis; presence is usually suggested by PE. When findings are indeterminate, diagnosis can be established by administration of 10–20 mg medroxyprogesterone acetate/day PO for 5 days or 100 mg progesterone in oil IM. If estrogen levels are adequate (and outflow tract is intact), menstrual bleeding should occur within 1 week of ending progestogen treatment, and hence diagnosis is *chronic anovulation with estrogen present*, usually *polycystic ovarian disease*. If no withdrawal bleeding occurs and the serum prolactin level is normal in the anovulatory woman with absent estrogen, plasma gonadotropins should be measured. If plasma gonadotropins are ↑, the diagnosis

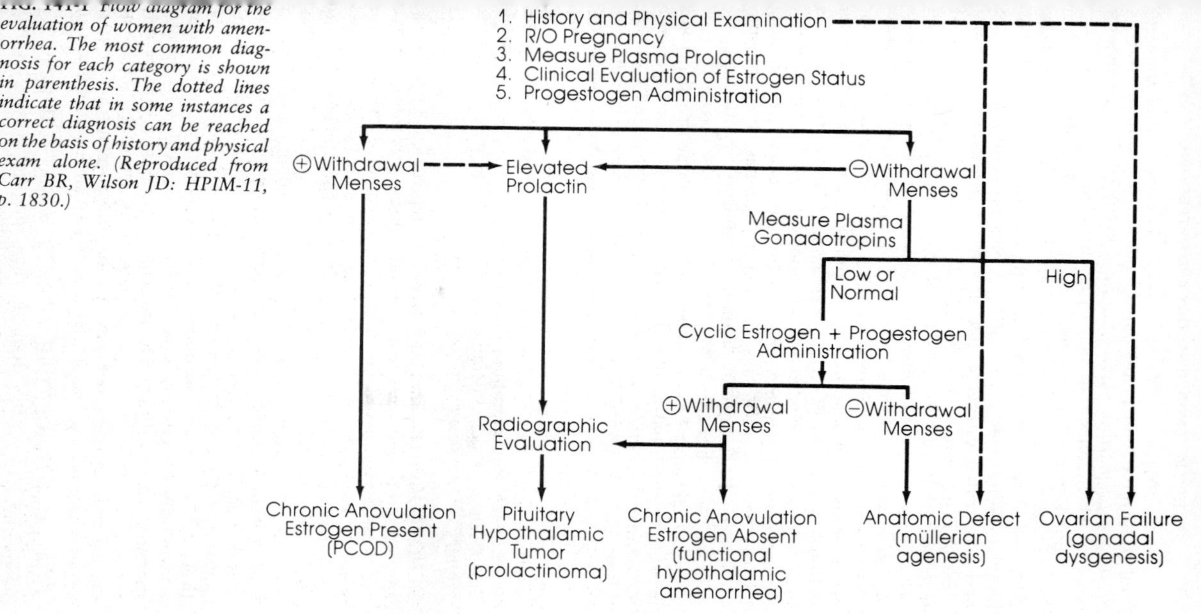

FIG. 141-1 *Flow diagram for the evaluation of women with amenorrhea. The most common diagnosis for each category is shown in parenthesis. The dotted lines indicate that in some instances a correct diagnosis can be reached on the basis of history and physical exam alone. (Reproduced from Carr BR, Wilson JD: HPIM-11, p. 1830.)*

is *ovarian failure*, i.e., *gonadal dysgenesis, resistant ovary syndrome*, or *premature ovarian failure*. Chromosomal karyotyping is useful when gonadal dysgenesis is suspected.

If gonadotropins are normal or ↓, the diagnosis is either *hypothalamic-pituitary disorder* or an anatomic defect of outflow tract (see above). When physical findings are not clear-cut, it is useful to administer cyclic estrogen plus progestogen (1.25 mg oral conjugated estrogens per day for 3 weeks with 10 mg medroxyprogesterone acetate added for the last 5–7 days of treatment) followed by 10 days of observation. If no bleeding occurs, the diagnosis of *Asherman's syndrome* or *other anatomic defects* of outflow tract is confirmed by hysteroscopy or hysterosalpingogram. If withdrawal bleeding occurs following estrogen-progesterone combination, the diagnosis is *chronic anovulation with estrogen absent (functional hypothalamic amenorrhea)*; causes include Kallman's syndrome (hypogonadotropic hypogonadism), extreme emotional stress, anorexia nervosa, chronic debilitating disease, pituitary adenomas, craniopharyngiomas, and panhypopituitarism. Radiologic evaluation of pituitary-hypothalamic region may be indicated.

Pelvic pain may be associated with normal menstrual periods as well as abnormal menstrual cycles. Many women experience abdominal discomfort with ovulation ("mittelschmerz"), a dull, aching pain at midcycle lasting minutes to hours. In addition, ovulatory women may experience somatic symptoms during the few days prior to menses, including edema, breast engorgement, abdominal discomfort, and a symptom of cyclic irritability, depression, and lethargy known as *premenstrual syndrome*. Severe or incapacitating cramping in women with ovulatory menses in the absence of demonstrable disorders of the pelvis is termed *primary dysmenorrhea*.

MENOPAUSE The interval between the reproductive years up to and beyond the last menstrual period. During this time there is a progressive loss of ovarian function accompanied by endocrine, somatic, and psychological changes. The same symptoms may result from surgical ablation of the ovaries and include those of vasomotor instability (hot flash), atrophy of urogenital epithelium and skin, decreased size of breasts, and osteoporosis. Additional symptoms include nervousness, anxiety, irritability, and depression. Plasma gonadotropins are elevated.

Estrogen therapy in menopause relieves vasomotor instability (hot flashes), prevents atrophy of urogenital epithelium and skin, and prevents osteoporosis. The risks of endometrial adenocarcinoma, venous thromboembolism, and hypertension may be minimized by low-dose cyclic estrogen administration (0.625 mg conjugated estrogen per day 25 days per month with daily progestogen for the last 10 days) and close clinical monitoring.

ORAL CONTRACEPTIVE AGENTS Widely used to prevent pregnancy and control dysmenorrhea and anovulatory bleeding. The ideal contraceptive contains the lowest amount of steroid to minimize side effects but sufficient to prevent pregnancy c breakthrough bleeding. Combination oral contraceptive agents contain synthetic estrogen (mestranol or ethinyl estradiol) and synthetic progestogen (norethindrone, norethindrone acetate, norethynodrel, norgestrel, or ethynodiol diacetate). Biphasic or triphasic formulations utilize different agents at different times of the cycle.

Despite overall safety, users are at risk for deep venous thrombosis, pulmonary embolism, thromboembolic stroke, hypertension, and cholelithiasis. Risks are increased with smoking and increasing age, and the drugs should be discontinued in women who experience visual complaints or headaches. Other side effects include minor dyspepsia, breast discomfort, weight gain, pigmentation of the face (chloasma), and psychological effects such as depression and changes in libido. Oral contraceptives are not associated with an increased incidence of cancer of the uterus, cervix, or breast.

Absolute contraindications to the use of oral contraceptives include previous thromboembolic disorders, cerebral vascular or coronary artery disease, known or suspected carcinoma of breasts or other estrogen-dependent neoplasia, undiagnosed genital bleeding, or known or suspected pregnancy. Relative contraindications include hypertension, migraine headaches, diabetes mellitus, uterine leiomyomas, sickle cell anemia, hyperlipidemia, and elective surgery.

For more detailed discussion of this topic, see Carr BR, Wilson JD: Disorders of the Ovary and Female Reproductive Tract, Chap. 333, in HPIM-11, p. 1818

---

142 DISORDERS OF THE BREAST

The breasts are the site of fatal and preventable disease in women and frequently provide clues to underlying systemic disease in both men and women. As a consequence, examination of the breasts is a vital part of the physical exam.

GALACTORRHEA Whereas small amounts of fluid can be commonly expressed from the breasts of parous women, secretions from the breasts of nulliparous women are always abnormal and require evaluation. Spontaneous leakage of milk is of particular concern. When secretion is milky or white, assume that it contains milk constituents; brown or green secretions rarely contain normal milk constituents. Bloody breast secretions suggest malignancy. Although enhanced prolactin secretion is necessary for initiation of milk production, the elevation need not be sustained in long-standing galactorrhea.

Galactorrhea is generally the result of failure of normal hypothalamic inhibition of prolactin release (sarcoidosis, craniopharyngioma, pinealoma, encephalitis, meningitis, hypothalamic tumors) or of autonomous secretion of prolactin (pituitary adenomas, hypothyroidism). Likewise, drugs (psychotropic agents, methyldopa, reserpine, antiemetics) may enhance prolactin release.

Once drug causes and hypothyroidism are excluded, workup of hyperprolactinemia is that of a pituitary tumor. *Treatment* is aimed at removing the source of elevated prolactin level, by resection or suppression of the pituitary tumor, withdrawal of causative drugs, or correction of hypothyroidism. Bromocriptine may cause disappearance of galactorrhea even when plasma prolactin levels are normal.

GYNECOMASTIA Growth of the breast in men and women is mediated by estrogen, and breast enlargement in men is believed to result from disturbances of the normal ratio of active androgen to estrogen or from increases in estrogen formation. In ≥50% of men with gynecomastia, no cause is found after extensive workup. Presumably, in these pts the elevation of estrogen is transient or remains unidentified, but in such cases the gynecomastia has no serious import for health. In other cases, gynecomastia results from major endocrine disturbances, including deficiency in testosterone production or action, increase in estrogen production, or drugs (Table 142-1).

Evaluation: (1) A careful drug history; (2) measurement and examination of testes (if both are small, a chromosomal karyotype should be obtained; if they are asymmetric, a testicular tumor should be considered); (3) evaluation of liver function; (4) measurement of plasma androstenedione or 24-h urinary 17-ketosteroids, plasma estradiol, plasma luteinizing hormone (LH), and plasma testosterone. If LH is ↑ and testosterone ↓, diagnosis is usually testicular failure; if both LH and testosterone are ↓, diagnosis is likely ↑ estrogen production; and if both LH and

TABLE 142-1 Differential diagnosis of gynecomastia

Physiologic gynecomastia:
Newborn
Adolescence
Aging
Pathologic gynecomastia:
Deficient production or action of testosterone:
Congenital anorchia
Klinefelter's syndrome
Androgen resistance
Defects in testosterone synthesis
Secondary testicular failure
Increased estrogen production:
Estrogen secretion:
True hermaphroditism
Testicular tumors
Carcinoma of the lung
Increased substate for peripheral aromatase:
Adrenal disease
Liver disease
Starvation
Thyrotoxicosis
Increase in peripheral aromatase
Drugs:
Estrogens
Gonadotropins
Inhibitors of testosterone synthesis and/or action
Unknown mechanisms
Idiopathic

Modified from Wilson JD: HPIM-11, p. 1839.

testosterone are ↑, diagnosis is either androgen resistance or a gonadotropin secreting tumor.

When primary cause of overestrogenization can be identified and corrected, breast enlargement usually subsides promptly and eventually disappears. *Indications for surgery* include severe psychological and/or cosmetic problems, continued growth, or suspected malignancy.

BREAST CANCER Breast cancer is a major disease. At particular risk are women whose mothers had breast cancer prior to menopause, women with first-degree relatives with postmenopausal breast cancer, nulliparous women above age 50, women whose first parity occurred after age 30, women with a history of chronic breast disease, women exposed to ionizing radiation, and obese women. Increased risk for breast carcinoma in men includes feminizing states (such as Klinefelter's syndrome) and testicular atrophy from viral orchitis or injury.

Breast cancer is frequently multicentric (13% of pts show microscopic foci in contralateral breast). Size of primary tumor can be estimated by palpitation combined with mammography. Tumor <2 cm in size are associated with most favorable outcome. Another prognostic factor is presence or absence of estrogen receptor (ER) and progesterone receptor (PR), the degree of positivity being proportional to cellular differentiation and responsiveness of tumor to hormonal deprivation.

Most breast masses are found by patient either accidentally or during self-examination. Annual mammograms are recommended for all women over 50 and for high-risk women ages 40–49. Disease usually presents with a hard, circumscribed mass in breast. Most lumps are benign, but if mass is fixed to skin or muscle or there is edema of skin or retraction of nipple, breast cancer is more likely. Once a mass is detected, metastatic disease should be searched for, and the mass should then be biopsied.

The current trend in management aims at minimal disfigurement by surgical or radiation therapy and control of metastatic disease with adjuvant systemic chemotherapy.

Skeletal metastases can cause both pain and fractures, including vertebral collapse. Limited-field irradiation of metastases and narcotics may be effective in control of pain. Hypercalcemia is also common in metastatic disease (see Chap. 143).

For more detailed discussion of these topics, see Henney JE, DeVita VT Jr.: Breast Cancer, Chap. 295, p. 1567; Wilson JD: Endocrine Disorders of the Breast, Chap. 332, p. 1837, in HPIM-11

143 HYPER- AND HYPOCALCEMIC DISORDERS

HYPERCALCEMIA

Primary hyperparathyroidism is a generalized disorder of bone metabolism that results from increased secretion of parathyroid hormone (PTH), because of either an adenoma (81%), carcinoma (4%) in a single gland, or hyperplasia of all 4 glands (15%). Familial hyperparathyroidism may be part of multiple endocrine neoplasia type I (MEN I), which also includes tumors of pituitary and pancreatic islets and hypergastrinemia with peptic ulcer disease (Zollinger-Ellison syndrome), or MEN II, in which hyperparathyroidism occurs with pheochromocytoma and medullary carcinoma of the thyroid.

Half or more of pts with hyperparathyroidism are asymptomatic. Specific manifestations involve primarily the kidneys (nephrolithiasis and nephrocalcinosis) and the skeletal system (commonly osteitis fibrosa cystica, in which normal cellular and marrow elements are replaced by fibrous tissue). Resorption of phalangeal tufts, subperiosteal resorption of bone in the digits, and tiny "punched out" lesions in the skull also may be present. Other symptoms are the result of hypercalcemia itself (see below).

Diagnosis is made on clinical grounds and confirmed by demonstration of an inappropriately ↑ PTH level for degree of hypercalcemia. Hypercalcemia may be intermittent or sustained. Serum K may be normal or low. Serum Cl is often ↑ with a reduced serum bicarbonate. An ↑ Cl and ↓ K (reflecting acidosis and renal phosphate wasting) can be a diagnostic clue. *Treatment* is usually surgical removal of involved gland or glands.

Hypercalcemia due to *malignancy* is common (involving 10–15% of tumors such as lung carcinoma), often severe, and difficult to manage. Malignancies may cause hypercalcemia by local bone destruction (myeloma, breast carcinoma), by increased synthesis of $1,25(OH)_2$ vitamin D (lymphoma), or by elaborating other humoral mediators of bone resorption (lung, kidney, squamous cell carcinomas).

Sarcoidosis and other granulomatous diseases (such as TBC and histoplasmosis) cause hypercalcemia by increasing the synthesis of $1,25(OH)_2$ vitamin D, thus enhancing calcium and phosphorus absorption from the gastrointestinal tract. Hypercalcemia also results from high bone turnover states such as *hyperthyroidism*, from *immobilization*, from *thiazide use*, and (rarely) from *vitamin A intoxication*. Secondary hyperparathyroidism may complicate end stage renal disease.

Hypercalcemia from any cause can cause fatigue, depression, mental confusion, anorexia, vomiting, constipation, renal tubular defects, increased urination, a short QT interval in the ECG, and cardiac arrhythmias. Symptoms are more common at Ca levels > 11.5–12.0 mg/dL. When Ca exceeds 13 mg/dL, nephrocalcinosis and renal insufficiency and calcification of skin, vessels, lungs, heart, and stomach may occur, particularly if blood phosphate is normal or high due to impaired renal function. Hypercalcemia > 15 mg/dL may cause coma and cardiac arrest.

Serum Ca levels can usually be reduced by 3–9 mg/dL by aggressive treatment. The first principle is to expand extracellular fluid volume with 2–3 L isotonic saline over several hours. Continued saline and furosemide administration will further enhance calcium excretion. Plicamycin (Mithramycin) may inhibit bone resorption in the hypercalcemia of malignancy. Glucocorticoids, indomethicin, and calcitonin may be useful in selective cases.

HYPOCALCEMIA

Can occur in the setting of low, normal, or increased levels of parathyroid hormone (Table 143-1). *Hypoparathyroidism* is usually the result of inadvertent removal of glands or compromise of blood supply to glands during thyroidectomy. Other causes include hemochromatosis and radiation damage. Also may occur as part of an autoimmune syndrome involving failure of adrenals, ovaries, and parathyroids in association with recurrent mucocutaneous candidiasis, alopecia, vitiligo, and pernicious anemia, the so-called autoimmune polyendocrine deficiency syndrome. Severe *hypomagnesemia* (<0.8 meq/L) causes hypocalcemia from both impaired secretion of PTH and ↓ responsiveness to its action. Repletion of Mg is the treatment.

Hypocalcemia also may result from *vitamin D deficiency* (inadequate dietary intake or malabsorption), abnormal metabolism of vitamin D (anticonvulsant therapy), or impaired production of

TABLE 143-1 Functionally based classification of hypocalcemia (excluding neonatal conditions)

- PTH absent:
  - Hereditary hypoparathyroidism
  - Acquired hypoparathyroidism
  - Hypomagnesemia
- PTH ineffective:
  - Chronic renal failure
  - Active vitamin D lacking:
    - ↓ dietary intake or sunlight
    - Defective metabolism:
      - Anticonvulsant therapy
      - Vitamin D–dependent rickets—type I
  - Active vitamin D ineffective:
    - Intestinal malabsorption
    - Vitamin D–dependent rickets—type II
  - Pseudohypoparathyroidism
- PTH overwhelmed:
  - Severe, acute hyperphosphatemia:
    - Tumor lysis
    - Acute renal failure
    - Rhabdomyolysis
  - Osteitis fibrosa after parathyroidectomy

Modified from Potts JT Jr.: HPIM-11, p. 1884.

$1,25(OH)_2D$ (as in renal failure). Hypocalcemia also occurs in *pseudohypoparathyroidism*, in which ↓ serum Ca and ↑ serum phosphorus occur in association with shortened metacarpals and metatarsals and osteodystrophy because of a deficient end-organ response to PTH. Immunoreactive PTH levels are ↑.

Transient hypocalcemia can occur in association with severe sepsis, burns, acute renal failure, or extensive transfusions with citrated blood. Heparin, protamine, and glucagon may cause transient hypocalcemia. Pts with acute pancreatitis may have hypocalcemia during acute phase. Hypoalbuminemia can cause decreased total Ca concentration, but free levels of Ca are usually normal.

Manifestations include muscle spasms, carpopedal spasm, facial grimacing, laryngeal spasm, convulsions, and respiratory arrest. Increased intracranial pressure and papilledema may occur in long-standing hypocalcemia. Other manifestations include irritability, depression, psychosis, intestinal cramps, and chronic malabsorption. Chvostek's or Trousseau's signs are frequently positive. The QT interval on ECG is prolonged.

Symptomatic hypocalcemia may be treated with IV calcium chloride or calcium gluconate. Treatment of chronic hypocalcemia generally involves administration of Ca and vitamin D.

For more detailed discussion of this topic, see Potts JT Jr.: Diseases of the Parathyroid Gland and Other Hyper- and Hypocalcemic Disorders, Chap. 336, in HPIM-11, p. 1870

OSTEOPOROSIS A reduction of bone density below level required for mechanical support. Remodeling of bone (formation and resorption) is continuous, and density decreases whenever rate of resorption exceeds formation. Vertebrae, wrist, hip, humerus, and tibia are particularly prone to fracture.

In *type I osteoporosis* disproportionate loss of trabeculae is associated with fractures of vertebrae and distal forearm in middle-aged, postmenopausal women. *Type II osteoporosis* occurs in men and women above age 75 and is associated with fractures of femoral neck, proximal humerus, proximal tibia, and pelvis.

Vertebral collapse is common in lower dorsal and upper lumbar regions after sudden bending, lifting, or jumping movements. Pain usually subsides after days, and patients may be ambulatory in 4–6 weeks. Collapse unassociated with pain can cause dorsal kyphosis and exaggerated cervical lordosis (widow's hump).

Blood levels of Ca, phosphorus, and alkaline phosphatase are normal. Mild hypercalciuria may be present. In absence of fractures, a 30% decrease in bone mass may not be evident on standard x-rays. More sensitive studies such as single and dual photon bone densitometry, quantitative CT, and neutron activation analysis may suggest whether pt is at risk for fracture.

Osteoporosis is common in Cushing's syndrome and with prolonged administration of corticosteroids. Additional predisposing conditions include hyperthyroidism, acromegaly, diabetes mellitus, Ca deficiency, malabsorption, and cigarette smoking. Other diseases known to reduce bone mass must be searched for, including hyperparathyroidism and malignancies such as multiple myeloma, lymphoma, leukemia, and carcinomas.

Treatment: Directed toward prevention of further loss of bone mass or to an increase in bone density. White postmenopausal women who are small, sedentary, and smokers are at high risk of developing osteoporosis. Estrogen administration to postmenopausal women decreases rate of bone resorption, but bone mass does not increase and eventually usually decreases. Oral Ca (1–1.5 g elemental Ca/day) also decreases bone resorption. Thiazide diuretics are useful in high-turnover osteoporosis with hypercalciuria and secondary hyperparathyroidism. Fluoride increases new bone formation. These therapies not only retard loss of bone density, but also result in decreased fracture rate in subjects at risk.

OSTEOMALACIA Defective mineralization of organic matrix of bone; may result from inadequate intake or malabsorption of vitamin D (chronic pancreatic insufficiency, gastrectomy, and steatorrhea of other causes), acquired or inherited disorders of vitamin D metabolism (anticonvulsant therapy or chronic renal failure), chronic acidosis (renal tubular acidosis, acetozolamide ingestion), renal tubular defects that produce hypophosphatemia

(Fanconi's syndrome), and chronic administration of aluminum-containing antacids.

Clinical manifestations: May be subtle in adults. Skeletal deformities may be overlooked until fractures occur after minimal trauma. Symptoms include diffuse skeletal pain and bony tenderness. Pain in hips may result in an altered gait. Proximal muscle weakness may mimic primary muscle disorders. Decrease in bone density is usually associated with loss of trabeculae and thinning of cortices. Characteristic x-ray finding is radiolucent bands (Looser's zones or pseudofractures) ranging from a few millimeters to several centimeters in length, usually perpendicular to surface of femur, pelvis, scapula, upper fibula, or metatarsals. Changes in serum Ca, phosphorus, 25(OH)D, and 1,25$(OH)_2$D vary with underlying causes.

Treatment: In osteomalacia due to vitamin D deficiency 2000–4000 IU/day vitamin D_2 (cholecalciferol) or D_3 (ergocalciferol) is given PO for 6–12 weeks, followed by daily supplements of 200–400 IU. Healing of pseudofractures may be evident within 3–4 weeks. Osteomalacia due to malabsorption requires large doses of vitamin D (up to 100,000 IU/day) and Ca (calcium carbonate 4 g/day). In pts on anticonvulsants, it is usually necessary to continue drugs while administering sufficient vitamin D to bring serum calcium and serum 25(OH)D to the normal range. Dihydrotachysterol (0.2–1.0 mg/day) or calcitrol (0.25 μg/day) are effective in treating hypocalcemia and osteodystrophy of chronic renal failure.

For more detailed discussion of this topic, see Krane SM, Holick MF: Metabolic Bone Disease, Chap. 337, in HPIM-11, p. 1889

145 DISORDERS OF LIPID METABOLISM

REGULATION OF PLASMA LIPIDS

LIPID TRANSPORT Exogenous pathway: In the intestinal wall, dietary triglycerides and cholesterol are incorporated into large lipoproteins (chylomicrons), which are transported via lymph to the circulation. Chylomicrons contain apoprotein CII, which activates lipoprotein lipase in capillaries, thus liberating fatty acids and monoglycerides from the chylomicron. Fatty acids pass through the endothelial cells into adipocytes or muscle. The chylomicron remnants in the circulation are taken up by liver. Net result is to deliver triglycerides to adipose tissue and cholesterol to the liver. **Endogenous pathway:** The liver synthesizes triglycerides and secretes them into the circulation together with cholesterol in the form of very low density lipoproteins (VLDL). VLDL particles are large, carry 5–10 times more triglycerides than cholesterol esters, and like other lipoproteins, are coated with apoproteins that direct them to tissues where lipoprotein lipase hydrolyzes triglycerides. VLDL remnants either return to the liver for reutilization or are processed to low-density lipoprotein (LDL). LDL supplies cholesterol to extrahepatic cells, such as adrenal cortex, lymphocytes, muscles, and kidney. LDL binds to specific receptors on cell surfaces and then undergoes endocytosis and digestion by lysosomes. The liberated cholesterol is used for membrane synthesis and metabolic requirements. In addition, some LDL is degraded by a scavenger system in phagocytic cells in the reticuloendothelial system. As cell membranes undergo turnover, unesterified cholesterol is released into plasma, where it initially binds to high-density lipoprotein (HDL) and is esterified with fatty acid by lecithin:cholesterol acyltransferase (LCAT). HDL cholesterol esters are transferred to VLDL and eventually to LDL. By this cycle LDL delivers cholesterol to cells and cholesterol returns from extrahepatic sites via HDL.

HYPERLIPOPROTEINEMIA (See Table 145-1.)

In adults, hyperlipoproteinemia is defined as plasma cholesterol > 240 mg/dL or triglyceride levels > 200 mg/dL. An isolated ↑ in plasma triglycerides indicates that chylomicrons, VLDL, and/or remnants are increased. An isolated ↑ of plasma cholesterol indicates ↑ LDL. Elevations of both triglycerides and cholesterol are caused by elevations in chylomicrons or VLDL, in which case the triglyceride/cholesterol ratio > 5:1. Alternatively, ↑ of both VLDL and LDL is associated with a triglyceride/cholesterol ratio < 5:1.

FAMILIAL LIPOPROTEIN LIPASE DEFICIENCY Rare autosomal recessive disorder that results from absence or deficiency in liproprotein lipase, which in turn retards metabolism of chylomicrons. Accumulation of chylomicrons in plasma causes recurrent bouts of pancreatitis, beginning usually in childhood. Eruptive

TABLE 145-1 Characteristics of the primary hyperlipoproteinemias

Disorder	Plasma lipoprotein elevation	Lipoprotein electrophoresis pattern	Serum findings	
			Cholesterol	Triglycerides
Familial lipoprotein lipase deficiency	Chylomicrons	1	N*	↑
Familial apoprotein CII deficiency	Chylomicrons and VLDL	1 or 5	N	↑
Familial dysbetalipoproteinemia	Remnants	3	↑	↑
Familial hypercholesterolemia	LDL	2a (rarely 2b)	↑	N
Familial hypertriglyceridemia	VLDL (rarely chylomicrons)	4 (rarely 5)	N	↑
Multiple lipoprotein-type hyperlipidemia (familial combined hyperlipidemia)	LDL and VLDL	2a, 2b, or 4 (rarely 5)	↑	↑

* N = normal.

Modified from Brown MS, Goldstein JL: HPIM-11, p. 1653.

xanthomas occur on buttocks, trunk, and extremities. Plasma is milky or creamy (lipemic). Symptoms and signs recede when patient is placed on a fat-free diet (<20 g/day). Accelerated atherosclerosis is not a feature.

FAMILIAL APOPROTEIN CII DEFICIENCY Rare autosomal recessive disorder due to absence of apoprotein CII, an essential cofactor for lipoprotein lipase. As a result, chylomicrons and triglycerides accumulate and cause manifestations similar to those in lipoprotein lipase deficiency. *Diagnosis* requires demonstration of absence of apoprotein CII by protein electrophoresis. *Treatment* involves the use of fat-free diet.

FAMILIAL DYSBETALIPOPROTEINEMIA Transmitted as a single-gene mutation, but expression requires additional environmental and/or genetic factors. Plasma cholesterol and triglycerides are ↑ due to accumulation of remnant-like particles derived from VLDL. Severe atherosclerosis involves coronary arteries, internal carotids, and abdominal aorta and causes premature MI, intermittent claudication, and gangrene. Cutaneous xanthomas are distinctive: xanthoma striata palmaris and tuberous or tuberoeruptive xanthomas. Plasma levels of triglyceride and cholesterol are similar (approximately 300 mg/dL). *Diagnosis* is established by finding of a broad beta band on lipoprotein electrophoresis. *Treatment* is either clofibrate or gemfibrozil. If present, hypothyroidism and diabetes mellitus must be treated.

FAMILIAL HYPERCHOLESTEROLEMIA Autosomal dominant disorder that affects 1 in 500 individuals. Heterozygotes manifest a 2- to 3-fold ↑ in plasma cholesterol and LDL. Accelerated atherosclerosis causes premature MI, particularly in men. Xanthomas of tendons and arcus cornea are common. Diagnosis is suggested by finding an isolated ↑ of plasma cholesterol with normal triglycerides. Every effort should be made to lower plasma cholesterol concentration to normal. *Treatment* is restriction of dietary cholesterol and bile acid–binding resins (cholestyramine or colestipol), with or without nicotinic acid.

FAMILIAL HYPERTRIGLYCERIDEMIA Autosomal dominant disorder in which ↑ of plasma VLDL causes plasma triglyceride concentration to range from 200–500 mg/dL. Obesity, hyperglycemia, and hyperinsulinemia are characteristic, and diabetes mellitus, ethanol consumption, oral contraceptives, and hypothyroidism may exacerbate the condition. Because atherosclerosis is accelerated, vigorous attempts should be made to control all exacerbating factors, and intake of saturated fat should be minimal. If dietary measures fail, clofibrate or gemfibrozil should be administered.

MULTIPLE LIPOPROTEIN-TYPE HYPERLIPIDEMIA Inherited disorder that can cause different lipoprotein abnormalities in affected subjects, including hypercholesterolemia (type 2a lipoprotein pattern), hypertriglyceridemia (type 4), or simultaneous hypercholesteremia and hypertriglyceridemia (type 2b). Atherosclerosis is accelerated. *Therapy* should be directed at predominant lipid abnormality. Restriction of dietary fat and cholesterol and avoidance of alcohol and oral contraceptives are appropriate for all patients. Triglyceride elevation may respond to clofibrate or gemfibrozil, and a bile acid–binding resin or nicotinic acid may be used when cholesterol is elevated.

SECONDARY HYPERLIPOPROTEINEMIAS Diabetes mellitus, ethanol consumption, oral contraceptives, and hypothyroidism can either cause secondary hyperlipoproteinemias or worsen prior hyperlipoproteinemic states. In either case, control of aggravating or inciting cause is essential for management.

For more detailed discussion of this topic, see Brown MS, Goldstein JL: The Hyperlipoproteinemias and Other Disorders of Lipid Metabolism, Chap. 315, in HPIM-11, p. 1650

HEMOCHROMATOSIS

Occurs when increased intestinal iron absorption causes Fe deposition, fibrosis, and organ failure of liver, heart, pancreas, and pituitary. Cause can either be a single-gene mutation, impaired hematopoiesis (as in sideroblastic anemia and thalassemia), or excessive Fe ingestion. Alcoholic liver disease also may be associated with a moderate increase in hepatic Fe and elevated body Fe stores. **Symptoms** include weakness, lassitude, weight loss, darkening of skin, abdominal pain, and loss of libido. Hepatomegaly occurs in 95% of pts, sometimes in the presence of normal LFTs. Other signs include bronze pigmentation, spider angioma, splenomegaly, arthropathy, ascites, cardiac arrythmias, CHF, loss of body hair, palmar erythema, gynecomastia, and testicular atrophy. The latter is due to pituitary involvement and gonadotropin deficiency. Diabetes mellitus occurs in about 65%, usually in pts with family history of diabetes.

Serum Fe, percent transferrin saturation, and serum ferritin levels are ↑. Liver biopsy is the definitive test and should be performed in suspected cases. Once diagnosis is established, family members at risk should be screened.

Treatment involves removal of excess body Fe, usually by intermittent phlebotomy. Since 1 unit of blood contains about 250 mg Fe, and since 25 g or more of Fe must be removed, phlebotomy is performed weekly for 2–3 years. Less frequent phlebotomy is then used to maintain serum Fe at < 150 μg/dL.

Causes of death in untreated patients include cardiac failure (30%), cirrhosis (25%), and hepatocellular carcinoma (30%); the latter may develop despite adequate Fe removal.

WILSON'S DISEASE

An autosomal recessive disorder that causes accumulation of copper in liver, brain, and other organs. Underlying defect is an inability to excrete Cu cleaved from ceruloplasmin into bile. Excessive Cu inhibits formation of ceruloplasmin from apoceruloplasmin and Cu, and when capacity to store Cu in liver is exceeded, it is released into blood and deposited in extrahepatic sites. Pathologic consequences in liver include necrosis, inflammation, fibrosis, and cirrhosis. On occasion, death can occur from the CNS effects when liver dysfunction is minimal.

Disease may present as acute hepatitis, cirrhosis, or asymptomatic hepatomegaly. Green or golden deposits in the cornea (Kayser-Fleischner rings) can be demonstrated by slit-lamp examination. Neurologic manifestations include resting and intention tremors, spasticity, rigidity, chorea, drooling, dysphagia, and dysarthria. Schizophrenia, manic depressive psychosis and neuroses may occur.

Diagnosis should be suspected in any pt $<$ age 40 with unexplained CNS disease, chronic active hepatitis, or cirrhosis of unknown etiology. Diagnosis is confirmed by demonstration of (1) a serum ceruloplasmin < 20 mg/dL and Kayser-Fleischner rings or (2) a serum ceruloplasmin < 20 mg/dL and a Cu level in a liver biopsy specimen > 250 μg/g dry weight.

Treatment is lifelong; penicillamine is given in an initial dose of 1 g PO before meals and at bedtime. WBC and platelet counts, UA, and body temperatures should be monitored several times weekly for the first month of therapy. Hypersensitivity reactions to penicillamine are common and should be treated with prednisone. Serum-free Cu should be kept < 10 μg/dL.

PORPHYRIAS

Result from any of several inherited or acquired disturbances in heme biosynthesis, each of which causes a unique pattern of overproduction, accumulation, and excretion of intermediates of heme synthesis. Manifestations include intermittent nervous system dysfunction and/or sensitivity of skin to sunlight.

ACUTE INTERMITTENT PORPHYRIA Characterized by recurrent attacks of colicky abdominal pain and neurologic and psychiatric abnormalities. Photosensitivity is not a feature. Both sensory and motor neuropathies occur, as may delerium, coma, and seizure. Manifestations may be precipitated by barbiturates, anticonvulsants, alcohol, estrogens, contraceptives, or prolonged fasting. Diagnosis is made by demonstration of large amounts of urine porphobilinogen (Watson-Swartz test). *Treatment* involves administration of IV glucose up to 20 g/h. If symptoms are not improved in 48 h, hematin, 4 mg/kg body weight, should be infused every 12 h for 3–6 days.

PORPHYRIA CUTANEA TARDA The most common porphyria; characterized by chronic skin lesions and (usually) hepatic disease. Common in alcoholics; due to deficiency (inherited or acquired) of uroporphyrinogen decarboxylase. Photosensitivity causes enhanced facial pigmentation, increased fragility of skin, erythema, and vesicular and ulcerative lesions, typically involving face, forehead, and forearms. Liver disease and hepatic siderosis may be related to alcoholism. Diabetes mellitus, SLE, and other autoimmune diseases may coexist. Urine uroporphyrin and coproporphyrin are increased. Abstinence from alcohol leads to improvement, and decrease in hepatic iron may ameliorate skin lesions. Chloroquine may be used in pts unable to undergo phlebotomy.

CONGENITAL ERYTHROPOIETIC PORPHYRIA A rare autosomal recessive defect that causes chronic photosensitivity, mutilating skin lesions, and hemolytic anemia. Death may occur in childhood. Exposure to sunlight should be avoided.

For more detailed discussion of these topics, see Powell LW, Isselbacher KI: Hemochromatosis, Chap. 310, p. 1632; Scheinberg IH: Wilson's Disease, Chap. 311, p. 1636; and Meyer UA: Porphyrias, Chap. 312, p. 1638, in HPIM-11

SECTION X
DERMATOLOGY

147 GENERAL EXAMINATION OF THE SKIN

Physical examination usually provides more useful information than history. Examination of skin with precise description of lesion(s) should generate a differential diagnosis regardless of Hx; narrowing the differential is then aided by pertinent facts from Hx. Examination of skin should take place in a well-illuminated room with pt completely disrobed. Ancillary helpful equipment includes a hand lens and a pocket flashlight to provide peripheral illumination of lesions.

GENERAL EXAMINATION **History:** Onset, duration, progression of lesions, prior treatment, allergies, personal or family Hx of atopic disease, occupation, predisposing or aggravating factors (including underlying diseases, exposure to cosmetics or irritating chemicals, etc.).

PHYSICAL EXAMINATION **Distribution:** Sun-exposed (SLE, photoallergic, phototoxic, polymorphous light eruption, porphyria cutanea tarda); dermatomal (herpes zoster); generalized (systemic diseases); extensor surfaces (elbows and knees in psoriasis); flexural surfaces (antecubiteal and popliteal fossae in atopic dermatitis). **Configuration:** *Linear*—contact dermatitis such as poison ivy or lesions that appear at sites of local skin trauma (Koebner phenomenon), such as psoriasis, lichen planus, and lichen nitidis; *annular*—"ring-shaped" lesion with an active border and central clearing (erythema chronicum migrans, erythema annulare centrificum, and tinea corporis); *circinate*—circular lesion (urticaria, herald patch of pityriasis rosea); *nummular*—"coin-shaped" (nummular eczema); *guttate*—"droplike" (guttate psoriasis); *morbilliform*—"measles-like" with small confluent papules coalescing into unusual shapes (measles, drug eruption); *reticulated*—"netlike" (livedo reticularis); *herpetiform*—grouped vesicles, papules, or erosions (herpes simplex); *iris or target lesion*—two or three concentric circles of differing hue (erythema multiforme).

PRIMARY LESIONS Cutaneous changes caused directly by disease process.

Macule—a flat circumscribed, lesion of a different color, allowing for differentiation from surrounding skin; *patch*—macule > 1 cm in diameter; *papule*—elevated, circumscribed lesion of any color < 1 cm in diameter, with the major portion of lesion projecting above surrounding skin; *nodule*—palpable lesion similar to a papule but > 1 cm in diameter; *plaque*—an elevated lesion > 2 cm in diameter; *vesicle*—sharply marginated elevated lesion < 1 cm in diameter filled with clear fluid; *bullae*—vesicular lesion > 1 cm in diameter; *pustule*—a well-marginated focal accumulation of inflammatory cells within skin; *wheal*—a transient elevated lesion due to accumulation of fluid in upper dermis; *cyst*—lesion consisting of liquid or semisolid material contained within limits of cyst wall (true cyst).

SECONDARY LESIONS Changes in area of primary pathology often due to secondary events, e.g., scratching, secondary infection, bleeding.

Scale—a flaky accumulation of excess keratin that is partially adherent to skin; *crust*—a circumscribed collection of inflammatory cells and dried serum on skin surface; *erosion*—a circumscribed, usually depressed, moist lesion resulting from loss of overlying epidermis; *ulcer*—a deeper erosion involving not only epidermis but also underlying papillary dermis; may leave a scar on healing; *atrophy:* (1) epidermal—thinning of skin with loss of normal skin surface markings, (2) dermal—depression of skin surface due to loss of underlying collagen or dermal ground substance; *lichenification*—thickening of skin with accentuation of normal skin surface markings most commonly due to chronic rubbing; *scar*—collection of fibrous tissue replacing normal dermal constituents.

OTHER DESCRIPTIVE TERMS: *Verrucous*—"wartlike"; *poikiloderma*—a combination of atrophy, hypo- and hyperpigmentation, and telangiectasia; *umbilicated*—containing a central depression; *color terms*—(i.e., violaceous, erythematous); *pedunculated*—on a stalk; *eczematous*—a crusted, weeping, erythematous, scaly patch with vesicles or erosions.

ROUTINE DIAGNOSTIC PROCEDURES **Potassium hydroxide preparation:** Useful for detection of dermatophyte or yeast. Scale is collected from advancing edge of a scaling lesion by gently scraping with side of a microscope slide. Nail lesions are best sampled by trimming back nail and scraping subungual debris. A drop of 10–15% potassium hydroxide is added to slide and cover slip is applied. The slide may be gently heated and examined under microscope. Positive preparations show translucent, septate branching hyphae among keratinocytes.

Tzanck preparation: Useful for determining presence of herpes viruses. Optimal lesion to sample is an early vesicle. Lesion is gently unroofed with no. 15 scalpel blade and base of vesicle is gently scraped with belly of blade (keep blade perpendicular to skin surface to prevent laceration). Scrapings are transferred to slide and stained with Wright's or Giemsa stain. A positive preparation has multinucleate giant cells.

For more detailed discussion of this topic, see Fitzpatrick TB, Haynes HA: Interpretation of Alterations in the Skin, Chap. 47, in HPIM-11, p. 226

PAPULOSQUAMOUS DISORDERS Disorders exhibiting papules and scale.

Psoriasis: A chronic, recurrent disorder. Classic lesion is a well-marginated, erythematous plaque with silvery-white surface scale. Distribution includes extensor surfaces (i.e., knees, elbows, and buttocks); may also involve palms and scalp (particularly anterior scalp margin). Associated findings include psoriatic arthritis and nail changes (oncholysis, pitting or thickening of nail plate with accumulation of subungual debris).

Pityriasis rosea: A self-limited condition lasting 4–8 weeks. Initially, there is a single round or oval erythematous to salmon-colored patch (herald patch) with a peripheral rim of scale. Within 5–7 days, a generalized eruption involves the trunk and proximal extremities. Individual lesions are similar to but smaller than the herald patch and are arranged in symmetric fashion with long axis of each individual lesion along skin lines of cleavage. Appearance may be similar to that of secondary syphilis.

Seborrheic dermatitis: A chronic noninfectious process characterized by erythematous patches with greasy yellowish scale. Lesions are generally on scalp, eyebrows, nasolabial folds, axillae, central chest, and posterior auricular area.

Dermatophyte infection: May involve any area of body; due to infection of stratum corneum, nail plate, or hair by a skin fungus. Appearance may vary from mild scaliness to florid inflammatory dermatitis. Classic lesion of tinea corporis ("ring worm") is an erythematous papulosquamous patch often with central clearing and scale along peripheral advancing border. Hyphae are seen on potassium hydroxide preparation.

ECZEMATOUS DISORDERS **Atopic dermatitis:** One aspect of atopic triad of hayfever, asthma, and eczema. Usually an intermittent, chronic, severely pruritic, eczematous dermatitis with scaly erythematous patches, vesiculation, crusting, and fissuring. Lesions are most commonly on flexures with prominent involvement of antecubital and popliteal fossae; generalized erythroderma in severe cases. Most pts with atopic dermatitis are chronic carriers of *Staphylococcus aureus* in anterior nares and on skin.

***Rhus* dermatitis (poison ivy, oak, sumac):** A common, vesicular, weeping, crusting dermatitis secondary to a delayed hypersensitivity reaction to resin of plants in the genus *Rhus*. Lesions occur at sites of contact with resin; linear arrangement of vesicles is common.

INFECTIONS AND INFESTATIONS **Impetigo:** A superficial infection of skin secondary to either *S. aureus* or more commonly beta-hemolytic streptococci (group A). The hallmark is an eruption that begins as small vesicles progressing to erosions covered by a "honey-colored" crust. A bullous variety is most often associated with *S. aureus* infection. Lesions may occur anywhere but commonly on face.

Erysipelas: Superficial cellulitis, most commonly on face, characterized by a bright red, warm plaque sharply demarcated from surrounding normal skin. Due to superficial location of infection and associated edema, surface of plaque may exhibit a *peau d'orange* (orange peel) appearance. Most commonly due to infection with gram-positive cocci (frequently beta-hemolytic streptococci) occurring at sites of trauma or other breaks in skin.

Scabies: A common infestation of children and adults due to the mite *Sarcoptes scabiei.* Often presents as pruritus, commonly worse at night. Typical lesions include burrows (short linear lesions often in web spaces of fingers) and small vesiculopapular lesions in intertriginous areas. Excoriations often with bleeding may be prominent.

Herpes simplex: Recurrent eruption characterized by grouped vesicles on an erythematous base that progress to erosions; often secondarily infected with staphylococci or streptococci. Tzanck preparation of an unroofed early vesicle reveals multinucleate giant cells.

Herpes zoster: Eruption of grouped vesicles on an erythematous base usually limited to a single dermatome; disseminated lesions also can occur, especially in immunocompromised patients. Tzanck preparation reveals multinucleate giant cells; indistinguishable from herpes simplex except by culture. Postherpetic neuralgia, lasting months to years, may occur, especially in elderly.

VASCULAR DISORDERS **Erythema nodosum:** Characterized by erythematous, warm, tender subcutaneous nodular lesions typically on anterior shins. Lesions are usually flush with skin surface but are indurated and have appearance of an erythematous/violaceous bruise. Commonly seen in sarcoidosis, leprosy, TBC, streptococcal infections, during treatment with some drugs (esp. oral contraceptives, sulfonamides, and estrogens); may be idiopathic.

Erythema multiforme: A reaction pattern of skin consisting of a variety of lesions but most commonly erythematous papules and bullae. "Target" or "iris" lesion is characteristic and consists of concentric circles of erythema and normal flesh-colored skin often with a central vesicle or bulla. Distribution of lesions classically acral, esp. palms and soles. Three most common causes include drug reaction (particularly penicillins and sulfonamides) or concurrent herpetic or *Mycoplasma* infection.

Urticaria: A common disorder, either acute or chronic, characterized by evanescent (individual lesions lasting < 24 h), pruritic, edematous, pink to erythematous plaques with a whitish halo around margin of individual lesions. Lesions range in size from papules (several mm in diameter) to giant coalescent lesions (10–20 cm in diameter). Often due to drugs, systemic infection, or foods (esp. shellfish). Food additives such as tartrazine dye (F.D.& C. yellow no. 5), benzoate, or salicylates also have been implicated. If individual lesions last > 24 h consider diagnosis of urticarial vasculitis.

Vasculitis: Palpable purpura (nonblanching, elevated lesions) is the cutaneous hallmark of vasculitis. Other lesions include petechiae (esp. early lesions), necrosis with ulceration, bullae, and urticarial lesions (urticarial vasculitis). Lesions usually most prominent on lower extremities. Pathogenic factors include bacterial infections, underlying collagen-vascular disease or malignancy, hepatitis B, drugs (esp. thiazides), and inflammatory bowel disease.

For more detailed discussion of these topics, see Fitzpatrick TB, Haynes HA: Interpretation of Alterations in the Skin, Chap. 47, p. 226; Fitzpatrick TB, Bernhard JD: Skin Lesions of General Medical Significance, Chap. 48, p. 232, in HPIM-11

---

149 SKIN CANCER

BASAL CELL CARCINOMA Most common form of skin cancer; most frequently on sun-exposed skin, esp. face.
Predisposing factors: Fair complexion, chronic UV exposure, exposure to inorganic arsenic (i.e., Fowler's solution or insecticides such as Paris green), or exposure to ionizing radiation.
General types:
• Superficial. • Nodular (most common). • Pigmented (may be mistaken for melanoma). • Sclerotic or infiltrative (most aggressive biological behavior).

Clinical appearance: Classically a pearly, translucent, smooth papule with rolled edges and surface telangiectasia.
Treatment: Local removal; metastases rare but may spread locally.

SQUAMOUS CELL CARCINOMA Less common than basal cell but more likely to metastasize.
Predisposing factors: Fair complexion, chronic UV exposure, previous burn or other scar (i.e., scar carcinoma), exposure to inorganic arsenic or ionizing radiation.
General types:

1 *Bowen's disease:* Erythematous patch or plaque, often with scale; noninvasive; involvement limited to epidermis and epidermal appendages.
2 *Scar carcinoma:* Suggested by sudden change in previously stable scar, esp. if ulceration or nodules appear.
3 *Verrucous carcinoma:* Most commonly on plantar aspect of foot; low-grade malignancy but may be mistaken for a common wart.

Clinical appearance: Hyperkeratotic papule or nodule; may be ulcerated.
Treatment: Local excision.
Prognosis: Favorable if secondary to UV exposure; less favorable if in sun-protected areas or associated with ionizing radiation.

MALIGNANT MELANOMA Most dangerous cutaneous malignancy; high metastatic potential; poor prognosis with metastatic spread.
Predisposing factors: Fair complexion, family history of melanoma, dysplastic nevus syndrome (autosomal dominant disorder with multiple nevi of distinctive appearance and cutaneous melanoma), and presence of a congenital nevus (esp. if > 10 cm in diameter).
Types:

1 *Superficial spreading melanoma:* Most common; begins with initial radial growth phase prior to invasion.
2 *Lentigo maligna melanoma:* Very long radial growth phase prior to invasion, lentigo maligna (Hutchinson's melanotic freckle) is

precursor lesions, most common in elderly and in sun-exposed areas (esp. face).

3 Acral lentiginous: Most common form in darkly pigmented pts; occurs on palms and soles, mucosal surfaces, in nail beds and mucocutaneous junctions; similar to lentigo maligna melanoma but with more aggressive biologic behavior.

4 Nodular: Generally poor prognosis because of invasive growth from onset.

Clinical appearance: Generally pigmented (rarely amelanotic); color of lesions varies, but red, white, and/or blue are common, in addition to brown and/or black. Suspicion should be raised by a pigmented skin lesion that is >6 mm in diameter, asymmetric, has an irregular surface or border, or has variation in color.

Prognosis: Best with thin lesions without evidence of metastatic spread; with increasing thickness or evidence of spread, prognosis worsens.

For more detailed discussion of these topics, see Haynes HA: Primary Cancer of the Skin, Chap. 301, p. 1593; Fitzpatrick TB, Sober AJ, Mihm MC Jr.: Malignant Melanoma of the Skin, Chap. 302, p. 1595, in HPIM-11

---

150 CUTANEOUS MANIFESTATIONS OF SYSTEMIC DISEASE

Many internal diseases have cutaneous presentations or manifestations which provide a clue to the underlying diagnosis.

COLLAGEN-VASCULAR DISORDERS **Systemic lupus erythematosus (SLE)** (Chap. 110): Mucocutaneous findings are common and include malar erythematous "butterfly" rash, photosensitivity, oral or nasal ulceration, alopecia, and rarely bullous lesions. Discoid lupus can present as a distinct entity or as a part of acute LE. *Active discoid* lesions are atrophic, scaly, erythematous plaques with sharp margination, prominent telangiectasia, and follicular plugging. *Inactive discoid* lesions become hypopigmented. Lesions most common on head and neck in sun-exposed distribution. *Subacute cutaneous LE* predominantly a sun-exposed eruption, esp. on arms (extensor area), upper back, chest, and face. Individual lesions may be annular or papulosquamous. Serum anticytoplasmic antibodies Ro (SS-A) or La (SS-B) are common. Discoid LE and subacute cutaneous LE have a better prognosis than SLE.

Dermatomyositis (Chap 169): May be a cutaneous marker of underlying malignancy. Classic cutaneous manifestations include violaceous heliotrope rash around eyes (esp. upper lids), Gottron's papules (erythematous, atrophic papules over extensor, interphalangeal joints of hands), telangiectasias, or poikiloderma (hyper- and hypopigmentation, atrophy, and telangiectasia). Cutaneous calcification may occur, but more commonly in children.

Progressive systemic sclerosis (Chap. 110): Skin typically indurated and thickened, esp. on face and hands. Sclerodactyly (atrophic, bound-down skin over digits) commonly associated with periungual telangiectasia. Tips of fingers often tapered due to either bone resorption or infarcts of finger pads secondary to associated Raynaud's phenomenon.

ENDOCRINE AND METABOLIC DISORDERS: **Diabetes mellitus** (Chap. 138): Cutaneous manifestations may occur and include:

- *Diabetic dermopathy* ("shin spots"): atrophic, circumscribed, pigmented lesions typically over anterior lower extremities.
- *Necrobiosis lipoidica diabeticorum:* one or more yellowish, atrophic, indurated plaques with a reddish border over pretibial areas primarily in female diabetics.
- *Dermal atrophy:* common at sites of insulin injection.
- *Ischemic ulcers:* usually on lower extremities; slow to heal due to underlying microvascular disease.
- *Acanthosis nigricans:* verrucous to velvety, dirty-appearing lesions on neck, dorsum of fingers, and axillae, esp. in insulin-resistant diabetics; may correlate with degree of insulin resistance.

Xanthomatous lesions: Dermal collections of lipid-containing cells classified on the basis of morphology and location:

- *Xanthelasma:* yellowish planar plaques on upper eyelids; usually associated with elevated cholesterol or type II hyperlipoproteinemia (HLP) (Chap. 145), or may be a normal variant.
- *Tuberous xanthomas:* yellow-orange papules on extensor surfaces, most frequently associated with type II HLP (but sometimes seen with type III HLP or others).
- *Eruptive xanthomas:* grouped inflammatory red to yellow papules that appear suddenly and usually in crops; lesions most closely correlated with elevated triglycerides (in HLP types I and IV).
- *Tendinous xanthomas:* nodular yellowish lesions involving tendons or fascia, esp. on feet, knees, elbows, or hands; most common in HLP type II.
- *Planar xanthomas:* yellow to tan plaques and papules common on palms but also on trunk, head, or extremities; associated with types III and IV HLP, but occasionally in patients with myeloma and secondary HLP.

Thyroid disease:

- *Hyperthyroidism* (Chap. 136): skin may have generalized velvety texture; there also may be distal onycholysis of nails, generalized pruritus, or diffuse alopecia with altered hair texture; pretibial "myxedema" may occur in true Graves' disease, usually with bilateral, symmetrical, diffuse, brawny, nonpitting edema over pretibial areas and dorsum of feet.
- *Hypothyroidism* (Chap. 136): generally skin is dry, cool, and pale; hair is dry, brittle, and coarse with outer third of eyebrows usually missing; myxedema may be present with puffy, edematous, but nonpitting appearance; macroglossia common; generalized pruritus also can occur.

Addison's disease (Chap. 137): Generalized hyperpigmentation is the hallmark with accentuation in scars, palmar creases, and other skin folds as well as on mucosal surfaces. Less than 15% of pts with primary adrenal failure may have vitiligo (patchy loss of pigment), esp. if other endocrine deficiencies are present (i.e., multiple glandular failure).

DISORDERS OF GI TRACT **Gluten-sensitive enteropathy** (Chap. 17): Some patients have dermatitis herpetiformis (DH) characterized by symmetric, grouped vesicles in an extensor distribution (esp. upper back, scalp, buttocks, elbows); lesions extremely pruritic.

Inflammatory bowel disease (Chap. 98): Both ulcerative colitis and Crohn's disease may exhibit similar skin lesions: erythema nodosum (Chap. 148), aphthous ulcers of the mouth, and/or pyoderma gangrenosum. Pyoderma gangrenosum is characterized by a papular lesion progressing to a pustule followed by ulceration. The ulcer border is usually undermined and appears violaceous. Healing progresses slowly, resulting in formation of a characteristic atrophic cribiform scar. Ulcer activity may or may not parallel that of underlying bowel disease.

Chronic liver disease (Chap. 105): Jaundice, when present, involves skin, sclera, and mucous membranes. Other cutaneous findings include vascular spider nevi (particularly on face and chest), palmar erythema, gynecomastia, and loss of secondary male hair growth. Purpuric lesions (ecchymoses) may be present due to hypoprothrombinemia. Nail changes include uniform opaque white color that obscures lunula and stops 1–2 mm from distal edge of nail, where there is a narrow pink transverse band (Terry's nails), paired, parallel white bands on the nail plate (Muehrke's lines), brittle nails (onychomadesis), and flat or spoon nails (koilonychia).

INFECTIOUS DISORDERS **Acquired immunodeficiency syndrome (AIDS)** (Chap. 109): Mucocutaneous findings are varied; may represent associated dermatologic findings or manifestations of opportunistic infection.

Associated findings:

- *Kaposi's sarcoma:* red to purplish nodules or verrucous lesions occurring anywhere on the body, including mucosal surfaces.
- *Seborrheic dermatitis:* similar appearance as seen in patients without AIDS (Chap. 148).
- *Granuloma annulare-like eruption:* multiple grouped papules on trunk and neck.

Infections: Virtually any opportunistic infection (particularly atypical mycobacteria, cryptococcus, and histoplasma) may occur. Other common infectious manifestations include:

- *Cutaneous herpetic infection:* either herpes simplex or herpes zoster (frequently disseminated).
- Other frequent cutaneous viral infections include *molluscum contagiosum* (small pink or flesh-colored, dome-shaped papules with soft central cores), *verruca vulgaris*, and *condyloma accuminata.*
- *Oral candidiasis* (thrush) and *candida intertrigo.*

Endocarditis (Chap. 63): Petechiae are most common skin finding; may occur anywhere on skin (particularly extremities) and on mucous membranes. Splinter hemorrhages (not specific) appear as small, linear, usually multiple subungual purpuric lesions. More specific lesions include Janeway lesions (painless purpuric macules most commonly located on proximal portion of hands) and Osler's nodes (painful urticarial-like nodules found on hands and feet, particularly in pulp of fingers and toes); most commonly associated with *Streptococcus viridans.*

Gonococcemia (Chap. 32): Cutaneous manifestations more common in females than males. Lesions usually few in number. Primary lesions may be pustular, vesicular, papular, or macular with associated purpura and usually periarticular, esp. on hands.

Lyme disease (Chap. 55): Erythema chronicum migrans (ECM) usually occurs at site of initial tick bite; although multiple similar-appearing lesions can occur elsewhere. ECM appears as an ad-

vancing ring of erythemas with central clearing and no appreciable scale.
Meningococcemia (Chap. 39)
Rocky Mountain spotted fever (Chap. 51)
Syphilis (Chap. 32):

- *Primary:* chancre is a clean, nonpainful indurated ulcer most frequently seen on the genitalia or in perianal area. *Secondary:* most commonly copper-colored macules and papules (often resembling pityriasis rosea) involving palms and soles; white patches ("mucous patches") on buccal mucosa and condyloma lata (moist smooth papules in anogenital area) may be seen, moth-eaten alopecia of scalp also characteristic.
- *Tertiary:* gummatous lesions are granulomatous nodular lesions, frequently exhibiting necrosis, that begin in subcutis and involve epidermis secondarily.

NEOPLASTIC DISEASES **Cutaneous metastases:** Hard dermal nodules with or without ulceration; frequently occur on scalp. Most common malignancies exhibiting cutaneous metastases include carcinomas of lung, breast, uterus, ovaries, GI tract (especially stomach), and malignant melanoma.
Leukemia (Chap. 130): Specific cutaneous lesions may be present in up to 50% of pts (monocytic greater than lymphocytic or granulocytic). All cutaneous leukemic infiltrates tend to exhibit a reddish-brown to purple color. *Monocytic types* present as plum-colored tumors or as purplish macules and papules. *Lymphocytic types* (ALL and CLL) present with lesions usually limited to face and extremities. Acute *granulocytic leukemia* may exhibit chloromas (soft tissue leukemic infiltrates; green in color due to presence of myeloperoxidase); often infiltrate bony periosteum (particularly orbital or cranial bones).
Lymphomas (Chap. 131): *B-cell lymphoma:* cutaneous lesions most common in histiocytic lymphoma; less frequent in lymphocytic, lymphoblastic, undifferentiated, and mixed types; rare in Hodgkin's disease. Lesions usually on head and neck are typically indurated; erythematous to purple dermal nodules that may be singular or multiple and occasionally may ulcerate.
T-cell lymphoma:

- *Mycosis fungoides:* a primary cutaneous form of lymphoma that frequently begins with eczematoid plaques and patches (except in the *d'emblée* form, where nodular tumors develop de novo); lesion proceeds from patch → plaque → tumor; latter characterized by thick, erythematous to violaceous plaques which frequently ulcerate.
- *HTLV I–associated T-cell lymphoma* often disseminated, maculopapular, or small nodular lesions or larger tumor nodules.

CUTANEOUS MANIFESTATIONS OF INTERNAL MALIGNANCY **Acanthosis nigricans** (Chap. 99): Not specific for internal malignancy, but when latter is present, most commonly seen with GI malignancies.

Acquired icthyosis: Dry, scaly, "fishlike" skin; most commonly seen with underlying lymphoproliferative disorders.
Clubbing of fingers and toes: Most commonly associated with carcinoma of lung (bronchogenic); also with chronic pulmonary infections such as bronchiectasis or lung abscess; may also be seen with mesothelioma, inflammatory bowel disease, or cirrhosis.
Erythema gyratum repens: Uncommon, dramatic, generalized serpiginous and circinate erythema with a "wood grain" appearance; almost always associated with internal malignancy.
Hypertrichosis lanuginosa acquisita: An acquired excessive growth of fine, downy (vellus) hairs beginning on face and ears; may spread to involve any hair-bearing skin; most commonly associated with adenocarcinomas.
Leukoderma: An acquired loss of pigment cells in an area of skin. Most common in persons with vitiligo, but may represent an underlying malignant melanoma. Suspect melanoma when leukoderma is not in typical distribution (around eyes, ears, nares, mouth, and genitalia) characteristic of vitiligo or when there is adenopathy or weight loss.
Pruritus: Generally nonspecific but may be associated with malignancy, most often lymphoma/leukemia, often with normal-appearing skin. Pruritus accentuated during bathing suggests underlying polycythemia rubra vera. May also occur with Hodgkin's disease, myeloma, gastric or pancreatic carcinoma.
Sweet's syndrome: Triad of fever, leukocytosis, and neutrophilic dermatosis characterized by erythematous, tender, often asymmetric plaques and nodules that occasionally exhibit surface pustules or vesicles. Most often seen with underlying leukemias, esp. acute granulocytic leukemia. Lesions most common on face and extremities.
Tylosis: An acquired, prominent, diffuse hyperkeratosis of soles and palms; most frequently seen with carcinoma of esophagus.

OTHER DISORDERS WITH PROMINENT CUTANEOUS MANIFESTATIONS **Amyloidosis of the skin** (Chap. 121): Skin manifestations usually only found in primary systemic amyloidosis and include purpura, patchy alopecia, flesh-colored waxy, or hemorrhagic papular lesions at various sites, including palms, tongue, and face. Macroglossia with glossitis and furrowing of tongue. Purpura, when present, often first noted in body folds or around eyes (periorbital purpura) or ears; later may involve other body surfaces. Lesions may vary from small petechiae to large purpuric lesions several centimeters in diameter.
Mastocytosis: Cutaneous lesions occur in one of three forms which all urticate with stroking (positive Darier's sign):

- *Solitary mastocytomas:* most common in children; single brownish macules or papules that may become vesicular or bullous with stroking.
- *Urticaria pigmentosa:* multiple brown, nonscaly, macular lesions usually limited to trunk and proximal extremities.
- *Telangiectasia macularis eruptiva perstans:* lesions similar to urticaria pigmentosa but exhibit fine telangiectasia.

Sarcoidosis (Chap. 112): Primary cutaneous lesions include granuloma formation in scars, annular plaques, nodules, psoriasiform plaques, and violaceous facial plaques and nodules of nose, cheeks, and ears (*lupus pernio*); erythema nodosum occurs in 10–20% of patients.

For more detailed discussion of these topics, see Fitzpatrick TB, Bernhard JD: Skin Lesions of General Medical Significance, Chap. 48, in HPIM-II, p. 232

SECTION XI
NEUROLOGY

151 THE NEUROLOGIC EXAMINATION

MENTAL STATUS EXAM Tests are designed to evaluate pt's attention, orientation, memory, insight, judgment, and grasp of general information. A series of numbers can be recited and the pt asked to respond every time a specific item recurs (attention). The pt should be asked about his or her name, the place, the day, and date. Retentive memory and immediate recall can be tested by determining the number of digits the pt can repeat in sequence. Recent memory is evaluated by testing recall of a series of objects after defined times (e.g., 5 and 15 minutes). More remote memory is evaluated by assessing pt's ability to provide a cogent chronologic history of his or her illness or personal life events. Recall of major historical events or dates or of major current events may provide insight into fund of general knowledge. Evaluation of language function should include assessment of spontaneous speech, naming, repetition, reading, writing, and comprehension. Additional tests such as ability to draw and copy, perform calculations, interpret proverbs or logic problems, identify right vs. left, name and identify body parts, etc. are also important.

CRANIAL NERVE (CN) EXAM **CN I:** Occlude each nostril sequentially and use a mild test stimulus, such as soap, toothpaste, coffee, or lemon oil, to see if pt can detect the odor and correctly identify it.

CN II: Check visual acuity with and without correction using a Snellen chart (distance) and Jaeger's test type (near). Map visual fields (VFs) by confrontation testing in each quadrant of visual field for each eye individually. The best method is to sit facing pt (2–3 ft apart), have him or her cover one eye gently, and fix uncovered eye on examiner's nose. A small white object (e.g., a cotton-tipped applicator) is then moved slowly from periphery of field toward center until pt appreciates its presence. The pt's VF should be mapped against examiner's for comparison. Formal perimetry and tangent screen exam are essential to identify and delineate small defects. Optic fundi should be examined with an ophthalmoscope and the color, size, and degree of swelling or elevation of the optic disc recorded. The retinal vessels should be checked for size, regularity, AV nicking at crossing points, hemorrhage, exudates, aneurysms, etc. The retina, including the macula, should be examined for abnormal pigmentation and other lesions.

CNs III, IV, VI: Describe size, regularity, and shape of pupils as well as their reaction (direct and consensual) to light and convergence of eyes. Check for lid drooping, lag, or retraction. Ask pt to follow your finger as you move it horizontally to left and right and vertically with each eye first fully adducted then fully abducted. Check for failure to move fully in particular directions and for presence of regular, rhythmic, involuntary oscillations of eyes (nystagmus). Test quick voluntary eye movements (saccades) as well as pursuit (e.g., follow the finger).

CN V: Feel the masseter and temporalis muscles as pt bites down and test jaw opening, protrusion, and lateral motion against resistance. Examine sensation over entire face as well as response to touching each cornea lightly with a small wisp of cotton.

CN VII: Look for asymmetry of face at rest and with spontaneous as well as emotion-induced (e.g., laughing) movements. Test eyebrow elevation, forehead wrinkling, eye closure, smiling, frowning, cheek puff, whistle, lip pursing, and chin muscle contraction. Look particularly for differences in strength of lower and upper facial muscles. Taste on the anterior two-thirds of tongue can be affected by lesions of the seventh CN proximal to the chorda tympani. Test taste for sweet (sugar), salt, sour (lemon), and bitter (quinine) using a cotton-tipped applicator moistened in appropriate solution and placed on lateral margin of protruded tongue about halfway back from tip.

CN VIII: Check ability to hear tuning fork, finger rub, watch tick, and whispered voice at specified distances with each ear. Check for air vs. mastoid bone conduction (Rinne) and lateralization of a tuning fork placed on center of forehead (Weber). Accurate, quantitative testing of hearing requires formal audiometry. Remember to examine tympanic membranes.

CNs IX, X: Check for symmetric evaluation of palate-uvula with phonation ("*ahh*"), as well as position of uvula and palatal arch at rest. Sensation in region of tonsils, posterior pharynx, and tongue also may require testing in specific pts. Pharyngeal ("gag") reflex is evaluated by stimulating posterior pharyngeal wall on each side with a blunt object (e.g., tongue blade). Direct examination of vocal cords by laryngoscopy is necessary in some situations.

CN XI: Check shoulder shrug (trapezius muscle) and head rotation to each side (sternocleidomastoid muscle) against resistance.

CN XII: Examine bulk and power of tongue. Look for atrophy, deviation from midline with protrusion, tremor, and small flickering or twitching movements (fibrillations, fasciculations).

MOTOR EXAM Power should be systematically tested for major movements at each joint (see Table 151-1). Strength should be recorded using a reproducible scale (e.g., 0 = no movement, 1 = flicker or trace of contraction with no associated movement at a joint, 2 = movement present but cannot be sustained against gravity, 3 = movement against gravity but not applied resistance, 4 = movement against some degree of resistance, and 5 = full power; values can be supplemented with the addition of + and − signs to provide additional gradations). The speed of movement, the ability to promptly relax contractions, and fatigue with repetition all should be noted. Loss in bulk and size of muscle

TABLE 151-1 **Muscles that move joints**

	Muscle	Nerve	Segmental innervation
Shoulder	Supra- and infra-spinati	Suprascapular n.	C4,5
	Deltoid	Axillary n.	C5,6
Forearm	Biceps	Musculocutanoeus n.	C5,6
	Brachioradialis	Radial n.	C5,6
	Triceps	Radial n.	C6,7,8
	Ext. carpi radialis	Radial n.	C5,6,7
	Ext. carpi ulnaris	P. interosseous n.	C6,7,8
	Ext. digitorum	P. interosseous n.	C6,7,8
	Flex. carpi radialis	Median n.	C6,7
	Flex. carpi ulnaris	Ulnar n.	C7,8,T1
	Supinator	Radial n.	C6,7
	Pronator teres	Median n.	C6,7
Hand	Lumbricals	Median + ulnar n.	C8,T1
	Interossei	Ulnar n.	C8,T1
Thumb	Opponens pollicis	Median n.	C8,T1
	Ext. pollicis	P. interosseous n.	C7,8
	Add. pollicis	Ulnar n.	C8,T1
	Flex. pollicis br.	Ulnar n.	C8,T1
Pelvis	Iliopsoas	Femoral n.	L1,2,3
	Glutei	Sup. + inf. gluteal n.	L4,5,S12
Thigh	Quadriceps	Femoral n.	L2,3,4
	Adductors	Obturator n.	L2,3,4
	Hamstrings	Sciatic n.	L5S12
Leg	Gastrocnemius	Tibial n.	S12
	Tibialis ant.	Deep peroneal n.	L4,5
	Peronei	Deep peroneal n.	L5S1
	Tibialis post.	Tibial n.	L4,5
Foot	Ext. hallucis l.	Deep peroneal n.	L5S1

(atrophy) should be checked for, as well as the presence of irregular involuntary contraction (twitching) of groups of muscle fibres ("fasciculations"). Involuntary movements should be looked for while pt is at rest, during maintained posture, and with voluntary action. Rhythmic involuntary movements are referred to as "tremors," whereas more irregular movements generally fall into categories of choreoathetosis, ballismus, myoclonus, or tics.

REFLEXES Important muscle-stretch reflexes to test routinely and the spinal cord segments involved in their reflex arcs include biceps C5,6, triceps C6,7,8, brachioradialis C5,6, patellar L2,3,4, Achilles L5,S1. A common grading scale is 0 = absent, 1 = present but diminished, 2 = normal, 3 = hyperactive, and 4 = hyperactive with clonus (repetitive rhythmic contractions with maintained stretch). The plantar reflex should be tested by using a blunt-ended object such as the point of a key to stroke the outer border of the sole of the foot from the heel toward the base of the great toe. An abnormal response (Babinski sign) is extension (dorsiflexion) of the great toe at the metatarsophalangeal joint. In some cases this may be associated with abduction (fanning) of other toes and variable degrees of flexion at ankle, knee, and hip.

(Normal response is slow plantar flexion of great toe.) Abdominal, anal, and sphincteric reflexes are important in certain situations, as are additional muscle stretch reflexes.

SENSORY EXAM For most purposes it is sufficient to test sensation to pinprick, touch, position, and vibration in each of the four extremities (see Figs. 151-1 and -2). Specific problems often require more painstaking evaluation. Pts with cerebral lesions may have abnormalities in "discriminative sensation" such as the ability to perceive double simultaneous stimuli, to localize stimuli accurately, to identify closely approximated stimuli as separate (two-point discrimination), to identify objects by touch alone (stereognosis), or to judge weights, evaluate texture, or identify letters or numbers written on the skin surface (graphesthesia).

FIG. 151-1 *(Reproduced from Asbury AK: HPIM-11, p 102.)*

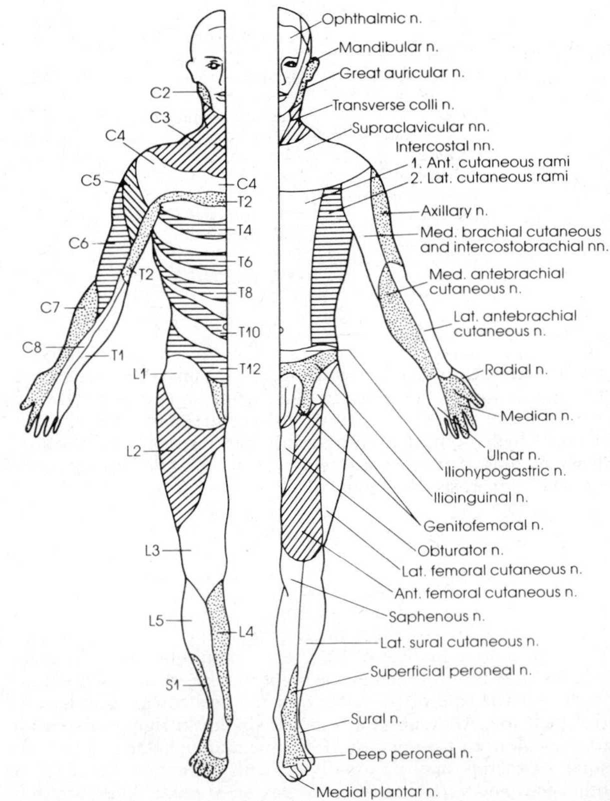

COORDINATION AND GAIT The ability to move the index finger accurately from the nose to the examiner's outstretched finger and the ability to slide the heel of each foot from the knee down the shin are tests of coordination. Additional tests (drawing objects in the air, following a moving finger, tapping with index finger against thumb or alternately against each individual finger) also may be useful in some pts. The pt's ability to stand with feet together and eyes closed (Romberg test), to walk a straight line (tandem walk), and to turn should all be observed.

For more detailed discussion of this topic, see Asbury AK: Numbness, Tingling, and Other Abnormalities of Sensation, Chap. 18, in HPIM-11, p. 99

FIG. 151-2 *(Reproduced from Asbury AK: HPIM-11, p 103.)*

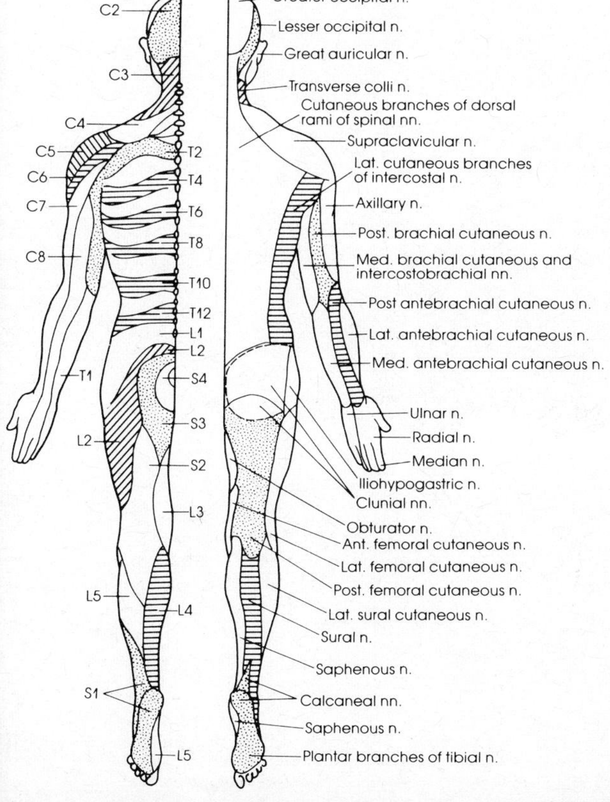

Laboratory procedures should follow clinical evaluation; in life-threatening emergencies, time may not permit detailed clinical observation. Because many methods are costly, time-consuming, and occasionally dangerous or painful, care should be taken to ensure that indications for test are clear and that information obtained will have important implications for diagnosis and treatment.

LUMBAR PUNCTURE **Indications:** (1) To obtain pressure measurements and secure a sample of CSF for cellular, chemical, and bacteriologic examination (see table of normal values in Chap. 190); (2) for administration of spinal anesthesia, antibiotics, or antitumor agents; and (3) to inject contrast agents for myelography. **Complications:** (1) Cerebellar or transtentorial herniation when performed in setting of markedly elevated intracranial pressure (ICP) or strategically placed space-occupying lesion. When the possibility of raised ICP exists, it is prudent to exclude a mass lesion by CT before obtaining CSF. In such cases, a fine-bore needle (no. 22 or 24), should be used, and if opening pressure > 400 mmHg the minimum amount of fluid required for examination is withdrawn, a unit of mannitol is given, and the manometer is left in place until pressure decreases. (2) Introduction of bacteria into CNS.

CT **Indications:** Without contrast, to differentiate epidural, subdural, and intracerebral hemorrhages and deformities of ventricular system from "mass" lesions; with contrast, to demonstrate tumors, abscesses, granulomas, sometimes large aneurysms or AV malformations; to identify areas of brain edema, infarction, hydrocephalus, and atrophy.
Complications: Allergic reaction to intravenous contrast dye; renal failure due to contrast administration in setting of preexisting renal disease or dehydration.

MRI **Indications:** For visualization of CNS lesions not evident on CT. Particularly useful for detection of tumors, lacunes, or demyelinating plaques < 1 cm; visualization of brainstem and cerebellum; imaging spinal cord and distinguishing intrinsic from extramedullary or epidural spinal cord lesions.

ANGIOGRAPHY May be intraarterial or digital subtraction venous angiography.
Indications: For diagnosis of vascular stenoses or occlusion, aneurysms, vascular malformations, assessment of vascular supply to tumors before surgery, and abscesses.
Complications: (1) Selective intraarterial injection: stroke from emboli dislodged from catheter tip, excessive bleeding or thrombotic occlusion at site of introduction of the arterial catheter; (2) digital subtraction venous angiography: renal insufficiency or congestive failure due to osmotic load of contrast dye (*note:* this method provides information only about extracranial vessels).

MYELOGRAPHY Either with iophendylate (Pantopaque) or water-soluble contrast (metrizamide); allows visualization of spinal canal and spinal cord to reveal tumors, ruptured disks, etc. Metrizamide can be used in conjunction with CT of spine to visualize transverse sections of spinal cord and subarachnoid space.
Complications: Arachnoiditis due to irritation from Pantopaque not removed during procedure; seizures due to lowering of threshold by metrizamide, especially after procedures in which dye moves above clinoid process. Prophylactic phenobarbital (60 mg qhs) is often given for two days before study.

ELECTROMYOGRAPHY (EMG) To aid in analysis of diseases affecting neuromuscular apparatus; to differentiate diseases of neuromuscular junction from primary myopathy or secondary to denervation. Studies usually include nerve conduction analyses (see Chap. 165).

ELECTROENCEPHALOGRAPHY (EEG) Used principally for diagnosis of seizure disorders, but also may be used to assess cerebral cortical disease or CNS effects of many medical illnesses.
Normal EEG rhythms in adults: Include *alpha*—8 to 12 Hz, 50 μV sinusoidal waves seen in occipital and parietal regions; *beta*—>13 Hz, 10–20 μV waves seen in frontal regions; in sleep, symmetric slowing with characteristic waveforms, e.g., vertex sharp waves and sleep spindles.
Abnormal EEG rhythms in adults: Awake recordings include: *theta*—4 to 7 Hz, 50–350 μV waves; *delta*—<4 Hz, 50–350 μV waves (the higher the voltage, the more abnormal are theta and delta slowing); spike or sharp waves—faster, higher-voltage waveforms which, when paroxysmal, are suggestive of epilepsy; characteristic epileptiform patterns such as the 3-Hz spike and wave complexes of absence (petit mal) seizures. The most pathologic finding of all is the disappearance of EEG pattern ("electrocerebral silence"), which, in the absence of extreme hypothermia (<70°F) or acute intoxication with anesthetic levels of drugs, is suggestive of "irreversible coma" or "brain death."

EVOKED RESPONSES Measures of electrical activity produced by groups of neurons within spinal cord, brainstem, thalamus, or cerebral hemispheres following sensory stimulation by visual, auditory, or tactile input. The amplitude of these potentials, recorded from scalp by ordinary EEG electrodes, ranges from 0.5 to 20 μV. The battery of tests includes *visual* (VERs), *brainstem auditory* (BAERs), and *somatosensory evoked responses* (SSERs). Can be used once for a single evaluation of lesions in these sensory pathways or over time as a quantitative method for following a pt's course or response to therapy.

PSYCHOMETRY, PERIMETRY, AUDIOMETRY, AND TESTS OF LABYRINTHINE FUNCTION Used in quantitating and defining nature of psychic or sensory deficits produced by disease of nervous system. Indications for obtaining these tests are to (1) confirm presence of a functional neurologic disorder and ascertain its nature, and (2) quantitate the deficit in order to determine, using repeated examination, the course of the illness (see Chap. 164).

For more detailed discussion of this topic, see Chiappa KH, Martin JB, Young RR: Diagnostic Methods in Neurology, Chap. 341, in HPIM-11, p. 1913

---

153 DISORDERS OF SLEEP

Continuous monitoring of EEG, EMG, and eye movements during sleep has revealed dynamic transitions from one stage of sleep to another. Slow wave sleep [non-rapid eye movement (NREM)] and REM sleep alternate 4–6 times during a normal period of night sleep. Abnormalities of onset, depth, duration, and transitions from one stage to another have been identified. The principal sleep disorders are described.

INSOMNIA A disorder in initiating or maintaining sleep; also describes pt's feeling of inadequate sleep, which may be due to an impairment in onset, depth, duration, or restorative properties of sleep. It may be a primary disorder or secondary to psychiatric illness, anxiety, drug use, or medical conditions. It may be a temporary problem or lifelong. Treatment is difficult when the condition is chronic. Avoid overuse of sedatives which may temporarily alleviate symptoms but over time may worsen the problem.

HYPERSOMNIAS Typified by inappropriate sleepiness leading to sleep when a patient wishes to be awake. Pt complains of an irresistable urge to sleep during the day or of decreased concentration. In clinical practice, two forms are likely to occur:

Sleep apnea syndrome: A sleep-induced respiratory impairment characterized by snoring, respiratory pauses lasting 10–120 s, and often respiratory obstruction. In severe cases, more than 500 episodes of sleep apnea may occur in a single night. During working hours, pt notes attacks of drowsiness, poor concentration, and headaches. Men are affected 20 times as frequently as women, usually in the 40–65 age range. About two-thirds of pts are obese. In obstructive apnea there is narrowing of the oral pharynx during respiration. A rare form of nonobstructive apnea is due to a central defect in respiratory control.

Treatment consists of weight loss and, in severe cases, positive pressure-assisted breathing or tracheostomy. Tricyclic antidepressants and progesterone are beneficial in some cases.

Narcolepsy-cataplexy: Characterized by recurrent episodes of irresistable daytime sleepiness associated with abnormal manifestations of REM sleep. Associated symptoms are cataplexy (brief episodes of muscular paralysis), often precipitated by emotional events, and hypnagogic hallucinations and sleep paralysis.

The disorder is not rare (prevalence 40/100,000 population); men and women are equally affected; onset is usually in adolescence or early adulthood. Sleep studies show the hallmark of disease to be rapid transition to REM sleep (shortened REM latency).

Treatment is a combination of stimulants and tricyclic antidepressants. Excessive hypersomnolence also can occur with metabolic or endocrine disorders—uremia, hypothyroidism, hypercalcemia, and chronic pulmonary disease (with hypercapnia).

For more detailed discussion of this topic, see Schwartz WJ, Stakes JW, Martin JB: The Sleep-Wake Cycle and Disorders of Sleep, Chap. 20, in HPIM-11, p. 109

Patients with disorders of language can present with several different syndromes.

GLOBAL APHASIA Etiology: Occlusion of internal carotid artery (ICA) or middle cerebral artery (MCA) supplying dominant hemisphere (less commonly hemorrhage, trauma, or tumor), resulting in a large lesion of frontal, parietal, and superior temporal lobes.
Clinical manifestations: All aspects of speech and language are impaired. Pt cannot read, write, or repeat and has poor auditory comprehension. Speech output is minimal and nonfluent. Usually hemiplegia, hemisensory loss, and homonymous hemianopsia are present.

BROCA'S APHASIA (motor or nonfluent aphasia) **Etiology:** Core lesion involves dominant inferior frontal convolution (Broca's area), although cortical and subcortical areas along superior sylvian fissure and insula are often involved. Commonly caused by vascular lesions involving the superior division of the MCA, less commonly due to tumor, abscess, metastasis, subdural hematoma, encephalitis.
Clinical manifestations: Speech output is sparse, slow, effortful, dysmelodic, poorly articulated, and telegraphic. Most pts have severe writing impairment. Comprehension of written and spoken language is relatively preserved. Pt is aware of and visibly frustrated by deficit.

With large lesions, a dense hemiparesis may occur and the eyes may deviate toward side of lesion. More commonly, lesser degrees of contralateral face and arm weakness are present. Sensory loss is rarely found, and visual fields are intact. Buccolingual apraxia is common, the pt having difficulty imitating movements with tongue and lips or performing these movements on command. An apraxia involving the ipsilateral hand may occur due to involvement of fibers in the corpus callosum.

WERNICKE'S APHASIA (sensory or fluent aphasia) **Etiology:** Embolic occlusion of inferior division of dominant MCA (less commonly hemorrhage, tumor, encephalitis, or abscess) involving posterior perisylvian region.
Clinical manifestations: Although speech sounds grammatical, melodic, and effortless ("fluent"), it is often virtually incomprehensible due to errors in word usage, structure, and tense and the presence of neologisms and paraphasia. Comprehension of written and spoken material is severely impaired, as are reading, writing, and repetition. Pt seems unaware of deficit. Associated clinical symptoms can include parietal lobe sensory deficits and homonymous hemianopsia. Motor disturbances are rare.

CONDUCTION APHASIA Comprehension of speech and writing is largely intact, and speech output is fluent, although paraphasia is common. *Repetition is severely affected.* Most cases are due to lesions involving supramarginal gyrus of dominant parietal lobe, dominant superior temporal lobe, or arcuate fasciculus. Lesions are typically due to an embolus to either the ascending parietal or posterior temporal branch of the dominant MCA. Associated symptoms include contralateral hemisensory loss and hemianopsia.

PURE WORD DEAFNESS Almost total lack of auditory comprehension with inability to repeat or write to dictation and relatively preserved spoken language and spontaneous writing. Comprehension of visual or written material is superior to that of auditory information. The lesion(s) are typically in or near the primary auditory cortex (Heschl's gyrus) in the superoposterior temporal lobe. Causes are infarction, hemorrhage, or tumor.

PURE WORD BLINDNESS Inability to read and often to name colors with preserved speech fluency, language comprehension, repetition, and writing to dictation (alexia without agraphia). Lesion usually involves left striate cortex and visual association areas as well as fibers in splenium of corpus callosum connecting right and left visual association areas. Most pts have an associated right homonymous hemianopsia, hemisensory deficit, and memory disturbance due to vascular lesions (involving the left PCA territory). Rarely tumor or hemorrhage may be the cause.

ISOLATION OF SPEECH AREA Hypotension, ischemia, or hypoxia may result in borderzone infarctions between the anterior cerebral–MCA–PCA territories which spare the sylvian region of the MCA. Pts are severely brain damaged and have parrot-like repetition of spoken words (echolalia) with little or no spontaneous speech or comprehension.

LABORATORY STUDIES IN APHASIA CT scan or MRI usually identify the location and nature of the causative lesion. Angiography helps in accurate definition of specific vascular syndromes.

THERAPY OF APHASIA Speech therapy may be helpful in treatment of certain types of aphasia.

For more detailed discussion of this topic, see Mohr JP, Adams RD: Disorders of Speech and Language, Chap. 22, in HPIM-11, p. 121

---

155 FOCAL CEREBRAL LESIONS

Patients with focal cerebral lesions often present with a characteristic set of signs and symptoms which enable the astute physician to (1) recognize that a brain disorder exists; (2) localize the disorder to a specific brain region; and (3) together with the clinical history, develop a differential diagnosis. A lesion causes focal symptoms and signs by disrupting functional centers or pathways that connect them.

FRONT LOBE (See Table 155-1.) Extensive anterior frontal lobe pathology may produce only subtle personality changes recognizable by family members or misdiagnosed as depression or thought disorder.

TABLE 155-1

Site of lesion	Signs
Primary and secondary motor cortex	Contralateral spastic paresis
Pre-motor cortex	Grasp reflex; left-sided lesions sometimes cause bilateral dyspraxia
Frontal eye fields	Gaze preference; eyes and sometimes head are turned toward the side of the lesion
Anterior (prefrontal)	May be relatively asymptomatic, but if large or bilateral damage, then cause lack of initiative, inappropriate jocularity, impulsivity, incontinence, perseveration
Prerolandic	Lesions on dominant side cause mutism, expressive aphasia, often with bilateral apraxia

TEMPORAL LOBE (See Table 155-2.) Temporal lobe centers are important for speech, memory, emotions. Left hemisphere coordinates speech in almost all right-handed and 60% of left-handed people.

TABLE 155-2

Site of lesion	Signs
Dominent superior convolution and adjacent inferior parietal convolution	Wernicke's receptive aphasia with jargon speech, inability to comprehend spoken or written language, often with agitation
Bilateral auditory cortex	Cortical deafness
Medial basal cortex	Emotional disorders, psychotic behavior; if bilateral, then Klüver-Bucy syndrome
Hippocampus	Short-term memory loss if dominant or bilateral

PARIETAL LOBE (See Table 155-3.) Parietal lobe lesions affect cortical sensation, i.e., two-point discrimination, ability to recognize objects by tactile cues (astereognosia), along with the more complicated sense of body's position in space.

TABLE 155-3

Site of lesion	Signs
Post-central sensory cortex	Extinction of double simultaneous stimulation, astereognosia, etc.
Dominant angular gyrus	Agraphia, acalculia, left-right disorientation, finger agnosia
Nondominant parietal	Contralateral visual inattention, neglect of contralateral side, constructional apraxia, lack of awareness for deficits

OCCIPITAL LOBE Occipital lobes deal primarily with visual processing. Lesions of inferior calcarine cortex (or temporal lobe lesions that affect optic radiations to this area) cause contralateral superior quadrantanopia. Damage to superior calcarine cortex or optic radiations through parietal lobe cause a contralateral inferior quadrantanopia. Bilateral lesions cause occipital blindness. Occasionally pt is unaware of his or her blindness.

THALAMUS All somatosensory input is processed in thalamus on way to cortical centers. Unilateral thalamic lesions often cause contralateral total hemianesthesia. A disabling delayed pain syndrome may follow. Many neural circuits involve loops through thalamus, so that aphasia, asterixis, choreoathetosis, and mental aberrations also can occur in pts with thalamic lesions. Pupils may be miotic.

BRAINSTEM (See Table 155-4.) All neural input and output must pass through compact brainstem. Relatively small lesions can be accurately diagnosed by neuroanatomic criteria.

TABLE 155-4

Site of lesion	Signs
Top of midbrain	Paralysis of upward gaze, convergence nystagmus, miosis, abulia, disorientation, third nerve palsy
Pontomedullary junction	Contralateral hemiplegia, sixth and seventh nerve palsy, ipsilateral loss of pain sense on face, contralateral sensory loss on body
Lateral medulla	Vertigo, nystagmus, ipsilateral ataxia, loss of facial pain, miosis, ptosis, anhidrosis, contralateral loss of pain sense on body

For more detailed discussion of this topic, see Adams, RD, Victor M: Syndromes Due to Focal Cerebral Lesions, Chap. 24, in HPIM-11, p. 135

ETIOLOGY Both seizure type and age of pt provide important clues to etiology. Important causes of seizures by age group include the following:

Infants: Hypoxia, ischemia, metabolic disorders, birth injury, infection.

Adolescents and young adults: Trauma, drug or alcohol withdrawal, AV malformation, tumors.

Older adults: Tumor, cerebrovascular disease, metabolic disorders.

HISTORY Seizures may begin in a localized area of cortex ("partial or focal") or diffusely ("generalized"). Partial seizures may be associated with loss or alteration in consciousness ("complex") or not affect mentation ("simple"). Simple partial seizures may be motor, sensory, autonomic, or psychic. In complex partial seizures there is alteration in consciousness coupled with automatisms (e.g., lip smacking, chewing, aimless walking, or other complex motor activities). Generalized seizures may result from secondary generalization of a partial seizure or as a primary disorder. Tonic-clonic seizures ("grand mal") result in sudden loss of consciousness, loss of postural control, tonic muscular contraction producing teeth-clenching and rigidity in extension (*tonic phase*), followed by rhythmic muscular jerking (*clonic phase*).

Recovery of consciousness is typically gradual with an intervening period of confusion and disorientation. Headache and somnolence are common postictal phenomena (see Chap. 7). Tongue biting and incontinence may occur during the seizure. In absence seizures ("petit mal") there is sudden cessation, without warning, of ongoing mental activity which rarely lasts longer than 30 seconds. Minor motor symptoms are common, but complex automatisms and clonic activity do not occur. Return of consciousness is abrupt, and there is no postictal somnolence or confusion. Other types of generalized seizures include atypical absence, infantile spasms, tonic, atonic, and myoclonic seizures.

PHYSICAL EXAMINATION Vital signs may provide a clue to malignant hypertension or infection. Gum hyperplasia suggests chronic phenytoin therapy. Skin lesions can occur in Sturge-Weber (port-wine facial nevus), tuberous sclerosis (adenoma sebaceum, shagreen patches), and neurofibromatosis (café-au-lait spots, neurofibroma). The general exam also may provide evidence of drug or alcohol abuse, trauma, hepatic or renal failure, or acute CNS infection. Asymmetries in the neurologic exam can suggest a brain tumor, stroke, or other focal lesion. During a generalized seizure, the pupils may be nonreactive, the corneal reflexes absent, and hyperreflexia and Babinski signs may be transiently present.

LABORATORY FINDINGS Serum glucose, electrolytes, and calcium should be obtained immediately. LFTs, BUN, CBC, toxic screen, and alcohol level can add valuable information in specific pts. If pt takes anticonvulsant medication, drug levels should be measured. CT scan should be obtained in all pts with an unexplained first seizure, and a follow-up study (at 3–6 months) is often advisable. An LP is indicated in all pts where infection is suspected. An EEG with activation procedures (hyperventilation, photic stimulation, sleep) often helps in diagnosis and classification of seizures.

THERAPY Acutely, pt should be placed in semiprone position, head down, to avoid aspiration. Oxygen should be given via face mask. Pt should not be forcibly restrained, and no attempt should be made to insert a tongue blade or other object between teeth. Reversible metabolic disorders (hypoglycemia, hyponatremia, hypertension, drug or alcohol withdrawal) should be promptly corrected. A general principle of drug therapy is that pts should be placed on a single anticonvulsant drug and its dose optimized by following serum levels. A second drug is added only after failure of high therapeutic levels of original drug to control seizures. If control is obtained after addition of a second drug, the original drug should be slowly tapered.

Suggested anticonvulsants for specific seizure types include: *partial seizures*: carbamazepine, phenytoin, phenobarbital, valproate; *tonic-clonic seizures*: carbamazepine, phenytoin, valproate, phenobarbital; *absence seizures*: ethosuzimide, valpropate. Typical therapeutic ranges (μg/mL): carbamazepine (4–12), ethosuximide (40–100), phenobarbital (10–50), phenytoin (10–20), valproate (50–100).

TREATMENT OF STATUS EPILEPTICUS (1) Assess patient carefully for evidence of respiratory or cardiovascular insufficiency. Intubate, establish IV, and administer 50 mL 50% dextrose in water, 100 mg thiamine, and 0.4 mg naloxone (Narcan). (2) Administer diazepam IV 10 mg over 2 minutes (see Table 156-1). (3) Administer 1 g phenytoin (15–20 mg/kg) IV slowly over 30 minutes. (4) If seizures continue and are life-threatening, repeat diazepam 10 mg IV slowly. (5) Then administer phenobarbital 300 mg IV over 30 minutes and repeat two or three times with careful attention to respiratory and cardiac function. Care must be taken to avoid overmedication of patients with seizures that are not life-threatening.

TABLE 156-1 **Treatment of status epilepticus**

Drug	Initial dose	Administration rate	Maximum per 24 h
Diazepam, IV adults	5–10 mg	1–2 mg/min	100 mg
Phenytoin, IV adults	15–20 mg/kg	30–50 mg/min	1.5 g
Phenobarbital, IV adults	300–800 mg	25–50 mg/min	1–2 g

For more detailed discussion of this topic, see Dichter MA: The Epilepsies and Convulsive Disorders, Chap. 342, in HPIM-11, p. 1921

157 CEREBROVASCULAR DISEASES

DEFINITION A focal neurologic injury of acute onset caused by a cerebrovascular disorder.

ETIOLOGY (1) *Atherothrombotic occlusion* of large and medium sized arteries subserving cerebral circulation; (2) *carotid dissection* with thrombosis (traumatic or associated with disease involving media of vessel); (3) *cerebral embolism* arising from heart (mural or valvular emboli), from an artery (artery-to-artery embolism), or due to fat or air emboli; (4) *small vessel disease* (arteriosclerosis, lipohyalinosis); (5) *systemic hypotension* in the presence of arterial stenosis (low flow); (6) *intracerebral hemorrhage*, associated with hypertension, rupture of aneurysm or AV malformation, amyloid angiopathy (in the elderly), hemorrhage into tumor, or with associated coagulopathy (warfarin, heparin, end-stage liver disease, thrombotic thrombocytopenic purpura, etc.); (7) *vasospasm* (4–14 days after subarachnoid hemorrhage, in hypoxia, during migraine attack); and (8) *arteritis* (meningovascular syphilis, bacterial and tuberculous meningitis, connective tissue disease, etc.).

CLINICAL PRESENTATION Abrupt, dramatic onset of focal neurologic symptoms. Temporal pattern is an indicator of underlying pathophysiology (see Table 157-1).

TABLE 157-1 **Anatomic localization of cerebral lesions in stroke**

Signs and symptoms	Structures involved
Cerebral hemisphere, lateral aspect (middle cerebral a.):	
Hemiparesis	Contralateral parietal and frontal motor cortex
Hemisensory deficit	Contralateral somatosensory cortex
Motor aphasia (Broca's)—hesitant speech with word-finding difficulty and preserved comprehension	Motor speech area, dominant frontal lobe
Central aphasia (Wernicke's)—anomia, poor comprehension, jargon speech	Central, perisylvian speech area, dominant hemisphere
Unilateral neglect, apraxias	Nondominant parietal lobe
Homonymous hemianopsia or quadrantanopsia	Optic radiation in inferior parietal or temporal lobe
Gaze preference with eyes deviated to side of lesion	Center for lateral gaze (frontal lobe)
Cerebral hemisphere, medial aspect (anterior cerebral a.):	
Paralysis of foot and leg with or without paresis of arm	Leg area with or without arm area of contralateral motor cortex
Cortical sensory loss over leg	Foot and leg area of contralateral sensory cortex
Grasp and sucking reflexes	Medial posterior frontal lobe
Urinary incontinence	Sensorimotor area, paracentral lobule
Gait apraxia	Frontal cortices

TABLE 157-1 **Anatomic localization of cerebral lesions in stroke (continued)**

Signs and symptoms	Structures involved
Cerebral hemisphere, inferior aspect (posterior cerebral a.):	
Homonymous hemianopsia	Calcarine occipital cortex
Cortical blindness	Occipital lobes, bilaterally
Memory deficit side	Hippocampus, bilaterally or dominant
Dense sensory loss, spontaneous pain dysesthesias, choreoathetosis	Thalamus plus subthalamus
Brainstem, midbrain (posterior cerebral a.):	
Third nerve palsy and contralateral hemiplegia	Third nerve and cerebral peduncle (Weber's syndrome)
Paralysis/paresis of vertical eye movement	Supranuclear fibers to third nerve
Convergence nystagmus, disorientation	Top of midbrain, periaqueductal
Brainstem, pontomedullary junction (basilar a.):	
Facial paralysis	Seventh nerve, ipsilateral
Paresis of abduction of eye	Sixth nerve, ipsilateral
Paresis of conjugate gaze	"Center" for lateral gaze, ipsilateral
Hemifacial sensory deficit	Tract and nucleus of V, ipsilateral
Horner's syndrome	Descending sympathetic pathways
Diminished pain and thermal sense over half body (with or without face)	Spinothalamic tract, contralateral
Ataxia	Middle cerebellar peduncle and cerebellum
Brainstem, lateral medulla (vertebral a.):	
Vertigo, nystagmus	Vestibular nucleus
Horner's syndrome (miosis, ptosis, decreased sweating)	Descending sympathetic fibers, ipsilateral
Ataxia, falling toward side of lesion	Cerebellar hemisphere or fibers
Impaired pain and thermal sense over half body with or without face	Contralateral spinothalamic tract

Stroke in evolution: A neurologic deficit that progresses or fluctuates while a pt is under observation. Possible mechanisms include (1) propagating thrombus obliterating collateral branches with enlarging territory of ischemic brain, (2) progressive narrowing of a vessel by thrombus, (3) cerebral edema, (4) enlarging intracerebral hematoma from continued hemorrhage, (5) emboli propagating, migrating, lysing, and dispersing, and (6) recurrent artery-to-artery embolization.

Completed stroke: A neurologic deficit that does not progress over several days after pt is under observation.

Transient ischemic attack (TIA): A focal neurologic deficit that resolves fully within 24 h. However, when a deficit persists beyond 1 h, some infarction of tissue has probably occurred. Repetitive, short-lived (<15 min), stereotyped focal neurologic deficits attributable to a vascular territory suggest a proximal vascular stenosis or occlusion with inadequate collateral circulation to maintain appropriate perfusion. A single episode of focal neurologic deficit persisting longer than 30 min but less than 24 h suggests an embolic TIA. Other causes of transient neurologic deficit (e.g., seizure manifestation or migraine accompaniment) should be ruled out by Hx or appropriate testing.

Ischemic stroke: A neurologic deficit produced by interruption of blood supply to a brain region due to an intravascular occlusion or low-flow state. Deficit is consistent with vascular territory supplied.

Embolic stroke: Suggested by abrupt appearance of a neurologic deficit that is maximal at onset.

Intracranial hemorrhage: Most common forms are *hypertensive* and *lobar* intracerebral hemorrhages (50%), ruptured saccular aneurysm, and ruptured AV malformation. Vomiting occurs in most cases and headache in about one-half. Signs and symptoms are not usually confined to a single vascular territory. Hypertensive hemorrhage typically occurs in the (1) putamen, adjacent internal capsule, and central white matter; (2) thalamus; (3) pons; and (4) cerebellum. A neurologic deficit that evolves relentlessly over 5–30 min is strongly suggestive of intracerebral bleeding. Ocular signs are important in the localization of these hemorrhages: (1) putaminal—eyes deviated to side opposite paralysis (toward lesion); (2) thalamic—eyes deviated downward, sometimes with unreactive pupils; (3) pontine—reflex lateral eye movements impaired and small (1–2 mm), reactive pupils; (4) cerebellar—eyes deviated to side opposite lesion (early on, in absence of paralysis).

Lacunar stroke: An infarct that can be pinpointed to an anatomic locus of up to 0.5–1.0 cm in diameter, resulting from local small vessel disease.

RISK FACTORS (1) Systemic atherothrombotic disease—ischemic stroke/TIA; (2) source of emboli (e.g., atrial fibrillation, valvular heart disease, MI, infective endocarditis, etc.)—embolic stroke/TIA; (3) severe hypertension—lacunar stroke with small vessel lipohyalinotic disease, atherothrombotic lesions of large and medium-sized vessels, and deep intracerebral hemorrhages; (4) smoking and familial hyperlipidemia—atherothrombotic ischemic stroke/TIA.

COMPLICATIONS (1) Occlusive atherothrombotic disease: increased risk of embolization from distal stump until endothelialization occurs; continued propagation of thrombus to occlude collateral circulation. (2) Embolic stroke: recurrent embolism. (3) Ischemic stroke: intracerebral hemorrhage, particularly in large strokes, as infarcted tissue undergoes necrosis; seizures in 5–10%. (4) Large cortical or cerebellar strokes: cerebral edema—this is particularly critical in cerebellar infarcts because expansion in the posterior fossa can rapidly cause brainstem compression and may require emergency cerebellectomy for lifesaving intervention; period of maximal risk is 12–72 h after infarct. (5) Intracerebral hemorrhage: in addition to cerebral edema, continued expansion of the hematoma with resultant compression; seizures (in < 10%, most likely when hemorrhage extends to the cortical–white matter junction).

LABORATORY EVALUATION **CT:** Should be obtained *without contrast* at time of initial evaluation. (1) To determine whether intracerebral lesion is hemorrhagic. *This is mandatory prior to placing a pt with suspected acute stroke or TIA on anticoagulants.* Rarely, the clinical presentation of TIA can be mimicked by subdural hematoma or tumor. (2) To detect the presence of prior infarcts that may or may not be clinically apparent and may yield clues to etiology.

MRI: Most useful for earlier detection of a cerebral infarct (within hours of onset of symptoms), higher resolution of small lacunes (2–7 mm), and localization of infarcts in the posterior fossa.

Noninvasive carotid tests: Ophthalmodynamometry, oculoplethysmography, directional supraorbital Doppler, carotid ultrasound techniques.

Cerebral angiography: By selective extracranial injection.

Intravenous digital subtraction angiography: For evaluation of stenosis or occlusion of large and medium-sized arteries subserving cerebral circulation; and angiographic detection of sacular aneurysm, AV malformation, or tumor in the case of intracerebral hemorrhage.

ECG, cardiac ultrasound, and 24-h Holter monitor: For evaluation of suspected embolic stroke/TIA.

Coagulation studies: To include PT and PTT, particularly in pts receiving anticoagulation therapy, as well as in cerebral hemorrhage.

TREATMENT **Ischemic stroke or TIA:** (1) When impending atherothrombotic vascular occlusion is suspected, particularly in ischemic stroke in evolution or in posterior circulation involvement, acute anticoagulation with IV heparin is advisable; (2) due to carotid stenosis below the siphon—surgical endarterectomy; (3) when surgery is not an option, atherothrombotic disease may be treated either with warfarin anticoagulation or antiplatelet agents; (4) due to cardiac embolism—anticoagulate (short term in uncomplicated MI, indefinitely in AF or valvular disease).

Lacunar stroke: Aggressive management of hypertension.

Intracerebral hemorrhage: (1) Aggressive correction of any coagulopathy; (2) neurosurgical evaluation for possible emergent evacuation of hematoma, especially in cases of cerebellar hemorrhage; (3) prophylactic anticonvulsant therapy in supratentorial hemorrhage, particularly when extending to cortical surface.

Fluid management in acute stroke: Governed by consideration of relative risk of developing cerebral edema or extending thrombotic occlusion (or propagation) by intravascular volume depletion. In general, restrict fluids and use isotonic IV maintenance fluids (with or without hyperosmotic agents) in cases of large supratentorial or cerebellar strokes (maintain serum osmolality of 290–310 mosmol/L); when basilar thrombosis is suspected, use only isotonic IV fluids; mild fluid restriction may be advisable if cerebellar infarction is present, but *avoid* intravascular volume depletion.

Blood pressure management in acute stroke: Adequate cerebral perfusion pressure must be maintained in face of a critical stenosis, vasospasm, or developing cerebral edema with increasing intracranial pressure; therefore, hypotension (and probably systolic BP < 140 mmHg) should be avoided; because of a risk of new or continued intracerebral hemorrhage, sustained systolic BP > 210 mmHg should be lowered with caution (usually gentle diuresis will suffice).

SUBARACHNOID HEMORRHAGE (SAH)

ETIOLOGY Most common causes (1) rupture of an intracranial aneurysm, (2) AV malformation. *Mycotic aneurysms* may occur in patients with infective endocarditis, systemic infection, or immunocompromise.

CLINICAL PRESENTATION Begins with rapid loss of consciousness in 45% of cases. In another 45%, the initial symptom is excruciating headache, often described as "the worst headache of my life." Vomiting is a prominent symptom and, in combination with severe headache, suggests SAH. A progressive third or sixth nerve palsy may herald SAH. Occasionally, an aneurysm may rupture into subdural space or into basal cisterns of subarachnoid space to form a clot large enough to produce focal neurologic symptoms by mass effect.

COMPLICATIONS (1) Communicating hydrocephalus; (2) recurrent rupture, especially in first 3 weeks after SAH; (3) cerebral ischemia and infarction due to vasospasm, usually 4–14 days after SAH, the major cause of delayed morbidity and death; (4) cerebral edema; (5) seizures; and (6) others: thrombophlebitis with pulmonary embolism, perforated stress-induced duodenal ulcer, ECG changes suggestive of MI or ischemia, cardiac arrhythmias, and hyponatremia due to inappropriate ADH secretion.

LABORATORY EVALUATION **CT:** Noncontrast first, to evaluate presence of blood in subarachnoid space; then with contrast in an effort to visualize an aneurysm or AVM. More than 75% of SAH cases are detectable by CT if obtained within the first 48 h.

Lumbar puncture: To demonstrate presence of blood in subarachnoid space; should be obtained only if CT fails to make diagnosis *and* shows no evidence of mass or obstructive hydrocephalus; CSF should be examined for xanthochromia.

Cerebral angiography: To establish diagnosis firmly, localize and characterize anatomy of aneurysm or AV malformation, and assess presence of vasospasm prior to surgery.

ECG: ST changes, prolonged QRS complex, increased QT interval, and prominent or inverted T waves are often secondary to the SAH rather than myocardial ischemia.

Serum electrolytes and osmolality: Should be followed because of hyponatremia secondary to inappropriate ADH secretion.

TREATMENT (1) *Strict bed rest* in a quiet room; stool softeners to prevent constipation, and analgesics to prevent rebleeding while awaiting surgery. (2) *Emergency surgical intervention* to evacuate intracerebral or subdural hematoma or to place intraventricular drains if obstructive or communicating hydrocephalus develops. (3) *Anticonvulsants* to prevent seizures. (4) *Assisted ventilation* for stuporous or comatose pt to control elevated intracranial pressure and ensure adequate oxygenation. (5) *Blood pressure* is monitored and controlled to maintain adequate cerebral perfusion pressure while avoiding excessive elevation. (6) *Aminocaproic acid (Amicar)* (antifibrinolytic therapy) to prevent rerupture; efficacy has not been established; reports suggest that it increases risk of ischemic complications of SAH. (7) *Symptomatic cerebral vasospasm*: increase cerebral perfusion pressure by increasing mean arterial pressure through plasma volume expansion and pressor agents. (8) *Surgical clipping of aneurysm and resection of AV malformation.* Surgery is typically delayed at least 10–14 days after SAH in an effort to stabilize pt and minimize risk of symptomatic vasospasm in postoperative period; however, surgery may be attempted within the first 48 h if pt is neurologically intact and aneurysm is easily accessible.

For more detailed discussion of this topic, see Kistler JP, Ropper AH, Martin JB: Cerebrovascular Diseases, Chap. 343, in HPIM-11, p. 1930

158 NEOPLASTIC DISEASES OF THE CENTRAL NERVOUS SYSTEM

Care of pts with primary or metastatic tumors in the CNS requires (1) accurate diagnosis of tumor and exclusion of other causes of symptoms (abscess, demyelinating and vascular disease); (2) proper use of CT scan, MRI, myelography, arteriography, and surgical biopsy; (3) control of edema and seizures; (4) exclusion of systemic malignancy prior to referring pt for intracranial biopsy; and (5) management of the medical complications of the tumor and its therapy.

SYMPTOMS AND SIGNS OF CNS TUMORS **Intracranial tumors:** Pts with intracranial tumors present because of nonfocal symptoms due to increased ICP (see Chap. 188) or focal symptoms that are dependent on location of the lesion (see Chaps. 155 and 170). Constant headache is common in pts with CNS tumors, especially if it worsens upon arising in morning or with coughing and sneezing. Papilledema and sixth nerve palsies occur frequently if ICP is elevated. Slow-growing tumors in relatively "silent" brain areas (unilateral prefrontal) can attain a large size with few symptoms. Occasionally, diencephalic and frontal or temporal lobe tumors present with prominent psychiatric disorders. New-onset epilepsy in adults often heralds the diagnosis of CNS malignancy. In such pts over 35 years of age MRI or CT scans every few months should be performed to document presence or absence of a tumor.

Tumors that occur in the third ventricle region include pituitary adenomas, craniopharyngiomas, germ cell neoplasms, pineal tumors, and astrocytomas. They give rise to neuroendocrine abnormalities, optic nerve or chiasmal compression, obstructive hydrocephalus, and Parinaud's syndrome (paralysis of upward gaze and accommodation with fixed pupils). Specific syndromes also are associated with acoustic nerve schwannomas (hearing loss, tinnitus, intermittent vertigo followed by facial weakness and facial sensory loss) and cerebellar hemangioblastomas (headache, head tilt, recurrent emesis, and ataxia, sometimes associated with polycythemia and renal tumors).

Spinal tumors: Spinal cord tumors can cause neurologic dysfunction due to direct compression of nerve tissue or interference with cord blood supply. Extramedullary tumors compress nerve roots, cause back and radicular pain, and produce spastic paresis with sensory loss below a spinal level. Bowel and bladder dysfunction also occur with loss of perineal sensation and rectal tone. Intramedullary tumors usually extend over many levels; their presentation is more varied, and they can be associated with syringomyelia.

Idiopathic syringomyelia, B_{12} deficiency, paraneoplastic syndromes, inflammatory myelitis, arachnoiditis, spinal AV malformation, and meningeal carcinomatosis may be difficult to distinguish from an intrinsic cord tumor on clinical grounds. Pts with slow-growing cord tumors who accumulate patchy cord deficits over time are often misdiagnosed as suffering from multiple sclerosis. Myelography, MRI, and CSF exam are essential for accurate diagnosis in many cases.

Melanoma, lymphoma, leukemia, and adenocarcinoma of breast, GI tract, and lung commonly invade the meninges. Leptomeningeal spread of tumor causes headache and cranial and spinal nerve root deficits, sometimes with spinal cord signs. The CSF shows an elevated protein, low glucose, and pleocytosis.

GENERAL AND RADIOLOGIC EVALUATION OF PATIENTS

Initial evaluation of pts suspected of having a brain tumor should include a search for a primary tumor; this should include careful examination for melanotic lesions, a search for enlarged lymph nodes, breast masses, bony tenderness, abdominal or rectal masses, and organomegaly. Urine and stool should be examined for occult blood. Chest films often reveal the site of primary or secondary tumor. CT scans with contrast will detect brain masses greater than 0.5 cm in diameter. Most tumors enhance after contrast administration. Low density surrounding the mass on CT scan usually represents edema; central low density indicates cavitation. Pts with tumors that shift midline structures to the opposite side or compress midbrain structures are prone to acute neurologic deterioration. MRI can define brainstem and intrinsic spinal cord tumors that are only poorly defined by CT scan. Angiography can show an abnormal vascular blush with early draining veins, characteristic of some tumors. It also provides important information to the neurosurgeon contemplating biopsy or resection. Myelography and CT scan after injection of metrizamide into the subarachnoid space are essential radiologic procedures in the diagnosis of spinal cord tumors; CT may detect deposits of tumor on nerve roots or on the cord itself in pts with leptomeningeal metastases. Repeated CSF examinations with cytologic study are often needed to establish meningeal spread of tumor.

MANAGEMENT **Initial management of intracranial tumors:** Dexamethasone, 32–48 mg per day, in 4 to 6 divided doses reduces cerebral edema due to tumor. Restriction of free water intake may be necessary to prevent edema formation. A mannitol infusion (1 g/kg) may be necessary if pt is deteriorating due to raised ICP (see Chap. 188). Anticonvulsants are sometimes used prophylactically. Surgical biopsy affords a definitive diagnosis of the tumor along with prognostically important pathologic features. Partial resection of large, surgically incurable tumors still enables decompression of intracranial contents and better seizure control.

Tumors that compress the pathway of CSF outflow can cause severe hydrocephalus. Urgent placement of a ventricular-atrial or ventricular-peritoneal shunt in such pts may be lifesaving. Shunts placed into expanding tumor cavities also can help decrease mass effect.

Cerebral metastases: Melanoma has the highest likelihood of any single tumor type to spread to the CNS. Lung and breast cancers are more prevalent and account for the largest percentage of CNS metastases. Pts with lung cancer should have a brain CT scan prior to undergoing curative pulmonary lobectomy. The surgical removal of a single brain metastasis may improve the quality of life for the cancer pt depending on the nature and stage of the systemic disease. Radiation therapy is often palliative and can cause neurologic improvement. Unfortunately, melanoma, GI tract, and lung cancer tend to be relatively resistant to the doses of radiation permissible in the CNS. Treatment of meningeal metastases requires combination of radiation and intrathecal chemotherapy.

Primary brain tumors: Malignant astrocytoma or glioblastoma accounts for 75% of adult glial tumors. Biopsy with resection of accessible tumors combined with radiation improves survival, but the gains are short-lived. Meningiomas are common benign tumors arising from cells of the pia-arachnoid. Schwannomas usually arise from cranial nerves close to their foramina. Resection can be curative for these benign tumors in addition to ependymomas, oligodendrogliomas, hemangioblastomas, and low-grade astrocytomas. Radiation can be reserved for a time of deterioration. Primary CNS lymphoma may be multifocal, simulating metastases or plaques of demyelination. Primary lymphoma is more frequent in pts with the combined immune deficiency syndrome, IgM or IgA deficiencies, or otherwise immunosuppressed. Marked shrinkage of the CNS lymphoma can occur after short courses of corticosteroids. Radiation is also effective in reducing tumor size. Unfortunately, recurrence and eventual therapeutic resistance are the common pattern.

Spinal cord tumors: Rapid radiologic diagnosis and treatment of cord compression are mandatory to avert permanent neurologic disability. Corticosteroids, radiation, and surgical decompression may prevent progression of deficits. Radiation therapy is palliative in some cases. Intrinsic cord tumors in children may be successfully resected even if they extend over multiple cord levels.

For more detailed discussion of this topic, see Hochberg F, Pruitt A: Neoplastic Disorders of the Central Nervous System, Chap. 345, in HPIM-11, p. 1968

---

159 BACTERIAL INFECTIONS OF THE CENTRAL NERVOUS SYSTEM

ACUTE BACTERIAL MENINGITIS

ETIOLOGY

- *Streptococcus pneumoniae* (see Chap. 34): 30–50% of cases in adults; ↑ risk: acute otitis media (25%), pneumonia (25%), head injury with CSF leak (10–20%), sickle cell, Hodgkin's, multiple myeloma, alcoholism.
- *Neisseria meningitidis* (see Chap. 39); most often children and adolescents; epidemics.
- *Haemophilus influenzae,* type B (see Chap. 40): most frequent meningeal infection between 2 months and 3 years; rare in adults except with anatomic defect (dermal sinus tract, skull fracture), immunodeficient, diabetes, alcoholism.
- *Staphylococcus aureus*: follows neurosurgery or penetrating head wound.
- *Staphylococcus epidermidis*: 75% of shunt infections.
- Gram-negative bacilli: associated with brain abscess, epidural abscess, neurosurgical procedures, cranial thrombophlebitis.
- *Listeria monocytogenes*: predisposed in elderly, debilitated, immunosuppressed, alcoholics, diabetics.

SYMPTOMATOLOGY

- Fever, headache, seizures, vomiting, impaired consciousness, stiff neck and back; 25% fulminant onset over 24 h; 50% over 1–7 days following respiratory symptoms.
- Children: onset often nonspecific with fever and vomiting, ↑ seizures.
- 50% with meningococcal meningitis have skin rash.

LABORATORY FINDINGS

• CSF leukocytes: 1000–100,000 (avg. 5–20,000); >50,000 suspicious for ruptured brain abscess; early ↑ PMNs with ↑ mononuclear cells as infection continues. • Pressure: consistently >180 mmH_2O. • Protein: average 150–500 mg/dL. • Sugar: usually <40% of blood sugar. • Gram's stain: + in three-quarters if untreated. • Cultures: + in 70–80%; in partially treated meningitis, latex agglutinin for *H. influenzae* type B. *S. pneumoniae*, meningococcus groups A, B, C, Y. • Blood cultures: + in 40–60% with *H. influenzae*, meningococcus, and pneumococcus.

TREATMENT

- Pneumococcal or meningococcal: penicillin G, 20–24 million U qd in 4–6 divided doses × 10 days or chloramphenicol 4–6 g qd IV in penicillin-allergic.
- *H. influenzae*: ampicillin 300–400 mg/kg qd in children or 12–18 g in adults + chloramphenicol 100–200 mg/kg qd or 4–6 g qd in adults (15–25% of isolates ampicillin-resistant).

- Community-acquired gram-negative: cefotaxime or moxalactam 2 g q 4 h; in hospital following head trauma or neurosurgery, ↑ risk *Pseudomonas aeruginosa* or *Acinetobacter*, add tobramycin 5 mg/kg qd IV and 8–10 mg intrathecally.
- *S. aureus*: Nafcillin or oxacillin 2.0 g q 4 h.
- Unknown etiology: adults—ampicillin 12 g qd; children—ampicillin 400 mg/kg + chloramphenicol 100–200 mg/kg qd; neonates—ampicillin 100–200 mg/kg qd + gentamicin 5 mg/kg qd.

SUBDURAL EMPYEMA

ETIOLOGY

• Primary from extension from sinuses. • Secondary from extension of osteomyelitis, brain abscess, neurosurgical drainage. • Usually polymicrobial: aerobic streptococci > staphylococci > microaerophillic and anaerobic streptococci > aerobic GNR > other anaerobes.

SYMPTOMATOLOGY Chronic sinusitis or otitis with recent flare → headache, fever, vomiting, depressed sensorium → focal motor seizures, hemiplegia, aphasia over several days; 50% papilledema.

DIAGNOSIS

• Laboratory: ↑ WBC and ESR. • LP contraindicated but if done, shows ↑ pressure, WBC of 50–1000, ↑ protein (75–300 mg/dL), normal sugar. • CT scan.

TREATMENT

• Early surgical drainage. • Empiric antibiotics: penicillin 20 million U qd + chloramphenicol 4 g qd × 3–6 weeks.

BRAIN ABSCESS

ETIOLOGY

• Most from chronic ear, sinus, or pulmonary infection. • Streptococci > *Bacteroides* > Enterobacteriaceae (ear infections) > *S. aureus* (penetrating head trauma or bacteremia).

CLINICAL MANIFESTATIONS

- Reactivation of chronic ear, sinus, or pulmonary infection → headache, vomiting, ↑ CSF pressure over < 2 weeks; fever > 50%.
- Frontal lobe: headache, drowsiness, inattention, hemiparesis, unilateral seizures.
- Temporal lobe: unilateral headache, aphasia, and anomia if in dominant hemisphere; homonymous upper quadrant field defect.
- Cerebellar: postauricular or suboccipital headache, nystagmus, gaze weakness, ipsilateral arm and leg weakness.

DIAGNOSIS

• Demonstration of infection in ears, sinuses, lungs or right-to-left cardiac shunt; ↑ ICP, focal cerebral or cerebellar signs. • LP dangerous; if suspect, get CT scan.

TREATMENT

- If focal cerebritis, may cure with antibiotics alone—penicillin 20–40 million U qd + chloramphenicol 4–6 g qd or cefotaxime 12 g qd + metronidazole 500 mg q 6 h × 6–8 weeks.
- Surgical drainage if encapsulated, multiple, deep, concomitant meningitis, or underlying debilitating disease → antibiotics alone.
- Control of ICP with urea, mannitol, or dexamethasone.

For more detailed discussion of this topic, see Harter DH, Petersdorf RG: Pyogenic Infections of the Central Nervous System, Chap. 346, in HPIM-11, p. 1980

160 VIRAL INFECTIONS OF THE CENTRAL NERVOUS SYSTEM, INCLUDING SLOW VIRUSES

ASEPTIC MENINGITIS

- *Epidemiology:* 90% < 30 years old; peak in late summer; majority by coxsackie- and echoviruses (see Chap. 46).
- *Clinical picture:* prodromal "flulike" illness; then intense headache, malaise, nausea, vomiting, photophobia, stupor rare; temperature 38–40°C; neck stiffness; parotitis → mumps; skin rash → consider coxsackie- or echovirus; herpangina (painful vesicles in posterior third of oropharynx) → Coxsackie.
- *Diagnosis:* CSF—10–100 WBCs, > ¾ lymphs, normal protein and glucose (glucose rarely ↓ with mumps, HSV); positive CSF cultures rare except mumps; diagnosis by serology.
- *Treatment:* symptomatic; fever usually resolves in 3–5 days; CSF WBC may be ↑ for several weeks.

VIRAL ENCEPHALITIS See Chap. 49.

MYELITIS

• Infection localizing to parenchyma of spinal cord. • Spinal paralytic disease: polio, cosackie- and echoviruses (see Chap. 46). • Herpes viruses: genital HSV → paralysis of sphincter tone, varicella-zostes virus → bilateral leg weakness with sphincter disturbances (see Chap. 47).

SUBACUTE SCLEROSING PANENCEPHALITIS

- *Epidemiology:* 80% < 11 years old; 3–10 times more likely in males; years after clinical measles.
- *Clinical picture:* well, then insidious mental deterioration → incoordination, ataxia → death.
- *Diagnosis:* abnormal EEG, ↑ measles antibody in CSF and serum; ? patients lack antibody to measles virus protein M.
- *Treatment:* none effective.

PROGRESSIVE MULTIFOCAL LEUKOENCEPHALOPATHY (PML)

- *Epidemiology:* ↑ risk—leukemia, lymphoma, carcinomatosis, AIDS.
- *Clinical picture:* insidious onset, organic mental changes, hemiplegia, hemianopsia, aphasia, visual field abnormalities; death in 1–6 months.
- *Diagnosis:* CSF normal; CT shows white matter destruction; brain biopsy → viral particles of JC virus (polyomavirus).

NEUROLOGIC CONDITIONS IN AIDS

- ↑ risk: herpes, CMV, PML.
- Human immunodeficiency virus may cause acute encephalopathy with recent seroconversion; AIDS dementia—insidious onset of

difficulty concentrating → gait unsteadiness, weakness; MRI shows patchy ↑ signal in central white matter.

CREUTZFELDT-JAKOB DISEASE

- *Etiology:* peak 55–75 years old; incubation as long as 20 years; transmission by corneal transplants, EEG electrodes, growth hormone from cadaveric pituitary glands; causative agent not identified.
- *Clinical picture:* gradual mental deterioration, disturbances of gait → myoclonic jerks, cortical blindness; majority die within 6 months.
- *Diagnosis:* distinct EEG; rapid progressive atrophic changes on CT suggestive; no serologic tests.

For more detailed discussion of this topic, see Harter DH, Petersdorf RG: Viral Diseases of the Central Nervous System: Aseptic Meningitis and Encephalitis, Chap. 347, in HPIM-11, p. 1987

---

161 MULTIPLE SCLEROSIS (MS)

PATHOLOGY Characterized pathologically by focal regions of demyelination ("plaques") of varying size and age scattered throughout the white matter of the CNS, with a propensity to involve the periventricular and subpial white matter of the cerebrum, the optic nerves, brainstem, cerebellum, and spinal cord.

CLINICAL MANIFESTATIONS Onset in third to fourth decades of recurrent attacks of focal neurologic dysfunction occurring at erratic and nonpredictable intervals, typically lasting weeks, and with subsequent variable recovery. Less commonly, slowly progressive neurologic deterioration occurs. Symptoms may be exacerbated by fatigue, stress, exercise, and heat. The manifestations of MS are protean but commonly include weakness and/or sensory symptoms involving a limb, visual difficulties, abnormalities of gait and coordination, and urinary urgency or frequency. Motor involvement can make a limb seem heavy, stiff, weak, or clumsy. Localized tingling, "pins and needles," or "deadness" are common sensory complaints. Optic neuritis can result in blurring or misting of vision, especially in the central visual field, often with associated retro-orbital pain accentuated by eye movement. Involvement of the brainstem may result in diplopia, nystagmus, vertigo, facial pain, and/or numbness, facial weakness, or hemispasm. Problems with coordination, ataxia, tremor, and dysarthria may reflect cerebellar disease.

PHYSICAL EXAMINATION Check for abnormalities in visual fields, loss of visual acuity, disturbed color perception, optic pallor or papillitis, abnormalities in pupillary reflexes, nystagmus, internuclear ophthalmoplegia (slowness or loss of adduction in one eye with nystagmus in the abducting eye on lateral gaze), facial numbness or weakness, dysarthria, incoordination, ataxia, weakness and spasticity, hyperreflexia, loss of abdominal reflexes, ankle clonus, upgoing toes, sensory abnormalities.

LABORATORY FINDINGS MRI scans are the most sensitive index of demyelinating lesions. CT scan, especially with high contrast doses and delayed imaging, also may show plaques. Visual, auditory, and somatosensory evoked response tests are of value in identifying lesions that are clinically silent. Abnormalities in the CSF may include oligoclonal bands, elevated IgG or myelin basic protein, mild lymphocytic pleocytosis, and slight elevation of total protein. Analysis of T-lymphocyte subpopulations in serum or CSF may demonstrate reduced numbers of cells with the "suppressor" phenotype during or immediately preceding attacks. Urodynamic studies often aid in investigation and management of bladder symptoms. CT scan, MRI, and myelography may help exclude other processes that can mimic MS.

TREATMENT No definitive therapy is currently available. Steroids (ACTH, prednisone) are of value in ameliorating the severity of acute attacks. Immunosuppressive therapy (cyclophosphamide) may decrease the frequency of attacks and stabilize progressive disease. Use of antibodies against specific lymphocyte subpopulations and other types of immunotherapy are subjects of active current research. Hyperbaric oxygen treatments are considered of value by some. Useful supportive therapy may include anticholinergics, smooth muscle relaxants, and self-catheterization for bladder symptoms; diazepam, baclofen, and dantrolene for spasticity and flexor spasms; and phenytoin and carbamazepine for dysesthesia. Clonazepam benefits some pts with intention tremor.

For more detailed discussion of this topic, see Antel JP, Arnason BGW: Demyelinating Diseases, Chap. 348, in HPIM-11, p. 1995

ETIOLOGY Degeneration of dopaminergic neurons of the substantia nigra. Parkinsonian syndromes may follow the use of major tranquilizers and other medications that interrupt dopaminergic functions (e.g., phenothiazines, reserpine, alpha-methyldopa), CO poisoning, intoxications with manganese and other heavy metals, and the use of illicit synthetic drugs (e.g., MPTP). Rare cases follow viral encephalitis or occur in association with focal lesions of substantia nigra and striatum. Parkinsonism also occurs in other degenerative neurologic disease (e.g., striatonigral degeneration, olivopontocerebellar atrophy, and progressive supranuclear palsy).

CLINICAL MANIFESTATIONS Onset between ages 40 and 70 with subsequent chronic progression. Presenting symptoms include tremor, stiffness and slowness of movement, loss of dexterity, deterioration in handwriting, difficulty arising from a chair or turning in bed, and abnormalities in gait and posture. Additional complaints may include excessive sweating and salivation, postural hypotension, subtle dementia, and depression.

PHYSICAL EXAMINATION Tremor at rest (4–7 Hz) is first noticed in the hands and fingers ("pill rolling") but later may involve legs, face, and tongue. A faster "action tremor" may be present. Slowness and poverty of movement (bradykinesia) can be detected by testing quick movements (e.g., "slap my hand!") and rapid alternating movements; the superimposition of tremor on passive movements creates a sense of "cogwheeling" most easily demonstrated at the wrist. Rigidity produces resistance to passive limb displacement. Postural abnormalities result in flexion of head and trunk, flexion of knees and elbows, and positional deformities of hands. Pts have infrequent eye blinking, a fixed, expressionless face ("masked"), and decreased spontaneous and associated movements (e.g., arm-swing while walking). Abnormalities of gait include short, shuffling steps, difficulty in getting started and in turning, festination, and frequent falls. Additional signs may include micrographia, hypophonia, hypometric saccades, drooling, excess salivation, and seborrhea. Some degree of intellectual deterioration is common in advanced cases. Paralysis, alterations in tendon reflexes, and objective sensory findings do not occur.

COMPLICATIONS Aspiration pneumonia, bedsores, and other problems secondary to inanition and general enfeeblement occur in advanced cases.

LABORATORY FINDINGS Diagnosis is based on typical history and clinical findings. CT scan, MRI, EEG, and CSF profile are typically normal. Neuropsychologic testing may help to define intellectual impairment. Recording of tremor rate, rhythm, and amplitude may be useful in some pts.

TABLE 162-1 **Doses of drugs used in Parkinson's disease**

Drug	Trade name	Dose	Side effects
Trihexyphenidyl	Artane	2–5 mg tid	Dry mouth, blurred vision, confusion
Benztropine	Cogentin	2 mg tid	Dry mouth, confusion
Procyclidine	Kemadrin	2–2.5 mg tid	Dry mouth, blurred vision, GI complaints
Carbidopa/levodopa	Sinemet	10/100 to 25/250 mg; increase slowly to tid or qid	Orthostatic hypotension, GI complaints, hallucinations, confusion, chorea
Amantadine	Symmetrel	100 mg bid	Depression, orthostatic hypotension, psychosis, urinary retention
Bromocriptine	Parlodel	10–100 mg daily in divided doses	Orthostatic hypotension, nausea and vomiting, hallucinations, psychosis

TREATMENT Drug-induced parkinsonism is treated by reducing dose of drug or by administrating an anticholinergic. Anticholinergics [e.g., trihexyphenidyl (Artane) or benztropine (Cogentin)] are used for treatment of mild cases of idiopathic Parkinson's disease to suppress resting tremor (see Table 162-1). Beta blockers (e.g., propranolol, metoprolol) are helpful for action tremor. Sinemet (carbidopa/levodopa) is the mainstay of therapy in most cases. Dopamine receptor agonists (e.g., bromocriptine) and amantadine are useful adjuncts. Stereotactic surgery to place lesions in the ventrolateral thalamus may be beneficial in cases of severe tremor.

For more detailed discussion of this topic, see Richardson EP Jr., Beal, MF, and Martin JB: Degenerative Diseases of the Nervous System, Chap. 350, in HPIM-11, p. 2012

163 ALZHEIMER'S DISEASE (AD) AND OTHER DEMENTIAS

ETIOLOGY About 70% of progressive dementias occurring in adults are due to AD. Other causes in descending order of frequency are multiinfarct dementia (MID), metabolic/nutritional/endocrine disorders (including Wernicke-Korsakoff syndrome), brain tumors, chronic CNS infection, and normal-pressure hydrocephalus (NPH). Less common causes are Huntington's disease (HD), Creutzfeldt-Jakob disease (see Chap. 160), and Pick's disease. AIDS encephalopathy is emerging as an important cause of dementia in groups at risk.

CLINICAL MANIFESTATIONS Dementia is defined as a decline from a former level of cognitive function. Although effects on memory (particularly recent memory) are usually prominent, all aspects of cortical functions may be affected, leading to disorientation, poor judgment, poor concentration, aphasia, apraxia, and alexia. Level of consciousness is usually normal, and hallucinations or agitated confusion should lead to consideration of toxic/metabolic/drug-related or infectious etiologies.

AD: Presents initially with memory loss, but soon also alters other cognitive functions with evidence of aphasia, apraxia, or impaired judgment. Pt's personality is preserved, and superficial assessment may miss extent of dementia. Symptoms are usually noted first by family members; pt is often unaware of serious degree of memory loss. Disease is characterized by neuropathologic changes of neurofibrillary tangles and senile plaques, found most prominently in hippocampus and association cortex. Familial AD (10%) is caused by a genetic defect on chromosome 21. Down's syndrome is also associated with neuropathologic changes identical to AD. The senile plaque contains an extracellular amyloid core formed by a protein encoded by a gene also on chromosome 21.

MID: Pts with hypertension, diabetes mellitus, and hypercholesterolemia are susceptible to multiple CNS infarcts of varying sizes. History of strokes, asymmetrical neurologic signs, and pseudobulbar palsy are clues to diagnosis. CT and MRI reveal multiple lesions.

Toxic/metabolic/nutritional: Pts should be assessed for systemic signs of vitamin deficiency (thiamine, B_{12}), for endocrine disturbance (hypothyroidism, hypercalcemia), and for history of drug use (iatrogenic or illicit). Pts with Wernicke's encephalopathy present with memory loss and confusion, abnormal eye movements (sixth nerve palsy, nystagmus), and ataxia. The persistent deficit in memory is called Korsakoff's syndrome. Pts with this condition have permanent inability to learn or memorize new material, show confabulation, but have near normal preservation of other higher cortical functions (language, calculations), etc.

Brain tumors (see chap. 158) **and subdural hematoma:** CT or MRI will clarify diagnosis.

CNS infections: Cryptococcus (torula), neurosyphilis, and other chronic infections can be sought by CSF examination. AIDS can present first as an aseptic meningitis followed by a progressive dementia. CSF is abnormal (WBC pleocytosis), and HIV can be cultured from CSF or brain.

NPH: Should be suspected in elderly patients with combination of gait disorder, dementia, and urinary incontinence. Diagnosis may be difficult in elderly pts with cortical atrophy and *hydrocephalus ex vacuo*. Diagnostic studies in hospital are required to make the diagnosis.

HD: An autosomal dominant disorder (gene on chromosome 4) that presents in pts aged 20–50, with depression, choreiform movements, and *subcortical* dementia—abulia, inattention, poor concentration, but less striking memory loss. Abnormal CT or MRI with caudate atrophy is found.

Limbic encephalitis: See Chap. 170.

Creutzfeldt-Jakob disease: See Chap. 160.

LABORATORY INVESTIGATION Pts with diagnosis of dementia should have (1) CBC, ESR; (2) serum calcium, electrolytes, B_{12}, and folate levels, and liver, renal, and thyroid function tests; (3) CT or MRI; (4) CSF examination for cell count, protein, and cytology; and (5) VDRL should always be measured; HIV antibody testing should be obtained when indicated.

DIFFERENTIAL DIAGNOSIS *Pseudodementia of depression* may be difficult to distinguish from true dementia. Pts over age 60 commonly complain of subtle memory loss—usually due to *benign senescent forgetfulness*. In both these cases, a clinical assessment of memory functions usually reveals no deficit. A useful test is the

TABLE 163-1 **Blessed dementia scale**

Item	Score
Name	0 1
Age	0 1
Time (hour)	0 1
Time of day	0 1
Day of week	0 1
Date	0 1
Month	0 1
Season	0 1
Year	0 1
Place:	
Name	0 1
Street	0 1
Town	0 1
Type of place (home, hospital, etc.)	0 1
Recognition of persons (any 2 available)	0 1 2
Personal memory:	
Date of birth	0 1
Place of birth	0 1
School attended	0 1
Occupation	0 1
Name of sibling or spouse	0 1
Name of any town where pt worked	0 1
Name of employer	0 1
Nonpersonal memory:	
Date WWI (1914–1918)	0 1
Date WWII (1939–1945)	0 1
President	0 1
Vice-President	0 1
5-Min recall:	
(Mr.) John Brown	0 1 2
42 West (Street)	0 1 2
Cambridge (MA)	0 1
Concentration	
Months backward	0 1 2
Counting 1–20	0 1 2
Counting 20–1	0 1 2

Blessed dementia scale (see Table 163-1), where each abnormal response is scored. Intact elderly individuals show scores of 0–2; scores >6 are associated with progressive dementia in most cases. Pts with Parkinson's disease (see Chap. 162) may become demented.

TREATMENT The treatable cases will emerge from the laboratory evaluation. NPH can be improved in two-thirds of cases by CSF shunting. Nontreatable causes of dementia include AD, HD, Creutzfeldt-Jakob.

For more detailed discussion of this topic, see Richardson EP Jr., Beal MF, Martin JB: Degenerative Diseases of the Nervous System, Chap. 350, in HPIM-11, p. 2011

OLFACTORY NERVE (I)

The sense of smell may be impaired by (1) interference with access of odorant to olfactory neuroepithelium (*transport loss*), e.g., by swollen nasal mucous membrane in URI, allergic rhinitis, or structural changes in naval cavity such as with a deviated septum, nasal polyps, or neoplasm; (2) injury to receptor region (*sensory loss*), e.g., destruction of olfactory neuroepithelium by viral infections, neoplasms, inhalation of toxic chemicals, or radiation to head; and (3) damage to central olfactory pathways (*neural loss*), e.g., by head trauma with or without fractures of cribriform plate, neoplasms of anterior cranial fossa, neurosurgical procedures, neurotoxic drugs, or congenital disorders such as Kallmann's syndrome.

OPTIC NERVE (II)

Visual disturbances may be localized upon examination of globe, retina, or optic disc or may require careful visual field testing to pinpoint. Retinal lesions cause arcuate, central, or centrocecal scotomas. Chiasmal lesions produce bitemporal hemianopsias. Homonymous hemianopsias arise behind the chiasm and, if complete, are of no further localizing value. When incomplete, an incongruous homonymous hemianopsia suggests a lesion in the tract or radiations (tract lesions may have associated optic atrophy and an afferent pupillary defect, whereas pupils in postgeniculate lesions are normal). A congruous (identical) homonymous hemianopsia implies a lesion in calcarine cortex.

AQUEOUS HUMOR AND GLAUCOMA Glaucoma is a condition in which elevated intraocular pressure (>22 mmHg) transmitted through aqueous humor damages the optic nerve. It is the leading cause of blindness in the U.S.

Open-angle glaucoma: Rarely causes ocular pain or corneal edema. Visual loss occurs first in the periphery, and visual acuity remains normal until late in the course. *Treatment*: topical cholinergic (pilocarpine or carbachol) and beta-blocking (timolol) agents with or without carbonic anhydrase inhibitors (acetazolamide or methazolamide).

Angle-closure glaucoma: May be precipitated by drugs to dilate the pupil. *Symptoms*: visual loss, pupillary dilation, pain, and when acute, erythema. This is a medical emergency, to be treated with IV mannitol, parenteral acetazolamide, and topical pilocarpine or timolol.

Congenital glaucoma: Rare.

Secondary glaucoma: May be associated with leukemia, sickle cell disease, Waldenström's macroglobulinemia, ankylosing spondylitis, RA, sarcoidosis, congenital rubella, onchocerciasis, amyloidosis, osteogenesis imperfecta, neoplastic metastases, neurofibromatosis, Sturge-Weber syndrome, chronic corticosteroid use, amphetamines, hexamethonium, reserpine, anticholinergics, ocular trauma, and dislocation of the lens (homocystinuria and Marfan's syndrome).

RETINA Causes of retinal disease include vasculopathies associated with major medical illnesses (e.g., hypertension, diabetes); central retinal artery occlusion (CRA) (with boxcar segmentation of blood flow in retinal veins, milky white retina, and cherry red spot from preserved vascularity of choroid) due to emboli, temporal arteritis, arteriosclerosis, collagen-vascular disease, hyperviscosity states; transient monocular blindness (amaurosis fugax) due to episodic retinal ischemia, usually associated with ipsilateral carotid artery stenosis or embolism of the retinal arteries; retinal degeneration due to retinitis pigmentosa and associated multisystem diseases; toxic effects of drugs, e.g., phenothiazines or chloroquin.

OPTIC NERVE **Retrobulbar optic neuropathy:** Characterized by rapid development (hours to days) of impaired vision in one or both eyes, usually due to acute optic nerve demyelination. Most cases occur in childhood, adolescence, or young adulthood. Total blindness is rare. PE: acutely, optic disc and retina are normal or there is papillitis; eye movement or pressure on globe produces pain; affects central more than peripheral vision, and the pupillary light reflex is impaired (swinging flashlight test). CSF is normal or has 10–20 WBCs/cm^3 with or without oligoclonal bands. 15–40% will develop signs of multiple sclerosis within 15 years. Other causes: postinfectious or disseminated encephalomyelitis, posterior uveitis, vascular lesions of the optic nerve, tumors (optic nerve glioma, neurofibromatosis, meningioma, metastases), and fungal infections.

Anterior ischemic optic neuropathy (AION): Caused by atherosclerotic or inflammatory disease of ophthalmic artery or its branches. Presents as acute painless monocular visual loss with an altitudinal defect. Optic disc is pale and swollen with splinter peripapillary hemorrhages and normal macula and retina. Evaluation should aggressively rule out temporal arteritis. Occasionally microemboli (e.g., following cardiac surgery) may cause AION.

Toxic or nutritional optic neuropathy: Presents as simultaneous impairment of vision in both eyes with central or centrocecal scotomas, developing over days to weeks. Agents: methyl alcohol intoxication, chloramphenicol, ethambutol, isoniazid, streptomycin, sulfonamides, digitalis, ergot, disulfiram, and heavy metal.

Bitemporal hemianopsia: Caused by suprasellar extension of a pituitary tumor or saccular aneurysm of circle of Willis, tuberculum sellae meningioma, or rarely, sarcoid, metastases, and Hand-Schüller-Christian disease.

OCULOMOTOR, TROCHLEAR, AND ABDUCENS NERVES (III, IV, VI)

Syndrome of ophthalmoplegia.

Isolated third or sixth nerve palsies: May be due to diabetes mellitus, neoplasm, increased ICP (sixth nerve), pontine glioma in

TABLE 164-1 **Cranial nerve syndromes**

Site	Cranial nerves involved	Usual cause
Sphenoid fissure (superior orbital)	III, IV, first division V, VI	Invasive tumors of sphenoid bone, aneurysms
Lateral wall of cavernous sinus	III, IV, first division V, VI, often with proptosis	Aneurysms or thrombosis of cavernous sinus, invasive tumors from sinuses and sella turcica, sometimes benign granuloma responsive to steroids
Retrosphenoid space	II, III, IV, V, VI	Large tumors of middle cranial fossa
Apex of petrous bone	V, VI	Petrositis, tumors of petrous bone
Internal auditory meatus	VII, VIII	Tumors of petrous bone (dermoids, etc.), infectious processes, acoustic neuroma
Pontocerebellar angle	V, VII, VIII, and sometimes IX	Acoustic neuroma, meningioma
Jugular foramen	IX, X, XI	Tumors and aneurysms
Posterior laterocondylar space	IX, X, XI, XII	Tumors of parotid gland, carotid body, and metastatic tumor
Posterior retroparotid space	IX, X, XI, XII and Horner syndrome	Tumors of parotid gland, carotid body, metastatic tumor, lymph node tumors, tuberculous adenitis

Modified from Victor M, Martin JB: HPIM-11, p 2037.

children or metastatic nasopharyngeal tumor in adults (sixth nerve), tumor at base of brain (third nerve), ischemic infarction of nerve, aneurysms in the circle of Willis. In compressive third nerve lesions the pupil is usually dilated, whereas pupils are spared in infarction of the nerve.

Third, fourth, and sixth nerve lesions: May occur at level of their nuclei, along their course from brainstem through subarachnoid space, cavernous sinus, or superior orbital fissure (see Table 164-1).

Tolosa-Hunt syndrome: Painful, combined unilateral palsies due to parasellar granuloma.

Pituitary apoplexy: Acute onset of uni- or bilateral ophthalmoplegia and visual field defect with headache and/or drowsiness.

Migrainous ophthalmoplegia: Attacks of ocular palsy in conjunction with typical migraine.

TRIGEMINAL NERVE (V)

Trigeminal neuralgia (tic douloureux): Frequent, excruciating paroxysms of pain in lips, gums, cheek, or chin (rarely in ophthalmic division of fifth nerve) lasting seconds to minutes. Appears in middle or old age. Pain is often stimulated at trigger points. Sensory deficit cannot be demonstrated. Must be distinguished from other forms of facial pain arising from diseases of jaw, teeth, or sinuses. Tic is rarely caused by herpes zoster or a tumor. *Treatment*: carbamazepine (1 to 1.5 g daily in divided doses) is effective in 75% of cases; follow CBC for rare complications of aplastic anemia. When medications fail, surgical gangliolysis or suboccipital craniectomy for decompression of trigeminal nerve are options.

Trigeminal neuropathy: May be caused by a variety of rare conditions, usually presenting with facial sensory loss or weakness of jaw muscles. These include tumors of middle cranial fossa, trigeminal nerve, or metastases to base of skull, lesions in cavernous sinus (affecting first and second divisions of fifth nerve) or superior orbital fissure (affecting first division of fifth nerve).

FACIAL NERVE (VII)

Lesions of the seventh nerve or nucleus produce hemifacial weakness that includes muscles of forehead and orbicularis oculi; if lesion is in middle ear portion, taste is lost over the anterior two-third of tongue and there may be hyperacusis; if lesion is at internal auditory meatus, there may be involvement of auditory and vestibular nerves, whereas pontine lesions usually affect abducens nerve and often corticospinal tract as well.

Bell's palsy: Most common form of facial paralysis, found in 23/100,000 annually. Weakness evolves over 12–48 h, sometimes preceded by retroaural pain. Fully 80% recover within several weeks or months. *Treatment:* involves protection of eye during sleep. Prednisone (60–80 mg qd over 5 days, tapered off over the next 5 days) may be beneficial, but this has not been firmly established.

Ramsay Hunt syndrome: Caused by herpes zoster infection of geniculate ganglion; distinguished from Bell's palsy by a vesicular eruption in pharynx, external auditory canal, and other parts of the cranial integument.

Acoustic neuromas: Often compress the seventh nerve.

Pontine tumors or infarcts: May cause a lower motor neuron facial weakness.

Bilateral facial diplegia: May appear in Guillain-Barré, sarcoidosis, Lyme disease, and leprosy.

Hemifacial spasm: May appear either as a result of Bell's palsy, with irritative lesions (e.g., acoustic neuroma, basilar artery aneurysm, or aberrant vessel compressing the nerve) or as an idiopathic disorder.

VESTIBULAR NERVE (VIII)

The eighth cranial nerve has a vestibular and an auditory component. Vertigo caused by a lesion of the vestibular nerve is discussed in Chap. 8. Lesions of the auditory nerve cause hearing impairment which can be either *conductive*, caused by structural abnormalities in external auditory canal or middle ear due to tumor, infection, trauma, etc., or *sensorineural*, due to damage to hair cells of the organ of Corti secondary to excessive noise, viral infections, ototoxic drugs, temporal bone fractures, meningitis, cochlear otosclerosis, Ménière's disease, or neural damage due largely to cerebellar angle tumors or vascular, demyelinating, or degenerative diseases affecting the central auditory pathways. Brainstem auditory evoked responses (BAERs) are a sensitive and accurate test for distinguishing sensory from neural hearing losses. Audiometry can distinguish conductive from sensorineural hearing losses. Most pts with conductive and asymmetric sensorineural hearing losses should have CT scans of the temporal bone. Those with sensorineural hearing losses should have the vestibular system evaluated with electronystagmography and caloric testing.

GLOSSOPHARYNGEAL NERVE (IX)

Glossopharyngeal neuralgia: Paroxysmal, intense pain in tonsillar fossa of throat that may be precipitated by swallowing. There is no demonstrable sensory or motor deficit. *Treatment* with carbamazepine or phenytoin is often effective, but surgical division of the ninth nerve near the medulla is sometimes necessary. Other diseases affecting this nerve include herpes zoster or compressive neuropathy when found in conjunction with vagus and accessory nerve palsies due to tumor or aneurysm in region of jugular foramen.

VAGUS NERVE (X)

Lesions of vagus nerve cause symptoms of dysphagia and dysphonia. Unilateral lesions produce drooping of soft palate, loss of gag reflex, and "curtain movement" of lateral wall of pharynx with hoarse, nasal voice. Diseases that may involve the vagus include diphtheria (toxin), neoplastic and infectious processes at the meningeal level, tumors and vascular lesions in the medulla, or compression of the recurrent laryngeal nerve by intrathoracic processes.

HYPOGLOSSAL NERVE (XII)

The twelfth cranial nerve supplies the ipsilateral muscles of the tongue. Lesions affecting the motor nucleus may occur in the brainstem (tumor, poliomyelitis, or motor neuron disease), during the course of the nerve in the posterior fossa, or in the hypoglossal canal.

For more detailed discussion of this topic, see Victor M, Martin JB: Diseases of the Cranial Nerves, Chap. 352, in HPIM-11, p. 2035

165 PERIPHERAL NEUROPATHIES

Any disorder of peripheral nerve; lesions may be primarily *axonal* (affecting metabolic function of the neuron distally) or *demyelinating* (with loss of myelin sheath). A wide array of processes can produce these lesions.

CLINICAL FEATURES Symmetric, distal sensorimotor neuropathy: Acquired toxic or metabolic neuropathies are typical. Initial symptoms tend to be sensory: tingling, prickling, burning, or bandlike, such as dysesthesias in distal extremities, first feet, later hands in a "stocking-glove" distribution. Onset is usually symmetric. If mild, sensorimotor signs may be absent. Worsening proceeds centripetally to muscle atrophy, pansensory loss, areflexia, motor weakness greater in extensor than corresponding flexor groups. In extreme cases, respiratory compromise or sphincteric dysfunction may develop. Time course, distribution, and severity vary widely with etiology.
Mononeuropathy: Confined to a single peripheral nerve. Raises possibility of mechanical entrapment which may require surgical release.
Mononeuropathy multiplex: Simultaneous or sequential involvement of isolated, noncontiguous nerve trunks. Raises possibility of a multifocal axonopathy (as in a vasculitis) or an acquired multifocal form of demyelinating neuropathy.
Polyneuropathy: A widespread process which is usually symmetric, distal, and graded, often a "stocking-glove" distribution. When *demyelinating:* acute, suggests Guillain-Barré syndrome (GBS); chronic, suggests immunoglobulin disorders (primary or associated with tumors). When *axonal*: subacute, suggests toxic exposure or associated systemic disease or alcoholism; chronic (years), suggests possible genetic/familiar disorder.

LABORATORY FINDINGS Begin with CBC, ESR, UA, CXR, blood glucose, B_{12} and folate levels, and serum protein electrophoresis. EMG and nerve conduction studies aid in further evaluation (see Tables 165-1 and -2).

SYSTEMIC DISEASES ASSOCIATED WITH POLYNEUROPATHY Diabetes mellitus, uremia, porphyria (three types), hypoglycemia, vitamin deficiencies (B_{12}, folate, thiamine, pyridoxine, pantothenic acid), chronic liver disease, primary biliary cirrhosis, primary systemic amyloidosis, hypothyroidism, chronic obstructive lung disease, acromegaly, malabsorption (sprue, celiac disease), carcinoma (sensory, sensorimotor, axonal, or demyelinating neuropathies), lymphoma, polycythemia vera, multiple myeloma, benign monoclonal gammopathy, macroglobulinemia, cryoglobulinemia.

DRUGS OR TOXINS ASSOCIATED WITH POLYNEUROPATHY Amiodarone, aurothioglucose, cisplatin, dapsone, disulfiram, hydralazine, isoniazid, metronidazole, misonidazole, perhexilene, phenytoin, thalidomide, vincristine, acrylamide (flocculant, grout-

TABLE 165-1 **Patterns of electrical activity in muscle**

	At rest	Slight contraction	Maximal contraction
Normal muscle	Short-lived activity after needle insertion	Bi–triphasic potentials, amplitude: 2–5 mV, duration: 2–10 ms	Continuous activity of multiple motor units ("full" interference pattern)
Denervated muscle	Prolonged insertional activity; fibrillation potentials	High-amplitude (5–15 mV) polyphasic potentials ("giant motor units")	Reduced interference pattern with gaps in activity
Myopathic muscle	Prolonged insertional activity; fibrillation potentials	Small-amplitude (0.2–0.5 mV) polyphasic potentials	"Full" interference pattern of small amplitude

ing agent), arsenic (herbicide; insecticide), buckthorn (toxic berry), carbon disulfide (industrial), diphtheria, dimethylamino propionitrile (industrial), γ-diketone hexacarbons (solvents), inorganic lead, organophosphates, thallium (rat poison), pyridoxine (vitamin).

GENETICALLY DETERMINED NEUROPATHIES Peroneal muscular atrophy (HMSN-I), peroneal muscular atrophy (HMSN-II), hereditary amyloid neuropathies, hereditary sensory neurop-

TABLE 165-2 **Nerve conduction studies**

	Conduction velocity	Distal latency
Normal motor nerve	42–74 m/s, depending on nerve	2–6 m/s, depending on nerve
Axonopathies with "dying back" or wallerian degeneration of selected fibers (diabetic, alcoholic, uremic, carcinomatous, nutritional neuropathies, etc.)	Mild slowing (35–40 m/s)	Prolonged
Axonopathies with segmental demeylination of all fibers (Guillain-Barré syndrome, diphtheria, metachromatic leukodystrophy, Krabbe's, Charcot-Marie-Tooth, etc.)	Marked slowing (10–15 m/s)	Prolonged
Focal compressive (entrapment) neuropathies (e.g., median n. in carpal tunnel syndrome)	Focal conduction slowing at site of compression	Prolonged (>4.5 m/s for median n.)

athy (HSN-I), porphyric neuropathy, hereditary liability to pressure palsy, Fabry's disease, adrenomyeloneuropathy, hereditary sensory neuropathy (HSN-III), Déjerine-Sottas (HMSN-III), Refsum's disease, ataxia-telangectasia, abetalipoproteinemia, giant axonal neuropathy, metachromatic leukodystrophy, globoid cell leukodystrophy, Friedreich's ataxia.

CAUSES OF MONONEUROPATHY Differential is implied by location of lesion as determined by PE and EMG (i.e., how distal to nerve root electrophysiologic abnormalities are first found). Considerations include nerve entrapment (carpal tunnel, meralgia paresthetica, etc.), direct trauma or dislocation, compression from tumor (Pancoast, in the case of brachial plexus; pelvic or retroperitoneal, in the case of lumbosacral plexus lesions), direct tumor infiltration of nerve sheath, compression from a retroperitoneal hematoma, plexitis, diabetes mellitus, peripheral nerve tumors, herpes zoster, Bell's palsy, sarcoidosis, leprous neuritis.

For more detailed discussion of this topic, see Asbury AK: Diseases of the Peripheral Nervous System, Chap. 355, in HPIM-11, p. 2058

CLASSIFICATION (1) Autoimmune: mysathenia gravis (MG), Lambert-Eaton (paraneoplastic) syndrome (LES); (2) toxic: botulism, drug-induced disorders; (3) congenital: familial infantile myasthenia, end-plate acetylcholinesterase (AChE) deficiency, slow-channel syndrome, end-plate acetylcholine receptor (AChR) deficiency.

ETIOLOGY Each disorder involves compromise of the generation of an adequate end-plate potential to trigger a propagated muscle fiber action potential.

1 *MG*: destruction of the AChR at motor end plate.

2 *LES*: associated with reduced probability of quantal release of acetylcholine (ACh) from nerve terminal with normal presynaptic stores and postsynaptic responses.

3 *Familial infantile myasthenia*: autosomal recessive, probably a presynaptic defect in ACh resynthesis of packaging.

4 *Congenital end-plate AChE deficiency*: sporadic, absence of AChE in the neuromuscular junction.

5 *Slow-channel syndrome*: autosomal dominant, overstimulation and destruction of the AChR due to slow ion-channel closure.

6 *Congenital end-plate AChR deficiency*: autosomal recessive.

7 *Botulism*: toxin from *Clostridium botulinum* interferes with calcium facilitation of ACh quantal release from the nerve terminal.

8 *Drug-induced myasthenic syndromes*: uncommon, usually associated with an overdose, or may unmask or worsen a preexisting myasthenic syndrome; drugs include tetracycline, polymyxin, and aminoglycoside antibiotics, antiarrhythmic agents (procainamide, quinidine), β-adrenergic blockers (timolol, propranolol), phenothiazines, lithium, trimethaphan, methoxyflurane, magnesium; poisoning by insecticides containing long-acting anticholinesterases.

CLINICAL FEATURES **MG:** May present at any age. Symptoms fluctuate throughout the day and are provoked by exertion, temperature extremes, infections, menses, or excitement. Early on, symptoms are purely ocular in 40% of pts, generalized in 40%, involve extremities in 10%, and involve only bulbar or bulbar and eye muscles in 10%. Symptoms remain ocular in only 16%. Typical symptoms: diplopia, ptosis, symmetric facial weakness, difficulty chewing, dysphagia, dysphonia, abnormal fatigability of proximal limb muscles with normally active deep tendon reflexes. Of MG pts, two-thirds have thymic hyperplasia, 10–15% have thymoma, 10% have other associated autoimmune diseases.

LES: Weakness of proximal limb and torso with relative sparing of oculobulbar muscles. Upon voluntary contraction, strength transiently increases then decreases. Tendon reflexes are hypoactive or absent. Autonomic dysfunction occurs in half of pts. Associated

with carcinoma (80%, small-cell lung) in 72% of male and 32% of female LES pts > age 40.
Botulism: In adults, begins with nausea, vomiting, diarrhea, abdominal cramps, dry mouth, blurred vision, meiosis. Weakness is initially oculobulbar and later involves limb and sometimes respiratory muscles.

LABORATORY **MG:** Edrophomium (Tensilon) test—1-mg test dose followed by 9 mg; look for improvement in muscle strength; serum AChR antibodies—80–90% positive in MG, but levels do not correspond to severity of disease; chest CT for thymoma.
MG and LES: EMG (including repetitive stimulation and single fiber recordings).
Botulism: Botulinum toxin in serum/feces.

TREATMENT **MG:** Anticholinesterases, immunosuppression (alternate-day prednisone, azathiaprine), plasmapheresis, thymectomy.
LES: Treatment of neoplasm, immunosuppression.
Botulism: Medical support, resolves as toxin is cleared.

COMPLICATIONS Most severe is respiratory compromise as thoracic and diaphragmatic musculature weakens; aspiration pneumonia when bulbar muscles are affected; cholinergic crisis in pts on anticholinesterases (neostigmine, Mestinon); acute exacerbation with intercurrent illness requiring therapy with drugs affecting the neuromuscular junction (see above).

For more detailed discussion of this topic, see Engel AG: Myasthenia Gravis and Other Disorders of Neuromuscular Transmission, Chap. 358, in HPIM-11, p. 2079

---

167 CHRONIC PROGRESSIVE MYOPATHIES AND MUSCULAR DYSTROPHIES

ETIOLOGY A disparate group of disorders that are all inherited progressive degenerations of muscle but vary widely in their clinical and pathologic features and mode of inheritance.

CLINICAL FEATURES OF INDIVIDUAL DISORDERS **Duchenne's dystrophy:** An X-linked recessive disorder that affects males almost exclusively. Onset, by age 5, of symmetric and relentlessly progressive weakness in hip and shoulder girdle muscles leading to difficulty in climbing, running, jumping, hopping, etc. By age 8–10, most children require leg braces; by age 12, the majority are nonambulatory. Survival beyond age 25 is rare.

Associated problems include tendon and muscle contractures (e.g., heel cords), progressive kyphoscoliosis, cardiomyopathy, and intellectual impairment. Muscle weakness is conjoined with palpable enlargement and firmness of some muscles (e.g., calves) resulting initially from hypertrophy and later from replacement of muscle by fat and connective tissue.

Laboratory findings include massive elevations of muscle enzymes (CK, aldolase), a myopathic pattern on EMG testing, and evidence of groups of necrotic muscle fibers with regeneration, phagocytosis, and fatty replacement of muscle on biopsy. ECG abnormalities (tall R in precordium, deep Q in limb leads) reflect the presence of cardiomyopathy.

Complications include respiratory failure and infections, aspiration, and acute gastric dilatation. CHF and cardiac arrhythmias may complicate the cardiomyopathy. Passive stretching of muscles, tenotomy, bracing, physiotherapy, mechanical assistance devices, and avoidance of prolonged immobility may all be of symptomatic benefit. New molecular biologic techniques are available for the detection of asymptomatic female carriers and for antenatal diagnosis.

Becker's dystrophy (benign pseudohypertrophic): A less severe and rarer dystrophy than Duchenne's with a slower course and later age of onset (5–15) but similar clinical and laboratory features.

Myotonic dystrophy: An autosomal dominant disorder in which weakness typically becomes obvious in the second to third decade and initially involves the muscles of the face, neck, and distal extremities. This results in a distinctive facial appearance ("hatchet face") characterized by ptosis, temporal wasting, drooping of the lower lip, and sagging of the jaw. Myotonia manifests as a pecular inability to rapidly relax muscles following a strong exertion (e.g., after tight hand grip), as well as by sustained contraction of muscles following percussion (e.g., of tongue or thenar eminence).

Associated problems can include frontal baldness, posterior subcapsular cataracts, gonadal atrophy, respiratory and cardiac problems, endocrine abnormalities, intellectual impairment, and hypersomnia.

Laboratory studies show normal or mildly elevated CK, characteristic myotonia and myopathic features on EMG, and a typical pattern of muscle fiber injury on biopsy. Cardiac complications, including complete heart block, may be life-threatening. Respiratory function should be carefully followed, as chronic hypoxia may lead to cor pulmonale. Phenytoin, procainamide, and quinine may help myotonia, but they must be used carefully in pts with heart disease.

Facioscapulohumeral dystrophy: Typically a slowly progressive, mild disorder with onset in the third to fourth decade. Weakness involves facial, shoulder girdle, and proximal arm muscles and can result in atrophy of biceps, triceps, scapular winging, and slope shoulders. Facial weakness results in inability to whistle and loss of facial expressivity. Foot drop and leg weakness may cause falls and progressive difficulty with ambulation.

Laboratory studies include normal or slightly elevated CK and mixed myopathic-neuropathic features on EMG and muscle biopsy. Orthoses and other stabilization procedures may be of benefit for selected patients.

LESS COMMON DYSTROPHIES **Scapuloperoneal dystrophy:** Clinical features are generally similar to facioscapuloperoneal dystrophy, although facial weakness does not occur and cardiomyopathy may be present. Most cases are of midlife onset and autosomal dominant inheritance, but an early-onset X-linked recessive form with prominent joint contractures and cardiomyopathy (Emery-Dreifuss type) can occur.

Oculopharyngeal dystrophy (progressive external ophthalmoplegia): Onset in the fifth to sixth decade of ptosis, limitation of extraocular movements, and facial and cricopharyngeal weakness. Cricopharyngeal muscle weakness results in achalasia, dysphagia, and aspiration. Chronic nature of the eye movement disorder rarely results in diplopia. Most pts are Hispanic or of French-Canadian descent.

Limb-girdle dystrophy: Probably a constellation of diseases with proximal muscle weakness involving the arms and legs as the core symptom. Age of onset, rate of progression, severity of manifestations, and associated complications (e.g., cardiac, respiratory) vary with the specific subtype of disease. Laboratory findings include elevated CK and myopathic features on EMG and muscle biopsy.

Distal dystrophy: A rare group of disorders with several variants that have differing ages of onset and patterns of inheritance. Typically there is weakness in the hands and feet with slow progression to more proximal muscle groups. CK is elevated, and EMG and muscle biopsy show myopathic features.

METABOLIC MYOPATHIES These disorders result from abnormalities in utilization by muscle of glucose or fatty acids as sources of energy. Pts present with either an acute syndrome of myalgia, myolysis, and myoglobinuria or chronic progressive muscle weakness. Definitive diagnosis requires biochemical-enzymatic studies

TABLE 167-1 **Toxic myopathies**

Focal myopathies:
- Pentazocine, meperidine

Generalized myopathies:
- Inflammatory:
  - Cimetidine, D-penicillamine, procainamide
- Muscle weakness and myalgias:
  - Chloroquine, clofibrate, colchicine, corticosteroids, emetine, ε-aminocaproic acid, labetalol, perhexiline, propranolol, vincristine
- Rhabdomyolysis and myoglobinuria:
  - Alcohol, azathioprine, heroin, amphetamine, clofibrate, ε-aminocaproic acid, phencyclidine, barbiturates
- Malignant hyperthermia:
  - Halothane, ethylene, diethyl ether, methoxylflurane, ethyl chloride, trichloroethylene, gallamine, succinylcholine, lidocaine, mepivacaine

Modified from Mendell JR, Griggs RC: HPIM-II, p. 2078.

of biopsied muscle. However, muscle enzymes, EMG, and muscle biopsy are all typically abnormal and may suggest specific disorders.

Infantile and childhood forms of glycogen storage disorders often have associated disorders of cardiac, hepatic, and endocrine function that overshadow the muscle disease. Childhood and adult forms can mimic muscular dystrophy or polymyositis. In some types the presentation is one of episodic muscle cramps and fatigue provoked by exercise. The ischemic forearm lactate test is helpful as normal postexercise rise in serum lactic acid does not occur. Disorders of fatty acid metabolism present with clinical pictures similar to those described above. In some pts, exercise-induced cramps, myolysis, and myoglobinuria are common; in others, the picture resembles polymyositis or muscular dystrophy. Some pts have benefited from special diets (medium-chain triglyceride-enriched), riboflavin, or steroids.

MISCELLANEOUS DISORDERS Myopathies may be associated with endocrine disorders, especially those involving hypo- or hyperfunction of the thyroid, parathyroid, and adrenal glands. Drugs (esp. steroids) and certain toxins (e.g., alcohol) are commonly associated with myopathies (see Table 167-1). In most cases weakness is symmetric and involves proximal limb girdle muscles. Weakness, myalgia, and cramps are common symptoms. Diagnosis often depends on resolution of signs and symptoms with correction of underlying disorder or removal of offending agent, as muscle enzymes, EMG, and even muscle biopsy may be unremarkable in individual pts.

For more detailed discussion of this topic, see Mendell JR, Griggs RC: Muscular Dystrophy and Other Chronic Myopathies, Chap. 357, in HPIM-11, p. 2072

168 AMYOTROPHIC LATERAL SCLEROSIS (ALS)

ETIOLOGY A disorder caused by degeneration of motor neurons at all levels of the CNS including anterior horns of the spinal cord, brainstem motor nuclei, and motor cortex. Syndromes clinically indistinguishable from classic ALS may result rarely from intoxication with mercury or lead and in hyperparathyroidism, thyrotoxicosis, paraproteinemias, and hexosaminidase A deficiency. Tumors near the foramen magnum, high spinal cord tumors, cervical spondylosis, chronic polyradiculopathies, polymyositis, spinal muscle atrophies, and diabetic, syphilitic, and postpolio amyotrophies can all produce signs and symptoms similar to those seen in ALS and should be carefully considered in differential diagnosis.

CLINICAL HISTORY Onset is usually midlife, with most cases progressing to death in 3–5 years. Common initial symptoms are weakness, muscle wasting, stiffness and cramping, and twitching in muscles of hands and arms. Legs are less severely involved than arms, with complaints of leg stiffness, cramping, and weakness common. Symptoms of brainstem involvement include dysarthria and dysphagia.

PHYSICAL EXAMINATION Lower motor neuron disease results in weakness and wasting that often first involves intrinsic hand muscles but later becomes generalized. Fasciculations occur in involved muscles, and fibrillations may be seen in the tongue. Hyperreflexia, spasticity, and upgoing toes in weak, atrophic limbs provide evidence of upper motor neuron disease. Brainstem disease produces wasting of the tongue, difficulty in articulation, phonation, and deglutition, and pseudobulbar palsy (e.g., involuntary laughter, crying). Important additional features that characterize ALS are preservation of intellect, lack of sensory abnormalities, and absence of bowel or bladder dysfunction.

LABORATORY FINDINGS EMG provides objective evidence of muscle denervation, as well as of involvement of muscles innervated by different peripheral nerves and nerve roots. Myelography, CT, or MRI may be useful to exclude compressive lesions. CSF is normal. Muscle enzymes (e.g., CK) may be elevated. Pulmonary function studies may aid in management of ventilation. Useful tests to exclude other diseases can include urine and serum screens for heavy metals, thyroid functions, serum immunoelectrophoresis, lysosomal enzyme screens, B_{12} levels, VDRL, CBC, ESR, and serum chemistries.

COMPLICATIONS Weakness of ventilatory muscles leads to respiratory insufficiency; dysphagia may result in aspiration pneumonia and compromised caloric intake.

TREATMENT There is no effective treatment. Options can include home care ventilation and pulmonary support, speech therapy, nonverbal, electronic or mechanical communication systems for anarthric patients, and dietary management to ensure adequate caloric intake. Attention to use of rehabilitative devices (braces, splints, canes, walkers, mechanized wheelchairs) is essential to improve care.

For more detailed discussion of this topic, see Richardson EP Jr., Beal MF, Martin JB: Degenerative Diseases of the Nervous System, Chap. 350, in HPIM-11, p. 2011

---

169 POLYMYOSITIS

DEFINITION Polymyositis is an inflammatory condition of skeletal muscle in which muscle tissue is involved predominantly by lymphocytic infiltration. When polymyositis is accompanied by a characteristic skin rash, the term *dermatomyositis* may be used. Approximately a third of cases are associated with connective tissue diseases such as RA, SLE, or scleroderma; 10% are associated with malignancy.

ETIOLOGY In most instances, the etiology is not known. There are likely a variety of causes. Myositis may follow certain viral and parasitic infections, and the disease may represent an immune-mediated response to viral antigens; alternatively, autoimmune processes may be operative.

CLASSIFICATION One commonly used classification is as follows:

- Group I: Primary idiopathic polymyositis
- Group II: Primary idiopathic dermatomyositis
- Group III: Dermatomyositis (or polymyositis) associated with neoplasia
- Group IV: Childhood dermatomyositis (or polymyositis) associated with vasculitis
- Group V: Polymyositis (or dermatomyositis) associated with collagen-vascular disease

CLINICAL MANIFESTATIONS

Group I: Primary idiopathic polymyositis:

- Approximately a third of all cases of polymyositis; onset and course usually insidiously progressive; 2:1 female:male predominance.
- Proximal muscle weakness first noted; difficulty climbing steps, combing hair, arising from squatting position; ocular muscles rarely affected.
- Some pts have aching muscle pain or tenderness.
- Dysphagia in 25%, cardiac abnormalities in 30%, respiratory involvement in 5%.

Group II: Primary idiopathic dermatomyositis:

- About 25% of all cases.
- Skin changes may precede or follow muscle findings; types of eruptions include (1) localized or diffuse erythema, (2) maculopapular eruption, (3) scaling eczematoid dermatitis, (4) exfoliative dermatitis, or (5) classic lilac-colored heliotrope rash on eyelids, nose, cheeks, forehead, trunk, extremities, nailbeds, knuckles.
- About 40% of all pts with myositis have dermatomyositis.

Group III: Polymyositis or dermatomyositis with neoplasia:

- About 8% of all myositis; skin and muscle changes indistinguishable from other groups.

- Malignancy may precede or follow onset of myositis by up to 2 years.
- Chiefly in older pts.
- Commonly associated malignancies include lung, ovary, breast, GI tract, and myeloproliferative disorders.

Group IV: Childhood polymyositis and dermatomyositis associated with vasculitis:

- About 7% of all myositis.
- Subcutaneous calcification common.
- Vasculitis may involve skin and visceral organs.

Group V: Polymyositis or dermatomyositis associated with a connective tissue disorder:

- About 20% of myositis cases.
- RA, scleroderma, SLE, MCTD most frequently associated; polyarteritis nodosa and rheumatic fever also seen.

OTHER DISORDERS ASSOCIATED WITH MYOSITIS Sarcoidosis, focal nodular myositis, infections (toxoplasma, coxsackievirus, trichinella, influenza), inclusion-body myositis.

DIAGNOSIS

- Typical clinical picture—weakness (proximal greater than distal), possible associated rash.
- Laboratory findings—elevated serum CK, aldolase, glutamic oxaloacetic transaminase (SGOT), lactic acid dehydrogenase (LDH), glutamic pyruvate transaminase (SGPT) levels; rheumatoid factor and ANA may be present; myoglobulinuria if muscle damage acute and extensive; elevated ESR.
- EMG—may show irritability and myopathic changes.
- ECG—abnormal in 5–10% at presentation.
- Muscle biopsy—usually diagnostic but may be normal in 10%.
- Workup for malignancy in older pts.

DIFFERENTIAL DIAGNOSIS Spinal muscular atrophies, amyotrophic lateral sclerosis, muscular dystrophies, metabolic myopathies, toxic myopathies, myasthenia gravis, Lambert-Eaton syndrome, Guillain-Barré syndrome, neurotoxin, enzyme-deficiency states, acute viral infections, polymyalgia rheumatica, fibrositis/fibromyalgia.

TREATMENT Corticosteroids are mainstay of therapy; improvement may occur promptly or may take up to 3 months. Cytotoxic drugs may be necessary when disease is severe, when corticosteroid response is inadequate, or when frequent relapses make steroid requirement excessive. Physiotherapy and rehabilitation are very important.

For more detailed discussion of this topic, see Bradley WG: Dermatomyositis and Polymyositis, Chap. 356, in HPIM-11, p. 2069

---

170 NEUROLOGIC MANIFESTATIONS OF SYSTEMIC NEOPLASIA

Patients with systemic neoplasia commonly develop neurologic disorders. These may result from local tumor (i.e., metastases, see Table 170-1) or leptomeningeal infiltration or follow compression or infiltration of cranial and peripheral nerves. Pts with systemic tumor are also at risk for *paraneoplastic syndromes* (see Table 170-2), disorders of central or peripheral nervous system structures that are distant from the tumor site.

TABLE 170-1 **Metastases**

Site	Clinical manifestations	Cancer	Evaluation
Cerebrum	Headache, focal signs, drowsiness papilledema, sixth nerve palsy, anisocoria	Breast, lung, GI tract, melanoma, treated ovarian	CT scan with contrast
Posterior fossa	Ataxia, headache, cranial nerve palsy, head tilt, emesis, obstructive hydrocephalus	Same as above	CT scan with contrast, MRI scan
Spinal cord	Sensory level, bowel and bladder dysfunction, back pain, corticospinal tract signs	As above; also lymphoma, prostate cancer	CT scan with metrizamide, myelography, spine films, MRI
Leptomeninges	Cranial or peripheral nerve lesions (often painful), spinal cord signs	Melanoma, lymphoma, glioblastoma, adenocarcinoma	CSF cytology, myelography

In addition to local tumor and paraneoplastic syndromes, delayed effects of radiation and chemotherapy can cause nervous system pathology.

TABLE 170-2 **Paraneoplastic syndromes**

Type	Clinical Manifestations	Cancer	Evolution
Limbic encephalitis	Confusional state, memory loss, dementia, anxiety	Oat cell, lung	Weeks to months
Photoreceptor degeneration	Visual loss	Oat cell, cervical	Weeks to months
Subacute cerebellar degeneration	Ataxia, dysarthria	Oat cell, ovarian, breast, Hodgkin's lymphoma	Weeks to months
Opsoclonus, myoclonus	Dancing eyes, ataxia (children)	Neuroblastoma, lung, breast	Weeks
Bulbar encephalitis	Nystagmus, diplopia, ataxia	Lung tumors	Days to weeks
Necrotizing myelopathy	Paraplegia, quadriplegia, sensory level	Oat cell, lymphoma	Hours to weeks
Subacute motor neuronopathy	Flaccid weakness, muscular atrophy	Non-Hodgkin's lymphoma	Weeks to months
Subacute sensory neuronopathy	Severe sensory loss	Oat cell	Weeks to months
Guillain-Barré	Weakness, areflexia, minimal sensory abnormalities	Hodgkin's lymphoma	Days to weeks
Sensory motor neuropathy	Distal motor and sensory loss, distal areflexia	Oat cell, myeloma	Weeks to months
Myasthenia gravis	Weakness, fatigability	Thymoma, breast, stomach	Weeks to months
Lambert-Eaton	Weakness, fatigability	Oat cell	Week to months
Polymyositis	Proximal muscle weakness, CHF, tender muscles	Breast, ovarian, lung, lymphoma	Months to years

For more detailed discussion of this topic, see Stefansson K, Arnason BGW: Neurologic Manifestations of Systemic Neoplasia, Chap. 304, in HPIM-11, p. 1600

171 SPINAL CORD COMPRESSION

SIGNS AND SYMPTOMS Principal clinical sign: loss of sensation below a horizontal meridian on trunk ("sensory level"), usually accompanied by weakness and spasticity of limbs.

Sensory symptoms: Often paresthesias; may begin in one or both feet and ascend. Sensory level correlates well with location of transverse lesion.

Motor impairment: Disruption of corticospinal and bulbospinal tracts at a single level causes quadriplegia or paraplegia with increased muscle tone, hyperactive deep tendon reflexes, and bilateral Babinski signs.

Autonomic dysfunction: Primarily urinary retention; must raise suspicion of spinal cord disease when associated with spasticity and/or a sensory level.

Pain: Midline back pain is of localizing value; interscapular pain may be first sign of midthoracic cord compression; radicular pain may mark site of more laterally placed spinal lesion; pain from lower cord (conus medullaris) lesion may be referred to low back.

Lesions at or below L1 vertebra: Compress cauda equina to produce flaccid, areflexic, asymmetric paraparesis with bladder and bowel dysfunction and sensory loss in saddle distribution up to L1; pain is common and projected to perineum or thighs.

Lesions at foramen magnum: Classically, weakness of shoulder and arm is followed by ipsilateral and then contralateral leg and finally contralateral arm; a Horner's syndrome suggests presence of a cervical lesion.

ETIOLOGY **Tumors of spinal cord:** Primary or metastatic, classified as extradural ("epidural") or intradural (either intra- or extramedullary). Most are epidural metastases from the adjacent vertebral column. Malignancies commonly responsible: prostate, breast, lung, lymphoma, and plasma cell dyscrasias. Initial symptom is usually back pain with local tenderness which may precede other symptoms by many weeks.

Transverse myelitis: Onset over days of sensory and motor symptoms, often with bladder involvement. May be first sign of multiple sclerosis. When severe, may lead to permanent, disabling paraplegia or quadriplegia.

Epidural abcess: Once neurologic signs appear, cord compression rapidly ensues. At first there may be only unexplained fever with a dull spinal ache and local tenderness, followed by radicular pain. Spinal osteomyelitis may be the nidus for abscess formation.

Spinal epidural hemorrhage and hematomyelia: Present as an acute transverse myelopathy evolving over minutes or hours accompanied by severe pain. Causes: minor trauma, lumbar puncture, anticoagulation, hematologic disorders, AV malformation, or hemorrhage into tumor. Most cases are idiopathic.

Acute disk protrusion: Lumbar disk herniation is discussed in Chap. 7. Thoracic and cervical disk herniation is less common and usually results from direct trauma to spinal column.

Acute trauma with spinal fracture/dislocation: Fracture with dislocation of vertebral column may not produce myelopathy until mechanical stress further displaces destabilized spinal column. It is imperative to support spine after trauma until careful radiographic evaluation is completed. Acutely, limbs in a transverse lesion may be flaccid rather than spastic due to "spinal shock."

LABORATORY EVALUATION Plain x-rays or CT of spine to assess presence of fractures and alignment of vertebral column or to detect possible metastases to vertebrae. In nontraumatic cases, metrizamide myelography with CT of spine. Increasingly, MRI of spine is used to evaluate cord compression, having the advantage of more rapid evaluation with better resolution of cord.

TREATMENT **Tumor-related compression:** For epidural metastases, high-dose steroids (to reduce edema) and local irradiation of metastasis, with or without chemotherapy; surgery is used when tumor is known to be insensitive to radiation or a maximal dose has already been delivered. Surgery is indicated for removal of neurofibromas, meningiomas, or other extramedullary tumors.
Epidural abcess: Usually requires emergency surgery for abscess drainage and culture of organism, followed by IV antibiotic course.
Epidural hemorrhage or hematomyelia: Where appropriate, emergency evacuation of clot. Bleeding dyscrasias should be identified and corrected. An AV malfunction may be diagnosed by MRI, myelography, or arteriography of segmental spinal arteries.
Acute disk protrusion or spinal fracture/dislocation: Requires surgical intervention.

COMPLICATIONS Damage to urinary tract due to urinary retention with bladder distention and injury to detrusor muscle; paroxysmal hypertension or hypotension with volume aberrations; ileus and gastritis; in high cervical cord lesions, mechanical respiratory failure; severe hypertension and bradycardia in response to stimuli or bladder or bowel distention; UTI; pressure sores; pulmonary emboli.

For more detailed discussion of this topic, see Ropper AH, Martin JB: Diseases of the Spinal Cord, Chap. 353, in HPIM-11, p. 2040

Global disruption of brain function occurs commonly in pts with serious medical illness. Such metabolic encephalopathies usually begin with an alteration in alertness (drowsiness), followed by agitation, confusion, delirium, or psychosis, and progressing to stupor and coma. These states are discussed in Chap. 9.

Evaluation of pt requires careful PE for underlying structural brain lesions, CNS infection, and general medical illness. Next, blood should be drawn, glucose and Narcan administered, and electrolytes, toxic screen, CBC, and renal, liver, and thyroid functions measured. A brain CT scan is sometimes necessary to exclude mass lesions, and spinal fluid examination should be done to exclude meningitis or encephalitis. Common causes of metabolic encephalopathy are listed below with their salient features.

ELECTROLYTE DISORDERS Hyponatremia is often associated with seizures if the serum $Na^+ < 120$. Too rapid or overcorrection of the serum Na^+ can cause central pontine myelinolysis. Extreme hyperosmolarity due to hypernatremia or hyperglycemia causes tremulousness, convulsions, and coma. Hypokalemia is associated with severe muscle weakness and confusion; hypercalcemia with inattentiveness, somnolence, and depression.

ENDOCRINE DISORDERS Confusional states, affective disorders, and psychosis occur commonly in *Cushing's disease* or in pts treated with corticosteroids. *Hyperthyroidism* causes restlessness, insomnia, tremor, and agitated delirium. A syndrome of lethargy and depression termed *apathetic hyperthyroidism* occurs in elderly pts. Slowed mentation, depression, dementia, and coma occur in *hypothyroidism* and *Addison's disease.* An inappropriate jocularity is sometimes seen in *dementia of hypothyroidism,* occasionally with paranoia and psychosis. *Hypoglycemia* causes convulsions and even focal neurologic findings if glucose falls below 25–30 mg/dL. Because of its variable clinical presentation and risk of permanent brain injury, hypoglycemia should be considered in all encephalopathies without known cause. Glucose level should be determined and IV dextrose administered.

MISCELLANEOUS ENCEPHALOPATHIES **Hypercapneic encephalopathy** is frequently accompanied by headache, asterixis, coarse muscular twitching, and sometimes papilledema.

Hepatic encephalopathy also causes asterixis sometimes with fluctuating rigidity, Babinski signs, and seizures. Paroxysms of triphasic slow waves may be found on the EEG. Chronic or recurrent hepatic encephalopathy can lead to hepatocerebral degeneration. *Reye's syndrome* is a special form of hepatic encephalopathy seen in children and characterized by brain swelling.

Anoxic-ischemic encephalopathy occurring after insults severe enough to cause loss of consciousness, is commonly seen after cardiorespiratory failure or arrest, CO poisoning, drowning, and asphyxia. If extreme and sustained, permanent brain injury will result. If brainstem reflexes and spontaneous respirations return, full recovery can occur. Incomplete recovery results in the postanoxic syndromes, i.e., persistent vegetative state, dementia, parkinsonism, cerebellar ataxia, intention myoclonus, Korsakoff's amnesia.

Renal disease with uremia leads to apathy, inattentiveness, and irritability progressing to delirium and stupor. There is usually myoclonus or seizures. Episodic encephalopathy with seizures, muscle cramps, and headache sometimes complicates hemodialysis. Dialysis dementia with prominent dysarthria, myoclonus, psychosis, and motor aphasia may be related to aluminum in the dialysate passing into the bloodstream.

Hypertensive encephalopathy with headache, retinopathy, and uremia can complicate pregnancy, renal failure, pheochromocytoma, or primary hypertension.

Nutritional encephalopathies occur in patients with B_{12}, thiamine, niacin, nicotinic acid, or pyridoxine deficiency. Peripheral neuropathy, spinal cord dysfunction, and mucocutaneous abnormalities are frequent accompaniments. Wernicke's encephalopathy is characterized by diplopia, nystagmus, and ataxia. Early treatment with thiamine can prevent a permanent Korsakoff's amnestic state. The encephalopathy of B_{12} deficiency is occasionally misdiagnosed as Alzheimer's dementia.

Toxic encephalopathies are common. A recent onset of an encephalopathic condition should lead to blood and urine screening for narcotics, salicylates, hypnotics, antidepressants, phenothiazines, lithium, anticonvulsants, amphetamines, alcohol, arsenic, lead, bismuth, and carbon monoxide.

Others: Illnesses that can present as encephalopathy include bacterial endocarditis, thrombotic thrombocytopenic purpura, multiple fat emboli, typhoid fever, AIDS, multiple intracerebral metastases, hepatic porphyria, collagen-vascular disorders, and hyperproliferative hematologic disorders.

For more detailed discussion of this topic, see Victor M, Martin JB: Nutritional and Metabolic Diseases of the Nervous System, Chap. 349, in HPIM-11, p. 2000

SECTION XII PSYCHIATRY

173 MAJOR AFFECTIVE DISORDERS AND PSYCHOSES

Primary disorders of affect and thought are considered psychobiologic manifestations of abnormal brain mechanisms. Pts also may present with depressive, manic, or psychotic disorders *secondary* to metabolic derangements, drug toxicity, focal cerebral lesions, epilepsy, or degenerative brain disease. Therefore, pts with newly diagnosed emotional or thought disorders should be carefully evaluated for underlying medical and neurologic illnesses. Pts with *primary* major affective disorders are divided into those with a history of depression alternating with mania (bipolar) and those with depression alone (unipolar). Schizophrenia is the major primary psychotic illness.

MAJOR DEPRESSION

DIAGNOSIS Dysphoric mood is always a feature in major depression but need not be the most prominent symptom. At least four of the following symptoms are also present: (1) change in appetite with corresponding change in weight; (2) insomnia (especially early morning awakening) or hypersomnia; (3) psychomotor retardation or its opposite, agitation; (4) loss of interest, pleasure, and decreased sexual drive; (5) loss of energy (fatigue); (6) feelings of worthlessness, self-reproach, or guilt; (7) complaints or evidence of diminished ability to concentrate and make decisions; (8) recurrent thoughts of death or suicide. Depression usually occurs in episodes lasting 5–12 months, and there is a tendency for periodicity and recurrence. Some pts are chronically depressed. Depressed pts commonly seek medical attention because of various subjective, unremitting somatic complaints, i.e., constant headache, diffuse achiness, fatigue. Some women note depressive symptoms prior to menses.

Pts with major depression often have disordered sleep patterns, abnormal monoamine neurotransmission, and abnormal neuroendocrine control. 10–50% of clinically depressed pts fail to suppress afternoon cortisol in response to a nighttime dose of 1 mg dexamethasone. Unfortunately, this test also may be abnormal in pts with obesity, anorexia, pregnancy, major medical illnesses, alcoholism, and malnutrition, as well as in the elderly.

PREVALENCE AND SUICIDE RISK Depression is common; it occurs in children as well as in adults. In the adult population, prevalence is 3% in men and twice that in women. Risk increases with age > 55. 30% of the 25,000 annual suicides in the U.S. occur in pts with major affective disorders. Many seek general medical attention just prior to their suicide attempt, so it is important that physicians directly question potentially depressed pts regarding suicide risk. Pts who have given detailed thought to possible methods of suicide, have concomitant alcoholism, are socially isolated, elderly males, or have serious medical illnesses have greater risk of suicide.

TREATMENT Pts with significant risk of suicide should be hospitalized. Antidepressants can produce remarkable amelioration of symptoms, usually over a period of weeks. The combination of psychotherapy with pharmacotherapy is significantly better than either alone. Electroshock therapy is used in those pts with life-threatening depression who require immediate benefit or in those refractory to antidepressants.

MANIC DISORDERS

DIAGNOSIS Pts with mania have elevated, expansive mood, although they are frequently hyperirritable. They experience (1) increase in activity or physical restlessness, (2) unusual talkativeness, (3) flight of ideas and the subjective impression that their thoughts are racing, (4) inflated self-esteem which may be delusional, (5) decreased need for sleep, (6) distractability, and (7) excessive involvement in risky activities, i.e., buying sprees, sexual indiscretion, foolish business investments.

TREATMENT Acutely manic pts may need hospitalization to reduce degree of environmental stimulation and to protect themselves and others from consequences of reckless behavior. Lithium therapy is the mainstay of treatment.

SCHIZOPHRENIA

DIAGNOSIS Schizophrenia usually presents in late teenage years or the third decade. Psychotic features last 6 months or more and include (1) bizarre delusions; (2) paranoid, jealous, somatic, grandiose, religious, nihilistic, or other delusions; (3) auditory hallucinations, often including a voice or voices maintaining a running commentary; and (4) incoherence, marked loosening of associations, markedly illogical thinking, inappropriate affect, delusions, hallucinations, and catatonic or grossly disorganized behavior. Pts with primary psychoses have normal memory, calculating abilities, and language function, but the insertion of bizarre thought may contaminate or even preclude accurate cognitive testing.

TREATMENT Acutely psychotic pts, especially those with violent "command hallucinations," may be dangerous to themselves or others. Such pts need psychiatric hospitalization. Antipsychotic medications are usually quite effective in ameliorating hallucinations and agitation.

For more detailed discussion of these topics, see Judd LL, Huey LY: Major Affective Disorders, Chap. 360, p. 2085; and Braff DL: Schizophrenic Disorders, Chap. 362, p. 2093, in HPIM-11

Anxiety refers to paroxysmal or persistent psychological feelings (dread, irritability, ruminations) and somatic symptoms (dyspnea, sweating, insomnia, trembling) which impair normal functioning. Such feelings and symptoms can be classified as (1) *anxiety states:* panic disorder, generalized anxiety disorder, obsessive-compulsive disorder, posttraumatic stress disorder, and (2) *phobic disorders:* agoraphobia (with and without panic attacks), social phobia, simple phobia.

ANXIETY STATES

PANIC DISORDER Characterized by sudden, unexpected, and overwhelming feeling of terror or apprehension with associated somatic symptoms. Estimated to occur in 1–2% of population with a female-male ratio of 2:1. Tends to be familial, and affective illness often coexists. The *Diagnostic and Statistical Manual,* third edition (DSM-III), developed by the American Psychiatric Association, lists specific criteria for diagnosis: (1) at least 3 panic attacks within 3 weeks in nonthreatening or nonexertional settings, which can be precipitated by other than circumscribed phobic stimuli; and (2) attacks manifested by discrete episodes of apprehension or fear and at least four of the following: dyspnea, palpitations, chest pain or discomfort, choking/smothering feelings, dizziness/vertigo/unsteady feelings, feelings of unreality, paresthesias, hot and cold flashes, sweating, faintness, trembling, and fear of dying, going crazy, or doing something uncontrolled during an attack.

Laboratory findings: IV lactate precipitates panic attacks in about half of afflicted individuals.

Differential diagnosis: The diagnostic challenge is to differentiate panic disorder from cardiovascular diseases it mimics. There may be an increased prevalence of mitral valve prolapse in pts with panic disorder. Symptoms associated with hyper- and hypothyroidism, pheochromocytoma, complex partial seizures, hypoglycemia, drug ingestions (amphetamines, cocaine, caffeine, sympathomimetic nasal decongestants), and drug withdrawal (alcohol, barbiturates, opiates, minor tranquilizers) may simulate panic attacks.

Treatment: Tricyclic antidepressants or monoamine oxidase inhibitors have an 80–90% effectiveness in treatment and prevention of spontaneous attacks. Alprazolam (Xanax) given in high dose (2–4 mg daily) is as effective as antidepressants with fewer side effects and works within 1 or 2 days. Other benzodiazepines have not proven effective. Beta blockers may reduce somatic symptoms but are ineffective in preventing psychic fear or panic.

GENERALIZED ANXIETY DISORDER These pts experience persistent anxiety, without the specific symptoms of phobic, panic or obsessive-compulsive disorders. Common signs are motor tension (shakiness, trembling, restlessness, easy startle, etc.), autonomic hyperactivity, apprehensive expectation (anxiety, fear, rumination, anticipation of misfortune, etc.), and vigilance (distractibility, poor concentration, insomnia, impatience, irritability). Prevalence is estimated at 2–3%. A familial or genetic basis has not been established. High-affinity, stereospecific benzodiazepine receptors, coupled to GABA receptors, have been defined through which the anxiolytic actions of benzodiazepines are mediated. This suggests that endogenous anxiogenic compounds may be found in the brain.

Differential diagnosis: Symptoms and signs resembling anxiety occur in coronary artery disease, thyroid disease, and drug intoxication or withdrawal. Anxiety may be present in depression, schizophrenia, and organic mental states.

Treatment: Supportive or intensive psychotherapy or behavioral modification therapy. When generalized anxiety is severe enough to warrant treatment with drugs, benzodiazepines are agents of choice. However, these should be given for a short time only, because such pts are particularly prone to drug dependence.

OBSESSIVE-COMPULSIVE DISORDER Characterized by recurrent obsessions (persistent intrusive thoughts) and compulsions (intrusive behaviors) which the pt experiences as involuntary, senseless, or repugnant. Common obsessions include thoughts of violence (e.g., killing a loved one), obsessive slowness, fears of germs or contamination, and doubt. Examples of compulsions include repeated checking to be assured that something was done properly, hand washing, extreme neatness, and counting rituals, as in numbering steps while walking.

Clinical features: Obsessive-compulsive disorder usually begins in adolescence, with 65% of cases manifest before age 25. It is rare in children. Clear precipitants are identified in 60% of cases. There are reports of an increased incidence of the disorder in monozygotic twins and first-degree relatives of probands. Most pts follow an episodic course with periods of incomplete remission.

Treatment: Behaviorally oriented psychotherapy and psychopharmacology can be helpful. Chronic administration of tricyclic antidepressants and monoamine oxidase inhibitors is relatively effective.

POSTTRAUMATIC STRESS DISORDER Refers to acute and chronic psychic distress following traumatic events. DSM-III criteria include (1) existence of a recognizable stress that would evoke significant symptoms of distress in almost everyone; (2) reexperiencing the trauma by recurrent intrusive recollections, recurrent dreams, or sudden acting or feeling as if the traumatic event were recurring; (3) numbing of responsiveness to or reduced involvement with the external world, beginning sometime after the trauma; and (4) presence of at least two of the following symptoms: hyperalertness or exaggerated startle, sleep disturbance, guilt about having survived when others have not or about behavior required for survival, memory impairment or trouble concentrating, avoidance of activities that arouse recollection of traumatic event, and

intensification of symptoms by exposure to events that symbolize or resemble traumatic event.
Treatment: Involves a combination of psychosocial support systems, psychotherapy, behavioral and conditioning techniques, and medications.

PHOBIC DISORDERS

This group has in common persistently recurring, irrational fear of specific objects, activities, or situations with secondary avoidance behavior of the phobic stimulus. The diagnosis is made only when avoidance behavior is a significant source of distress to the individual or interferes with social or occupational functioning.

AGORAPHOBIA Fear of being alone or in public places. May occur in absence of panic disorder but is almost invariably preceded by that condition.

SOCIAL PHOBIAS Persistent irrational fear of and need to avoid any situation where there is risk of scrutiny by others, embarrassment, or humiliation. Common examples include excessive fear of public speaking or any public performance.

SIMPLE PHOBIAS Persistent irrational fears and avoidance of specific objects. Common examples include fear of heights (acrophobia), closed spaces (claustrophobia), and animals.
Treatment: *Social and simple phobias:* behavioral modification and relaxation techniques, systematic desensitization. Propranolol and/or alprazolam may be helpful in treating social phobias. *Agoraphobia:* as in treatment of panic disorder.

For more detailed discussion of this topic, see Britton KT, Risch SC, Gillin JC: Anxiety Disorders, Chap. 361, in HPIM-11, p. 2089

---

175 PSYCHOTROPIC DRUGS

The four major classes of psychotropic drugs are (1) antidepressants, (2) anxiolytics, (3) antipsychotics, and (4) other mood-normalizing medications.

GENERAL PRINCIPLES OF DRUG ADMINISTRATION

1 Nonpsychiatric physicians should familiarize themselves with *one* drug in each of the four classes, so that it can be tried first and its indications, efficacy, and side effects are well known.
2 Avoid polypharmacy or drug combinations.
3 Previous history of positive response to a drug is usually an indication that positive response to the same drug will occur again.
4 Two common errors in prescribing psychotropic drugs are *undermedication* and *impatience;* effects from proper dosage levels may take weeks or months.

TABLE 175-1 **Commonly used antidepressants**

Drug	Daily oral therapeutic dose range, mg
Tricyclic derivatives:	
Amitriptyline (Elavil, etc.)	150–300
Nortriptyline (Aventyl, etc.)	50–150
Imipramine (Tofranil, etc.)	150–300
Desipramine (Norpramin)	150–250
Doxepin (Sinequan, etc.)	150–300
Monoamine oxidase inhibitors:	
Phenelzine (Nardil)	45–90
Tranylcypromine (Parnate)	10–30
Isocarboxazid (Marplan)	10–30

Reproduced from Judd LL: HPIM-11, p. 2100.

TABLE 175-2 **Common side effects of tricyclic antidepressants**

Anticholinergic (atropine-like) responses:
Dry mouth*
Nausea and vomiting*
Constipation*
Urinary retention
Blurred vision (mydriasis and cycloplegia)
Cardiovascular effects:
Postural hypotension*
Tachycardia
Cardiotoxic side effects—can induce an arrythmia
Obstructive jaundice—more rare; is reversible when drug is removed
Drowsiness and sleepiness—may want to avoid driving a car until this diminishes
Fine rapid tremor*
Dizziness, ataxia
Hematologic effects:
Leukopenia

* Side effects seen most commonly.
Reproduced from Judd LL: HPIM-11, p. 2100.

5 Pharmacokinetics of psychotropic drugs in elderly pts are different, with longer biologic half-lives.
6 Failure to respond to one drug in a class does not mean that pt will not respond to another drug in same class.
7 The physician should never withdraw a psychotic drug abruptly; taper over 2–4 weeks.
8 Physicians who only infrequently prescribe psychotropic drugs should review the side effects each time a drug is prescribed; pts and family members should be informed of potential side effects.

ANTIDEPRESSANTS See Tables 175-1, 175-2, and 175-3.

TABLE 175-3 **Selected second-generation antidepressants**

Drug	Daily oral therapeutic dose range, mg
Tricylic derivatives:	
Trimipramine (Surmontil)	100–250
Amoxapine (Asendin)	150–300
Tetracyclic derivatives:	
Mianserin (Bolvidon)	50–150
Maprotiline (Ludiomil)	150–300
Derivatives of other chemical classes:	
Nomifensine (Merital)	100–200
Trazodone (Desyrel)	100–600
Alprazolam (Xanax)	0.75–4
Bupropion (Wellbutrin)	350–750

Reproduced from Judd LL: HPIM-11, p. 2100.

ANXIOLYTICS See Table 175-4.

TABLE 175-4 **Commonly used benzodiazepines**

Drug	Daily oral dose range, mg	Half-life, h*
Anxiolytics:		
Chlordiazepoxide (Librium)	20–100†	7–28*
Diazepam (Valium)	5–40	20–90*
Lorazepam (Ativan)	1–10‡	10–20
Oxazepam (Serax)	30–120‡	3–20
Prazepam (Centrax)	20–60	40–70*
Alprazolam (Xanax)	0.75–4‡	12–15
Sedative-hypnotic:		
Flurazepam (Dalmane)	15–30§	24–100*
Temazepam (Restoril)	30§	8–10
Triazolam (Halcion)	0.5–1.0§	2–5

* Indicates long-active active metabolites.
† Prescribed in a qd or bid regimen.
‡ Prescribed in a tid or qid regimen.
§ Prescribed in a qd or qhs regimen.
Reproduced from Judd LL: HPIM-11, p. 2103.

ANTIPSYCHOTICS See Table 175-5.

TABLE 175-5 **Some of the more commonly used antipsychotic medications**

Drug	Average daily oral dose range, mg	Potency ratio compared to 100 mg chlorpromazine
Phenothiazines:		
Aliphatics:		
Chlorpromazine (Thorazine)	400–800	1:1
Piperazines:		
Fluphenazine (Prolixin)	4–20	1:50
Fluphenazine enanthate or decanoate	25–100*	
Perphenazine (Trilafon)	8–32	1:10
Trifluoperazine (Stelazine)	6–20	1:20
Piperidines:		
Thioridazine (Mellaril)	200–600	1:1 (approx)
Butyrophenones:		
Haloperidol (Haldol)	8–32	1:50
Thioxanthenes:		
Chlorprothixene (Taractan)	400–800	1:1
Thiothixene (Navane)	15–30	1:25
Oxoindoles:		
Molindone (Moban, Lidone)	40–200	1:10
Dibenzoxazepines:		
Laxapine (Loxitane, Daxolin)	60–100	1:10

* IM injection, long-acting, q 1 to 3 weeks.
Reproduced from Judd LL: HPIM-11, p. 2105.

OTHERS **Lithium:** The administration of lithium is monitored by serum levels, best obtained in the morning approximately 10 h after the last dose of lithium. In treatment of acute mania, therapeutic efficacy is achieved at serum levels between 0.8 and 1.5 meq/L. There is rarely necessity for pts to be treated at serum levels above 1.5 meq/L. Oral dose range to sustain therapeutic serum levels ranges from 600 mg to approximately 3000 mg daily.

For more detailed discussion of this topic, see Judd LL: Use of Psychotropic Medications, Chap. 364, in HPIM-11, p. 2099

ALCOHOLISM

DEFINITION Regular and excessive use of alcohol with associated psychologic dependence on its use during daily life which results in social and occupational problems and physical impairment.

HISTORY Pts typically present with marital difficulties, job problems (including absenteeism), legal problems resulting from driving while intoxicated, disorderly behavior, etc. Medical Hx should be reviewed for presence of alcohol-related physical problems, which can be neurologic (blackouts, seizures, delirium tremens, Wernicke-Korsakoff's, cerebellar degeneration, neuropathy, myopathy), gastrointestinal (esophagitis, gastritis, pancreatitis, hepatitis, cirrhosis, GI hemorrhage), cardiovascular (hypertension, cardiomyopathy), hematologic (macrocytosis, folate deficiency, thrombocytopenia, leukopenia), endocrine (testicular atrophy, amenorrhea, infertility), skeletal (fractures, osteonecrosis), or infectious.

CLINICAL MANIFESTATIONS Behavioral, cognitive, and psychomotor changes may occur at blood alcohol levels of 20–30 mg/dL. Incoordination, tremor, ataxia, confusion, stupor, coma, and even death can occur at progressively higher blood alcohol levels. Signs of alcohol withdrawal may include tremulousness ("shakes" or "jitters"), autonomic hyperactivity (sweating, hypertension, tachycardia, tachypnea, fever), insomnia, nightmares, anxiety, and GI upset. Psychotic symptoms can include visual, auditory, tactile, and olfactory hallucinations. Seizures can occur ("rum fits"). Delirium tremens ("DTs") is a severe withdrawal syndrome characterized by extreme confusion, agitation, vivid delusions and hallucinations, and profound autonomic hyperactivity.

LABORATORY FINDINGS Clues to occult alcoholism include mild anemia with macrocytosis, folate deficiency, thrombocytopenia, granulocytopenia, abnormal LFTs (e.g., elevated γ-glutamyl transferase), hyperuricemia, elevated triglycerides. Decreases in serum K, Mg, Zn, and P levels are common. Diagnostic studies such as GI radiology or endoscopy, abdominal ultrasound or CT, liver-spleen scan, liver biopsy, ECG, echocardiogram, cranial CT, EEG, and nerve conduction studies may show evidence of alcohol-related organ dysfunction.

THERAPY Alcohol withdrawal is treated with thiamine (50–100 mg IV daily for 5 days), multivitamins, short-acting CNS depressant drugs (e.g., oxazepam, lorazepam), and in some cases, anticonvulsants. Fluid and electrolyte status and blood sugar levels should be closely followed. Cardiovascular and hemodynamic monitoring is crucial, because deaths have resulted from hemodynamic collapse and cardiac arrhythmias. Care should be taken to search for evidence of trauma or infection that may be masked by prominent withdrawal symptoms. Treatment of chronic alcoholism depends on recognition of the problem by pt. Rehabilitation programs and support groups (e.g., Alcoholics Annonymous) may be of value.

Disulfuram, a drug that inhibits aldehyde dehydrogenase and results in toxic symptoms (nausea, vomiting, diarrhea, tremor) if pt consumes alcohol is used in some centers.

For more detailed discussion of this topic, see Schuckit MA: Alcohol and Alcoholism, Chap. 365, in HPIM-11, p. 2106

---

177 NARCOTIC ABUSE

Opioid addiction creates major social and medical problems. Three groups of abusers can be identified: (1) patients with chronic pain syndromes, (2) medical staff with easy access to narcotics, and (3) street abusers.

PHYSICAL ADDICTION AND THE OPIATE ABSTINENCE SYNDROME

Opiate tolerance, dependence, and withdrawal symptoms are considered to be related phenomena with common underlying mechanisms. The euphoric, analgesic, or anxiolytic effects of opioids initially attract the user. Family history of substance abuse and a variety of psychologic factors influence the development of drug dependence. Acute, uncomfortable abstinence syndromes begin to occur as the opiate effects wane. The former include diarrhea, coughing, lacrimation, rhinorrhea, diaphoresis, twitching muscles, piloerection, fever, tachypnea, hypertension, diffuse body pain, insomnia, and yawning. Relief of these exceedingly unpleasant symptoms by narcotic administration leads to more frequent narcotic use. Eventually, chronic addiction is established, and all the person's efforts are consumed by drug-seeking behavior.

TREATMENT OF THE ABSTINENCE SYNDROME Pts who present with any manifestation of drug abuse should be examined for signs of the life-threatening complications listed above. Effective treatment of withdrawal requires admitting pt to hospital or drug withdrawal center for initial administration of opiates followed by gradual reduction over 5–10 days. Long-acting oral methadone is most convenient: 1 mg methadone is equivalent to 3 mg morphine, 1 mg heroin, or 20 mg meperidine. Most pts receive 10–25 mg methadone twice daily, and higher doses are given if withdrawal symptoms break through. Clonidine is effective in decreasing sympathetic nervous system hyperactivity. Withdrawal syndromes in newborns of street abusers are fatal in 3–30%.

EFFECTS OF NARCOTIC ABUSE ON BODY SYSTEMS

Opioid effects on the CNS can result in sedation, euphoria, decreased pain perception, decreased respiratory drive, and vomiting. The adulterants added to "cut" street drugs (quinine, phenacetin, strychnine, antipyrine, caffeine, powdered milk) may contribute to more permanent neurologic damage, including peripheral neuropathy, amblyopia, and myelopathy. The shared use of contaminated needles is a major cause of brain abscess, in addition to acute endocarditis, hepatitis B, AIDS, septic arthritis, and soft tissue infections. At least 25% of street abusers die within 10–20 years of active abuse.

TREATMENT

OVERDOSE High doses, taken in suicide attempt or accidentally if the potency is misjudged, are frequently lethal. Toxic syndrome occurs immediately after IV administration, with a variable delay after oral ingestion. Symptoms include miosis, shallow respirations, bradycardia, hypothermia, and stupor or coma; less commonly pulmonary edema. Treatment requires cardiorespiratory support and administration of the opiate antagonist naloxone (0.4 mg IV and repeated in 3 minutes if no or partial response). Because effects of naloxone diminish in 2–3 h compared to longer-lasting effects of heroin (up to 24 h) or methadone (up to 72 h), it is important to observe these pts for reappearance of toxic state.

PATIENT WITH CHRONIC PAIN Physicians should avoid establishing narcotic addiction in pts with chronic pain syndromes. If physical dependence is established, then abstinence syndromes will intensify the pain and confuse an already difficult problem. Drugs should be used to minimize effects of pain on function and not to abolish pain. Oral administration of the least potent drug able to take the edge off the pain should be used. Nonmedicinal approaches to pain control should be part of the pt's program.

MEDICAL STAFF Doctors are advised never to prescribe opiates for themselves or members of their families. Medical organizations need to identify and rehabilitate substance-impaired physicians before problems escalate to the point of licensure revocation.

THE STREET ABUSER Identification of any chronic narcotic user is possible by blood and urine screens or the opiate antagonist challenge test (0.4 mg naloxone given slowly IV over 5 minutes, after which the patient is observed for 1–2 h for signs of withdrawal). For any realistic expectation of rehabilitation, the pt must be motivated to make a long-term commitment to a drug-free lifestyle. Special vocational, counseling, and peer programs are often helpful. Chronic use of opiate antagonists (naltrexone, 50–100 mg per day) blocks the "high" of moderate doses of narcotics and is sometimes helpful. Addicts who fail drug-free programs and who still wish to improve function within the family, social structure, etc. can do so on chronic methadone treatment. A relatively low dose (30–40 mg per day) may control abstinence symptoms and help curb drug-seeking behavior. The drug is administered orally at a program center.

For more detailed discussion of this topic, see Schuckit MA, Segal DS: Opioid Drug Use, Chap. 366, in HPIM-11, p. 2111

SECTION XIII
NUTRITION

178 ASSESSMENT OF NUTRITIONAL STATUS

Malnutrition and obesity are usually recognized by history and physical examination, but subtle forms of undernutrition may be overlooked, particularly in the presence of edema. Quantitative assessment of nutritional status (Table 178-1) reveals life-threatening undernutrition and allows measurement of progress once repletion is begun. Objective indicators of nutritional status correlate with morbidity and mortality, but no single measurement is of predictive value in individual patients.

NITROGEN BALANCE Estimation of nitrogen balance (nitrogen intake minus nitrogen excretion) effectively evaluates adequacy of nutritional support (Table 178-1). After growth ceases, rates of anabolism and catabolism are normally in equilibrium (nitrogen balance of zero). In catabolic states (trauma, infection, burns), increased protein losses and negative nitrogen balance ensue. Nitrogen intake is protein intake divided by 6.25. Normally, 95% of nitrogen is excreted in urine as urea, the remainder (about 2.5 g) in stool and skin. Hence, total daily nitrogen excretion equals 24-h urine nitrogen + 2.5 g. Nitrogen balance assessments give information about nutritional status during periods of observation but not about caloric or protein stores, e.g., duration of malnutrition or overnutrition.

LEAN BODY MASS (LBM) In the absence of edema, body weight as percent of ideal is a useful indicator of adipose tissue plus LBM. Ideal body weight can be estimated from a standardized height/weight table (Table 178-2) or as follows: women, 45 kg for first 152 cm of height + 0.9 kg for each cm above 152; men, 48 kg for first 152 cm + 1.1 kg for each cm above 152. Reduction of body weight/ideal body weight ratio to ≤80% usually indicates protein-calorie undernutrition.

Skeletal muscle comprises about 30% of LBM. Anthropometric measurements of LBM require only calipers and tape measure. In the nondominant arm, triceps skinfold is pulled away from triceps muscle midway between the acromial and olecranon processes. Skinfold is then measured with calipers (mm). Midarm muscle circumference is estimated from midarm circumference and skinfold thickness by the formula in Table 178-1. Normal ranges for skin thickness and muscle circumference are so wide that measurements are most useful as baselines for individual pts.

Since creatinine excretion is a function of the amount of skeletal muscle, size of muscle mass can be estimated by comparing ratio

TABLE 178-1 **Measures of nutritional status**

	Normal	Deficiency		
		Mild	Mod	Severe
Nitrogen balance (g/24 h): $\frac{\text{Protein intake (g)}}{6.25}$ − 24-h urine urea nitrogen (g) + 2.5	0–3	−1	−2	−3
Body weight: $\frac{\text{Actual body weight}}{\text{Ideal body weight}} \times 100$	100	80	70–80	<70
Adipose tissue: Triceps skin fold (mm)	Men 8–23 Women 10–30			
Lean body mass: Arm muscle circumference (cm) Arm circumference − 0.314 × triceps skinfold	Men 25.3 Women 23.2			
24-h urinary creatinine/height index (mg/cm)	Men 10.5 Women 5.8	8.4–9.5 4.6–5.2	7.4–8.4 4.1–4.6	<7.4 <4.1
Visceral protein compartment: Serum transferrin (0.8 × TIBC) − 43 (mg/dL)	200–260	180–200	160–180	<160
Serum albumin (g/dL)	4.0	3.5–3.9	2.5–3.0	<2.5
Immune function: Total lymphocyte count/mm^3	>1800	1500–1800	900–1500	<900
Skin test (mm induration) (Tuberculin/PPD, Candida, Streptokinase/Streptodornase, Mumps)	>10	5–10	0–5	0

TABLE 178-2 **Desirable weights of adults age 25 or over**

Height, cm (in shoes)	Clothed weight, kg Small frame	Medium frame	Large frame
Men			
158	51–54	54–58	57–64
160	52–56	55–60	58–65
163	54–57	56–62	60–67
165	55–58	58–63	61–69
168	56–60	59–65	63–71
170	58–62	61–67	64–73
173	60–64	63–69	67–75
175	62–66	64–71	68–77
178	64–68	66–73	70–79
180	65–70	68–75	72–81
183	67–72	70–77	74–84
185	69–74	72–79	76–86
188	71–76	74–82	78–88
190	73–78	76–84	81–90
193	74–79	78–86	83–92
Women			
147	42–44	44–48	47–54
150	43–46	45–50	48–55
152	44–47	46–51	49–57
155	45–48	47–53	51–58
158	46–50	48–54	52–59
160	48–51	50–55	54–61
163	49–53	51–57	55–63
165	50–54	53–59	57–64
168	52–56	54–61	58–66
170	54–58	56–63	60–68
173	55–59	58–65	62–70
175	57–61	60–67	64–72
178	59–64	62–68	66–74
180	61–65	64–70	68–76
183	63–67	65–72	69–78

Source: Weights of insured persons in the United States associated with lowest mortality. Stat Bull Metropol Life Ins Co, Nov 1959, p. 40.

of urinary creatinine excretion (g/day) either to height (cm) or to ideal urinary creatinine excretion (23 mg/kg body weight/day for men and 18 mg/kg body weight/day for women) with normal values.

THE VISCERAL COMPARTMENT The visceral compartment comprises 20% of LBM. When nutrition is inadequate, protein synthesis declines, and metabolic pathways are altered; when malnutrition is severe, the immune system becomes impaired. Serum albumin and transferrin are sensitive indicators of status of visceral protein pool. Transferrin has an average half-life of 8 days, and its measurement provides a sensitive indicator of protein repletion after refeeding.

Immune competence requires normal protein nutrition. Lymphocyte depletion and anergy to skin antigens (*Candida albicans,* mumps, streptokinase/streptodornase, and tuberculin/PPD) are associated with increase in morbidity and mortality. When abnormal, these parameters may revert to normal within weeks of initiating protein-calorie repletion.

Once refeeding is initiated in the malnourished pt, weekly monitoring of weight, albumin, creatinine excretion, midarm circumference, skin thickness, and immune function should be performed.

For more detailed discussion of this topic, see Rudman D: Assessment of Nutritional Status, Chap. 71, in HPIM-11, p. 390

---

179 NUTRITIONAL DEFICIENCY STATES

Malnutrition is significant among alcoholics and the poor, elderly, and chronically ill. In hospitalized pts, common deficiency states are protein-calorie undernutrition, beriberi, and scurvy.

PROTEIN AND ENERGY UNDERNUTRITION Progressive loss of lean body mass (LBM) and adipose tissue results from insufficient consumption of protein and energy. Overt clinical deficiency develops when hypermetabolism, catabolism, anorexia, infection, or other illness supervene. Two syndromes of protein-calorie malnutrition are: (1) *marasmus* (calorie deficiency), evident as stunted growth (children), loss of adipose tissue, generalized wasting of LBM without edema; and (2) *kwashiorkor* (protein deficiency), evident as hypoalbuminemia, generalized edema, "flaky paint" dermatosis, enlarged, fatty liver, and relative preservation of adipose tissue. These syndromes rarely present in pure form and generally overlap.

The manifestations are often apparent on examination. A history of inadequate calorie and protein intake is elicited. Listlessness, easy fatigability, swollen ankles, and cracked, dry skin may be accompanied by temporal wasting, exaggerated intercostal spaces, and dyspigmentation of skin and hair. In advanced cases, decubitus ulcers, hypothermia, and terminal infection may supervene. Midarm and midarm muscle area and the ratio of 24-h urinary creatinine/height are decreased. Serum albumin, transferrin, and Hct are low. Immune function is impaired, and T-lymphocyte function is decreased, as evidenced by cutaneous anergy and lymphopenia (absolute lymphocyte count < 1200 cells/mm^3).

Mortality rate varies from 15–40%, and institution of nutritional replacement is a medical emergency. Stupor, jaundice, petechiae, hyponatremia, and hypovitaminosis A are ominous signs. Death may be due to electrolyte imbalance, infection, hypothermia, or circulatory failure.

THIAMINE DEFICIENCY (BERIBERI) Thiamine deficiency occurs in alcoholics and food faddists or after chronic peritoneal dialysis, refeeding (without adequate thiamine) after starvation, or administration of glucose to asymptomatic thiamine-depleted pts. Clinical manifestations develop in only a fraction of subjects at risk, and genetic factors may be involved in susceptibility. Major manifestations involve the cardiovascular and nervous systems.

Beriberi heart disease comprises three derangements: (1) peripheral vasodilation leading to a high-output state, (2) biventricular myocardial failure, and (3) edema. Peripheral vasodilatation leads to increased AV shunting of blood (increased cardiac output), rapid circulation time, tachycardia, and a venous congestive state. Temporary hypertension after thiamine repletion is due to closing of AV shunts in presence of volume overload. In acute fulminant cardiovascular (shoshin) beriberi, the myocardial lesion may lead to severe dyspnea, restlessness, acute cardiovascular collapse, and death within hours to days.

In dry beriberi, peripheral neuropathy may or may not be painful and is characterized by symmetric impairment of sensory, motor, and reflex function that is more severe in distal segments of limbs. *Wernicke's encephalopathy* develops in an orderly sequence and consists of vomiting, nystagmus, palsies of the rectus muscles leading to ophthalmoplegia, fever, ataxia, and mental deterioration, eventuating in a global confusional state and even coma or death. Improvement occurs after thiamine replacement, although *Korsakoff's syndrome* may supervene, consisting of retrograde amnesia, impaired learning ability, and (usually) confabulation.

The best laboratory test is a depressed erythrocyte transketolase. Another diagnostic clue is the response to thiamine administration. In wet beriberi, blood pressure and heart rate may improve within 12 h of start of therapy.

Prompt administration of thiamine is indicated when beriberi is diagnosed or suspected. A dose of 50 mg/day should be given IM for several days, after which 2.5–5.0 mg/per day can be administered PO.

ASCORBIC ACID DEFICIENCY (SCURVY) Scurvy now occurs for the most part in areas of urban poverty. Many features result from defective collagen synthesis, including perifollicular hyperkeratotic papules in which hairs become fragmented and buried; purpura beginning on the backs of the lower extremities coalescing to ecchymoses; hemorrhage into muscles of the extremities with secondary phlebothromboses; hemorrhages into joints; splinter hemorrhages in nailbeds; swelling, friability, bleeding, and secondary infection of gums and loosening of the teeth. Terminally, icterus, edema, and fever are common; and convulsions, shock, and death may occur abruptly.

If diagnosis is suspected, blood should be obtained for measurement of platelet ascorbate levels (if available), and ascorbic acid should be administered promptly. The usual dose in adults is 100 mg three to five times a day PO until 4 g has been administered, then 100 mg/day. Spontaneous bleeding, muscle and bone pain, and gums begin to improve within 2–3 days, and large ecchymoses resolve in 10–12 days.

For more detailed discussion of this topic, see Rudman D: Protein and Energy Undernutrition, Chap. 72, p. 393; and Wilson JD: Vitamin Deficiency and Excess, Chap. 76, p. 410 in HPIM-11

180 ANOREXIA NERVOSA AND BULIMIA

Anorexia nervosa and bulimia are eating disorders in young women who develop a paralyzing fear of becoming fat. In anorexia nervosa, this fear causes radical restriction of caloric intake, the end result being emaciation. In bulimia, massive binge eating is followed by self-induced vomiting and laxative abuse. The features of anorexia nervosa and bulimia overlap, and the separation of the two is not always clearcut.

ANOREXIA NERVOSA While hypothalamic dysfunction (impaired regulation of gonadotropins, partial diabetes insipidus, and abnormal thermoregulation) is common in anorexia, most investigators favor a psychiatric cause. Interpersonal communication among family members tends to be inadequate, and there is a pathologic focus within family on food and eating behavior. Anorexia nervosa usually becomes apparent before or shortly after puberty. Despite emaciation, patients deny hunger, thinness, or fatigue. Amenorrhea is common and may precede anorexia. Body fat may be undetectable, but breast tissue is often preserved. Parotid gland enlargement and edema may be accompanied by anemia, leukopenia, hypokalemia, and hypoalbuminemia. Basal luteinizing hormone (LH) and follicle-stimulating hormone (FSH) are low, accounting for the amenorrhea. Menses usually return with weight gain.

BULIMIA In bulimics episodic ingestion of large amounts of food in uncontrollable fashion is associated with an awareness that the eating pattern is abnormal, a fear that the eating cannot be stopped voluntarily, and feelings of depression after the act. Eating episodes are followed by induced vomiting, with or without ingestion of laxatives. Secrecy about the eating/vomiting sequence is characteristic. Weight loss is not as profound as with anorexia, and half continue to menstruate. Hypokalemia and metabolic alkalosis may be present.

COURSE The course of anorexia and bulimia is variable. Mortality is about 5–6%, major causes of death being starvation and suicide. Poor prognostic signs include older age at onset (after age 20), longer duration of illness, prominent vomiting, extreme weight loss, and significant depression.

THERAPY No specific therapy exists. Supportive treatment involves a combination of psychotherapy, family counseling, and hospitalization for nutritional support if malnutrition is severe or if hypokalemia, hypotension, or prerenal azotemia is present. Antidepressants may be used with some success. Treatment is a long-term proposition, rife with failure, and requires perseverance by subject, family, and physician.

For more detailed discussion of this topic, see Foster DW: Anorexia Nervosa and Bulimia, Chap. 73, in HPIM-11, p. 397

181 OBESITY

Obesity implies ≥20% excess above ideal body weight, and a fifth of men and a third of women are obese. Mild obesity may not impart significant risk, but men who weigh 150–300% of ideal body weight have mortality rates 12 times those of nonobese men.

Excess weight can be assessed by comparison with standard tables for height and weight (see Table 178-2) or by calculation of body mass index (body weight in kg/height in meters). More precise estimates of adiposity may be obtained by skinfold measurements with skin calipers (see Table 178-1).

Most obesity is due to overeating. Genetic, environmental, and social factors are involved, but ultimately regulation of eating depends on interaction between hunger and satiety centers of hypothalamus, modulated by input from cerebral cortex. When caloric intake exceeds expenditure, excess calories are stored in adipose tissue; if net positive caloric balance is prolonged, obesity results.

Several disorders can cause secondary obesity. *Hypothyroidism* may cause obesity secondary to diminished caloric needs. *Cushing's disease* causes obesity involving centripetal fat stores, the face, and cervical or supraclavicular fat deposits. *Insulinoma* may cause obesity from increased caloric intake secondary to recurrent hypoglycemia.

Obesity causes morbidity and mortality primarily through cardiovascular complications and sudden death. Impaired glucose tolerance and fasting hyperlipidemia may occur. Morbid obesity also produces mechanical and physical stresses that predispose to or aggravate osteoarthritis, thromboembolism, cholelithiasis, hypertension, hypoventilation, and hypoxemia.

Caloric restriction is the cornerstone of weight reduction. Hyperinsulinemia, insulin resistance, diabetes, hypertension, and hyperlipidemia are ameliorated following weight loss. By estimating daily caloric needs (approximately 33 kcal/kg), one can calculate the daily deficit needed to achieve a given rate of weight loss, which should be targeted at 0.5–1 kg per week. Low-calorie diets should be balanced in protein, carbohydrate, and fat and should provide minerals and vitamins. Pts should be monitored closely while on weight-loss regimens (Table 181-1). Drugs are both ineffective in promoting weight loss and produce serious side effects and hence have no role in treatment.

Surgical treatment should be reserved for pts who have failed standard weight-reduction regimens and maintain a weight 50–100% over ideal body weight. Small-bowel bypass is effective in achieving weight reduction in such pts, but complications are common. Gastroplasty establishes a small upper gastric remnant attached to a larger gastric pouch by a 1.0–1.5 cm channel and thus delays gastric emptying. Weight loss with this procedure is without severe metabolic consequences.

A major problem in treatment is maintenance of reduced weight following weight loss. Techniques of behavior modification are sometimes useful.

TABLE 181-1 **Complications of therapy for obesity**

Treatment	Complication
Dietary:	
Total starvation	Anemia, hyperuricemia, gout, ketosis, potassium depletion, cardiac arryhthmias, sudden death
Carbohydrate depletion	Excessive water excretion, acidosis, ketosis, bone demineralization, cardiac arrhythmias, hypokalemia, hyperlipidemia
High protein	Hypokalemia, cardiac arrhythmias
Drug:	
Diuretics	Hypokalemia, volume depletion, metabolic alkalosis
Laxatives	Hypokalemia, metabolic acidosis
Anorexiants	Cardiac arrhythmias, anxiety
Thyroid supplements	Cardiac arrhythmias, anxiety
Surgery:	
Jejunoileal bypass	Diarrhea, electrolyte disturbances, hepatic cirrhosis, urinary calculi, arthritis, cholelithiasis
Gastroplasty	Gastric outlet obstruction

For more detailed discussion of this topic, see Olefsky JM: Obesity, Chap. 317 in HPIM-11, p. 1671

182 DIET THERAPY

Diet prescription is essential for all hospitalized pts (Table 182-1), recognizing that for most a regular hospital diet containing about 2000–2200 kcal and fed in three meals of ⅕, ⅖, and ⅖ proportion will suffice. Daily caloric requirements can be estimated with the Harris-Benedict equation for basal energy expenditure (BEE):

Men, kcal/day

$$\text{BEE} = 66 + 13.8W + 5H - 6.8A$$

Women, kcal/day

$$\text{BEE} = 665 + 9.6W + 1.8H - 4.7A$$

where W = weight in kg, H = height in cm, and A = age in years.

Average energy expenditure is 1.37 BEE − 312. For usual pt, recommended intake should equal energy expenditure. To maintain a positive caloric balance when energy expenditure is increased (burns, infection, trauma, surgery, hyperthyroidism), energy intake should be 1.5–2 × this value.

In healthy adults, recommended protein intake is 0.8 g/kg body weight/day, but under conditions of stress, requirement may increase to 2–4 g/kg body weight/day. Optimal ratio of kcal to g protein intake in the healthy individual is 150:1, and intermediate ratios may be appropriate in conditions of altered growth or repair needs.

Needs for special restrictions and/or additions to diet depend on diagnosis (Table 182-1). Administration can be *oral intake, tube feeding,* or *parenterally.* For oral intake, consistency can vary from clear liquid to pureed or soft to regular, and for tube feedings and parenteral formulas, concentration and osmolality must be specified.

TUBE FEEDING When oral intake is inadequate or the GI tract is incapable of absorbing sufficient nutrients, enteral feeding may be indicated (Table 182-2). Such situations include anorexia, neurologic disorders such as dysphagia or cerebrovascular accidents, and malignancy. Enteral routes include nasogastric and

TABLE 182-1 **Principles of diet prescription**

Assess caloric and protein needs
Designate route of administration:
oral intake, tube feeding, parenteral nutrition
Select texture and/or concentration
Specify frequency and/or rate of feeding
Designate special restrictions:
Na, Ca, K, fluid, gastric irritants, fiber, residue, gluten, fat, carbohydrate, protein, purine, tyronine, galactose, sucrose, oxalate, lactate
Designate special additions:
fiber, medium chain triglycerides, vitamins, prepared nutritional supplements

TABLE 182-2 **Examples of formulas for tube feeding**

Example	Osmolality mosmol/kg	kcal/ mL or g	Volume for 100% RDA,* mL/day	Composition, g/1000 kcal			Electrolytes, mg/1000 kcal	
				Protein/ amino acids	Carbohydrate	Fat	Na	K
Elemental:								
Vivonex HN	810	1	3000	46	210	1	529	1173
Vital	460	1	1500	42	188	11	383	1167
Travasorb HN	560	1	2000	45	175	13	920	1170
Polymeric:								
Sustacal	625	1	1080	60	138	23	920	2060
Osmolite HN	300	1	1400	44	131	47		
Ensure	450	1.1	1900	35	135	35	708	1179
Isocal	300	1.1	1900	32	125	42	500	1250
Ensure Plus	600	1.5	1920	37	133	35	704	1267
Two Cal HN	750	2	960	40	200	90		
Modular								
Polycose†	850	2	NA	0	250	0	290	100
Casec†	NA	3.7	NA	230	0	5	408	0
MCT oil†	NA	7.7	NA	0	0	120	0	0
Product 80056	NA	4.9	NA	0	146	46	147	688

* Recommended daily needs.
† Do not contain vitamins.

nasoduodenal tubes, jejunostomy tubes, and gastrostomy tubes placed by percutaneous endoscopy. Small-bore Silastic or polyurethane tubes are associated with low rates of nasopharyngitis, rhinitis, otitis media, and stricture formation.
Elemental formulas: Composed of di- and tripeptides and/or amino acids, glucose oligosaccharides, and vegetable oils or medium-chain triglycerides. Residue is minimal, and little digestion is required. Such formulas may be of use in pts with short bowel syndrome, partial small bowel obstruction, pancreatic insufficiency, inflammatory bowel disease, radiation enteritis, or bowel fistula.
Polymeric formulas: Contain complex nutrients and can be used in most pts with a functional GI tract.

SINGLE-NUTRIENT MODULES FOR PROTEIN, CARBOHYDRATE, AND FAT. Can be combined to create formulas for specialized requirements, e.g., a high-caloric, low-protein, low-sodium formula for a cachetic cirrhotic patient with ascites and encephalopathy.

PARENTERAL NUTRITION When pts cannot eat or deteriorate on oral feeding, partial or complete nourishment via the parenteral route is needed. Indications for total parenteral nutrition (TPN) include malnourished pts who cannot tolerate oral feedings; bowel rest in pts with regional enteritis; well-nourished pts who require 10–14 days of abstinence from oral intake; prolonged coma when tube feeding is not possible; nutritional support in pts with hypercatabolism such as sepsis, burns, or trauma; pts receiving chemotherapy that precludes oral intake; and prophylactic use in malnourished pts undergoing surgery.

TPN should generally provide 32–40 kcal/kg body weight and basal water intake of 1.2 mL/kcal per day. To this should be added a volume equivalent to losses from diarrhea, stomal output, nasogastric suction, and fistula drainage (Table 182-3). In oliguric pts, a basal intake of 750–1000 mL fluid should be given, plus a volume equal to urine and other losses. In edematous pts, Na intake should be limited to 20–40 meq/day.

Positive nitrogen balance can usually be achieved by infusing 0.5–1.0 g amino acids per kg of body weight/day, together with

TABLE 182-3 **Representative daily protocols for total parenteral nutrition**

Components	Fat free	50% Lipid	85% Lipid
Amino acids, g	60	60	75
Glucose, g	750	375	187
Lipids, g	0	100	150
Electrolyte mix, mL	60	60	60
Trace element mix, mL	5	5	5
Vitamins, mL	10	10	10
Na^+, mg	125	125	132
K^+, mg	81	80	87
Total kcal	2550	2375	2286
Total volume, mL	3075	2775	3075

Modified from Jeejeebhoy KN, Baker JP: HPIM-11, p. 408.

nonprotein calories. The protein-sparing effect of carbohydrate and fat is maximal at around 55–60 kcal/kg ideal body weight/day. Carbohydrates and lipids can be infused with amino acids to provide sufficient nonprotein calories using a Y connector. A mixture in which lipid provides half the calories simulates the normal diet, causes neither hyperinsulinemia nor hyperglycemia, and eliminates the need for exogenous insulin.

Complications related to catheter insertion include pneumothorax, thrombophlebitis, catheter embolism, and hyperglycemia (from hypertonic glucose infusions). Disseminated candidiasis may occur after prolonged nutritional support. Hypokalemia, hypomagnesemia, and hypophosphatemia may result in disorientation, convulsions, and coma. Hyperchloremic acidosis may occur with inadequate sodium acetate supplementation.

For more detailed discussion of these topics, see Rudman D: Diet Therapy, Chap. 74, p. 400; and Jeejeebhoy KN, Baker JP: Parenteral Nutrition, Chap. 75, p. 406 in HPIM-11

SECTION XIV
MEDICAL EMERGENCIES

183 POISONING AND ITS MANAGEMENT

A common problem, responsible for more than 10,000 deaths/year in the U.S.

DIAGNOSIS Should be considered in pts with coma, convulsions, acute hepatic, renal, and bone marrow failure. Ask pt, relatives, and acquaintances about possible poisons. Specimens of blood, urine, vomitus, and gastric aspirate should be sent immediately for analysis and "toxic screen." Obtain consultation from nearest poison information center if necessary. If poison is identified, estimate total ingested and relate to minimum lethal dose.

TREATMENT (Table 183-1)
1 *Evacuation of stomach*—useful even several hours following ingestion; avoid following ingestion of corrosives; *emesis* (E) may be induced in conscious pts who are not postictal; syrup of ipecac (15–30 mL) followed by 120 mL H_2O; may repeat dose; *gastric*

TABLE 183-1 **Treatment of acute chemical poisoning**

Prevention of further absorption of ingested poison:
- Emptying the stomach:
  - Induction of vomiting
  - Gastric lavage
- Minimizing gastrointestinal absorption:
  - Adsorption
  - Catharsis

Removal of absorbed poisons from body:
- Detoxification
- Biliary excretion—interruption of enterohepatic circulation
- Urinary excretion:
  - Forced diuresis
  - Alteration of urinary pH
- Dialysis:
  - Peritoneal dialysis
  - Hemodialysis
- Charcoal or resin hemoperfusion
- Exchange transfusion
- Chelation and chemical binding

Supportive therapy

Administration of systemic antidotes:
- Chemical agents
- Pharmacologic antagonists

Modified from Friedman PA: HPIM-11, p. 839.

lavage (GL) is more predictable; every effort must be made to avoid aspiration by endotracheal tube in stuporous pts.

2 *Minimize absorption* with 60–100 g activated charcoal (AC) after E or in lavage fluid.

3 *Catharsis* with 10% $MgSO_4$, 2–3 mL/kg.

4 *Enhance renal excretion*—forced diuresis (saline + IV furosemide); alkaline diuresis useful for salicylates and long-acting barbiturates; acid diuresis for acetaminophen.

5 *Hemodialysis or hemoperfusion* used for dialyzable toxins not tissue- or protein-bound (e.g., ethylene glycol, methanol, paraquat, salicylates) in pts suspected of having ingested lethal quantities.

Supportive therapy: (1) Maintenance of ventilation when CNS is depressed; (2) anticonvulsants (e.g., IV diazepam) in pts with convulsions; (3) cerebral edema caused by several poisons (e.g., lead or CO) should be treated with IV corticosteroids and/or IV hypertonic mannitol; (4) all pts should be evaluated and treated for frequent concomitants of poisoning, which should be specifically sought, including hypovolemia (saline), hypotension (pressors), cardiac arrhythmias (antiarrhythmics, cardioversion), pulmonary edema (diuretics, ↑ O_2 under positive pressure), hypoxia (treatment depends on etiology), acute renal failure, acute hepatic failure, and disturbances of electrolytes and pH.

COMMON POISONS

ACETAMINOPHEN Toxic dose > 8 g; plasma concentration > 200 μg/mL causes lethargy, nausea, vomiting. Hepatotoxicity occurs after 1–2 days. Other hazards include acute tubular necrosis, hypoglycemia.

Treatment: E or GL with AC. N-Acetylcysteine (Mucomyst) to supply sulfhydryl groups decreases hepatotoxicity if given < 10 h after ingestion (140 mg/kg followed by 70 mg/kg IV q 4 h for 3 days).

ANTIMUSCARINIC COMPOUNDS (atropine, belladonna, and synthetics such as benztropine) Prior hepatic and renal failure increase susceptibility to these agents; causes dryness of mucous membranes, xerophthalmia, hypertension, tachycardia, fever, urinary retention, toxic psychosis, confusion, delirium, lethargy, and somnolence.

Treatment: E or GL with AC; ↓ body temp.; catheterize bladder; treat excitement with sedatives, coma with physostigmine.

CARBON MONOXIDE (CO) An odorless, nonirritating gas; causes tissue hypoxia because of CO affinity for hemoglobin; increasing concentrations cause headache, cherry red skin and mucous membranes, irritability, confusion, nausea, exertional syncope, coma, convulsions, respiratory failure, and death.

Treatment: Ventilation with 100% O_2 and transfusion with blood and packed RBCs.

CHLORINATED INSECTICIDES Ingredients of DDT, lindane, and chlorinated polycyclics (e.g., aldrin); cause nausea and vom-

iting, excitement, tremors, CNS hyperexcitability and convulsions → CNS depression, paralysis, coma, and hepatic damage.
Treatment: E or GL with AC; catharsis; cholestyramine to increase excretion; treat with anticonvulsants, artificial ventilation; avoid sympathomimetics.

CHOLINESTERASE INHIBITOR INSECTICIDES (organic phosphates, e.g., parathion) Toxicity results from acetylcholine → convulsions, coma, respiratory depression, nausea and vomiting, diarrhea, muscle twitching, weakness.
Treatment: E or GL with AC; catharsis; atropine 2 mg IM q 10 min; 1 g pralidoxime IV q 12 h may relieve muscle weakness; also use artificial ventilation with suction and treatment with anticonvulsants.

CYANIDE (CN) May result from inhalation of hydrocyanic acid or from ingestion of inorganic CN or CN-releasing substances, including nitroprusside; toxicity results from CN reaction with cytochrome oxidase; causes, in sequence, hyperventilation, headache, nausea and vomiting, dyspnea, hypotension, coma, convulsions, and death; "bitter almond" odor on breath useful in diagnosis.
Treatment: Amyl nitrite (1 perle q 2 min), followed by 10 mL 3% $NaNO_2$ in 3 min (IV norepinephrine may be necessary to maintain BP), followed by 50 mL 25% Na thiosulfate IV in 10 min; artificial respiration with 100% O_2.

DETERGENTS AND SOAPS *Common soaps and household detergents* cause nausea and vomiting and diarrhea, but no serious effects; no treatment is usually necessary. *Cationic detergents,* e.g., benzalkonium Cl, may cause oral and esophageal corrosion, nausea and vomiting, coma, convulsions, and death.
Treatment: E or GL with AC with ordinary soap (which inactivates cationic detergents).

ETHYLENE GLYCOL Used in antifreeze; often drunk intentionally by alcoholics; manifestations resemble alcohol intoxication; stupor, coma, anisocoria, convulsions, bradycardia, hypothermia, respiratory failure.
Treatment: IV ethanol to blood level of 100 mg/dL and thiamine 100 mg qd; dialysis is quite effective.

HALOGENATED HYDROCARBONS (CCl_4, trichlorethyl, methyl halides, etc.) Used as solvents, refrigerants, fumigants, household cleansers, and floor waxes; cause CNS depression, hepatic, renal, and myocardial toxicity; immediate nausea and vomiting, dizziness, confusion, headache, stupor, coma, convulsions, respiratory failure, hypotension, and death; severe and often fatal hepatic and renal tubular damage may occur in survivors.
Treatment: E or GL with AC and catharsis; very early hemodialysis and hemoperfusion may remove halogenated hydrocarbons from body; hemodialysis may be helpful if renal failure occurs late.

IODINE Causes brown staining of oral mucous membranes, corrosion of GI tract, nausea and vomiting, and bloody diarrhea.
Treatment: Ingestion of milk, starch, or activated charcoal; catharsis; oral and IV Na thiosulfate.

METHYL ALCOHOL (METHANOL) Used as solvent, antifreeze, or denaturant of ethyl alcohol; metabolic products (formaldehyde and formic acid) are toxic and lead to blindness, metabolic acidosis, CNS depression, respiratory failure, visual disturbances.
Treatment: E or GL; $NaHCO_3$ IV then PO; IV ethanol (1 g/kg in 30 min followed by 10 g/h); hemodialysis if methanol > 50 mg/dL.

MUSHROOMS Poisoning usually due to *Amanita* species; causes parasympathetic stimulation, lacrimation, salivation, nausea and vomiting, diarrhea, wheezing, dyspnea, tremors, confusion, and delirium; later hepatic, renal, and CNS damage.
Treatment: Atropine 2 mg IM; treat hypoglycemia, fluid and electrolyte imbalance; hemoperfusion may be useful very early.

NICOTINE An important component of insecticides; causes nausea and vomiting, diarrhea, headache, tachypnea, sweating and salivation, irritability, convulsions, coma, and cardiac arrest.
Treatment: E or GL with AC; catharsis; lavage with K permanganate; atropine 2 mg and phentolamine 5 mg; artificial respiration with 100% O_2; and IV beta blockers.

PHOSPHORUS Used in rodent and insect poisons and fireworks; causes hepatotoxicity; first causes nausea and vomiting, diarrhea, and coma; later, hepatomegaly, jaundice, hypotension, oliguria, convulsions, and coma.
Treatment: E or GL with AC, osmotic cathartic, calcium gluconate.

SALICYLATES Toxic doses range from 3–10 g; mild toxicity (salicylism): vertigo, tinnitus, nausea and vomiting, diarrhea; severe toxicity: confusion, excitement, convulsions, coma, hyperventilation, respiratory alkalosis; later, respiratory and metabolic acidosis occurs.
Treatment: E or GL with AC; catharsis; treat acid-base and electrolyte disturbances and hypoglycemia; use artificial ventilation with 100% O_2; diazepam for convulsions; raise urine pH > 7 with IV $NaHCO_3$ + furosemide to ↑ renal clearance of salicylates.

SMOKE Causes CO toxicity and irritant fumes → chemical burns of upper respiratory tract and skin; can cause severe coughing with later dyspnea and cyanosis → pulmonary edema.
Treatment: Same as for CO; also 100% O_2 and IV glucocorticosteroids.

For more detailed discussion of this topic, see Friedman PA: Poisoning and Its Management, Chap. 171, in HPIM-11, p. 838

DROWNING

EPIDEMIOLOGY 7000 fatalities per year; second most common cause of accidental death between 5 and 44 years of age.

PATHOPHYSIOLOGY 10–20% of deaths due to asphyxia. Most important is anoxia or hypoxia, also bronchospasm, laryngospasm, aspiration of particulate matter. Aspiration of salt H_2O → pulmonary edema → intrapulmonary right-to-left shunt. Aspiration of fresh H_2O → alveolar collapse → altered ventilation-perfusion ratio → hypoxia. Hemolysis is rarely important.

CLINICAL MANIFESTATIONS Cough, tachypnea, pulmonary edema, ARDs, CNS—organic brain syndromes; fever < 24 h following aspiration; later, complicating infections.

LABORATORY FINDINGS ABGs show ↓ P_{O_2}, acidosis; CXR: 25% normal; perihilar infiltrates → pulmonary edema; increased WBC; decreased Hct; look for bleeding.

THERAPY

- On scene: mouth-to-mouth respiration; closed chest massage.
- Do not waste time draining H_2O from lungs.
- Establish airway, 100% O_2 stat and continuously.
- In hospital, ABGs, pH, hemogram, electrolytes, CXR.
- If alert, observe for several hours.
- Treat metabolic acidosis with $NaHCO_3$ and supplemental O_2.
- If pulmonary edema and no response to $F_{IO_2} \geq 40\%$, intubate and use PEEP; continue PEEP until ABGs stable (48–72 h).
- Comatose pts often have ICP > 15–20 mmHg; institute cerebral resuscitation (controlled hyperventilation, hypothermia, barbiturates, steroids, and osmotic and loop diuretics).
- Other measures: treat pulmonary infection; maintain fluid and electrolyte balance; plasma expanders (if ↓ BP); transfusion if blood volume ↓.

PROGNOSIS Depends on hypoxia, CNS status; good if CXR normal and pt alert.

For more detailed discussion of the this topic, see Wallace JF: Drowning and Near Drowning, Chap. 175, in HPIM-11, p. 861

185 TRANSFUSION REACTIONS

Transfusion reactions may be classified as *immune* or *nonimmune*.

IMMUNOLOGICALLY MEDIATED REACTIONS

Reaction may be directed against red or white blood cells, platelets, or IgA; in addition, other, less well characterized reactions may occur.

Intravascular hemolysis: Usually due to ABO incompatibility; very rapid and massive hemolysis; symptoms and signs may include restlessness, anxiety, flushing, chest or back pain, tachypnea, tachycardia, nausea, shock, renal failure, coagulation disorders (including DIC).

Extravascular hemolysis: Usually due to antibodies of Rh system, but antibodies of Kell, Duffy, and Kidd systems may also be involved; clinical manifestations are less severe, often simply with malaise and fever; shock and renal failure are rare; initial red cell survival may be normal followed by delayed destruction in RE system.

LABORATORY INVESTIGATION OF IMMUNE-MEDIATED REACTIONS

- Careful check on identity of donor and recipient; samples of recipient blood to blood bank for analysis and further cross-matching.
- Documentation of hemolysis—plasma and urine hemoglobin, haptoglobin, Hct, bilirubin.
- Check renal status—UA, BUN, creatinine.
- Check coagulation status—platelet count, PT, PTT.

TREATMENT

- Avoid further transfusion unless absolutely necessary.
- Management of shock and renal failure in intravascular hemolysis; osmotic diuresis and volume expansion may be indicated in certain cases; if renal failure ensues, adjust drug doses and closely monitor fluid/electrolyte status.
- Factor replacement if needed to control coagulation abnormalities; platelet infusion if thrombocytopenia severe.

NONIMMUNE REACTIONS

- *Circulatory overload*—especially in infants and patients with renal or cardiac insufficiency.
- *Effects of massive transfusion*—hyperkalemia, ammonia and citrate toxicity, dilutional coagulopathy, thrombocytopenia.
- *Infection*—hepatitis, syphilis, CMV, malaria, babesiosis, toxoplasmosis, brucellosis, AIDS can all be transmitted by transfused blood.
- *Iron overload*—with repeated transfusions; may require chelation therapy.

- *Complications related to intravenous access*—air embolism, thrombophlebitis.

For more detailed discussion of this topic, see Giblett ER: Blood Groups and Blood Transfusion, Chap. 282, in HPIM-11, p. 1483

SNAKE BITE

EPIDEMIOLOGY AND ETIOLOGY

- In U.S., poisonous snakes are coral snake, rattle snake, water moccasin, copperhead.
- 8000 snake bites/year; most in S.E. and Gulf States (esp. Texas); <20 fatal.
- Factors affecting severity of snake bite: age, size, health; location (trunk, face worse than extremities), size of snake, bacteria (*Clostridium*) in mouth of snake, exercise after bite (running promotes absorption of toxin).

SIGNS AND SYMPTOMS Burning at site, local swelling, gangrene of skin. Systemic—fever, nausea and vomiting, circulatory collapse, bleeding, muscle cramping, pupillary constriction, delirium, convulsions.

LABORATORY FINDINGS If severe, anemia, ↑ WBC, ↓ platelets, DIC.

THERAPY Verify fang marks, local edema.
First aid: Rest, immobilize limb, tourniquet, linear incision over fang mark → suction.
Hospital care: Antivenin vital in severe bites. In treatment with polyvalent crotaline antivenin, reconstitute 1 vial with 10 mL H_2O; 5 vials usually sufficient; test for horse serum sensitivity.
No antivenin except above available in U.S., but antiserum against various types available at Oklahoma Zoo and Poison Info Center [(405) 271 5454].
Other: Maintain respiration; provide tetanus toxoid or TIG, antibiotics for wound infection (gram-negative pathogens), debridement (fasciotomy), pain relief; combat shock and bleeding; steroids may or may not be useful.

PREVENTION Long pants, gloves. For first aid, carry sharp knife, constriction band, suction bulb, antiseptic, antivenin.

LIZARD BITE

Epidemiology and etiology: Only poisonous lizards are Gila monster and Mexican beaded lizard.
Signs and symptoms: Tissue injury, pain, edema, erythema, nausea, vomiting, blurred vision, dyspnea, dysphonia, weakness.
Therapy: Constriction band, incision, suction, cooling of bitten area; prevent or treat infection; provide pain relief.

SPIDER BITES

WIDOW SPIDER In U.S., black widow spider; bites between April and October; victims often males using privies; after bite, cramping pain from extremities → trunk (boardlike abdomen); pain is severe.

Treatment: Relieve pain, give antivenin, 10 mL of 10% calcium gluconate for cramps; if severe 1 vial (2.5 mL) *Latrodectus* antivenin in 50 mL saline over 15 min IV.

LOXOSCELES SPIDER In the South and Southwest as well as California; bite—initially mild burning → severe pain → necrosis and bullae formation; some pts have systemic symptoms.
Treatment: If pain is not intense and there are no bullae, no treatment; if pain is severe, provide steroids, Dapsone (experimental), debridement.

OTHER ANIMALS

SCORPIONS One dangerous species (*Centruroides*) in Arizona, New Mexico, southern California, Texas; most mild; rarely fatal: numbness → hyperexcitable state → coma and convulsions → death.
Treatment: Cold compresses and mild analgesics; severe: goat serum antivenin, diazepam; combat shock and dehydration.

BEE STINGS, WASPS, HORNETS, YELLOW JACKETS

- Most severe and lethal reactions: allergic.
- Symptoms: sharp pain → wheal and erythema → itching.
- Danger if bee swallowed or inhaled → edema of glottis or larynx.
- In hypersensitive → acute anaphylaxis or serum sickness.
- Treatment: Remove stinger, apply tourniquet, icepacks.
- Anaphylaxis: Epinephrine 0.3–0.5 mL 1:1000 q 20–30 min, airway, vasopressors, O_2 as needed.

TICK BITE

- Vectors for Rocky Mountain spotted fever, Q fever, tularemia, borreliosis, babesiosis, Lyme disease.
- Local: papule, nodule.
- Remove tick intact.

Tick paralysis: Ascending, flaccid paralysis; victims mainly young girls with tick hidden in hair.

- Differential diagnosis: Poliomyelitis, diphtheria, Guillain-Barré, Eaton-Lambert, myasthenia gravis, botulism.
- Treatment: Remove tick.

MARINE ANIMALS

- Portuguese man-of-war and jellyfish: Local pain, swelling, erythema → muscle cramps, nausea and vomiting. *Treat* with saltwater bath, scrape off tentacles.
- Paralytic and neurotoxic shellfish: Coastal waters, "red tide"; humans infected by ingestion. *Treat* with purgation.

VENOMOUS FISH Dorsal fins of bullhead sharks, dogfish, ratfish, catfish. *Treat* by immersion in hot water. Most common in U.S. is tail of stringray resulting in local pain and occasional systemic absorption. *Treat* with constriction band, saltwater syringing of wound.

For more detailed discussion of this topic, see Wallace JF: Disorders caused by Venoms, Bites, and Stings, Chap. 170, in HPIM-11, p. 831

187 HYPER- AND HYPOTHERMIA

DISORDERS ASSOCIATED WITH HIGH TEMPERATURES

Heat cramps

- Most with benign heat syndrome.
- Painful spasms in voluntary muscles after strenuous exercise.
- Therapy: NaCl and H_2O.
- If abdominal muscles in spasm, do not operate!

Heat exhaustion

- High external temperatures.
- Occurs in elderly receiving diuretics.
- Weakness, vertigo, anorexia, nausea; vomiting and faintness may precede collapse.
- Onset sudden; duration brief.
- Color gray; skin cold and clammy; BP low; body temp. normal or ↓.
- Therapy: Remove to cool place; recumbency.
- IV fluids rarely necessary.

Exertional heat injury

- Due to exertion at hot ambient temps. (≥80°F) when relative humidity is high (≥60%).
- Common in runners who are insufficiently acclimatized, conditioned, and hydrated, or who are overweight.
- In contrast to heat stroke, these patients sweat freely and their temps. are low (102–104°F).
- Symptoms: headache, gooseflesh, chills, hyperventilation, nausea, vomiting, muscle cramps, ataxia, incoherent speech.
- PE: Tachycardia, hypotension, sometimes loss of consciousness.
- Laboratory findings: ↑ Hct, ↑ Na^+, ↑ liver and muscle enzymes, ↓ Ca^{2+}, ↓ PO_4.
- Rarely, there are DIC, rhabdomyolysis, myoglobinemia.
- Therapy: Lower core temp to 100–104°F (wet sheets); massage extremities to improve blood flow; infuse hypotonic glucose/saline.
- Prevention for runner: Run races early in morning; enter race well-hydrated; place aid stations at intervals; do not increase pace at end; avoid alcohol before race.

Heat stroke

- Elderly, preexisting chronic disease; diuretics.
- Sometimes military recruits.
- Cardinal signs and symptoms: Hyperpyrexia (≥106°F) and prostration.
- Skin hot and dry; sweating ceases.
- Pulse rapid; respirations rapid and weak; BP low.
- Hemoconcentration; WBC ↑, BUN ↑; protein and casts in urine; respiratory alkalosis followed by metabolic acidosis.
- Lactic acidemia; ↓ Ca^{2+}, ↓ PO_4.

- ECG abnormal.
- Clotting abnormalities that may culminate in DIC.
- Early death or pt may die of acute complications such as renal failure.
- Therapy: *Emergency*—place pt in cool area; remove clothing; immerse in ice water bath without delay; massage skin; phenothiazine to reduce shivering; Swan-Ganz catheter; ensure airway; avoid epinephrine and narcotics; hydrate but do not overhydrate.

Malignant hyperthermia

- Episodic rapid increase in temp. in response to inhalational anesthetic (halothane, methoxyflurane, or muscle relaxants such as succinyl choline).
- In genetic form, 50% have ↑ CK.
- In another (King syndrome) in young boys there are a number of other congenital abnormalities.
- Symptoms: Decreased relaxation during induction of anesthesia; muscle fasciculations with succinyl choline, rapid rise in temp., muscle rigidity; hypotension and cyanosis.
- Laboratory findings: Respiratory and metabolic acidosis, ↑ K^+, ↑ Mg, ↑ blood lactate and pyruvate.
- Therapy: *Medical emergency*—stop surgery; cool with ice; 100% O_2; induce diuresis; give dantrolene sodium (1 mg/kg) rapidly IV until symptoms stop—up to maximum single dose of 10 mg/kg.
- Prevention: Family Hx; monitor temp. during anesthesia; prophylactic dantrolene ineffective.

Neuroleptic malignant syndrome (NMS)

- Muscular rigidity, hyperthermia, altered consciousness; autonomic dysfunction.
- Leukocytosis (15,000–30,000); ↑ CK.
- Occurs after neuroleptics (haloperidol, thiothixene, or piperazine phenothiazine) in therapeutic doses.
- Primarily young adult males.
- Lasts 5–10 days after administration of neuroleptics is discontinued.
- Therapy: None; try dantrolene as in malignant hyperthermia.

DISORDERS ASSOCIATED WITH LOW TEMPERATURES

Accidental hypothermia

- Winter months; after exposure; in alcoholics.
- Diagnosis often not made because thermometers do not register ≤95°F; use incubator thermometer or thermocouple.
- Associated with myxedema, pituitary insufficiency, adrenal insufficiency, cerebrovascular disease, drug or alcohol ingestion.
- Pts appear cold, pale, stiff.
- If temp. < 80°F, patients are unconscious.
- Hemoconcentration, azotemia, metabolic acidosis (lactic acid).

- Therapy: *Medical emergency*—maintain airway; oxygenate well; monitor blood gases; expand blood volume; monitor K^+; watch for arrhythmias; give $NaHCO_3$ if pH ≤ 7.25; if severely hypothermic, rewarm in bath or Hubbard tank (104–108°F).
- Watch for rewarming shock and treat with hemo- or peritoneal dialysis.
- Pneumonia common; treat with antibiotics.
- Do not cease resuscitation even in the face of asystole until pt has been rewarmed to 96.8°F and remains unresponsive to CPR at that temperature.

Hypothermia of acute illness

- Differs from above in that it occurs at ambient temperatures.
- Degree of hypothermia modest (92–93°F).
- Associated with CHF, uremia, diabetes mellitus, drug overdose, respiratory failure.
- Characterized by severe metabolic acidosis, cardiac arrhythmias, and loss of consciousness.
- Usually responds to rewarming with circulating blanket; otherwise, treat as above.

Immersion hypothermia

- Due to immersion in cold water for prolonged periods.
- Therapy: Rewarming in warm water.

Local cold injuries

- Frostnip (earlobes, nose, fingers, and toes).
- Immersion foot (feet wet but not freezing for prolonged periods; symptoms vary from ischemia to hyperemia); for ischemia, need to rewarm slowly (note: overheating of tissue may lead to gangrene); hyperemia requires careful cooling.
- Frostbite (differs from immersion foot because blood vessels are involved); rewarm frostbitten limb carefully in water at 50–59°F and increase temperature every 5 minutes by 5°F to maximum of 104°F; once rewarming has taken place, treatment is bed rest, elevation of injured part, tetanus toxoid, antibiotics, debridement of blebs and bullae, local antiseptic washes, early physiotherapy.
- Amputation usually not necessary; IV dextran of possible value; sympathectomy or intraarterial reserpine may decrease vasospasm.

For more detailed discussion of this topic, see Petersdorf RG, Root RK: Disturbances of Heat Regulation, Chap. 8, in HPIM-11, p. 43

---

188 INCREASED INTRACRANIAL PRESSURE AND TRAUMA TO THE CNS

INCREASED INTRACRANIAL PRESSURE

A limited volume of extra tissue, blood, CSF, or edema fluid can be added to the intracranial contents without raising the intracranial pressure (ICP). Pts will deteriorate and may die when ICP reaches levels that compromise cerebral perfusion or causes a shift in intracranial contents that distorts vital brainstem centers.

CLINICAL MANIFESTATIONS Symptoms that occur in pts with high ICP include headache (especially a constant ache that is worse upon awakening), nausea, emesis, drowsiness, diplopia, and blurred vision. Papilledema and sixth nerve palsies are common. If not controlled, then pupillary dilatation, coma, decerebrate posturing, abnormal respirations, systemic hypertension, and bradycardia may result.

A posterior fossa mass, which may initially cause ataxia, stiff neck, and nausea, is especially dangerous because it can compress vital brainstem structures and cause obstructive hydrocephalus. Masses that cause raised ICP also displace brain tissue against fixed intracranial structures and into spaces not normally occupied. These herniation syndromes include (1) medial cortex displaced under the midline falx → anterior or posterior cerebral artery occlusion and stroke; (2) uncus displaced through the tentorium, compressing the third cranial nerve and pushing the cerebral peduncle against the tentorium, → ipsilateral pupillary dilatation and contralateral hemiparesis; (3) cerebellar tonsils displaced into the foramen magnum, causing medullary compression, → cardiorespiratory collapse; and (4) downward displacement of the diencephalon through the tentorium causing miotic pupils and drowsiness.

MANAGEMENT Cerebral perfusion pressure (CPP) = BP − ICP. Global cerebral ischemia occurs when CPP < 45 mmHg. Hypertension should be treated carefully, if at all. Careful intubation (without causing gagging or coughing) allows controlled hyperventilation to lower ICP quickly. The arterial P_{CO_2} should be maintained around 30 mmHg. Mannitol (1 g/kg) lowers ICP by decreasing interstitial brain fluid. Lasix is somewhat less effective. Free H_2O should be restricted. Pt's head should be elevated to 45 degrees.

EVALUATION OF PATIENT After stabilization and initiation of the above therapies, a CT scan is performed to delineate the cause of the elevated ICP. Emergency surgical intervention is sometimes necessary to decompress the intracranial contents. Hydrocephalus, cerebellar stroke with edema, surgically accessible cerebral hemorrhage or tumor, and subdural or epidural hemorrhage often require lifesaving neurosurgery. ICP monitoring can guide medical and surgical decisions in pts with cerebral edema due to stroke, head trauma, Reye's syndrome, and intracerebral hemorrhage.

High doses of barbiturates may decrease ICP in otherwise refractory pts, and in these pts ICP monitoring is obligatory.

TRAUMA TO THE CENTRAL NERVOUS SYSTEM

Head trauma can cause immediate loss of consciousness. If transient and unaccompanied by other serious brain pathology, it is called *concussion*. Prolonged alterations in consciousness may be due to parenchymal, subdural, or epidural hematoma or to diffuse shearing of axons in the white matter. Skull fracture should be suspected in pts with CSF rhinorrhea, hemotympanum, and periorbital or mastoid ecchymoses. Spinal cord trauma can cause transient loss of function or a permanent myelopathy with loss of motor, sensory, and autonomic function below the damaged spinal level.

MANAGEMENT The neck should be immobilized and spine kept straight; vital functions should be stabilized. An initial neurologic exam should determine the level of consciousness, visual acuity, cranial nerve palsies, gross motor and sensory deficits, presence of blood in the middle ear, visible evidence of head trauma, and presence of pain over spine. Cervical spine films should be evaluated before neck is freed. Dysfunction below a spinal level suggests cord injury; lesions at the C5 level or above can threaten respiratory function. If x-rays show aberration of vertebral alignment, then reduction should be quickly undertaken. Spinal CT scan, MRI, or myelography may show evidence of reversible cord compression.

The pt with minor head injury who is alert and attentive after short period of unconsciousness (<1 min) sometimes has headache with a single episode of emesis or mild vertigo. Head injury of intermediate severity causes more prolonged loss of consciousness followed by persistent emesis and change in mental state. CT scan is required to exclude subdural or epidural hematoma and to define extent of contusions and posttraumatic edema. CT scan may be normal in comatose pts with axonal shearing lesions in cerebral white matter. Pts with intermediate head injury require medical observation to detect increasing drowsiness, respiratory dysfunction, and pupillary enlargement, as well as to ensure fluid restriction. Management of pts with raised ICP due to head injury is outlined above.

For more detailed discussion of this topic, see Ropper AH: Trauma of the Head and Spinal Cord, Chap. 344, in HPIM-11, p. 1960

SECTION XV

189 ADVERSE DRUG REACTIONS

Adverse drug reactions are among the most frequent problems encountered clinically and represent a common cause for hospitalization. They are caused by

1 Errors in self-administration of prescribed drugs (quite common in the elderly).
2 Exaggeration of intended pharmacologic effect (e.g., hypotension in a pt given antihypertensive drugs).
3 Concomitant administration of drugs with synergistic effects (e.g., aspirin and warfarin).
4 Cytotoxic reactions (e.g., hepatic necrosis due to acetaminophen).
5 Immunologic mechanisms (e.g., quinidine-induced thrombocytopenia, hydralazine-induced SLE).
6 Genetically determined enzymatic defects (e.g., primaquine-induced hemolytic anemia in G6PD deficiency).
7 Idiosyncratic reactions (chloramphenicol-induced aplastic anemia).

Table 189-1 lists a number of clinical manifestations of adverse effects of drugs. It is not designed to be complete or exhaustive.

TABLE 189-1 Clinical manifestations of relatively common adverse reactions to drugs

Multisystem

Fever
- Penicillins
- *p*-Aminosalicylic acid
- Amphotericin B
- Antihistamines
- Cephalosporins
- Barbiturates
- Phenytoin
- Quinidine
- Sulfonamides
- Iodides
- Thiouracil
- Methyldopa
- Bleomycin
- Procainamide

Drug-induced lupus erythematosus
- Acebutolol
- Hydralazine
- Procainamide
- Isoniazid

Serum sickness
- Aspirin
- Penicillins
- Streptomycin
- Sulfonamides
- Prophylthiouracil

Anaphylaxis
- Penicillins
- Cephalosporins
- Streptomycin
- Dextran
- Iron dextran
- Procaine
- Insulin
- Demeclocyline
- Iodinated drugs or contrast media
- Lidocaine

Endocrine

Disorders of thyroid function tests
- Oral contraceptives
- Phenindione
- Iodides
- Tolbutamide
- Chlorpropamide
- Lithium
- Gold salts

TABLE 189-1 Clinical manifestations of relatively common adverse reactions to drugs (continued)

Dimercaprol
Phenothiazines
Phenylbutazone
Sulfonamides
Phenytoin

Gynecomastia
Estrogens
Testosterone
Spironolactone
Digitalis
Methyldopa
Isoniazid

Galactorrhea (may also cause amenorrhea)
Methyldopa
Phenothiazines
Reserpine
Tricyclic antidepressants

Metabolic

Hyponatremia
1 Dilutional
Vincristine
Cyclophosphamide
Chlorpropamide
Diuretics
2 Salt wasting
Diuretics
Corticosteroid (withdrawal)

Hyperkalemia
Spironolactone
Triamterene
Amiloride
Cytotoxics
Corticosteroid (withdrawal)
Succinylcholine
Digitalis overdose
Potassium salts of drugs
Lithium

Hypokalemia
Diuretics
Laxative abuse
Corticosteroids
Amphotericin B
Alkali-induced alkalosis
Insulin
Osmotic diuretics

Metabolic acidosis
Paraldehyde (degraded)
Phenformin
Acetazolamide
Spironolactone
Salicylates

Hypercalcemia
Antacids with absorbable alkali
Vitamin D
Thiazides

Hyperuricemia
Thiazides
Chlorthalidone
Ethacrynic acid
Furosemide
Aspirin
Cytotoxics

Hyperglycemia
Corticosteroids
Oral contraceptives
Chlorthalidone
Ethacrynic acid
Thiazides
Furosemide
Diazoxide
Growth hormone

Porphyria exacerbation
Barbiturates
Chlordiazepoxide
Meprobamate
Sulfonamides
Estrogens
Oral contraceptives
Chlorpropamide

Dermatologic

Exfoliative dermatitis
Penicillins
Sulfonamides
Barbiturates
Phenytoin
Phenylbutazone
Gold salts
Quinidine

Toxic epidermal necrolysis (bullous)
Barbiturates
Phenylbutazone
Phenytoin
Sulfonamides
Phenolphthalein
Penicillins
Allopurinol
Iodides
Bromides

Erythema multiforme or Steven-Johnson syndrome
Sulfonamides
Barbiturates
Phenylbutazone
Chlorpropamide
Thiazides
Sulfones
Phenytoin
Salicylates
Tetracyclines
Codeine

TABLE 189-1 Clinical manifestations of relatively common adverse reactions to drugs (continued)

Penicillins

Erythema nodosum
- Penicillins
- Sulfonamides
- Oral contraceptives

Fixed drug eruptions
- Phenolphthalein
- Barbiturates
- Sulfonamides
- Salicylates
- Phenylbutazone
- Quinine
- Captopril

Photodermatitis
- Tetracyclines, particularly demeclocycline
- Griseofulvin
- Sulfonamides
- Sulfonylureas

Urticaria
- Aspirin
- Penicillins
- Sulfonamides
- Barbiturates

Nonspecific rashes
- Ampicillin
- Barbiturates
- Allopurinol
- Phenytoin
- Methyldopa

Pigment changes (hyperpigmentation)
- ACTH
- Busulfan
- Phenothiazines
- Hypervitaminosis A
- Oral contraceptives
- Gold salts

Alopecia
- Cytotoxics

Eczema (contact dermatitis)
- Topical antimicrobials
- Topical local anesthetics
- Topical antihistamines

Hematologic

Pancytopenia (aplastic anemia)
- Chloramphenicol
- Phenytoin
- Mephenytoin
- Trimethadione
- Phenylbutazone
- Oxyphenbutazone
- Gold salts
- Quinacrine
- Sulfonamides
- Cytotoxics

Agranulocytosis (see also pancytopenia)
- Chloramphenicol
- Sulfonamides
- Phenylbutazone
- Oxyphenbutazone
- Gold salts
- Indomethacin
- Propylthiouracil
- Methimazole
- Carbimazole
- Phenothiazines
- Cytotoxics
- Tolbutamide
- Tricyclic antidepressants
- Captopril

Thrombocytopenia platelet dysfunction (see also pancytopenia)
- Quinidine
- Quinine
- Furosemide
- Chlorthalidone
- Thiazides
- Gold salts
- Aspirin
- Indomethacin
- Phenylbutazone
- Oxyphenbutazone
- Chlorpropamide
- Acetazolamine
- Phenytoin and other hydantoins
- Methyldopa
- Carbamazepine
- Digitoxin
- Novobiocin
- Carbenacillin

Megaloblastic anemia
- Folate antagonists
- Cotrimoxazole
- Phenytoin
- Primidone
- Phenobarbital
- Triamterene
- Trimethoprim
- Oral contraceptives

Hemolytic anemia
- Methyldopa
- Levodopa
- Mefenamic acid
- Melphalan
- Isoniazid
- Rifampin
- Sulfonamides
- Penicillins
- Cephalosporins

TABLE 189-1 Clinical manifestations of relatively common adverse reactions to drugs (continued)

Insulin
Quinidine
Chlorpromazine
Phenacetin
p-Aminosalicylic acid
Dapsone
Procainamide
Hemolytic anemia (in G6PD deficiency)
Antimalarials, e.g., primaquine
Chloramphenicol
Dapsone
Naldixic acid
Nitrofurantoin
Sulfonamides
Aspirin
Phenacetin
p-Aminosalicylic acid
Quinidine
Vitamin C
Vitamin K
Lymphadenopathy
Phenytoin
Primidone
Cardiovascular
Exacerbation of angina
Vasopressin
Oxytocin
Ergotamine
Methysergide
Propranolol withdrawal
Excessive thyroxin
Alpha blockers
Hydralazine
Cardiomyopathy
Emetine
Sympathomimetics
Phenothiazines
Lithium
Sulfonamides
Daunorubicin
Adriamycin
Pericarditis
Procainamide
Hydralazine
Methysergide
Emetine
Fluid retention or CHF
Estrogens
Steroids
Carbenoxolone
Phenylbutazone
Indomethacin
Propranolol
Diazoxide
Minoxidil
Verapamil
Arrhythmias
Sympathomimetics
Thyroid hormone
Digitalis
Quinidine
Procainamide
Verapamil
Atropine
Propranolol
Guanethidine
Emetine
Propellants in aerosols
Tricyclic antidepressants
Phenothiazines, particularly thioridazine
Lithium
Anticholinesterases
Papaverine
Daunomycin
Adriamycin
Lincomycin (intravenous)
Hypotension (see also arrhythmias)
Nitroglycerin
Phenothiazines
Morphine
Diuretics
Citrated blood
Levodopa
Nifedipine
Verapamil
Hypertension
Oral contraceptives
Sympathomimetics
Monoamine oxidase inhibitors with sympathomimetics
Tricyclic antidepressants with sympathomimetics
Corticosteroids
ACTH
Phenylbutazone
Thromboembolism
Oral contraceptives
Respiratory
Nasal congestion
Guanethidine
Isoproterenol
Oral contraceptives
Decongestant abuse
Respiratory depression
Aminoglycosides
Polymixins
Trimethaphan
Opiates
Sedatives

TABLE 189-1 **Clinical manifestations of relatively common adverse reactions to drugs (continued)**

Hypnotics

Airway obstruction (bronchospasm, asthma; see also anaphylaxis)

Beta blockers
NSAIDs, e.g., aspirin, indomethacin
Cholinergic drugs
Tartrazine
Penicillins
Cephalosporins
Streptomycin
Pentazocine

Pulmonary infiltrates

Amiodarone
Nitrofurantoin
Methysergide
Bleomycin
Chlorambucil
BCNU
Procarbazine
Busulfan
Melphalan
Cyclophosphamide

Pulmonary edema

Heroin
Methadone
Hydrochlorthiazide
Propoxyphene
Contrast media

Gastrointestinal

Dental discoloration

Tetracycline

Gingival hyperplasia

Phenytoin

Oral ulceration

Aspirin
Isoproterenol (sublingual)
Cytotoxics

Taste disturbances

Penicillamine
Biguanides
Griseofulvin
Lithium
Rifampin
Captopril

Peptic ulceration or hemorrhage

Aspirin
Phenylbutazone
Indomethacin
Ethacrynic acid

Intestinal ulceration

Enteric-coated potassium chloride

Nausea or vomiting

Digitalis
Opiates
Estrogens
Levodopa
Potassium chloride
Ferrous sulfate

Diarrhea or colitis

Lincomycin
Clindamycin
Broad-spectrum antibiotics
Magnesium in antacids
Guanethidine
Methyldopa
Digitalis
Colchicine

Constipation or ileus

Ganglionic blockers
Tricyclic antidepressants
Phenothiazines
Opiates
Aluminum hydroxide
Calcium carbonate
Barium sulfate
Ion exchange resins
Ferrous sulfate

Malabsorption

Broad-spectrum antibiotics
Neomycin
Cholestyramine
Colchicine
p-Aminosalicylic acid

Pancreatitis

Corticosteroids
Thiazides
Azathioprine
Oral contraceptives
Sulfonamides
Opiates
Furosemide
Ethacrynic acid

Diffuse hepatocellular damage

Halothane
Methoxyflurane
Methyldopa
Isoniazid
Rifampin
Aminosalicylic acid
Ethionamide
Phenytoin and other hydantoins
Acetaminophen (paracetamol)
Salicylates
Allopurinol
Sulfonamides
Tetracyclines
Erythromycin estolate
Ketoconazole
Propylthiouracil

TABLE 189-1 Clinical manifestations of relatively common adverse reactions to drugs (continued)

Methimazole
Methotrexate
Pyridium
Propoxyphene
Monoamine oxidase inhibitors
Sodium valproate
Nitrofurantoin

Cholestatic jaundice
Phenothiazines
Androgens
Anabolic steroids
Oral contraceptives
Erythromycin estolate
Chlorpropamide
Gold salts

Renal

Nephrotic syndrome
Penicillamine
Gold salts
Phenidione
Probenecid
Captopril

Tubular necrosis
Amphotericin B
Aminoglycosides
Polymixins
Cephaloridine
Tetracyclines
Colistin
Sulfonamides
Radioiodinated contrast medium
Cyclosporin

Interstitial nephritis
Penicillins, particularly methicillin
Sulfonamides
Phenindione
Furosemide
Thiazides
Allopurinol

Nephropathies
Due to analgesics (e.g., phenacetin)

Concentrating defect with polyuria (or nephrogenic diabetes insipidus)
Vitamin D
Lithium
Demeclocycline
Methoxyflurane

Renal tubular acidosis
Degraded tetracycline
Amphotericin B
Acetazolamide

Calculi
Acetazolamide
Vitamin D

Obstructive uropathy
Intrarenal: cytotoxics
Extrarenal: methysergide

Hemorrhagic cystitis
Cyclophosphamide

Bladder dysfunction
Anticholinergics
Monoamine oxidase inhibitors
Tricyclic antidepressants
Disopyramide

Genital (see also endocrine)

Vaginal carcinoma
Diethylstilbestrol (administered to mother)

Impairment of spermatogenesis or oogenesis
Cytotoxics

Neurologic

Peripheral neuropathy
Isoniazid
Hydralazine
Nitrofurantoin
Vincristine
Mustine
Streptomycin
Polymixin, colistan
Tricyclic antidepressants
Chloramphenicol
Procarbazine
Ethambutol
Ethionamide
Glutethimide
Demeclocycline
Nalidixic acid
Tolbutamide
Chlorpropamide
Methysergide
Phenytoin
Metronidazole
Clofibrate
Chloroquine
Perhexiline
Disopyramide

Exacerbation of myasthenia
Aminoglycosides
Polymixins

Extrapyramidal effects
Butyrophenones, e.g., haloperidol
Phenothiazines
Tricyclic antidepressants
Methyldopa
Levodopa

TABLE 189-1 Clinical manifestations of relatively common adverse reactions to drugs (continued)

- Reserpine
- Metoclopramide
- Oral contraceptives

Seizures
- Amphetamines
- Analeptics
- Phenothiazines
- Isoniazid
- Lidocaine
- Theophylline
- Penicillins
- Nalidixic acid
- Physostigmine
- Tricyclic antidepressants
- Vincristine
- Lithium

Stroke
- Oral contraceptives

Pseudotumor cerebri (or intracranial hypertension)
- Corticosteroids
- Oral contraceptives
- Tetracyclines
- Hypervitaminosis A

Headache
- Hydralazine
- Bromides
- Glyceryl trinitrate
- Ergotamine (withdrawal)
- Indomethacin

Ocular

Corneal opacities
- Vitamin D
- Chloroquine
- Indomethacin

Corneal edema
- Oral contraceptives

Cataracts
- Phenothiazines
- Corticosteroids
- Busulfan
- Chlorambucil

Glaucoma
- Mydriatics
- Sympathomimetics

Retinopathy
- Chloroquine
- Phenothiazines

Optic neuritis
- Clioquinol
- Chloramphenicol
- Streptomycin
- Isoniazid
- Ethambutol
- Quinine
- Phenothiazines
- Penicillamine
- PAS
- Phenylbutazone

Ear

Vestibular disorders
- Aminoglycosides
- Quinine

Deafness
- Aminoglycosides
- Ethacrynic acid
- Furosemide
- Quinine
- Bleomycin
- Chloroquine
- Aspirin
- Nortriptyline

Musculoskeletal

Myopathy or myalgia
- Corticosteroids
- Chloroquine
- Clofibrate
- Oral contraceptives
- Amphotericin B
- Carbenoxolone

Bone disorders

1 Osteoporosis
- Corticosteroids
- Heparin

2 Osteomalacia
- Anticonvulsants
- Glutethimide
- Aluminum hydroxide

Psychiatric disorders

Schizophrenic-like or paranoid reactions
- Amphetamines
- Lysergic acid
- Levodopa
- Tricyclic antidepressants
- Monoamine oxidase inhibitors
- Bromides
- Corticosteroids

Depression
- Centrally acting antihypertensives (reserpine, methyldopa, clonidine)
- Propranolol
- Corticosteroids
- Amphetamine withdrawal
- Levodopa

Hypomania, mania, or excited reactions
- Levodopa

TABLE 189-1 Clinical manifestations of relatively common adverse reactions to drugs (continued)

Sympathomimetics
Corticosteroids
MAO inhibitors
Tricyclic antidepressants

Hallucinatory states
Amantadine
Narcotics
Pentazocine
Propranolol
Levodopa
Tricyclic antidepressants
Meperidine

Delirious or confusional states
Digitalis
Anticholinergics
Bromides
Sedatives and hypnotics
Phenothiazines
Antidepressants
Corticosteroids
Isoniazid
Levodopa
Amantadine
Penicillins
Aminophylline
Methyldopa

Sleep disturbances
Anorexiants
Levodopa
Monoamine oxidase inhibitors
Sympathomimetics

Drowsiness
Anxiolytic drugs
Major tranquilizers
Tricyclic antidepressants
Antihistamines
Methyldopa
Clonidine

Modified from Wood AJJ, Oates, JA: HPIM-11, pp. 355–358.

For more detailed discussion of this topic, see Wood AJJ, Oates JA: Adverse Reactions to Drugs, Chap. 65, in HPIM-11, p. 352

SECTION XVI

190 LABORATORY VALUES OF CLINICAL IMPORTANCE

The following laboratory values are a selection of those which have particularly frequent clinical relevance. Values in SI units appear in brackets after values in traditional units. For a more complete listing, please consult the Appendix of HPIM-11, pp. A-1 to A-10.

BODY FLUIDS AND OTHER MASS DATA

Body fluid, total volume: 50% (in obese) to 70% (lean) of body weight
 Intracellular: 30–40% of body weight
 Extracellular: 20–30% of body weight
Blood:
 Total volume:
  Males: 69 mL/kg body weight
  Females: 65 mL/kg body weight
 Plasma volume:
  Males: 39 mL/kg body weight
  Females: 40 mL/kg body weight
 RBC volume:
  Males: 30 mL/kg body weight (1.15–1.21 liters/m^2 of body surface area)
  Females: 25 mL/kg body weight (0.95–1.00 liters m^2 of body surface area)

$$\text{Body surface area } (m^2) = \frac{(\text{wt in kg})^{0.425} \times (\text{ht in cm})^{0.725}}{139.315}$$

CSF

Glucose	40–70 mg/dL
Total protein	20–45 mg/dL
CSF pressure	50–180 mmH_2O
Leukocytes:	
Total	<4 per mm^3
Differential:	
Lymphocytes	60–70%
Monocytes	30–50%
Neutrophils	1–3%

CHEMICAL CONSTITUENTS OF BLOOD

Albumin, serum: 3.5–5.5 g/dL [35–55 g/liter]
Aldolase: 0–8 U/liter [0–130 nmol/s per liter]

Aminotransferases, serum:
 Aspartate (AST, SGOT): 10–40 Karmen units/mL; 6–18 U/liter; [100–300 μmol/s per liter]
 Alanine (ALT, SGPT): 10–40 Karmen units/mL; 3–26 U/liter [50–430 μmol/s per liter]
Ammonia, whole blood, venous: 80–110 μg/dL [47–65 μmol/liter]
Amylase, serum: 60–180 Somogyi units per dL; 0.8–3.2 U/liter [13–53 nmol/s per liter]
Arterial blood gases:
 [HCO_3^-]: 21–28 meq/liter [21–28 mmol/liter]
 P_{CO_2}: 35–45 mmHg
 pH: 7.38–7.44
 P_{O_2}: 80–100 mmHg at sea level
Bilirubin, total, serum (Malloy-Evelyn): 0.3–1.0 mg/dL [5.1–17 μmol/liter]:
 Direct, serum: 0.1–0.3 mg/dL [1.7–5.1 μmol/liter]
 Indirect, serum: 0.2–0.7 mg/dL [3.4–12 μmol/liter]
C-reactive protein, serum: 7–820 μg/dL
Calcium, ionized: 2.3–2.8 meq/liter; 4.5–5.6 mg/dL [1.1–1.4 mmol/liter]
Calcium, plasma: 4.5–5.5 meq/liter; 9–10.5 mg/dL [2.2–2.6 mmol/liter]
Carbon dioxide content, plasma (sea level): 21–28 meq/liter; 50–70 vol% [21–28 mmol/liter]
Chlorides, serum: 98–106 meq/liter [98–106 mmol/liter]
Complement, serum:
 Total hemolytic (CH_{50}): 150–250 U/mL
 C3: 55–120 mg/dL [0.55–1.20 g/liter]
 C4: 20–50 mg/dL [0.20–0.50 g/liter]
Creatinine phosphokinase, serum (total):
 Females: 10–70 U/mL [0.17–1.18 mmol/s per liter]
 Males: 25–90 U/mL [0.42–1.51 mmol/s per liter]
 Isoenzymes, serum: fraction 2 (MB) $< 5\%$ of total
Digoxin, serum:
 Therapeutic level: 1.2 ± 0.4 ng/mL [1.54 ± 0.5 nmol/liter]
 Toxic level: >2.4 ng/mL [>3.2 nmol/liter]
Ferritin, serum: 15–200 ng/mL [15–200 μg/liter]
γ-Glutamyl transferase (transpeptidase), serum: 4–60 U/liter [0.07–1.00 μmol/s per liter]
Glucose (fasting), plasma:
 Normal: 75–115 mg/dL [4.2–6.4 mmol/liter]
 Diabetes mellitus: >140 mg/dL (on more than one occasion) [>7.8 mmol/liter]
Glucose, 2-h postprandial, plasma:
 Normal: <140 mg/dL [<7.8 mmol/liter]
 Impaired glucose tolerance: 140–200 mg/dL [7.8–11.1 mmol/liter]
 Diabetes mellitus: >200 mg/dL [>11.1 mmol/liter] (on more than one occasion)

Hemoglobin, blood (sea level):
- Males: 14–18 g/dL [8.7–11.2 mmol/liter]
- Females: 12–16 g/dL [7.4–9.9 mmol/liter]
- Hemoglobin A_{1c}: Up to 6% of total hemoglobin

Immunoglobulins, serum:
- IgA: 90–325 mg/dL [0.9–3.2 g/liter]
- IgD: 0–8 mg/dL [0–0.08 g/liter]
- IgE: <0.025 mg/dL [<0.00025 g/liter]
- IgG: 800–1500 mg/dL [8.0–15.0 g/liter]
- IgM: 45–150 mg/dL [0.45–1.5 g/liter]

Iron, serum:
- Males and females (mean ± 1 SD): 105 ± 35 μg/dL [19 ± 6 μmol/liter]

Iron-binding capacity, serum (mean ± 1 SD): 305 ± 32 μg/dL [55 ± 6 μmol/liter]
- Saturation: 20 to 45%

Lactate dehydrogenase, serum:
- 200–450 U/mL (Wrobleski)
- 60–100 U/mL (Wacker)
- 25–100 U/liter [0.4–1.7 μmol/s per liter]

Lipase, serum: 1.5 U (Cherry-Crandall)

Magnesium, serum: 1.3–2.1 meq/liter, 2 to 3 mg/dL [0.8–1.3 mmol/liter]

5′-Nucleotidase, serum: 0.3–2.6 Bodansky units per dL [27–233 nmol/s per liter]

Osmolality, plasma: 285–295 mosmol/kg of serum water

Phosphatase, acid, serum: 0.2–1.8 IU [3 to 30 nmol/s per liter]

Phosphatase, alkaline, serum: 21–91 IU/liter at 37°C [0.4–1.5 μmol/s per liter]

Phosphorus, inorganic, serum: 1–1.5 meq liter; 3–4.5 mg/dL [1.0–1.4 mmol/liter]

Potassium, serum: 3.5–5.0 meq/liter [3.5–5.0 mmol/liter]

Proteins, total, serum: 5.5–8.0 g/dL [55–80 g/liter]

Protein fractions, serum:
- Albumin: 3.5–5.0 g/dL (50–60%) [35–55 g/liter)
- Globulin: 2.0–3.5 g/dL (40–50%) [20–35 g/liter]
- $Alpha_1$: 0.2–0.4 g/dL (4.2–7.2%) [2–4 g/liter]
- $Alpha_2$: 0.5–0.9 g/dL (6.8–12%) [5–9 g/liter]
- Beta: 0.6–1.1 g/dL (9.3–15%) [6–11 g/liter]
- Gamma: 0.7–1.7 g/dL (13–23%) [7–17 g/liter]

Sodium, serum: 136–145 meq/liter [136–145 mmol/liter]

Urea nitrogen, serum: 10–20 mg/dL [3.6–7.1 mmol/liter]

Uric acid, serum:
- Men: 2.5–8.0 mg/dL [0.15–0.48 mmol/liter]
- Women: 1.5–6.0 mg/dL [0.09–0.36 mmol/liter]

FUNCTION TESTS

Circulation

Cardiac output (Fick): 2.5–3.6 liter/m^2 of body surface area per min

Left ventricular ejection fraction, stroke volume/end-diastolic volume (SV/EDV): Normal range: 0.55–0.78, average 0.67
Pulmonary vascular resistance: 20–120 (dyn·s)/cm^5 [2–12 kPa·s/liter]
Systemic vascular resistance: 770–1500 (dyn·s)/cm^5 [77–150 kPa·s/liter]

Gastrointestinal

D-Xylose absorption test: After an overnight fast, 25 g xylose is given PO in aqueous solution; urine collected for the following 5 h should contain 5–8 g [33–53 mmol] (or >20% of ingested dose); serum xylose should be 25 to 40 mg per 100 mL 1 h after the oral dose [1.7–2.7 mmol/liter].
Gastric juice:
Volume:
24 h: 2–3 liters
Nocturnal: 600–700 mL
Basal, fasting: 30–70 mL/h
pH: 1.6–1.8
Acid output:
Basal:
Females (mean ± 1 SD) 2.0 ± 1.8 meq/h [0.6 ± 0.5 μmol/s]
Males (mean ± 1 SD) 3.0 ± 2.0 meq/h [0.8 ± 0.6 μmol/s]
Maximal (after subcutaneous histamine acid phosphate 0.004 mg/kg and preceded by 50 mg promethazine; or after betazole 1.7 mg/kg or pentagastrin 6 μ/kg):
Females: 16 ± 5 meq/h [4.4 ± 1.4 μmol/s]
Males: 23 ± 5 meq/h [6.4 ± 1.4 μmol/s]
Secretin test (pancreatic exocrine function: 1 U/kg of body weight, IV):
Volume (pancreatic juice): > 2.0 mL/kg in 80 min
Bicarbonate concentration: >80 meq/liter [>80 mmol/liter]
Bicarbonate output: >10 meq in 30 min [>10 mmol in 30 min]

Metabolic and endocrine

Cortisol:
8 A.M. 5–25 μg/dL [138–691 nmol/liter]
4 P.M. 3–12 μ/dL [82–331 nmol/liter]
Adrenal steroids, urinary excretion:
Aldosterone: 5–19 μg/day [14–53 nmol/day]
Cortisol, free: 20–100 μg/day [54–276 mnol/day]
17-Hydroxycorticosteroids: 2–10 mg/day [5.4–28 μmol/day]
17-Ketosteroids:
Men: 7–25 mg/day [24–88 μmol/day]
Women: 4–15 mg/day [14–52 μmol/day]
Estradiol:
Women: 20–60 pg/mL [0.07–0.22 nmol/liter], higher at ovulation
Men: <50 pg/mL [<0.18 nmol/liter]
Progesterone:
Men, prepubertal girls, preovulatory women, and postmenopausal women: <2 ng/mL [<6 nmol/liter]

Women, luteal, peak: >5 ng/mL [>16 nmol/liter]
Testosterone:
Women: <100 ng/dL [<3.5 nmol/liter]
Men: 300–100 ng/dL [10–35 nmol/liter]
Prepubertal boys and girls: 5–20 ng/dL [0.17–0.7 nmol/liter]
Thyroid function tests:
Radioactive iodine uptake, 24 h: 5–30% (range varies in different areas due to variations in iodine intake)
Resin T_3 uptake: 25–35% (varies among laboratories)
Thyroid-stimulating hormone (TSH): <5 μU/mL [<5 mU/liter]
Thyroxine (T_4), serum radioimmunoassay: 5–12 μg/dL [64–154 nmol/liter]
Triiodothyronine (T_3), plasma: 70–190 ng/dL [1.1–2.9 nmol/liter]

Renal

Clearances (corrected to 1.72 m^2 body surface area):
Inulin clearance (mean ± 1 SD):
Males: 124 ± 25.8 mL/min [2.1 ± 0.4 mL/s]
Females: 119 ± 12.8 mL/min [2.0 ± 0.2 mL/s]
Endogenous creatinine clearance: 91–130 mL/min [1.5–2.2 mL/s]
Concentration and dilution test:
Specific gravity of urine:
After 12-h fluid restriction: 1.025 or more
After 12-h deliberate water intake: 1.003 or less

HEMATOLOGIC EXAMINATIONS (See also Chemical Constituents of Blood)

Carboxyhemoglobin:
Nonsmoker: 0–2.3%
Smoker: 2.1–4.2%
Haptoglobin, serum (mean ± 2SD): 128 ± 15 mg/dL [1.3 ± 0.2 g/liter]
Sedimentation rate:
Westergren, <50 years of age:
Males: 0–15 mm/h
Females: 0–20 mm/h
Westergren, >50 years of age:
Males: 0–20 mm/h
Females: 0–30 mm/h
Wintrobe:
Males: 0–9 mm/h
Females: 0–20 mm/h
Bleeding time:
Ivy method, 5-mm wound: <9 min
Duke method: <4 min
Simplate: <7 min
Fibrinogen: 200–400 mg/dL
Fibrin split products: <10 μg/mL
Platelets: 130,000–400,000/mm^3

URINE

Creatinine: 1.0–1.6 g in 24 h [8.8–14 mmol/day]
Protein: <150 mg in 24 h [<0.05 g/day]
Potassium: 25–100 meq in 24 h (varies with intake) [25–100 mmol/day]
Sodium: 100–260 meq in 24 h (varies with intake) [100–260 mmol/day]

GLOSSARY

A_2	aortic second sound
ABGs	arterial blood gases
ACTH	adrenocorticotrophic hormone
ADH	antidiuretic hormone
AF	atrial fibrillation
AIDS	acquired immunodeficiency syndrome
ALS	amyotrophic lateral sclerosis
AMI	acute myocardial infarction
ANA	antinuclear antibody
ARDS	acute respiratory distress syndrome
ARF	acute renal failure
ATN	acute tubular necrosis
AV	atrioventricular
AVP	arginine vasopressin
BC	blood culture
BP	blood pressure
CBC	complete blood count
CF	complement fixation
CHF	congestive heart failure
CIE	counterimmunoelectrophoresis
CK	creatinine phosphokinase
CLL	chronic lymphocytic leukemia
CML	chronic myeloid leukemia
CMV	cytomegalovirus
CNS	central nervous system
CSF	cerebrospinal fluid
CT	computerized tomography
Cu	copper
CVA	costovertebral angle
CVP	central venous pressure
CXR	chest x-ray
DC	discontinue
$D_{L_{CO}}$	diffusing capacity of lung for carbon monoxide
DIC	disseminated intravascular coagulation
DU	duodenal ulcer
DVT	deep venous thrombosis
Dx	diagnosis
EBV	Epstein Barr virus
ECG	electrocardiogram
EEG	electroencephalogram
EMG	electromyogram
ENT	ear, nose, and throat
EOM	extraocular movement
ERCP	endoscopic retrograde cholangiopancreatography
ESR	erythrocyte sedimentation rate
Fe	iron
FEV_1	forced expiratory volume in 1st second
FSH	follicle-stimulating hormone
FVC	forced vital capacity
GFR	glomerular filtration rate
GI	gastrointestinal
G6PD	glucose 6-phosphate dehydrogenase

Hb	hemoglobin
Hct	hematocrit
hs	at bedtime
Hx	history
IBD	inflammatory bowel disease
ICP	intracranial pressure
ICU	intensive care unit
Ig	immunoglobulin
IM	intramuscular
IV	intravenous
IVC	inferior vena cava
IVP	intravenous pyelogram
JVP	jugular venous pressure
LA	left atrium
LAD	left axis deviation
LBBB	left bundle branch block
LFT	liver function test
LH	luteinizing hormone
Li	lithium
LLQ	left lower quadrant
LP	lumbar puncture
LUQ	left upper quadrant
LV	left ventricle
MCA	middle cerebral artery
MRI	magnetic resonance imaging
NG	nasogastric
NPO	nothing by mouth
NSAIDs	nonsteroidal anti-inflammatory drugs
P	pulse
P_2	pulmonic second sound
Pa_{CO_2}	partial pressure of CO_2 in arterial blood
Pa_{O_2}	partial pressure of O_2 in arterial blood
pc	after meals
PE	physical examination
PFTs	pulmonary function tests
PMNs	polymorphonuclear cells or leukocytes
PO	by mouth
PO_4	phosphate
PPD	purified protein derivative
PR	per rectum (rectal instillation)
prn	when necessary
pt	patient
PT	prothrombin time
Pth	pathology
PTT	partial thromboplastin time
qd	every day
qh	every hour
q 2 h	every 2 hours
qhs	every bedtime
qod	every other day
qs	a sufficient quantity
R	respiratory rate/min
RA	rheumatoid arthritis
RBBB	right bundle branch block
RBC	red blood (cell) count
RLQ	right lower quadrant
RUQ	right upper quadrant
RV	right ventricle
S_1	first heart sound
S_2	second heart sound
S_3	third heart sound
S_4	fourth heart sound
SC	subcutaneous
SL	sublingual
SLE	systemic lupus erythematosus
STD	sexually transmitted diseases

STS serologic test for syphilis
SVC superior vena cava
Sx signs and symptoms

T_3 tri-iodothyronine
T_4 thyroxine
TBC tuberculosis
TIA transient ischemic attack
TLC total lung capacity

UA urinalysis
URI upper respiratory infection
UTI urinary tract infection
UV ultraviolet

VDRL Venereal Disease Research Laboratory (test for syphilis)
VF ventricular fibrillation
VPC ventricular premature contractions

WBC white blood (cell) count

INDEX

Main discussion is indicated by **boldface** page numbers.

D

I

J

K

L

P

U

V

W

X

Y

Z

FREQUENTLY USED PHONE NUMBERS

Name	Number

Name **Number**

Name	Number

Name Number

Name	Number

Name

Number